Novel Pathogenesis and Treatments for Cardiovascular Disease

Edited by David C. Gaze

Published in London, United Kingdom

Novel Pathogenesis and Treatments for Cardiovascular Disease
http://dx.doi.org/10.5772/intechopen.101292
Edited by David C. Gaze

Contributors
Robert Lust, Katie Lovell, Greyson Keel, Julia Cook, Megan Goins, Francesco Gallo, Enrico Forlin, Alberto Barolo, Marco Barbierato, Fathia Mghaieth Zghal, Abdeljelil Farhati, Mohamed Sami Mourali, Omigbile Olamide, Oni Adebayo, Abe Emmanuel, Lawal Eyitayo, Oyasope Beatrice, Mayaki Tomisin, Saritphat Orrapin, Ahmed Tijani Bawah, Abdul-Malik Bawah, Ruhaima Issah Zorro, Angela Young, Ankur Wadhwa, Anwer Zohaib Siddiqi, Massimiliano Mulè, Giulia Passaniti, Daniela Giannazzo, Angel Martin Castellanos, Asma S. Alonazi, Anfal F. Bin Dayel, Tahani K. Alshammari, Nouf M. Alrasheed, Brandon S. Shaw, Gavin R.H. Sandercock, Anneke Van Biljon, Ina Shaw, Melisa Rivera, Blanca Frisia Morales-López, José Heriberto López-Beltrán, Mabitsela Hezekiel 'Pitso' Mphasha, Mitsuru Seki, Md. Shah Amran, Nasiba Binte Bahar, Shopnil Akash, Thang Nguyen, Suol Thanh Pham, Thi Anh Nguyen, Nghia Minh Tran, Hoang Thi Kim Cao, Khanh Kim Le, Chu Xuan Duong, Thao Huong Nguyen, Katja Taxis, Khanh Duy Dang, Jennifer C. Caroline Van Wyk, Pedro Felipe Parra Velasco, Valeh Mirzazada, Sadagat Sultanova, Natavan Ismailova, Aygun Huseynova, Gulnara Nurmamadova, Aygun Aliyeva, Sevil Ismailova, Bruno Papelbaum, Andre Sbaraini Brambilla, Bruno Kioshi Kimura Numata, Joshua Chadwick, Balasubramanian Ganesh, Lokesh Shanmugam, Jake J. Wen, Ravi S. Radhakrishnan, Shubham Barik, Aritra Mukherjee, Boda Karunakar, Angelina Job Kolady, Tony Grace, Pavol Svorc, Pavol Svorc Jr, David C. Gaze, Gabriela Silvia Gheorghe, Andreea Simona Hodorogea, Andrei Cristian Dan Gheorghe, Ana Ciobanu, Azin Alizadehasl, Haniye Hajiali Fini, Zahra Mortezaei, Narges Hosseini

First published in London, United Kingdom, 2023 by IntechOpen
IntechOpen is the global imprint of INTECHOPEN LIMITED, registered in England and Wales, registration number: 11086078, 5 Princes Gate Court, London, SW7 2QJ, United Kingdom

British Library Cataloguing-in-Publication Data
A catalogue record for this book is available from the British Library

Additional hard and PDF copies can be obtained from orders@intechopen.com

Novel Pathogenesis and Treatments for Cardiovascular Disease
Edited by David C. Gaze
p. cm.
Print ISBN 978-1-80356-116-5
Online ISBN 978-1-80356-117-2
eBook (PDF) ISBN 978-1-80356-118-9

For EU product safety concerns:
IN TECH d.o.o., Prolaz Marije Krucifikse Kozulić 3, 51000 Rijeka, Croatia,
info@intechopen.com or visit our website at intechopen.com.

Meet the editor

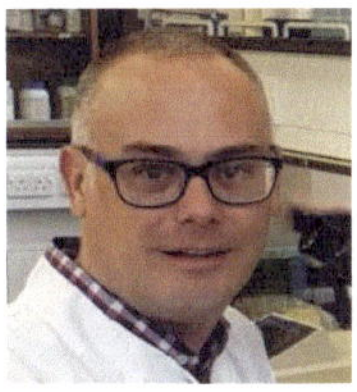

Dr. David C. Gaze is a Senior Lecturer in Chemical Pathology, Director of Employability, and Course Leader for the MSc Biomedical Science programme at the University of Westminster, London, UK. His academic research interests are in the development and clinical utility of cardiac biomarkers for the detection of cardiovascular diseases. Dr. Gaze has authored and co-authored more than 150 peer-reviewed papers and 200 abstracts. He has contributed five book chapters to cardiovascular textbooks as well as authored a textbook on cardiac troponin. He is a peer reviewer for twenty-five medical journals and writes regularly for the scientific forum The Conversation. Dr. Gaze is the commissioning editor for review articles for the *Annals of Clinical Biochemistry & Laboratory Medicine* and is co-editor in chief of *Practical Laboratory Medicine*.

Contents

Preface

This is the latest book in a series of related texts covering concepts of cardiovascular diseases (CVD) and associated conditions. The latest volume is divided into three sections: "Cardiovascular Pathophysiology", "Cardiovascular Diagnostics", and "Cardiovascular Treatments".

Section 1, "Cardiovascular Pathophysiology," approaches subjects related to disease development. The chapters investigate the role of obesity in CVD, the emergence of cardiotoxicity, and the role of cardio-oncology, especially in light of the COVID-19 pandemic, which disrupted many routine but essential treatment options for cancer patients. Other topics discussed are the role of adiponectin in preeclampsia, CVD in Kawasaki disease, Takayasu arteritis in pediatrics, and stress-induced cardiomyopathy.

Section 2, "Cardiovascular Diagnostics," concentrates on modalities for detecting CVD including anthropometric measurements, echocardiography in pulmonary hypertension, assessment of hair cortisol and cardiometabolic risk, and cardiac troponin in postmortem samples obtained at autopsy.

Section 3, "Cardiovascular Treatments," focuses on interventional strategies to prevent or treat CVD, including discussions of the value of resistance exercise training, adherence to medical prescriptions for CVD, Treatment of type II diabetes mellitus, diagnosis and management of acute ischemic stroke, surgical interventions for valvular prosthesis, and cryoablation and transcatheter treatments for aortic valve disease.

This book is designed for general medical and biomedical students at both undergraduate and postgraduate levels. It offers insightful updates on recent advances in the understanding of the pathophysiology of cardiac diseases and new techniques added to the medical armamentarium to improve outcomes and prevent mortality; thus it is also of interest to those working in academic research and within the field of healthcare science. Finally, my thanks go to the authors of each chapter who have provided excellent scientific content and responded to editorial changes at speed. I also acknowledge the help and support of the book management team at IntechOpen.

Dr. David C. Gaze
School of Life Sciences,
Biomedical Sciences,
University of Westminster,
London, UK

Dedication

Dedicated to Edward (Ted) N. Flint

25th December 1930 – 10th September 2022

The kindest man I have ever known, my grandfather.

Section 1

Cardiovascular Pathophysiology

Chapter 1

Perspective Chapter: Physiology and Pathology of the Cardiovascular System

Md. Shah Amran, Nasiba Binte Bahar and Shopnil Akash

Abstract

The cardiovascular system (CVS) is made up of the heart, blood vessels, and blood. The fundamental function of CVS is to transport substances to and from all parts of the body. The heart is the major pumping organ, pressurizing blood for circulation through the blood vessels; blood is propelled away from the heart in the arteries and returns to the heart through the veins. Cardiovascular disease (CVD) is an umbrella term for a number of inter-linked diseases, generally defined as coronary artery disease, cerebrovascular disease, high blood pressure, peripheral arterial disease, rheumatic and congenital heart diseases, arrhythmia, etc. Globally, CVDs are the leading cause of deaths, and according to the estimation of the World Health Organization (WHO), about 17.9 million people died from CVDs in 2019, accounting for 32% of all global deaths. About 75% of CVD deaths occur in low- and middle-income countries. This burden of CVDs can be decreased by careful risk reduction (such as lifestyle modification, smoking and alcohol cessation, weight optimization, physical exercise), and proper medical treatments, including herbal components. The prevention of CVDs can reduce the occurrence of major cardiovascular events, thereby reducing premature disability, morbidity, and mortality, while prolonging survival and quality of life.

Keywords: cardiovascular system (CVS), heart, coronary artery disease (CAD), physiology, pathology, cardiovascular drugs, herbal components

1. Introduction

The cardiovascular system acts as the engine that drives the human body. It is responsible for transporting oxygen, nutrients, hormones, and enzymes throughout the body, as well as removing carbon dioxide and other waste products from it [1]. This cardiovascular system is mainly separated into two parts—(i) the pulmonary circulation and (ii) the systemic circulation, which are supplied by the right and left ventricles of the heart, respectively [2]. Each of these circulations is constituted of the respective heart pump, the microcirculation, the arteries, and the veins. Basically, the cardiovascular system is a well-regulated carrier syntax of the body that allows the circulation of blood throughout an intact system under varying pressure gradients, generated by the pumping mechanism, with the heart serving as the core pumping unit [3]. This heart is a super sophisticated and highly developed organ that integrates a diverse range of anatomical and functional features to fulfill its fundamental pumping function. It is not just a sophisticated information processing and encoding center [4], but it also functions as an endocrine gland that is capable of generating and releasing its hormones and neurotransmitters [5–8]. The heart is positioned in the center of the chest, between the lungs in humans. An average human heart measures around the size of a clenched fist and its mass falls within the range of 250–350 grams, with a typical beating of around 100,000 times per day (approximately 72 beats per minute (bpm)) [9]. The interior anatomy of the heart exposes four myocardial chambers—two atria and two ventricles. The two atria are the upper chambers that primarily serve as the collecting chambers; whereas the two ventricles are the lower chambers that primarily function as the blood-pumping chambers [10]. A healthy heart has a set of four valves that keep blood flowing in one direction to prevent backflow. The rate and strength of the heart's contractions dictate cardiac functioning [4]. The cardiovascular system entails the blood vessels as well, which circulate the blood pumped by the heart throughout the body. Since the heart and blood vessels are integral parts of the cardiovascular system, any damage or dysfunction of the heart or blood vessels can have catastrophic repercussions, leading to severe cardiovascular diseases (CVDs) and even death [11].

CVDs encompass a wide spectrum of disorders, including diseases of the heart muscle and the vascular system that supplies the brain, heart, and other vital organs with blood and oxygen. CVDs are the preeminent cause of death worldwide, claiming the lives of an estimated 17.9 million people annually [12], with the majority (80%) of these deaths occurring in developing nations [13]. The prevalence of CVDs is projected to increase as their risk factors become more pervasive in formerly low-risk countries. The death toll from CVD is currently three times higher in developing countries than that in developed ones [14]. According to the estimation of the World Health Organization (WHO), more than 75% of premature CVDs are avertible and the mitigation of the risk factors can assist to deal with the rising burden of CVDs [15]. Moreover, WHO has emphasized the importance of lifestyle factors such as unhealthy diet habits, tobacco use, psychological stress, and physical inactivity contributing to the rise of CVD, and according to the estimation of WHO, three-quarters of deaths caused by CVDs might be avoided with united efforts [16]. Furthermore, an early diagnosis of CVDs is pivotal for reorienting the focus of therapy toward prevention rather than treatment [17]. However, in recent years rapid progress is being made in the treatment of heart diseases. Several therapeutic choices are constantly being presented to cardiologists caring for patients with CVDs . The most frequently prescribed drugs for CVDs include beta-blockers, angiotensin-converting enzyme (ACE) inhibitors, angiotensin II receptor blockers (ARB), alpha-adrenoceptor blockers, adrenergic receptor blockers, antihypertensive drugs, vasodilators, nitrates, calcium channel blockers, potassium channel activators, diuretics, positive inotropic drugs, antiarrhythmic drugs, sympathomimetic drugs, anticoagulants and protamine sulfate, antiplatelet drugs, fibrinolytic drugs and lipid-lowering agents etc. [18]. According to the Bangladesh Unani, Ayurvedic and Herbal pharmacopeia, a lot of plant-derived medications are also applied for the treatment of these ailments.

This book chapter aims to present a succinct and simplistic review of the basic physiological and anatomical aspects as well as the pathological information regarding the cardiovascular system. Additionally, this chapter includes information on the diagnosis, treatment, and prevention of CVDs.

2. Cardiovascular system

Every living body relies on a functioning cardiovascular system, which is a complex and multifaceted physiological system with numerous regulatory sub-systems controlled by the central and peripheral autonomic nervous systems as well as humoral factors [19]. The cardiovascular system is primarily responsible for supplying the body's cells with the materials they require to function properly and for removing the waste products that they make as a result of their metabolic processes. It is responsible for transporting blood throughout the body. It is controlled by numerous stimuli, including sympathetic and parasympathetic nervous systems, changes in blood volume, electrolytes, hormones, osmolarity, adrenal glands, kidneys, medications etc. [20–23].

The fundamental role of the cardiovascular system is to meet the metabolic requirements of the body as well as transporting carbon dioxide and other wastes out of the body. This function is accomplished in two ways—by maintaining a healthy circulatory system and by keeping blood pressure at an optimum level.

2.1 Divisions of the cardiovascular system

The circulatory system has two functionally opposite divisions through which blood flows—systemic circulation and pulmonary circulation as shown in **Figure 1**.

2.1.1 Systemic circulation

This circulation is more generally referred to as greater or superior circulation with a highly elevated resistance circuit [3]. It commences at the left ventricle and terminates in the right atrium [3]. The left ventricle pumps blood which is traveled through a set of blood vessels known as the arterial system [24]. At the capillaries, blood and tissue exchange a variety of substances. Following such exchange, blood turns back to the right atrium of the heart via the venous system. After that, the right ventricle receives blood from the right atrium. As a consequence of this systemic circulation, the oxygenated blood from the heart travels to the tissues, while venous blood from the tissues returns to the heart [3].

2.1.2 Pulmonary circulation

This circulatory system is known as the lesser circulatory system with a lower resistance circuit [3]. Such circulation begins at the right ventricle and terminates in the left atrium [3]. At first, the right ventricular blood flows to the lungs via the pulmonary artery [24]. By means of the pulmonary capillaries, the exchange of gases takes place between the circulating blood and the lungs' alveoli [24]. Once the blood has been oxygenated, it returns to the left atrium via the pulmonary veins.

2.2 Components of the cardiovascular system

The cardiovascular system is primarily composed of—(i) heart and (ii) blood vessels (i.e. capillaries, arteries, and veins).

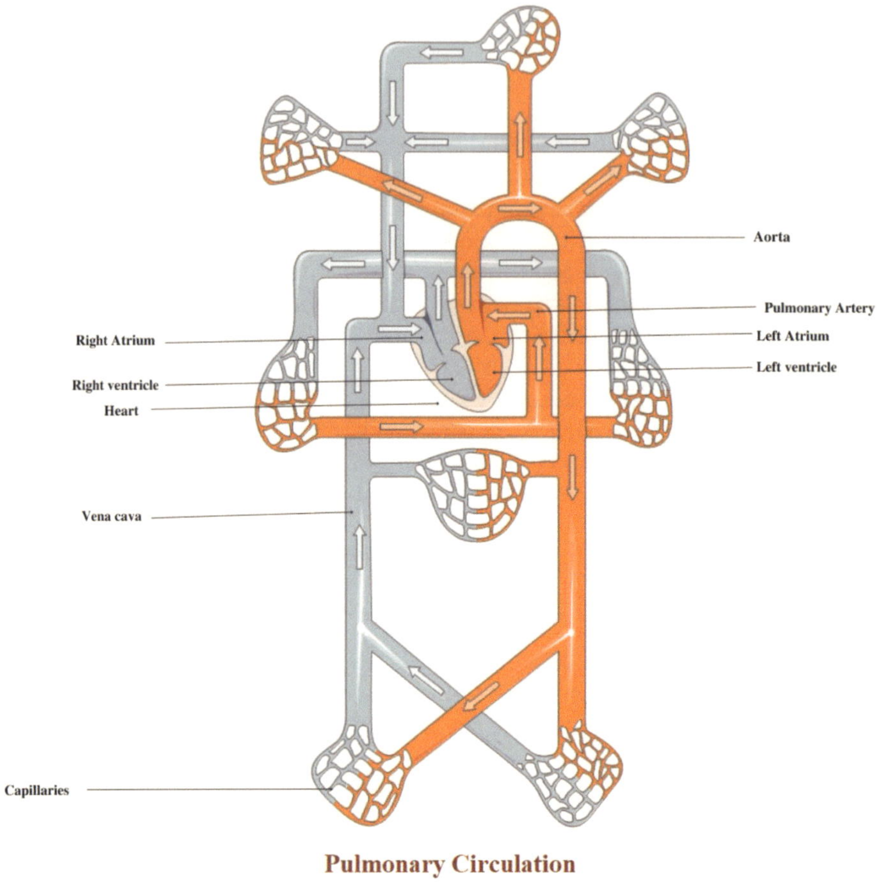

Figure 1.
Circulatory system of a heathy heart (designed with biorender).

3. Healthy heart

A healthy heart serves as the chief pumping unit of the cardiovascular system. In a healthy state, the muscular heart performs two key functions. Firstly, a healthy heart takes oxygen-depleted blood from the tissues and pumps it to the lungs, where the lungs pick up oxygen and discharge carbon dioxide. The second function of a healthy heart is to draw oxygen-rich blood from the lungs and deliver it throughout the body. The heart also removes interstitial fluid from the bloodstream and transports it to the extracellular space through systemic circulation.

4. Anatomical and physiological aspects of a healthy human heart

4.1 Structural features and anatomical position of healthy heart

The structure of a healthy human heart roughly resembles the shape of the heart on a playing card (**Figure 2A**) [3], with around two-thirds of its mass located to the left of the midline [10]. The human heart lies obliquely in the thorax which shields the

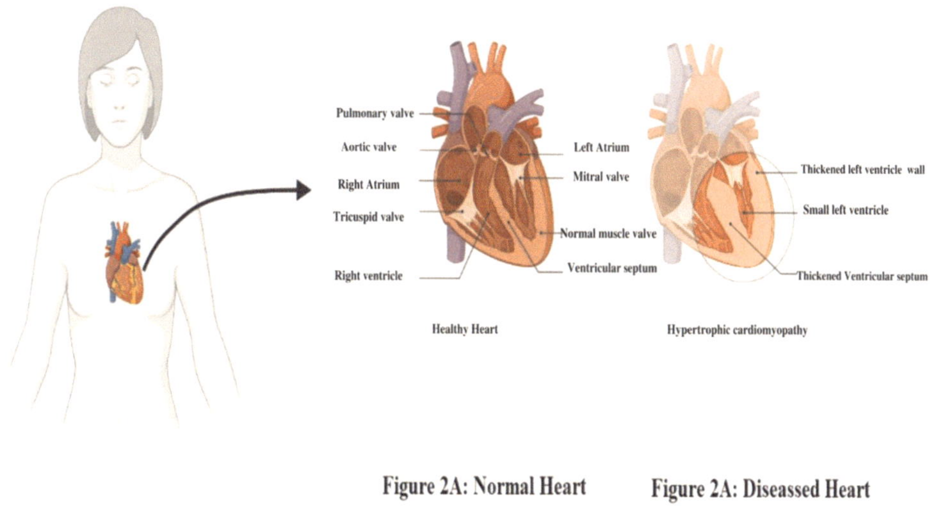

Figure 2.
Healthy heart (A) vs. diseased heart (B) (designed with biorender).

delicate anatomical structure of the heart. It is positioned roughly on a plane that spans from the right shoulder to the left nipple of the body [10]. Its anterior surface confronts the sternum, whereas its posterior surface confronts the vertebral column. However, the inferior surface of the heart is supported by the superior surface of the diaphragm. The human heart is housed in an enclosed region within the pleural cavities known as the middle mediastinum, which refers to the inner space of the pericardium, the protective sac that covers and cushions the heart as well as keeps the heart separated from other parts of the chest, including the lungs [9]. This pericardium is a serous membrane, which consists of a fibrous thick outer layer (the parietal pericardium) and an inner layer (visceral pericardium) separated by a lubricating substance known as the "serous fluid" (∼25–35 ml), that aids to "glide" the inner visceral pericardium against the outer parietal one [2, 10]. This pericardium serves to limit the heart's ability to expand excessively.

4.2 Layers of the heart wall

There are three distinct layers that make up the walls of a healthy human heart (as illustrated in **Figure 3**). These are—(i) Superficial Epicardium (ii) Middle Myocardium, and (iii) Inner Endocardium.

i. Superficial Epicardium: This layer is the most external to the heart. It is the visceral layer of the pericardial sac, which constitutes the innermost layer of the serous pericardium. An exterior layer of flat mesothelial cells forms this epicardium, with a layer of adipose and connective tissue lying beneath [25]. This inner layer shields the heart and it directly connects the epicardium to the muscular myocardium. This epicardium houses the blood vessels and nerves that furnish the heart [25]. At the base of the great vessels, the epicardium extends as the pericardial sac, composing an enclosed pericardial cavity.

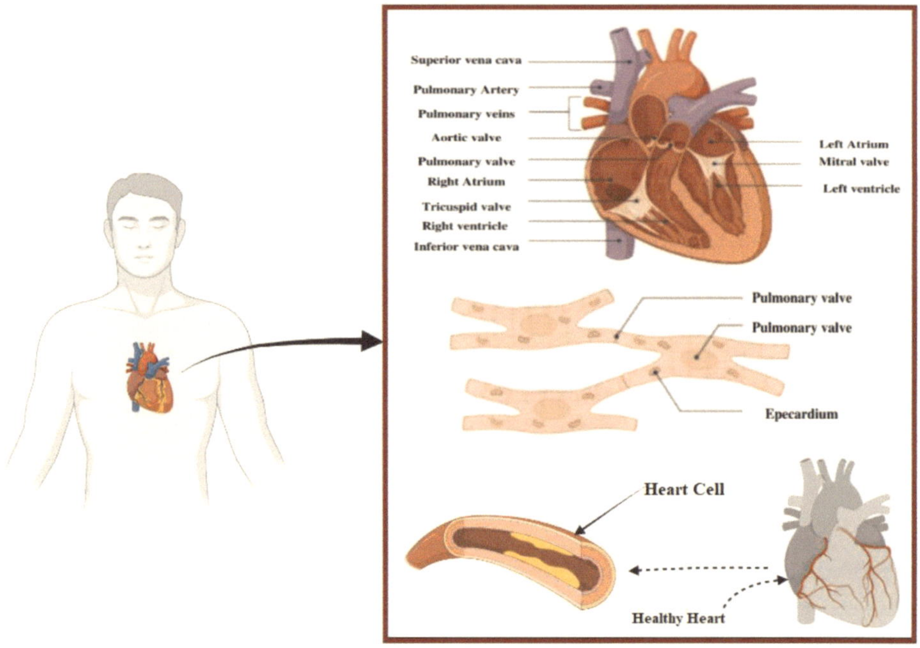

Figure 3.
Physiology of healthy human heart (designed with biorender).

ii. Middle Myocardium: The myocardium is the thickest of the three heart layers and it is the primary functioning component of the heart. The pumping action of the heart is made possible by this layer, which allows the heart to contract. This layer is primarily made up of capillaries, collagen fibers, and cardiomyocytes. The cardiomyocytes are arranged in a spiral pattern in the myocardium to press the blood into an appropriate trajectory throughout the heart [10]. These cardiomyocytes possess a high concentration of mitochondria and glycogen deposits, which has a tremendous functional eminence since this layer is contracting persistently, requiring a lot of energy all the time.

iii. Inner Endocardium: It is the inner layer of the heart wall. This layer is a smooth, thin gleaming membrane. This endocardium consists of an endothelium that is connected to the endothelium of blood vessels and connective tissue that fuses with the muscular myocardium [10, 24]. This layer forms the heart valves and serves as the lining of heart chambers.

4.3 Chambers of the heart

A healthy human heart is composed of four chambers—right atrium, right ventricle, left atrium, and left ventricle (**Figure 3**). Therefore, humans have two sides of their hearts—the right and left parts.

4.3.1 The right part of the heart

This section is made up of the right atrium and the right ventricle. The wall of the right atrium is quite thin, and this chamber remains under low pressure [24]. The right atrium carries the pacemaker called the SA (sinoatrial) node, which generates cardiac impulses, as well as the AV (atrioventricular) node, which transmits electrical signals to the ventricles [22]. This right atrium collects the deoxygenated (venous) blood from the whole body via the superior and inferior vena cava and the coronary sinus [3]. This right atrium is connected to the right ventricle via the tricuspid valve, through which deoxygenated blood enters the right ventricle from the right atrium. The pulmonary trunk, which originates in the right ventricle, transports the deoxygenated blood from the right ventricle to the lungs, where it is oxygenated [24]. The right ventricle has a thicker wall than that of the right atrium, but it's less muscular compared to the left ventricular wall.

4.3.2 Left part of the heart

This part is made up of the left atrium and the left ventricle. The left atrium is a low-pressure and thin-walled chamber [24]. Pulmonary veins deliver the oxygenated blood from the lungs to the left atrium, from where the blood moves to the left ventricle via the bicuspid or mitral valve [24]. The arterial blood is pumped by the left ventricle throughout the body via the systemic aorta.

However, the two right chambers are detached from the left ones by a constant divider, the ventricular section of which is known as the interventricular septum whereas the atrial portion is called the interatrial septum [3]. The interatrial septum is fibrous in nature, but the interventricular septum possesses dual structural characteristics, with the upper one-fourth segment being fibrous and the lower three-fourth section being muscular.

4.4 Valves of the heart

The human heart possesses four valves, each with a distinct function. Two of them are situated within the junction of the atria and the ventricles. These two valves are termed as the atrioventricular valves. On the other hand, the remaining two valves are located at the aperture of blood vessels originating from the ventricles, i.e., the pulmonary trunk and systemic aorta. These two valves are termed as semilunar valves. Four of these heart valves ensure the unidirectional flow of blood across the heart [26].

4.4.1 Atrioventricular valves

The right atrioventricular orifice is shielded by the tricuspid valve, which is composed of three cusps or flaps, i.e., infundibular or anterior cusp, medial or septal cusp, and marginal or posterior cusp [3]. Conversely, the left atrioventricular orifice is protected by the bicuspid valve, which is composed of two valvular cusps, namely, the anterior cusp and the posterior cusp [3]. This bicuspid valve is also known as the mitral valve because of its similarity to the miter of a bishop. The cusps of both of these valves are triangular in appearance and are linked to the edges of the fibrous or dense connective tissue surrounding the atrioventricular openings.

4.4.2 Semilunar valves

The aperture within the pulmonary artery and the right ventricle is guarded by the pulmonic semilunar valve, while the opening between the systemic aorta and the left ventricle is guarded by the aortic semilunar valve that is stronger and larger compared to the other one [3]. Both of these valves have a shape that resembles a half moon, because of which these are referred to as semilunar valves. These valves are composed of three cusps. The pulmonary semilunar valve is composed of the left anterior cusp, right posterior, and left posterior cusp; whereas the aortic semilunar valve is made up of the right anterior cusp, right posterior, and left posterior cusps, respectively [3].

4.5 Special junctional tissues of the healthy heart

A healthy heart muscle is primarily made up of some specialized structures that play critical roles in commencing and transmitting impulses at a rate that is significantly faster than that of the remaining muscles. These structures are inclusively termed as the "Junctional Tissues of the Heart". They consist of the following structures—(i) S.A. (sino-atrial) node, (ii) A.V. (atrioventricular) node, (iii) Bundle of His, (iv) Bundle branch, (v) Purkinje fibers. A brief description is given below:

i. S.A. node: It is located in the right atrium of the heart at the intersection of the right auricular appendage and superior vena cava [3]. It is wider at the top and tapers toward the bottom, measuring approximately 5 × 20 mm. It functions as the heart's natural pacemaker and produces impulses at a rate of 70–80 bpm in adults [3, 24, 26]. The rhythm initiated from the S.A. node is commonly referred to as the sinus rhythm.

ii. A.V. node: It is located in the right atrium, near the opening of the coronary sinus, in the posterior portion of the interatrial septum [3]. It has a measurement of approximately 2 × 5 mm. It serves as the reserve pacemaker of the heart. It accepts the impulses generated by the SA node and conducts it to the ventricles at a rate of 40–60 bpm via the bundle of His [24, 26]. The rhythm emerging from this node is termed as the nodal rhythm.

iii. Bundle of His: The main trunk of this bundle is continuous with the A.V. node and passes upwards until it reaches the posterior margin of the membranous part of the interventricular septum and then forwards below it [3]. It is approximately 20 mm in length.

iv. Purkinje fibers: The branches of the bundle of His give rise to these fibers, which travel through the papillary muscle and lateral ventricular walls, eventually terminating in the subendocardial network of the heart [3]. The primary function of these fibers is to instantly transmit impulses to all parts of the ventricular muscle fiber. Atrioventricular dissociation can cause these fibers to fire at a rate of 30–35 bpm [3, 24, 27].

v. Bundle branch: Immediately above the muscular portion of the septum, two branches (right and left) of the bundle are visible. Both of these branches remain just below the endocardium [3]. The right branch of the bundle travels along the right side of the septum and is comparatively longer than its left counterpart. On the contrary, the left bundle branch travels along the left side of the septum, bifurcating into inferior and superior sections, and culminates in the Purkinje system, which is located within the ventricular subendocardial tissue [3]. The atrial impulse is normally carried to the ventricles by these bundle branches. These branches can generate cardiac impulses at a rate of 36 beats/min in the event of failure of the S.A. and A.V. nodes.

5. Physiological properties of heart muscle

Heart muscle possesses certain special features. These include:

i. Rhythmicity

ii. Conductivity

iii. Contractility

iv. Excitability

v. All or None Law

vi. The Staircase Phenomenon

vii. Refractory Period

viii. Tone

A summary of all these properties is given below:

i. Rhythmicity: It is the capacity of a cardiac tissue to generate its own impulses regularly. This property is also known as self-excitation or autorhythmicity. All of the tissues of the heart own this feature. However, in the human heart, there is an exclusive excitatory structure that produces rapid electrical impulses. This exclusive structure is termed as the "pacemaker of the heart". The sinoatrial node (SA node) serves the purpose of the pacemaker in the mammalian heart. From this node, the impulses propagate to other portions of the heart through a specific conductive system. Moreover, the AV node, the atria, and the ventricles of the heart are also capable of generating impulses and can perform as pacemakers. In spite of this, SA node is referred to be the pacemaker because of its high rate of impulse generation capacity compared to others.

   The rhythmicity of different portions of a healthy human heart is shown in **Table 1**.

ii. Conductivity: The human heart possesses a unique conducting system, which is constructed by specialized cardiac muscle fibers known as internodal fibers. These fibers are responsible for the quick transmission of impulses from the SA node to other parts of the heart. The fundamental elements of the conductive system in the heart include—the AV node, Purkinje fibers, right and left bundle branches, and bundle of His. These conductive tissues are also referred to as the junctional tissues of the human heart. The conductivity of the heart muscle is maintained in the following way:

Portions of human heart	Rhythmicity
SA node	70–80 bpm
AV node	40–60 bpm
Purkinje fibers	30–35 bpm
Atrial muscle	40–60 bpm
Ventricular muscle	20–40 bpm

Table 1.
Rhythmicity of different portions of a healthy human heart.

Components of conductive system	Velocities of impulses
SA node	0.05 m/s
AV node	0.1 m/s
Purkinje fibers	1 m/s
Bundle of His	1 m/s
Ventricular muscle fibers	0.4 m/s

Table 2.
The velocities of impulses at various portions of the conductive system.

At first, the AV node receives the impulses from the SA node through the internodal fibers. The AV node then sends these impulses to the ventricles via the bundle of His and its branches. The Purkinje fibers further carry these impulses from the top of the heart down to the base.

The velocities of impulses at various portions of the conductive system of the heart are given in **Table 2**.

iii. Contractility: Contractility of the heart muscle refers to its ability to shorten or contract in length in response to a stimulus. Myofibril is the core contractile unit of the heart muscle, which is made up of actin and myosin. These two units are linked together under the presence of ATP during contraction, which causes the fiber to be shortened. However, at the time of rest, these two units become dissociated as the ATP is resynthesized.

As it pertains to contractility, Starling's Law of the heart or Frank-Starling Law has been codified. This law states that the heart has the ability to modify its stroke volume and force of contraction in response to changes in venous return.

iv. Excitability: It is the capacity of the cardiac muscle to generate a propagated action potential in response to a stimulation that is sufficiently strong.

v. All or None Law: The cardiac muscle strictly obeys this law. In accordance with this law, whenever a stimulus is provided, regardless of its strength, the entire heart muscle either responds to it at its maximum capacity or there is no response at all.

vi. The Staircase Phenomenon: When the heart muscle is excited with sequential maximal stimuli, the initial few contractions display a progressive increase in magnitude, which is referred to as a staircase. Following that, the strength of contraction stabilizes at its regular level.

Refractory Period: The refractory period of the heart is the duration of time during which a typical cardiac impulse cannot re-excite a section of cardiac muscle that has already been stimulated or excited. It is of two types: absolute refractory period and relative refractory period.

Absolute Refractory Period: In the absolute refractory period, the muscle does not respond at all, no matter how strong the stimulus is. The reason is that depolarization is taking place at the time. As a result, there cannot be a second depolarization.

Relative Refractory Period: During this period, the muscle responds if the power of stimulus is maximum. At this point, the muscle is in a repolarizing state.

The comparative refractory periods of different portions of the heart muscle are given in **Table 3**.

vii. Tone: The heart muscle of humans has tone. This tone is nerve-independent and adjustable. This allows the heart to keep reasonably constant tension on its different contents.

6. Cardiac cycle of healthy heart

A single cardiac cycle consists of two primary phases- diastole and systole. The term "diastole" denotes relaxation, and the term "systole" refers to contraction [3].

6.1 Diastole

During the diastolic phase, blood flows into the right atrium from the superior and inferior vena cava, which elevates the internal pressure of the right atrium. When the right atrial pressure surpasses the right ventricular pressure, the tricuspid valve passively opens, enabling the blood to move toward the right ventricle. Simultaneously, the oxygen-rich blood from the lungs returns to the left atrium, resulting in an

Portions of heart muscle	Refractory period
SA node	Highest
AV node	Lower than S.A node
Ventricular muscle fibers	Lower than nodal
Atrial muscle fibers	Lower than ventricular
Purkinje fibers	Lower than ventricular

Table 3.
The comparative refractory periods of different portions of the heart muscle.

escalation in left atrial pressure. This leads to the opening of the bicuspid valve, which allows the passage of blood from the left atrium to the left ventricle.

6.2 Systole

During systole, the right and left ventricles contract and discharge blood into the pulmonary trunk and the aorta respectively. At this time the pulmonic and aortic heart valves open to allow the passage of blood into the pulmonary artery and aorta. However, the bicuspid and tricuspid atrioventricular valves remain closed during this period. But during the closure of these two valves, the first cardiac sound, i.e. the "lub" sound is generated at the beginning of the ventricular systole; and at the end of the ventricular systole, the second heart sound, i.e. the "dub" sound is generated due to the closure of the pulmonic and aortic valves.

So, each cardiac cycle comprises the full contraction and relaxation of both the atria and ventricles and lasts around 0.8 s.

The time periods of the atrial and ventricular events of the cardiac cycle are given below:

Atrial events	• Atrial systole • Atrial diastole	0.1 s 0.7 s
Ventricular events	• Ventricular systole • Ventricular diastole	0.3 s 0.5 s

7. Cardiac output of heart

The volume of blood that a healthy heart pumps in 1 min is termed as the cardiac output of the heart. Logically, the cardiac output (CO) is equal to the product of the stroke volume (SV) and heart rate (HR). It is expressed in l/min.

$$\mathrm{CO\ (ml/\ min\ )} = \mathrm{SV\ (ml/beat)} \times \mathrm{HR\ (beats/\ min\ )}$$

8. Pathology of cardiovascular system

8.1 Diagnosis of cardiovascular diseases

Diagnosis of CVDs is often conducted by the following approach

i. Assessment of risk factors, medical, and family history of the patient.

ii. Physical Examination: Physical examinations can assist in evaluating an individual's risk of developing heart disease. Complete cholesterol testing is the most generally recommended physical examination to determine susceptibility of CVDs.

iii. Electrocardiogram (ECG): ECG helps to monitor the electrical activity of the heart painlessly. The activities of the heart are recorded on graph paper via a portable small machine. ECG aids in detecting the incidence of arrhythmias, angina, and heart attacks.

iv. Echocardiogram: It is a type of ultrasonography of the heart. It creates an image of the heart using sound waves. It may be used by doctors to examine the conditions of the heart muscles and heart valves of the patient.

v. Chest X-ray: In this test small doses of radiation are used to provide high-resolution pictures of the chest and heart. The causes of chest discomfort can be identified with the help of this test.

vi. Magnetic Resonance Imaging (MRI) of the Heart: An MRI uses radio waves and large magnets to produce internal images of the body. During this test, a technician generates images of the heart and blood vessels as it beats. The captured pictures can help doctors in diagnosing diseases of the coronary artery and heart muscle.

8.2 Risk factors of cardiovascular diseases

The risk factors of CVDs can be categorized into two classes: non-modifiable and modifiable risk factors (**Figure 4**). Non-modifiable risk factors are those that cannot be altered or controlled. These include- ethnicity, race, age, gender, and genetic factors of an individual. On the contrary, modifiable risk factors are those that can be altered or controlled by modifying the lifestyle of an individual. For

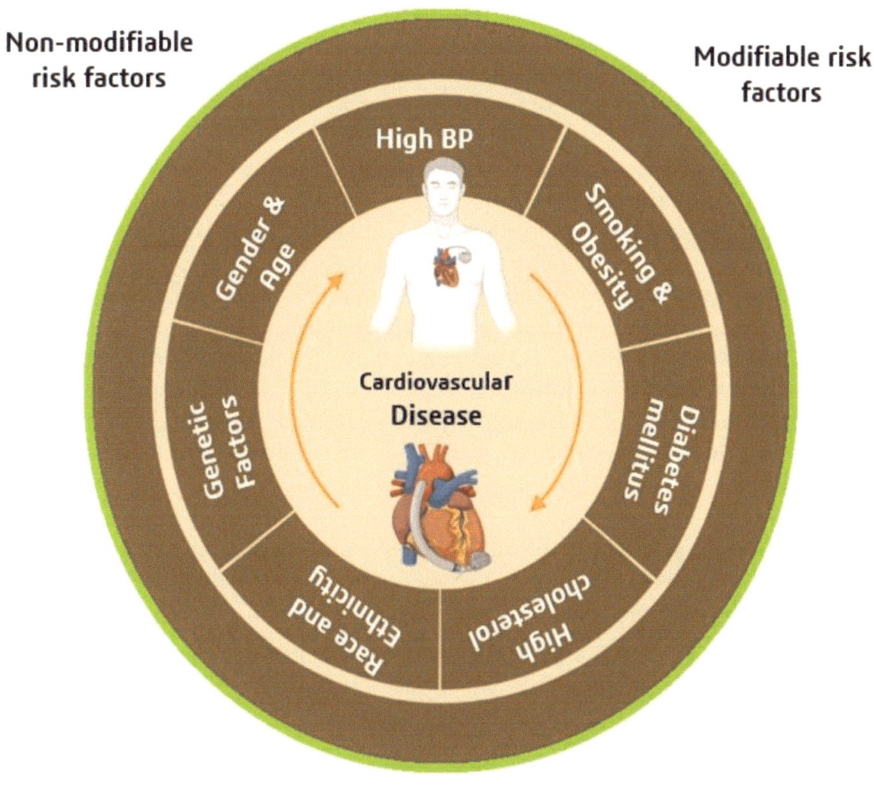

Figure 4.
Risk factors of cardiovascular diseases (designed with biorender).

example—smoking cessation, weight control, proper maintenance, and control of lifestyle diseases (e.g. diabetes, hypertension) can significantly reduce the risk of CVDs.

8.3 Classification of cardiovascular diseases

Heart disease is of basically two types

i. Coronary Artery Diseases (CAD) and

ii. Arrhythmia.

iii. Brief descriptions of both of these diseases are given below:

8.3.1 Coronary artery diseases (CADs)

Coronary artery disease (CAD) or coronary heart disease (CHD) is one of the most pervasive forms of CVD which is considered to be the preeminent cause of mortality in both first-world and third-world countries [28]. According to the estimation from a study, CAD accounts for 32.7% of overall CVDs and 2.2% of the total burden of maladies worldwide [29]. CAD is an inflammatory atherosclerotic disease [27]. It is a multifarious human disorder in which there is an insufficient transmission of oxygen and blood to the cardiac muscle, resulting from a blockage of the coronary arteries. It is often characterized by plaque deposition within the lumens of coronary arteries, which obstruct blood flow [30]. Hence CADs are linked to impaired circulation to the heart via the coronary artery. There are various forms of CAD. Among these are:

a. Myocardial Ischemia and Reperfusion: Ischemia and reperfusion is a diseased state marked by a temporary reduction in blood flow to an organ, followed by a successive restoration of perfusion and accompanying reoxygenation [31]. Myocardial ischemia develops when the oxygen requirements of the heart muscle are greater than the amount of oxygen that is available to the heart. Unless this situation is remedied, cell damage is likely to occur. Ischemic myocardial cells can have their oxygen and energy substances restored when the ischemic myocardium is repercussed [32] during procedures such as coronary artery bypass surgery, thrombolysis, or angioplasty. However, this process may create another form of myocardial damage, which is referred to as "reperfusion injury".

b. Angina Pectoris: Angina pectoris is caused by a lack of oxygen supply in the myocardium. There are three clinically distinct types of angina pectoris, each with its own pathogenesis:

- Stable or typical angina
- Prinzmetal's variant angina and
- Unstable or crescendo angina.

A brief description of each type is given below:

- Stable or typical angina: It is the most typical form of angina. It is marked by the sudden attack of chest pain or bouts of discomfort after emotional stimulation or physical activity, which are assuaged by rest. The pathogenesis of such a situation lies in atherosclerosis which is chronically stenosing the coronary arteries and thereby preventing the heart muscle from receiving adequate blood supply when the heart's workload rises [33].

- Prinzmetal's variant angina: Pain at rest characterizes this type of angina, which is unrelated to physical exertion. The specific cause of prinzmetal's angina is still a mystery to scientists. Atherosclerosis-induced sudden coronary vasospasm or mast cell-stimulated release of humoral vasoconstrictors in the coronary adventitia may be to blame for this phenomenon [33].

- Unstable or crescendo angina: It is the most severe form of angina. It is marked by a greater recurrence of pain onsets that last longer and occur more frequently during rest [33]. Therefore, it may be a warning sign of an oncoming myocardial attack and should be handled seriously.

c. Myocardial infarction (MI): It refers to the occurrence of a heart attack. MI takes place when the blood ceases to flow adequately to a segment of the heart, causing injury to the heart muscle due to a deficit of oxygen delivery, when one of the coronary vessels that supply the heart with blood becomes blocked due to an unstable deposition of cholesterol, white blood cells, plaques, and fat [34]. When the situation becomes more critical, it is referred to as acute myocardial infarction (AMI).

d. Coronary Sclerosis or Atherosclerosis: Accumulation of plaque in the inner lining of artery results in a condition known as arterial hardening or thickening. When fatty materials, calcium, and fibrous elements build up in the intima of an artery, it is known as atherosclerosis or coronary sclerosis.

8.3.2 Arrhythmia

Cardiac arrhythmias are a form of irregular heartbeats that are either too slow (i.e. bradycardia) or too fast (i.e. tachycardia). Arrhythmia attacks can be triggered by even a slight shift in the morphology or dynamics of the electrocardiogram (ECG), resulting in shortness of breath, chest pain, exhaustion, and even unconsciousness due to reduced heart pumping capacity [35].

8.3.2.1 Mechanisms of cardiac arrhythmias

Cardiac arrhythmias are caused by three basic mechanisms:

- Abnormal Automaticity

- Triggered Electrical Activity

- Reentry

Brief descriptions of these mechanisms are given below:

- Abnormal Automaticity: Premature heartbeats are caused by abnormal automaticity, which happens when non-pacemaker cells initiate spontaneous firing. Ventricular tachycardia, atrial tachycardia, accelerated idioventricular rhythm, and premature beats are examples of arrhythmias caused by abnormal autorhythmicity.

- Triggered Electrical Activity: Although activated once, cardiac cells contract twice in response to triggered activity. This is frequently brought on by events known as early after-depolarizations (EADs) or delayed after-depolarizations (DADs), which are attributable to electrical instability in the cell membrane of the heart. Torsade de Pointes is a typical example of this phenomenon.

- Reentry: Following normal activation of the heart, when a propagating impulse does not die out, reentry occurs, leading to re-excitation of the heart and causing it to beat faster after the refractory period has expired. Many forms of arrhythmias are brought about by this mechanism. Wolff-Parkinson-White syndrome, atrial flutter, atrioventricular nodal reentry, and bundle branch reentry are some examples of reentry-based cardiac arrhythmias.

8.3.2.2 Types of cardiac arrhythmias

Arrhythmias come in many varieties, which are associated to origination of impulses in the S.A. node and their consequent distribution to every portion of the heart. Some of the most notable forms of arrhythmias are mentioned in **Table 4** along with their morphology and characteristic features.

Besides these two major cardiovascular problems, there are a number of other critical heart ailments. These include:

8.3.3 Hypertension

Hypertension or high blood pressure occurs when the blood exerts an excessive force against the walls of the blood vessels. In other terms, a persistently elevated blood pressure of more than 140 mmHg over 90 mmHg (i.e. a systolic pressure greater than 140 or diastolic pressure greater than 90) is considered to be hypertension. The most severe form of hypertension is chronic hypertension, which is an asymptomatic "silent" illness. It can lead to alterations in the retinal blood vessels, brain damage, kidney failure, and atypical thickening of the cardiac muscle.

8.3.4 Cor pulmonale

Cor pulmonale is the medical term for cardiac disease affecting the right side of the heart as a result of respiratory issues [33]. More specifically, cor pulmonale is defined as an anomaly in the structure and performance of the right ventricle of the heart owing to an ailment in the primary respiratory system that results in pulmonary hypertension. Hypertrophy, right ventricular dilatation or both are hallmarks of this condition [33].

Types of arrhythmia	Morphology	Characteristic features	References
Sinus Tachycardia	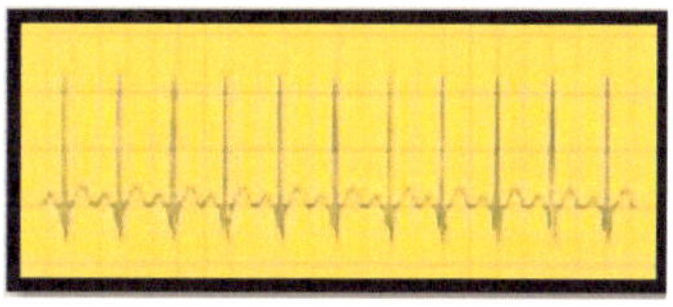	• Increased impulse release from the SA node causes an abnormal elevation in heart rate which may rises up to 150 bpm; • ECG exhibits short R-R interval due to elevated heart rate	[24, 36]
Sinus Bradycardia	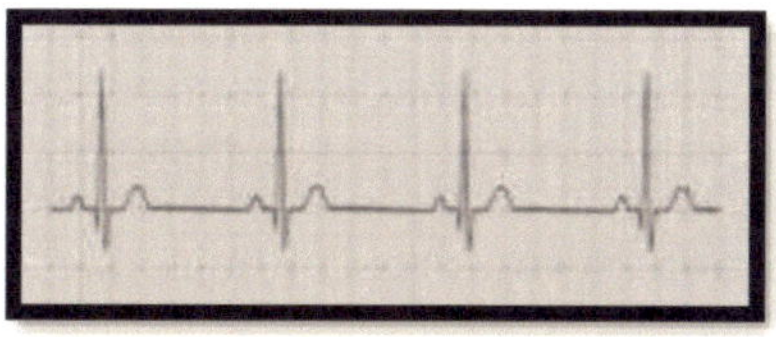	• Decrease in heart rate which is less than 60 bpm; • Extended R-R intervals on ECG.	[24, 37]
Sinus Disrhythmia	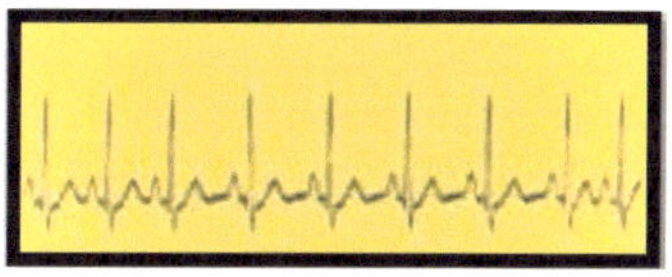	• Periodic rise (during inspiration) and fall (during expiration) in heart rate associated with respiration; • Shortened R-R intervals during inspiration and prolonged R-R intervals during expiration.	[19, 36, 37]
Atrial Tachycardia	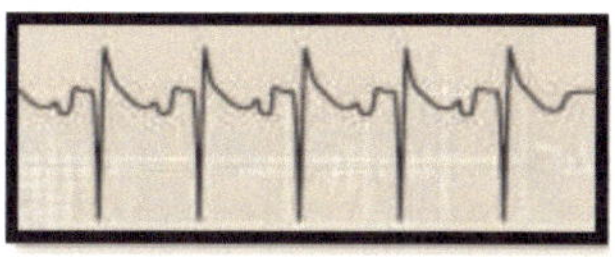	• Atria beat at a rate of 300 bpm; • Characteristic sawtooth pattern observed in the intervals between the QRS complexes on ECG.	[38]
Ventricular Tachycardia	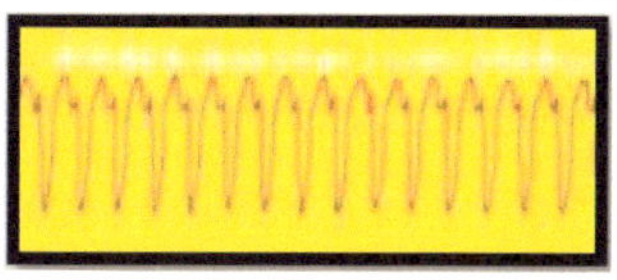	• Three or more consecutive abnormal heartbeats in a row beating faster than 100 bpm.	[38]
Atrial Fibrillation	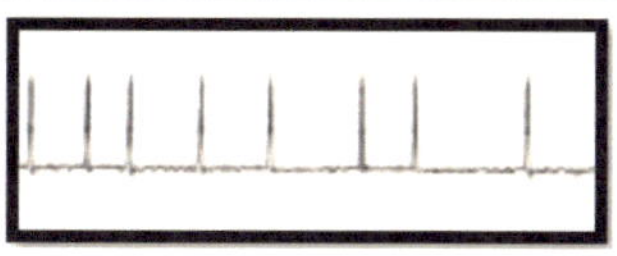	• Irregular and rapid contractions of atria at a rate of 300–400 bpm; • ECG shows no P wave.	[24, 39]
Ventricular Fibrillation	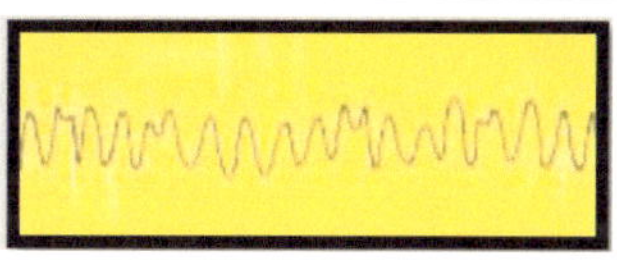	• Irregular and rapid ventricular twitching at a rate of 400–500 bpm.	[24, 40]

Types of arrhythmia	**Morphology**	**Characteristic features**	**References**
Premature Supraventricular Contractions	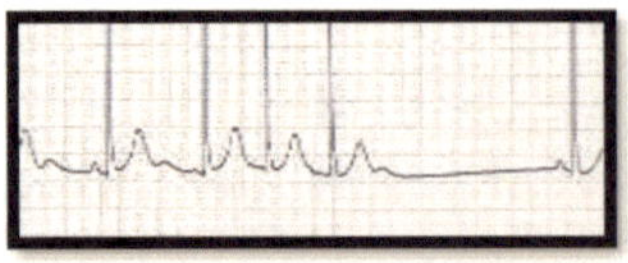	• Premature actuation of the atria originating from a site except for the S. A. node.	[41]
Paroxysmal supraventricular tachycardia (PSVT)	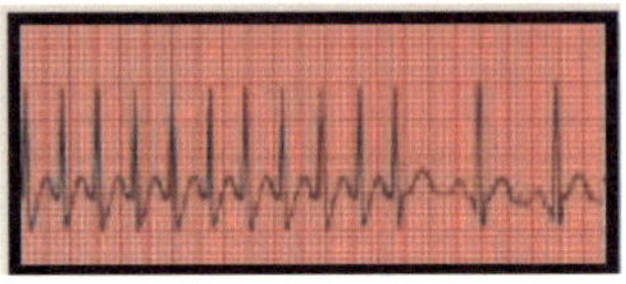	• Events of rapid heart rate (150–250 bpm) originating in a portion of the heart above the ventricles; • ECG shows a narrowed QRS complex with regular rhythm.	[42]
Premature Ventricular Contractions (PVCs)	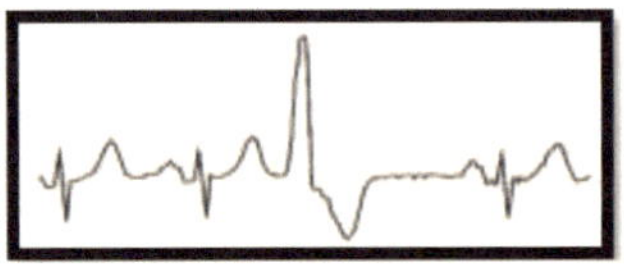	• The heartbeat is generated by the purkinje fibers instead of the S.A. node; • With each PVC, there is an additional pause in the heart's regular rhythm; • PVCs may appear singly or repeatedly in a pattern.	[43]
Wolff-Parkinson-White Syndrome	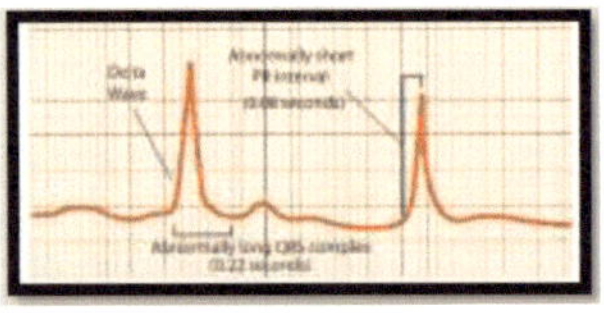	• Marked by frequent attacks of AV nodal paroxysmal tachycardia in those with bundle of Kent; • ECG exhibits shortened P-R interval with normal T wave and QRS complex.	[24, 44]
Heart Block	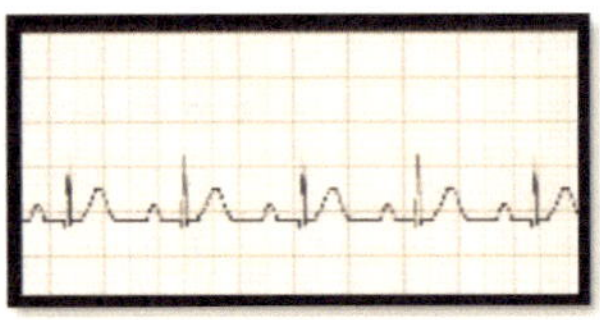	• Partial or complete blockade of electrical signals controlling heartbeat, leading to an obstruction in transmission of impulses from atria to ventricles	[45]
Torsade de Pointes	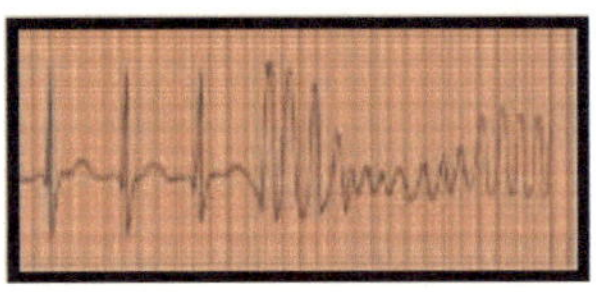	• Each subsequent QRS complex has a different shape than the preceding one; • Twisted QRS complex is observed around the baseline on ECG surface;	[46]

Types of arrhythmia	Morphology	Characteristic features	References
		• Multiform and queer shaped QRS complexes with unidirectional sharp points for a short duration; • Extremely rare arrhythmia that may be caused by prolonged QT complexes.	

Table 4.
Different forms of arrhythmias with their morphology and characteristic features.

8.3.5 Heart failure

Heart failure is characterized as a pathophysiologic condition in which the defective heart function is incapable of maintaining optimal circulation for the metabolic demands of the body's tissues [33]. Heart failure may be chronic or acute.

8.3.6 Valvular heart disease

It develops when the valves of the heart become impaired or defective. Valvular heart diseases are of two types:

- Stenosis and

- Regurgitation.

- Stenosis: Stenosis refers to the inability of the heart valve to completely open during diastole, which obstructs the blood flowing in a forward direction [33]. Aortic and mitral stenosis are the most prevalent types of valvular stenosis.

- Regurgitation: Regurgitation of blood occurs when a valve fails to close perfectly during systole, causing regurgitation or backflow of blood [33]. Aortic and mitral regurgitation are the two most common types of valvular regurgitation.

8.3.7 Inflammatory heart disease

Inflammatory heart disease (IHD) refers to a set of conditions that include myocarditis, pericarditis, and endocarditis [47].

- Myocarditis: It is an inflammation or infection that develops inside the heart muscle prompted by viruses like specific immunological conditions and sarcoidosis [48, 49].

- Pericarditis: It refers to the inflammation or infection of the pericardium [48].

- Endocarditis: This condition is brought on by an infection of the inner lining of the heart (i.e. endocardium), which causes severe inflammation [48].

8.3.8 Rheumatic heart disease

It is a nonsuppurative, post-streptococcal, systemic, inflammatory disorder that mostly affects the central nervous system, heart, skin, joints, and subcutaneous tissues. The chronic episode of RF affects all layers of the heart (pancarditis), resulting in significant cardiac consequences known as rheumatic heart disease (RHD).

8.3.9 Stroke

According to the definition of World Health Organization (WHO), stroke can be defined as- "rapidly developing clinical signs of focal (or global) disturbance of cerebral function, with symptoms lasting 24 h or longer or leading to death, with no apparent cause other than of vascular origin [50].

8.3.10 Peripheral arterial disease (PAD)

It is a chronic atherosclerotic condition that leads to the narrowing of the peripheral artery vasculature, primarily in the lower extremities [50]. This usually restricts blood supply to the extremities, resulting in calf or thigh pain while exertion or walking. It has an estimated global incidence of up to 10%, rising to approximately 30% in patients older than 50 years [51].

8.3.11 Cardiomyopathy

It is a pathological and anatomic condition related to electrical or muscular malfunction of the heart [49]. In other terms, cardiomyopathies constitute a varied category of disorders that frequently result in progressive heart failure and substantial morbidity and mortality. Cardiomyopathies can be either primary (i.e., inherited, acquired, or mixed) or secondary (e.g., infammatory, toxic, infltrative) [52]. Hypertrophic cardiomyopathy, dilated cardiomyopathy, arrhythmogenic right ventricular cardiomyopathy, and restrictive cardiomyopathy are the most prevalent forms of cardiomyopathy.

8.3.12 Congenital heart disease

The malformation of the heart that is apparent at birth is referred to as congenital heart disease [30]. The condition affects roughly 0.5% of all newborns and is the most common kind of congenital cardiac disease. Premature newborns have a higher risk of congenital heart disease. Some notable forms of congenital heart diseases include—congenital long QT syndrome (LQTS), congenital short QT syndrome (SQTS) etc.

- Congenital LQTS: An inherited heart condition known as congenital long QT syndrome (LQTS) is attributable to a prolonged QT interval at rest and a significant risk of life-threatening arrhythmias [53]. Nearly one in every 2500 live newborns is estimated to be affected by the disease.

- Congenital SQTS: This condition is characterized by an unusually short QT interval, potentially fatal ventricular arrhythmias, and paroxysmal atrial fibrillation. Children and young adults can be affected by this autosomal dominant condition; often a family history of cardiac abrupt death is revealed [54].

- Andersen-Tawil Syndrome: It is a congenital heart disorder in which irregular heartbeats (arrhythmia), muscle weakness (periodic paralysis), and developmental anomalies are common occurrences. The paralysis episodes generally begin in early infancy and last from a few hours to several days.

9. Management of cardiovascular diseases

CVDs can be managed by following two approaches

- Non-pharmacological approach

- Pharmacological approach

Brief descriptions of both of these approaches are presented below:

9.1 Non-pharmacological management of cardiovascular diseases

The recommendations for the management of heart failure developed by the European Society of Cardiology (ESC) contain a number of tips and advice that should be included in patient education. These tips and advice are intended for patients who have chronic heart diseases [55]. In patients suffering from heart disease, the following are some of the most important aspects of non-pharmacological therapy and treatment plans -.

9.1.1 Diet modification

Diet modification is of utmost significance for persons suffering from chronic heart diseases to maintain their disease conditions [55, 56]. These may include:

i. Control of Salt Intake: Chronic cardiovascular patients should intake less than 2000 mg salts per day [57]. It is important for patients with advanced heart failure to keep their daily salt intake under 2000 mg, and these patients should also be encouraged to limit their fluid intake between 1500 and 2000 ml [58]. It should also be pointed out that salt replacements need to be used with extreme care since potassium might be included in them. They have the potential to cause hyperkalemia when consumed in significant doses in conjunction with medications that inhibit angiotensin-converting enzymes (ACEs) [59].

ii. Inhibition of Alcohol Consumption: In patients with a diagnosis alcoholic cardiomyopathy, drinking alcohol is strictly restricted; nevertheless, in other situations, drinking alcohol in moderation is acceptable [60].

iii. Smoking Cessation: For smoker cardiac patients, quitting smoking is the most successful course of therapy. It greatly curtails the fatality rates of cardiac patients compared to any other form of intervention or treatment [61–63]. Cardiac patients who cease the habit of smoking minimize their possibilities for prospective diseases and fatality by one-third two years later [62, 64].

iv. Intake of Calorie Restricted Diets: Calorie-restricted diet consumption may lead to modest loss of weight and reduction in blood pressure in overweight hypertensive individuals.

9.1.2 Rest and exercise

Patients diagnosed with heart failure were traditionally counseled for engaging in physical activity in the hopes of preventing their condition from deteriorating. Numerous investigations have reported that physical rest has come to be recommended only in cases of acute heart failure or instability in chronic heart failure [58]. Physical exercise is critical for reducing obesity, overweight and is also useful for chronic cardiovascular suffering. Even if no weight is lost, exercise can help reduce the risk factors for CVDs and assist weight loss efforts for those who are overweight and have type 2 diabetes.

9.1.3 Ventilatory support: oxygen and non-invasive ventilation

Oxygen has been utilized extensively outside of hospitals as well as in emergency rooms due to the widespread belief that it may alleviate breathlessness and increase myocardial oxygenation, regardless of the fact that oxygen saturation levels should be maintained and available for heart patients. On the other hand, supplementary oxygen and supported breathing such as ventilation should be stored or reserved for cardiac patients who are experiencing hypoxemia. Several research findings have comprehensively evaluated the effects of elevating fraction of inspired oxygen (FiO2), oxygen deficiency produces a decline in cardiac output as well as enhances systemic vascular resistance (SVR), and ventricular filling pressures [65].

9.2 Pharmacological management of cardiovascular diseases

Pharmacological management involves two approaches –

i. Treatment with Allopathic Medicines

ii. Treatment with Herbal Medicines

9.2.1 Treatment with allopathic medicines

Different types of medications are recommended for cardiac patients depending on their disease conditions. In **Table 5**, major classes of cardiovascular drugs are presented along with their mechanisms of action.

Different classes of cardiovascular drugs	Mechanism of actions	Examples of drugs	References
Beta-adrenoceptor Antagonists	Block beta-adrenoceptors in heart and inhibit the actions of epinephrine and norepinephrine, leading to a deceleration in heart beat and a reduction in blood pressure (**Figure** 5).	• Propranolol (non-selective) • Timolol (non-selective) • Atenolol (selective) • Metoprolol (selective)	[67]
Angiotensin Converting Enzyme (ACE) Inhibitors	Inhibit the conversion of angiotensin I to angiotensin II (**Figure** 5).	• Captopril • Enalapril	[68]
Angiotensin II Receptor Antagonists	Selectively block the action of angiotensin II by competitively antagonizing the angiotensin II receptors, specially AT1 receptors and aid in dilating the arteries and veins to reduce elevated blood pressure (**Figure 5**).	• Losartan • Valsartan • Candesartan	[69, 70]
Alpha-Adrenoceptor Blocking Drugs	Block alpha receptor in heart.	• Prazosin • Doxazosin	[71]
Adrenergic Receptor Blocking Drugs	Block adrenergic neurons and prevent the release of noradrenaline from postganglionic adrenergic neurons.	Guanethidine	[72]
Vasodilator Antihypertensive Drugs	Dilate the constriction or narrowing of blood vessels.	• Diazoxide • Minoxidil • Hydralazine	[73]
Centrally Acting Antihypertensive Drugs	Regulate and control impulses along certain nerve pathways.	• Clonidine • Methyldopa	[74]
Ganglionic Blocking Drugs	Inhibit transmission of impulses at both sympathetic and parasympathetic ganglia	• Pempidine • Trimetaphan • Mecamylamine • Hexamethonium	[75]
Nitrates	Coronary vasodilation (**Figure 6**)	• Nitroglycerine • Isosorbide Dinitrate	[76]
Calcium Channel Blockers	Blocks inward movement of calcium ions (**Figure 5, Figure 6**).	• Verapamil • Diltiazem • Nifedipine • Nicardipine	[77, 78]
Potassium Channel Activators	Dilates veins and arteries.	• Nicorandil	[79]
Cerebral and Peripheral Vasodilators	Dilates blood vessels	• Cilostazole • Niftidrofuryln	[80, 81]
Potassium Channel Inhibitor	Block efflux of potassium ions through the cell membranes, resulting in a prolongation in action potentials.	• Satolol • Amiodarone • Amifampridine	[82]
Potassium-sparing Diuretics	Act either by disrupting the exchange of sodium-potassium in the distal convoluted tubule or as an aldosterone receptor antagonist (**Figure** 7).	• Amiloride • Eplerenone • Triamterene • Spironolactone	[83, 84]

Different classes of cardiovascular drugs	Mechanism of actions	Examples of drugs	References
Thiazide Diuretics	Reduce sodium and fluid reabsorption (**Figure** 7).	• Metolazone • Chlorthalidone	[85]
Loop Diuretics	Inhibit the luminal Na-K-Cl cotransporter in the thick ascending limb of the loop of Henle (**Figure** 7).	• Furosemide • Bumetanide	[86]
Osmotic Diuretics	Elevate the osmolality of blood plasma (**Figure** 7).	• Mannitol • Isosorbide	[87]
Inotropic Sympathomimetic Drugs	Directly stimulate beta-1 receptors of the heart to increase myocardial contractility and stroke volume, resulting in increased cardiac output.	• Dobutamine • Dopamine • Isoprenaline	[88]
Vasoconstrictors	Indirectly stimulate the adrenergic receptor system by enhancing the activity of norepinephrine.	• Ephedrine • Methoxamine	[89]
Drugs for Cardiopulmonary Resuscitation	Relax the muscles in the airways and tightens the blood vessels.	• Epinephrine • Norepinephrine	[90]
Parenteral Anticoagulants	Produce antithrombotic effect by binding to antithrombin III.	• Heparin • Fondaparinux	[91]
Oral Anticoagulants	Block one of the enzymes (proteins) that uses vitamin K to produce clotting factors.	• Dabigatran • Rivaroxaban	[92]
Anti-heparin Agent	Form a complex by binding with high affinity heparin and rapidly reverse the anticoagulant effects.	Protamine Sulphate	[93]
Antiplatelet Drugs	Irreversibly blocks prostaglandin H synthase in platelets and prevent platelet aggregation by inhibiting the synthesis of thromboxane A2.	• Clopidogrel • Aspirin	[94]
Fibrinolytic Drugs	Act with plasminogen to produce an “activator complex” that converts plasminogen to the proteolytic enzyme plasmin.	• Anistreplase • Urokinase	[95]
Antifibrinolytic Drugs and Hemostatic	Act by inhibiting the breakdown of blood clots, which prevents bleeding.	Aminocaproic acid	[96]
Anion Exchange Resins	Reduce high cholesterol levels in the blood.	• Cholestipol • Cholestyramine	[97]
Fibrates	Decrease the levels of triglycerides and increase HDL cholesterol levels.	• Clofibrate • Fenofibrate	[98]
Statins	Block 3-hydroxy-3-methylglutaryl-coenzyme A (HMG-CoA) reductase (**Figure 8**).	• Atorovastatin • Fluvastatin • Simvastatin	[100]
Nicotinic Acid Derivatives	Reduce plasma viscosity and platelet aggregation.	Inositol nicotinate	[101]

Table 5.
Major classes of cardiovascular drugs and their mechanisms of actions with examples of each class.

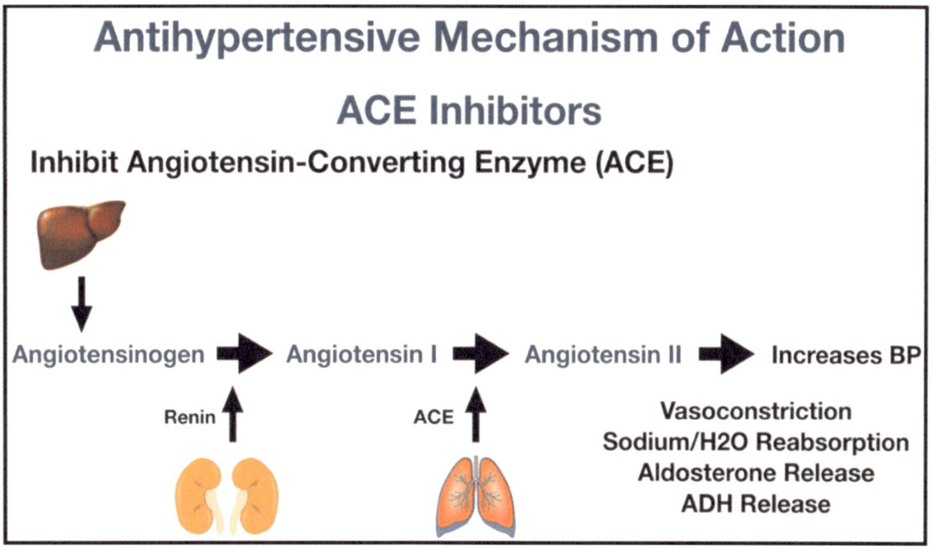

Figure 5.
General mechanism of antihypertensive drugs (significantly modified as per study design) [66].

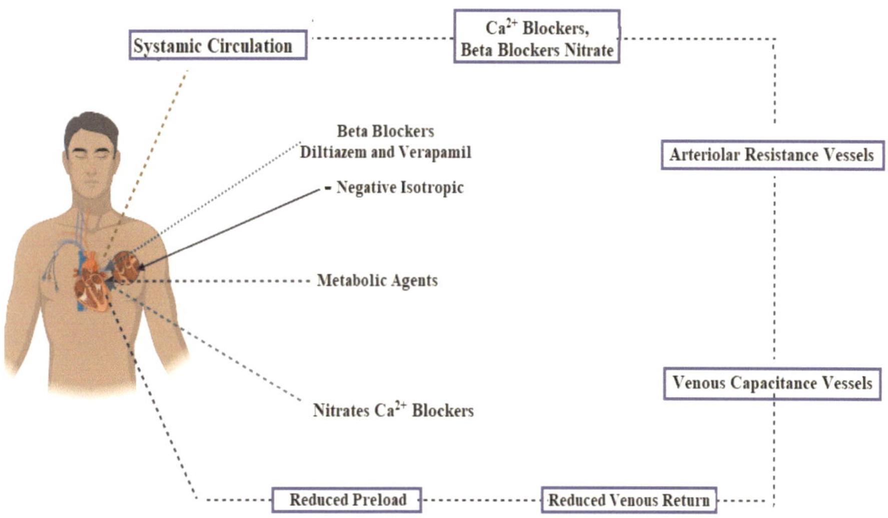

Figure 6.
Proposed anti-anginal mechanism for nitrates, beta-blockers and calcium channel blockers (designed with biorender).

9.2.2 Treatment with herbal medicines

Various herbal drugs are also utilized for the management of cardiovascular diseases (**Table 6**).

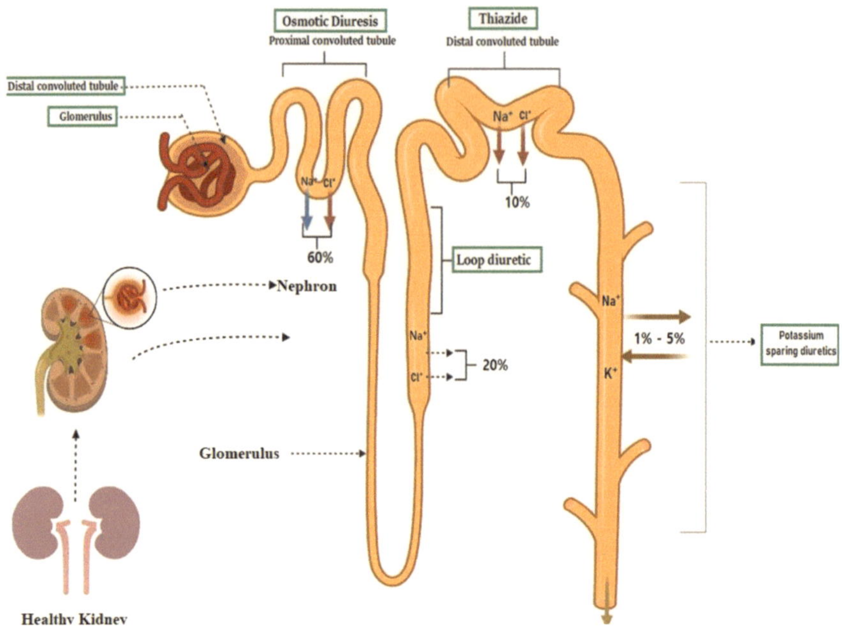

Figure 7.
General mechanism of action of diuretics (designed with biorender).

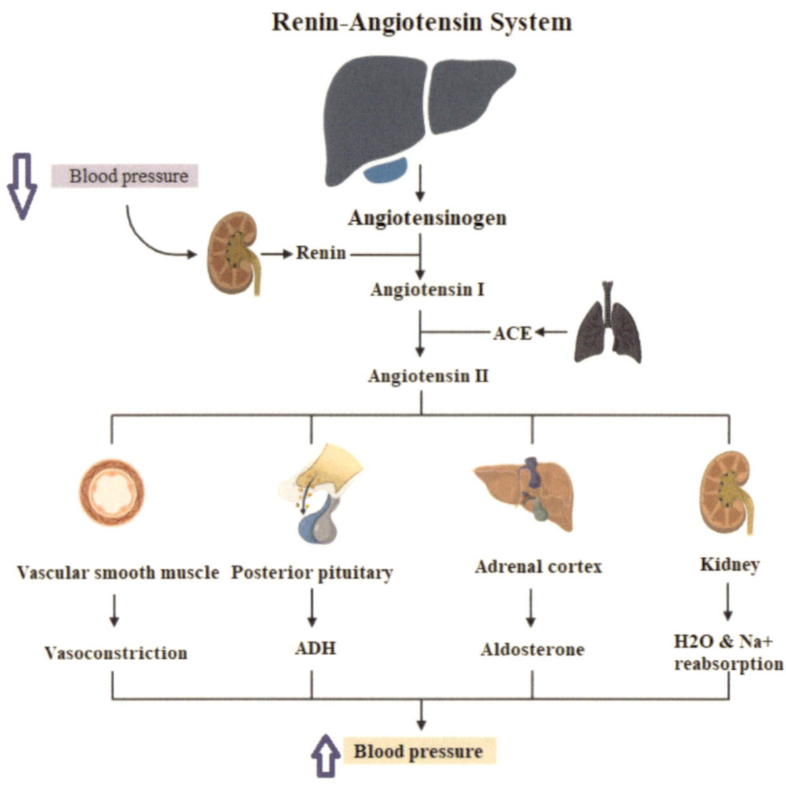

Figure 8.
Mechanism of action of statins [99].

Herbal drugs	Treated diseases	References
Anthocyanidin	Coronary heart disease Ischemia–reperfusion injury	[100]
Citrus fruits	Ischemia–reperfusion	[101]
Peanuts, red wine,	Hypertension Ischemia–reperfusion	[102]
Rhizoma coptidis	Hypertension	[103]
Rhizome of a turmeric plant	Hypertension	[104]
Crocus sativus L.	Heart failure	[105]
Angelica sinensis	Heart failure	[106]
Sophora flavescens	Arrhythmia	[107]
Dendrobium nobile	Acute myocardial infarction Ischemia–reperfusion	[108]
Glycine max	Acute myocardial infarction	[109]
Allium in *Liliaceae*	Hypertension	[110]
Tea	Hypertension	[110]
Carthamus tinctorius L.	Acute myocardial infarction	[111]
Panax ginseng	Coronary heart disease Ischemia–reperfusion injury	[112]

Table 6.
Lists of herbal drugs and treated cardiovascular disorders.

10. Conclusion

This review shines a spotlight on the physiology, pathology, and management of the cardiovascular system. The cardiovascular system simultaneously eliminates waste products from the tissues and delivers fresh oxygen and nutrients to the tissues and cells of the body. The heart and blood vessels are the fundamental components of this cardiovascular system, with the heart serving as the core pumping unit. The heart is composed of two atria and two ventricles. It has been considered that the right side of the heart receives blood that is depleted in oxygen but rich in carbon dioxide. This blood is then pushed into the pulmonary veins and finally travels back to the left side of the heart, where the blood is oxygenated by the lungs, which removes carbon dioxide from the blood. The left ventricle is responsible for ejecting blood from the heart and distributing it to the rest of the body. During each phase of the cardiac cycle, the atria compress while the ventricles remain relaxed, and then the process is reversed. However, any dysfunction of this precious organ can have disastrous consequences, leading to serious cardiovascular ailments and even death. These cardiovascular ailments are the greatest cause of morbidity and mortality in both developing and developed countries, with CADs and arrhythmias being the most prominent. These CVDs can be triggered by a variety of risk factors that can be either modifiable or nonmodifiable, including age, gender, ethnic background, smoking, physical inactivity, high cholesterol, and blood pressure etc. The treatment of these cardiovascular ailments requires the administration of certain allopathic drugs and herbal medications based on disease conditions and progression, as well as adherence to specified non-pharmacological interventions, which will significantly help in reducing the morbidity associated with severe cardiovascular events.

Acknowledgements

We would like to thank all the authors of the books and articles we have cited. We also express our gratitude to the authority of the Department of Pharmaceutical Chemistry for using their computer of the Molecular and Herbal Drug research Laboratory established under the HEQEP Project.

Conflict of interest

The authors declare no conflict of interest.

Author details

Md. Shah Amran[1*], Nasiba Binte Bahar[2] and Shopnil Akash[3]

1 Faculty of Pharmacy, Molecular Pharmacology and Herbal Drug Research Laboratory, Department of Pharmaceutical Chemistry, University of Dhaka, Dhaka, Bangladesh

2 Faculty of Pharmacy, Department of Pharmacy, University of Dhaka, Dhaka, Bangladesh

3 Faculty of Allied Health Sciences, Department of Pharmacy, Daffodil International University, Dhaka, Bangladesh

*Address all correspondence to: amranms@du.ac.bd

References

[1] Lanir Y. Multi-scale structural modeling of soft tissues mechanics and mechanobiology. Journal of Elasticity. 2017;**129**:7-48

[2] Thiriet M, Parker KH. Physiology and pathology of the cardiovascular system: a physical perspective. In: *Cardiovascular Mathematics*. Springer; 2009. pp. 1-45

[3] John NA. *CC Chatterjee's Human Physiology*. India: CBS Publishers & Distributors Private Limited; 2018

[4] Armour JA, Ardell JL. *Basic and Clinical Neurocardiology*. England: Oxford University Press; 2004

[5] Cantin M, Genest J. The heart as an endocrine gland. Scientific American. 1986;**254**:76-81

[6] Huang M-H, Friend DS, Sunday ME, Singh K, Haley K, Austen KF, et al. An intrinsic adrenergic system in mammalian heart. The Journal of Clinical Investigation. 1996;**98**: 1298-1303

[7] Mukoyama M, Nakao K, Hosoda K, Suga S, Saito Y, Ogawa Y, et al. Brain natriuretic peptide as a novel cardiac hormone in humans. Evidence for an exquisite dual natriuretic peptide system, atrial natriuretic peptide and brain natriuretic peptide. The Journal of Clinical Investigation. 1991;**87**: 1402-1412

[8] Islam M, Rahman M, Ahasan M, Sarkar N, Akash S, Islam M, et al. The impact of mucormycosis (Black fungus) on SARS-Cov-2-infected patients: At a glance. Environmental Science and Pollution Research. 2022;**29**:69341-69366

[9] Shaffer F, McCraty R, Zerr CL. A healthy heart is not a metronome: An integrative review of the heart's anatomy and heart rate variability. Frontiers in Psychology. 2014;**5**:1040

[10] Weinhaus AJ, Roberts KP. Anatomy of the human heart. In: *Handbook of Cardiac Anatomy, Physiology, and Devices*. Springer; 2005. pp. 51-79

[11] Somers VK, White DP, Amin R, Abraham WT, Costa F, Culebras A, et al. Sleep apnea and cardiovascular disease: An American heart association/ American college of cardiology foundation scientific statement from the American heart association council for high blood pressure research professional education committee, council on clinical cardiology, stroke council, and council on cardiovascular nursing in collaboration with the national heart, lung, and blood institute national center on sleep disorders research (national institutes of health). Journal of the American College of Cardiology. 2008;**52**:686-717

[12] Kaufman-Shriqui V, Navarro DA, Salem H, Boaz M. Mediterranean diet and health–a narrative review. Functional Foods in Health and Disease. 2022;**12**:479-487

[13] ATF Members, Perk J, De Backer G, Gohlke H, Graham I, Reiner Z, et al. 'European Guidelines on cardiovascular disease prevention in clinical practice (version 2012)' The Fifth Joint Task Force of the European Society of Cardiology and Other Societies on Cardiovascular Disease Prevention in Clinical Practice (constituted by representatives of nine societies and by invited experts)* Developed with the special contribution of the European Association for Cardiovascular Prevention & Rehabilitation (EACPR). [Eur Heart J 2012; 33: 1635–1701, doi:

10.1093/eurheartj/ehs092]. European Heart Journal. 2012;**33**:2126-2126

[14] Beaglehole R. *The World Health Report 2003: Shaping the Future*. World Health Organization; 2003

[15] W. H. Organization. the Challenge of Cardiovascular Disease—Quick Statistics. WHO; 2016

[16] Who J, Consultation FE. Diet, nutrition and the prevention of chronic diseases. World Health Organization Technical Report Series. 2003;**916**:1-149

[17] Basson M. Cardiovascular disease. Nature. 2008;**451**:903-903

[18] Laste NJ. Cardiovascular pharmacotherapy: Hemodynamic drugs and antiarrhythmic agents. Veterinary Clinics of North America: Small Animal Practice. 2001;**31**:1231-1252

[19] Berntson GG, Quigley KS, Norman GJ, Lozano DL. "Cardiovascular Psychophysiology". Cambridge University Press. 2017:183-216

[20] Chaudhry R, Miao JH, Rehman A. Physiology, Cardiovascular. In: *StatPearls [Internet]*. StatPearls Publishing; 2021

[21] Polak-Iwaniuk A, Harasim-Symbor E, Gołaszewska K, Chabowski A. How hypertension affects heart metabolism. Frontiers in Physiology. 2019;**10**:435

[22] Huang Y, Hu D, Huang C, Nichols CG. Genetic discovery of ATP-sensitive K^+ channels in cardiovascular diseases. Circulation. Arrhythmia and Electrophysiology. 2019;**12**:e007322

[23] Tsibulnikov SY, Maslov LN, Gorbunov AS, Voronkov NS, Boshchenko AA, Popov SV, et al. A review of humoral factors in remote preconditioning of the heart. Journal of Cardiovascular Pharmacology and Therapeutics. 2019;**24**:403-421

[24] Sembulingam K, Sembulingam P. Essentials of Medical Physiology. Tamil Nadu, India: JP Medical Ltd; 2012

[25] Varga I, Kyselovič J, Galfiova P, Danisovic L. The non-cardiomyocyte cells of the heart. Their possible roles in exercise-induced cardiac regeneration and remodeling. Exercise for Cardiovascular Disease Prevention and Treatment. 2017:117-136

[26] Hall JE. Guyton and Hall Textbook of Medical Physiology, Jordanian Edition E-Book. Jackson, Mississippi: Elsevier Health Sciences; 2016

[27] Rahman MM, Islam MR, Akash S, Harun-Or-Rashid M, Ray TK, Rahaman MS, et al. Recent advancements of nanoparticles application in cancer and neurodegenerative disorders: At a glance. Biomedicine & Pharmacotherapy. 2022;**153**:113305

[28] Feigin VL, Abajobir AA, Abate KH, Abd-Allah F, Abdulle AM, Abera SF, et al. Global, regional, and national burden of neurological disorders during 1990–2015: A systematic analysis for the global burden of disease study 2015. The Lancet Neurology. 2017;**16**:877-897

[29] Shahjehan RD, Bhutta BS. Coronary artery disease. In: *StatPearls [Internet]*. StatPearls Publishing; 2021

[30] Ross R. Atherosclerosis—An inflammatory disease. New England Journal of Medicine. 1999;**340**:115-126

[31] Eltzschig HK, Eckle T. Ischemia and reperfusion—From mechanism to

translation. Nature Medicine. 2011;**17**: 1391-1401

[32] Baker J, Felix C, Olinger G, Kalyanaraman B. Myocardial ischemia and reperfusion: Direct evidence for free radical generation by electron spin resonance spectroscopy. Proceedings of the National Academy of Sciences. 1988; **85**:2786-2789

[33] Mohan H. Textbook of Pathology. Chandigarh, India: Jaypee Brothers Medical Publishers; 2018

[34] Lu L, Liu M, Sun R, Zheng Y, Zhang P. Myocardial infarction: Symptoms and treatments. Cell Biochemistry and Biophysics. 2015;**72**: 865-867

[35] Anwar SM, Gul M, Majid M, Alnowami M. Arrhythmia classification of ECG signals using hybrid features. Computational and Mathematical Methods in Medicine. 2018;**2018**:1-8

[36] Li H, Boulanger P. A survey of heart anomaly detection using ambulatory electrocardiogram (ECG). Sensors. 2020; **20**:1461

[37] Sotoodehnia M, Payandemehr P. A 58-year-old woman with weakness and shortness of breath. *Advanced Journal of Emergency Medicine*. 2018;**2**

[38] Williams M, McCarthy D, Foster A, Yednock SF, Rydel R, Messersmith E, et al. Comprehensive Medicinal Chemistry II Volume 6: Therapeutic Areas I: Central Nervous System, Pain, Metabolic Syndrome, Urology, Gastrointestinal and Cardiovascular. Elsevier Science Limited; 2007

[39] Heijman J, Guichard J-B, Dobrev D, Nattel S. Translational challenges in atrial fibrillation. Circulation Research. 2018;**122**:752-773

[40] Jalife J. Ventricular fibrillation: mechanisms of initiation and maintenance. Annual review of physiology. 2000;**62**:25

[41] Meijborg VM, Conrath CE, Opthof T, Belterman CN, de Bakker JM, Coronel R. Electrocardiographic T wave and its relation with ventricular repolarization along major anatomical axes. Circulation: Arrhythmia and Electrophysiology. 2014;**7**:524-531

[42] Introduction to Pediatric Paroxysmal Supraventricular Tachycardia (PSVT). Website: Available from: https://www.rnceus.com/psvt/psvtintro2021.html. Vol. 7. p. 12. Accessed: October 29, 2022

[43] Ghanbari H. "Premature Ventricular Contractions Could Lead to a More Serious Heart Condition. https://healthblog.uofmhealth.org/heart-health/premature-ventricular-contractions-could-lead-to-a-more-serious-heart-condition, 2016

[44] Heart Block. 2011. Available from: https://matthewheron.wordpress.com/tag/heart-block/. Accessed: October 29, 2022

[45] Torsade de Pointes. Available from: https://www.rnceus.com/ekg/ekgtp.html. Accessed October 29, 2022

[46] Hall JE, Granger JP, do Carmo JM, da Silva AA, Dubinion J, George E, et al. Hypertension: Physiology and pathophysiology. Comprehensive Physiology. 2012;**2**:2393-2442

[47] WMPP Investigators. The World Health Organization MONICA project (monitoring trends and determinants in cardiovascular disease): A major international collaboration. Journal of Clinical Epidemiology. 1988; **41**:105-114

[48] Mascarenhas JV, Albayati MA, Shearman CP, Jude EB. Peripheral arterial disease. Endocrinology and Metabolism Clinics. 2014;**43**:149-166

[49] Kumer A, Chakma U, Matin MM, Akash S, Chando A, Howlader D. The computational screening of inhibitor for black fungus and white fungus by D-glucofuranose derivatives using in silico and SAR study. Organic Communications. 2021;**14**:305-322

[50] Wexler R, Elton T, Pleister A, Feldman D. Cardiomyopathy: An overview. American Family Physician. 2009;**79**:778

[51] Crotti L, Celano G, Dagradi F, Schwartz PJ. Congenital long QT syndrome. Orphanet Journal of Rare Diseases. 2008;**3**:1-16

[52] Crotti L, Taravelli E, Girardengo G, Schwartz PJ. Congenital short QT syndrome. Indian Pacing and Electrophysiology Journal. 2010;**10**:86

[53] Swedberg K, Cleland J, Dargie H, Drexler H, Follath F, Komajda M, et al. Guidelines for the diagnosis and treatment of chronic heart failure: Executive summary (update 2005) the task force for the diagnosis and treatment of chronic heart failure of the European Society of Cardiology. European Heart Journal. 2005;**26**: 1115-1140

[54] Adams KF, Lindenfeld JA, Arnold JMO, Baker DW, Barnard DH, Baughman KL, et al. Executive summary: HFSA 2006 comprehensive heart failure practice guideline. Journal of Cardiac Failure. 2006;**12**:10-38

[55] Cappuccio FP. Cardiovascular and other effects of salt consumption. Kidney International Supplements. 2013;**3**: 312-315

[56] Jaarsma T. Non-pharmacological management and patient education in heart failure patients. European Cardiovascular Disease. 2006;**17**:108-110

[57] Hunt SA, Baker DW, Chin MH, Cinquegrani MP, Feldman AM, Francis GS, et al. ACC/AHA guidelines for the evaluation and management of chronic heart failure in the adult: Executive summary: A report of the American College of Cardiology/ American Heart Association Task Force on practice guidelines (committee to revise the 1995 guidelines for the evaluation and management of heart failure) developed in collaboration with the international society for heart and lung transplantation endorsed by the heart failure society of america. Journal of the American College of Cardiology. 2001;**38**:2101-2113

[58] Maisch B. Alcoholic cardiomyopathy. Herz. 2016;**41**:484-493

[59] Critchley JA, Capewell S. Mortality risk reduction associated with smoking cessation in patients with coronary heart disease: A systematic review. JAMA. 2003;**290**:86-97

[60] van Domburg RT, op Reimer WS, Hoeks SE, Kappetein AP, Bogers AJ. Three life-years gained from smoking cessation after coronary artery bypass surgery: A 30-year follow-up study. American Heart Journal. 2008;**156**: 473-476

[61] Wilson K, Gibson N, Willan A, Cook D. Effect of smoking cessation on mortality after myocardial infarction: Meta-analysis of cohort studies. Archives of Internal Medicine. 2000;**160**:939-944

[62] Frothingham SM, Smith PO, Payne TJ, Meadows SE. "How Much Does Smoking Cessation Cut CHD Risk?".

Family Physicians Inquiries Network. 2008

[63] Felker GM, Mentz RJ, Cole RT, Adams KF, Egnaczyk GF, Fiuzat M, et al. Efficacy and safety of tolvaptan in patients hospitalized with acute heart failure. Journal of the American College of Cardiology. 2017;**69**:1399-1406

[64] Panoulas VF, Metsios GS, Pace A, John H, Treharne G, Banks M, et al. Hypertension in rheumatoid arthritis. Rheumatology. 2008;**47**:1286-1298

[65] Conolly ME, Kersting F, Dollery CT. The clinical pharmacology of beta-adrenoceptor-blocking drugs. Progress in Cardiovascular Diseases. 1976;**19**: 203-234

[66] Antihypertensive Medication Chart: Drug List, Classes, and Examples. 2022. Available from: https://www.ezmedlearning.com/blog/antihypertensive-medication-drug-list. Accessed: 29 October, 2022

[67] Burnier M, Brunner H. Angiotensin II receptor antagonists. The Lancet. 2000;**355**:637-645

[68] Dina R, Jafari M. Angiotensin II-receptor antagonists: An overview. American Journal of Health-System Pharmacy. 2000;**57**:1231-1241

[69] Reid JL, Vincent J. Clinical pharmacology and therapeutic role of prazosin and related alpha-adrenoceptor antagonists. Cardiology. 1986;**73**:164-174

[70] Glaubiger G, Tsai BS, Lefkowitz RJ, Weiss B, Johnson EM. Chronic guanethidine treatment increases cardiac β-adrenergic receptors. Nature. 1978;**273**: 240-242

[71] Gille J, Seyfarth H-J, Gerlach S, Malcharek M, Czeslick E, Sablotzki A. Perioperative anesthesiological management of patients with pulmonary hypertension. Anesthesiology Research and Practice. 2012;**2012**:1-16

[72] Webster J, Koch H. Aspects of tolerability of centrally acting antihypertensive drugs. Journal of Cardiovascular Pharmacology. 1996;**27**: S49-S54

[73] Schiff J. Drugs affecting nicotinic receptors. In: *Pharmacology and Therapeutics for Dentistry*. St. Louis, Missouri: CV Mosby; 1995

[74] Mehta JL. Endothelium, coronary vasodilation, and organic nitrates. American Heart Journal. 1995;**129**: 382-391

[75] Eisenberg MJ, Brox A, Bestawros AN. Calcium channel blockers: An update. The American Journal of Medicine. 2004;**116**:35-43

[76] Elliott WJ, Ram CVS. Calcium channel blockers. The Journal of Clinical Hypertension. 2011;**13**:687

[77] Longman SD, Hamilton TC. Potassium channel activator drugs: Mechanism of action, pharmacological properties, and therapeutic potential. Medicinal Research Reviews. 1992;**12**: 73-148

[78] Goldsmith DR, Wellington K. Naftidrofuryl. Drugs & Aging. 2005;**22**: 967-977

[79] Cook P, James I. Cerebral vasodilators. New England Journal of Medicine. 1981;**305**:1560-1564

[80] Post JM, Hume JR, Archer SL, Weir EK. Direct role for potassium channel inhibition in hypoxic pulmonary vasoconstriction. American Journal of

Physiology-Cell Physiology. 1992;**262**: C882-C890

[81] Investigators R. Effectiveness of spironolactone added to an angiotensin-converting enzyme inhibitor and a loop diuretic for severe chronic congestive heart failure (the Randomized Aldactone Evaluation Study [RALES]). The American Journal of Cardiology. 1996; **78**:902-907

[82] Horisberger J-D, Giebisch G. Potassium-sparing diuretics. Kidney and Blood Pressure Research. 1987;**10**: 198-220

[83] Sica DA, Carter B, Cushman W, Hamm L. Thiazide and loop diuretics. The Journal of Clinical Hypertension. 2011;**13**:639-643

[84] Roush GC, Kaur R, Ernst ME. Diuretics: A review and update. Journal of Cardiovascular Pharmacology and Therapeutics. 2014;**19**:5-13

[85] Gennari FJ, Kassirer JP. Osmotic diuresis. New England Journal of Medicine. 1974;**291**:714-720

[86] Nakashima M, Maeda K, Sekiya A, Hagino Y. Effect of hypothyroid status on myocardial responses to sympathomimetic drugs. The Japanese Journal of Pharmacology. 1971;**21**: 819-825

[87] Naftalin LW, Yagiela JA. Vasoconstrictors: Indications and precautions. Dental Clinics. 2002;**46**: 733-746

[88] Gueugniaud P-Y, David J-S, Chanzy E, Hubert H, Dubien P-Y, Mauriaucourt P, et al. Vasopressin and epinephrine vs. epinephrine alone in cardiopulmonary resuscitation. New England Journal of Medicine. 2008;**359**: 21-30

[89] Garcia DA, Baglin TP, Weitz JI, Samama MM. Parenteral anticoagulants: Antithrombotic therapy and prevention of thrombosis: American College of Chest Physicians evidence-based clinical practice guidelines. Chest. 2012;**141**: e24S-e43S

[90] Garcia D, Libby E, Crowther MA. The new oral anticoagulants. Blood, The Journal of the American Society of Hematology. 2010;**115**:15-20

[91] Lindblad B. Protamine sulphate: A review of its effects: Hypersensitivity and toxicity. European Journal of Vascular Surgery. 1989;**3**:195-201

[92] Schrör K. Antiplatelet drugs. Drugs. 1995;**50**:7-28

[93] Squizzato A, Manfredi E, Bozzato S, Dentali F, Ageno W. Antithrombotic and fibrinolytic drugs for retinal vein occlusion: A systematic review and a call for action. Thrombosis and Haemostasis. 2010;**103**:271-276

[94] Slaughter TF, Greenberg CS. Antifibrinolytic drugs and perioperative hemostasis. American Journal of Hematology. 1997;**56**:32-36

[95] Taylor NS, Bartlett JG. Binding of Clostridium difficile cytotoxin and vancomycin by anion-exchange resins. Journal of Infectious Diseases. 1980;**141**: 92-97

[96] Jun M, Foote C, Lv J, Neal B, Patel A, Nicholls SJ, et al. Effects of fibrates on cardiovascular outcomes: A systematic review and meta-analysis. The Lancet. 2010;**375**:1875-1884

[97] Maji D, Shaikh S, Solanki D, Gaurav K. Safety of statins. Indian Journal of Endocrinology and Metabolism. 2013;**17**:636-646

[98] Lee HC, Aarhus R. A derivative of NADP mobilizes calcium stores insensitive to inositol trisphosphate and cyclic ADP-ribose. Journal of Biological Chemistry. 1995;**270**:2152-2157

[99] Savoiu-Balint G, Petrus A, Mihaescu R, Ionescu D, Citu C, Marincu I, et al. Role of atorvastatin ((3R, 5R)-7-[2-(4-fluorophenyl)-3-phenyl-4-(phenylcarbamoyl)-5-propan-2-ylpyrrol-1-yl]-3, 5-dihydroxyheptanoic acid) on endothelial function in patients with Dyslipidemia. Revista de Chimie. 2015;**66**:833-836

[100] Goetz ME, Judd SE, Safford MM, Hartman TJ, McClellan WM, Vaccarino V. Dietary flavonoid intake and incident coronary heart disease: The REasons for Geographic and Racial Differences in Stroke (REGARDS) study. The American Journal of Clinical Nutrition. 2016;**104**:1236-1244

[101] Di Majo D, Giammanco M, La Guardia M, Tripoli E, Giammanco S, Finotti E. Flavanones in Citrus fruit: Structure–antioxidant activity relationships. Food Research International. 2005;**38**:1161-1166

[102] King RE, Bomser JA, Min DB. Bioactivity of resveratrol. Comprehensive Reviews in Food Science and Food Safety. 2006;**5**:65-70

[103] Luo S, Kan J, Zhang J, Ye P, Wang D, Jiang X, et al. Bioactive compounds from coptidis rhizoma alleviate pulmonary arterial hypertension by inhibiting pulmonary artery smooth muscle cells. Proliferation and Migration. 2021;**78**:253-262

[104] Zahra SK, Aslam B, Javed I, Khaliq T, Khan JA, Raza A. Hematopoietic potential of polysaccharides isolated from *Angelica sinensis* against ACE inhibitor induced anemia in albino rats. Pakistan Veterinary Journal. 2016;**36**:11-15

[105] Dai S, Chan M-Y, Lee S-S, Ogle CW. The antiarrhythmic effects of *Sophora flavescens* Ait. in rats and mice. The American Journal of Chinese Medicine. 1986;**14**:119-123

[106] Sun Y, Geng J, Wang D. Cardioprotective effects of ginsenoside compound-Mc1 and Dendrobium Nobile Lindl against myocardial infarction in an aged rat model: Involvement of TLR4/ NF-κB signaling pathway. European Journal of Inflammation. 2021;**19**: 20587392211000577

[107] Kingsley UI, Steven OO, Agu CE, Orji OC, Chekwube BE, Nwosu TF. Anti-hyperlipidemic effect of crude methanolic extracts of Glycine max (soy bean) on high cholesterol diet-fed albino rats. Journal of Medical & Allied Sciences. 2017;**7**:34

[108] Bahmani M, Zargaran A, Rafieian-Kopaei M, Saki K. Ethnobotanical study of medicinal plants used in the management of diabetes mellitus in the Urmia, Northwest Iran. Asian Pacific Journal of Tropical Medicine. 2014;**7**: S348-S354

[109] Landazuri P, Chamorro N, Cortes B. Medicinal plants used in the management hypertension. Journal of Analytical & Pharmaceutical Research. 2017;**5**:00134

[110] Yang Y-C, Lu F-H, Wu J-S, Wu C-H, Chang C-J. The protective effect of habitual tea consumption on hypertension. Archives of Internal Medicine. 2004;**164**:1534-1540

[111] Han S-Y, Li H-X, Ma X, Zhang K, Ma Z-Z, Jiang Y, et al. Evaluation of the anti-myocardial ischemia effect of individual and combined extracts of

Panax notoginseng and Carthamus tinctorius in rats. Journal of Ethnopharmacology. 2013;**145**:722-727

[112] Kim J-HJ. Cardiovascular diseases and Panax ginseng: A review on molecular mechanisms and medical applications, Journal of Ginseng Research. 2012;**36**:16

Chapter 2

Rat Electrocardiography and General Anesthesia

Pavol Svorc Jr and Pavol Svorc

Abstract

General anesthesia is an established and well-known factor with a significant impact on cardiac parameters, which can be a problem in the final evaluation of changes in the individual electrophysiological myocardial parameters after various interventions. The present chapter provides a composite review of published data on electrocardiographic parameters (heart rate, PR interval, P wave duration, P wave amplitude, QRS complex, QT and QTc interval duration, and R wave and T wave amplitude) for *in vivo* rat experiments under general anesthesia from 130 articles, which were retrieved from a search of the Web of Science database, for articles published mainly between 2000 and 2021. ECG parameters reported as baseline or control values were summarized, and averages with ranges were calculated. It is important to be cautious in interpreting the results of such studies and discussions addressing the mechanisms underlying a given type of arrhythmia, it is important to acknowledge that initial ECG parameters may already be affected to some extent by general anesthesia as well as by sex and the time of day the experiments are performed. Although it is not an original research work, researchers working with rats in the laboratory, who routinely perform anesthesia, can use this as a reference to look into while analyzing their data.

Keywords: ECG parameters, general anesthesia, sex, chronobiology, rat

1. Introduction

In vivo experimental animal models are often used to elucidate or, at least clarify, specific mechanisms and/or to identify interrelationships between monitored functions that cannot be observed directly in humans. The results of such studies are often approximated to preclinical or clinical research and, can thus, have a significant scientific impact on a more detailed understanding of the monitored system.

A specific feature of *in vivo* experimental animal models is the fact that experiments are usually performed with the animals under general anesthesia, in which homeostatic regulatory mechanisms are not removed and the animal responds to various interventions. Undoubtedly, this also applies to experiments in which changes in electrocardiographic (ECG) parameters are monitored after various interventions or after the administration of specific agents to assess the basis of the origin and development of heart rhythm disorders. However, different anesthetics may have varying impacts on myocardial electrophysiology. Thus, the extent to which ECG parameters are altered from normal after anesthetic administration can become a confounder—if not a problem—even before assessing the effects of the intervention itself.

The second problem is that many published methodologies do not describe the synchronization of the animals to the light-dark (LD) cycle, mainly in studies based on rat models. The LD cycle is the strongest synchronizer for this type of laboratory animal, and it is known that all measurable cardiovascular parameters oscillate depending on the LD cycle. Moreover, even when this synchronization is described, the time of day at which the experiments are performed is often not reported. In common practice, experiments are performed during regular work hours (i.e., during the day); therefore, after synchronization of rats, for example, to the LD cycle (12 h: 12 h), these experiments are essentially being performed on "sleeping" animals during their naturally inactive period. The question then becomes, what are the oscillations of ECG parameter values during a 24-h period (i.e., spanning the light [inactive] and dark [active] period) in healthy, sexually mature rats?

Another possible problem in the correct evaluation of changes in myocardial electrophysiology in rats may be sex. Sex is not typically considered in *in vivo* cardiovascular and toxicological experiments involving rats, although this type of experimental model animal is commonly used to examine normal and pathological physiology. In the majority of experimental studies, only male rats are used; however, there is another sex (i.e., female) in which differences in the essence of functional systems and response(s) to the same interventions are different from males. The study of sex differences is also a driving force of development and, in many cases, the basis of health and medicine. However, there are opinions that the study of sex differences is ineffectual and does not merit extensive research [1]. One of the reasons why both sexes are not used in experiments is the simple fact that males and females are biologically different and these differences increase the range of variability. However, if sex differences are documented and accounted for in experimental studies, these must be respected. As such, future studies should address these questions and attempt to include females in experiments where possible.

This review aims to highlight the fact that there are differences in baseline or control values, which are, nevertheless, used as reference values in individual studies. However, they are impacted by the type of anesthesia used, and all the above-mentioned confounders/problems can significantly affect the correct interpretation of the results obtained.

2. Evaluation of ECG parameters

The methodologies of studies that performed *in vivo* rat cardiovascular or toxicological experiments were retrieved from a search of the Web of Science database for articles published mainly between 2000 and 2021; in total, 130 articles were retrieved. ECG parameters reported as baseline or control values were summarized and averages with ranges were calculated. Not all ECG parameters were described and evaluated in each study and, in some studies, two to three control values were reported. A relatively high number of studies described only changes in ECG parameters, in terms of lengthening and shortening, and these changes were directly indicated in graphs without reporting numerical baseline values.

Because each ECG parameter has diagnostic significance, we focused on commonly evaluated ECG parameters, including the following: heart rate (HR), atrial complex (PR interval, P wave duration, and P wave amplitude), and ventricular complexes (QRS complex, QT and QTc interval duration, and R wave and T wave amplitude).

Tables consider studies (although there were only one or two), which also suggest a possible sex difference with regard to the LD cycle on the monitored parameter. The figures show the ranges of the monitored parameter from at least three baseline or control values.

3. Prognostic significance of changes in HR in arrhythmogenesis

HR is an easily measurable parameter of cardiac activity, and alterations in HR can have a direct effect on the cardiovascular system. Caetano and Alves [2] reported that increased resting HR is an independent predictor of cardiovascular and overall mortality in the general population. Thus, the occurrence of arrhythmias is often associated with baseline HR, which has prognostic significance. In a review article titled "Arrhythmias and heart rate: Mechanisms and significance of a relationship", Zaza et al. [3] describe, in detail, the mechanisms influencing arrhythmogenesis according to HR, in which the authors focused on several factors related mainly to electrical stability of the myocardium. HR also reflects autonomic balance, which also affects myocardial stability. The prognostic significance of the relationship between arrhythmias and HR may vary depending on the substrate present in a specific case and should be considered. In rats, electrical stability of the heart has been shown to be greatest at increased HRs in the dark (i.e., active) part of the regimen day, when myocardial vulnerability to ventricular arrhythmias decreases [4].

It has been found that tachycardia may provide greater electrical stability to the myocardium; however, if an abnormal substrate is present, it may trigger arrhythmia [5]. Severe bradycardia, in contrast, can trigger life-threatening arrhythmias, thus reflecting its destabilizing effect on repolarization. Zaza et al. [3] remained cautious, arguing that, from a mechanistic perspective in assessing the relationship between HR and arrhythmias, the question should be "what is the appropriate sinus rate for autonomic balance?" and not "what is the high (or low) heart rate?" Thus, it can be assumed that baseline HR in *in vivo* cardiovascular studies can significantly affect the results obtained during experimentation. The considerations mentioned above are also generally valid for rats. However, it is interesting that the effect of some interventions on HR is monitored and the impact of this change on myocardial electrophysiology is not further analyzed [6–8].

3.1 Telemetry and HR

To establish reference values for HR, as well as other ECG parameters, logically, the most suitable method is using telemetry studies, in which rats are not placed under general anesthesia and ECG can be recorded continuously throughout the day. Telemetry studies help to reveal very important information about fluctuations in myocardial electrophysiological parameters during the day. Currently, however, relatively few telemetry studies have analyzed ECG parameters in rats under *in vivo* conditions, and did not address circadian dependence and the dependence on sex.

Sex can also be a confounder. Nevertheless, several experimental rat studies [9] did not report any sex differences in heart repolarization, or that there is little clear evidence supporting sex differences in ventricular repolarizations *per se*, in which there is only a short estrous cycle lasting only 4 days [10]. Although no sex differences were found in the repolarization of isolated ventricular myocytes, they were associated with excitation and contraction [11]. Sex differences were not found in APD90 between isolated ventricular myocytes, in external K^+ currents, Ipk and Isus, in internal rectification current IK1, or ICa [11, 12]. While less information is available from animal models, sex differences in the ionic basis of the effective refractory period in the atria and atrioventricular node may also contribute to sex differences in the incidence of atrial fibrillation and supraventricular tachycardias. Nevertheless, the physiological significance of sex differences has yet to be fully determined; as such, further studies are needed to clarify the basic mechanisms.

Baseline HR analysis from telemetry studies involving non-anesthetized rats, in which a chronobiological approach was applied, indicates that there is a circadian rhythm in HR among rats, with a higher HR during the active (i.e., dark) period of the regimen day and not only in males [13–17] but also in females [15, 18]. If HR exhibits circadian fluctuations, then when it is evaluated, it can be problematic.

The question is whether there are also sex differences in single-lighted periods. Telemetry studies have revealed that among females, HR values are lower in both light periods (**Table 1**). The averaged results of baseline HR values indicate that sex differences are exhibited in both the light and dark periods of the rat regimen day; however, more experimental studies are needed to confirm these data. In female rats, changes in HR depended on the LD cycle; however, LD differences were modified by the anesthetic used [19, 20]. Although the adaptation of animals to the LD cycle was described in the Methods sections, it is not clear from the methodologies whether the values of the presented HRs were average values from the entire 24-h period, or the current baseline value only from certain time intervals before the intervention itself when the measurements were performed or recorded.

Anesthesia	**Not specified**		**Light period**		**Dark period**	
	Female	**Male**	**Female**	**Male**	**Female**	**Male**
Telemetry studies	460 432–488 (n = 1)	346 310–362 (n = 16)	316 307–325 (n = 2)	349 340–357 (n = 5)	371 345–397 (n = 2)	390 382–398 (n = 5)
Pentobarbital	—	374 359–389 (n = 22)	346 315–377 (n = 1)	—	369 328–410 (n = 1)	—
Thiopental	—	349 332–366 (n = 13)	-	—	-	—
Phenobarbital	—	368 340–396 (n = 1)	-	—	-	—
Nembutal	—	—	—	—	—	—
Ketamine/xylazine	331 304–257 (n = 2)	288 239–293 (n = 18)	230 207–253 (n = 1)	—	276 247–305 (n = 1)	—
Ketamine/medetomidine	-	165 146–184 (n = 1)	-	—	-	—
Ketamine/diazepam	-	330 298–361 (n = 2)	-	—	-	—

Anesthesia	Not specified		Light period		Dark period	
	Female	Male	Female	Male	Female	Male
Ketamine/midazolam	-	414 375–453 (n = 1)	-	—	-	—
Urethane	—	378 352–403 (n = 14)	—	—	—	—
Isoflurane	—	408 400–416 (n = 5)	—	—	—	—
Desflurane	—	441 429–453 (n = 1)	—	—	—	—
Chloralose	-	418 404–431 (n = 2)	-	-	-	-
Tribromoethanol	—	393 387–399 (n = 1)	—	—	—	—
Ether	—	366 343–388 (n = 6)	—	—	—	—
Isolated heart	—	368 ± 14 354–382 (n = 1)	—	—	—	—

Data presented as average heart rate (beats/min) (range); (n, number of baseline or control values from which heart rate was evaluated). Not specified—the methodology did not specify the lighted period when the experiments were performed.

Table 1.
Heart rate under individual types of anesthesia according to sex and light cycle (light [inactive]) versus dark [active]).

3.2 General anesthesia and HR

The question is what are the reference values for HR in the rat under normal circumstances? Based on the values reported in **Table 1**, is clear that HR varies depending on the type of general anesthesia, which can be problematic in evaluating changes in HR after an intervention. Other factors, in addition to general anesthesia, that may directly or indirectly affect the initial HR can be the methodology used to determine HR, the time of day (or part of the rat regimen day) at which the experiments are performed, or the fact that the majority of ECGs are evaluated only in male rats; as such, there is little-to-no information about HR in females.

Evaluation of HR in telemetry studies involving male rats [21–31] reported a mean HR of 347 beats/min, with a range of 303 beats/min up to 362 beats/min without taking into account the evaluation methodologies and the time of day the experiments were performed.

If we consider that the average HR value with the range reported in telemetry studies involving male rats is our desired reference value, then a slightly increased average HR in pentobarbital (approximately 28 beats/min.) [32–51], and urethane anesthesia (approximately 32 beats/min) [52–60]. In female rats under pentobarbital anesthesia, baseline HR values were reported in only one study, depending on the LD cycle [20]. Even with pentobarbital anesthesia, although nonsignificant, there were LD differences. In female Wistar rats, pentobarbital probably only modifies circadian rhythms, but does not disturb them. Thiopental anesthesia [31, 61–71] did not alter HR from the mean HR reported in telemetry studies.

A significant tachycardic effect was found under isoflurane (approximately 62 beats/min) [72–75], desflurane (approximately 95 beats/min) [72], and chloralose (approximately 72 beats/min) [76, 77] anesthesia in male rats.

Under ketamine/xylazine anesthesia [45, 78–92], HR was drastically reduced in males and reduced values were also recorded in females [93, 94]. In females have been preserved significant LD differences [19].

The effect of phenobarbital [95], ketamine/medetomidine [96], ketamine/midazolam [97], and ketamine/diazepam [96, 98] on anesthesia could not be assessed as valid because there was only one study.

Although ether is no longer used to induce general anesthesia, some works used this type of light anesthesia needed to perform ECG recordings [99–104]. However, ether anesthesia had virtually no effect on HR. One study describing HR in isolated rat hearts did not reveal any significant deviation, in terms of tachycardia or bradycardia [105]. Interesting differences were also found between young and old rats under tribromoethanol anesthesia, where higher values prevailed in older rats (405 ± 11 beats/min vs. 381 ± 1 beats/min) [106]. Unfortunately, these comparisons are only from males and without a description of the adaptation of the animals to the LD cycle.

From **Table 1** and **Figure 1**, it is evident that for different types of general anesthesia, baseline or control HR values can differ significantly compared to the mean baseline HR from telemetry studies, which can logically be considered as a reference value. There is very little information about HR in females and almost none of the studies took circadian fluctuations into account.

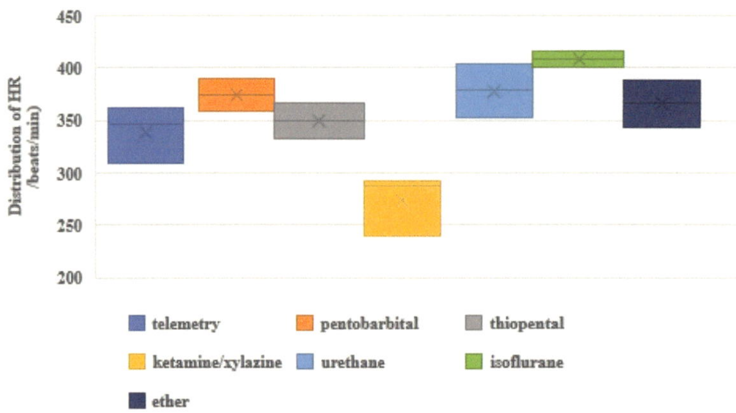

Figure 1.
Distribution of average values and ranges of heart rate (HR) from telemetry studies and under different types of general anesthesia in rat males without taking into account the light periods of the rat regimen day when the experiments were performed. Only HR ranges from at least three studies where HR has been evaluated are shown in the figure. Telemetry studies (n = 16), pentobarbital anesthesia (n = 22), thiopental anesthesia (n = 13), ketamine/xylazine anesthesia (n = 18), isoflurane anesthesia (n = 5), ether anesthesia (n = 6), urethane anesthesia (n = 14). (n—number of baseline or control values from which heart rate [HR] was evaluated).

4. Prognostic significance of changes in the atrial complex in arrhythmogenesis

4.1 PR (PQ) interval

The PR (PQ) interval is measured from the beginning of the P wave to the beginning of the QRS complex. This interval reflects the time that the electrical impulse passes from the SA node through the AV node. The PR interval provides information about the time required for the transmission of the electrical impulse from the atria through the AV node, His bundle, Tawar's branches, and Purkinje fibers to the start of ventricular muscle depolarization [107–109].

A prolonged PQ interval reflects a longer time of transmission of the impulse from the atrium to the ventricles in disorders of the conductive system of the AV node [110, 111]. A shortened PQ interval means that the impulse was transmitted to the ventricular conductive system earlier than normal; thus, it is likely that it passes around the AV node through abnormal connections of the conductive system [111–113]. The duration of the PR interval is a crucial marker in the diagnosis of atrioventricular blocks. However, it appears that the PR interval in rats also appears to be dependent on the type of anesthesia, and we have practically no information about sex differences and changes dependent on the LD cycle.

Although mean values of the duration of the PR (PQ) interval were comparable among the different types of anesthesia and did not exhibit significant differences (**Table 2**, **Figure 2**), the shortest duration was found with nembutal anesthesia [114]. With this type of anesthesia, there is a problem with the validity of this value because it is from only one study. The situation is similar with desflurane [72], ketamine/

Anesthesia	Not specified		Light period		Dark period	
	Female	Male	Female	Male	Female	Male
Telemetry Studies	42.23 41.5–42.96 (n = 1)	49.26 47.51–50.88 (n = 10)	-	-	-	-
Pentobarbital	—	47.53 45.35–49.71 (n = 18)	44.16 36.46–51.86 (n = 1)	—	45.3 40.6–50 (n = 1)	—
Thiopental	—	48.35 46.52–50.18 (n = 6)	-	—	-	—
Phenobarbital	—	—	—	—	—	—
Nembutal		42 41–43 (n = 1)				
Ketamine/Xylazine	44 34–54 (n = 1)	44.77 41.02–45.42 (n = 13)	47 35.7–58.3 (n = 1)	—	36.5 30.7–42.3 (n = 1)	—

Anesthesia	Not specified		Light period		Dark period	
	Female	Male	Female	Male	Female	Male
Ketamine/ Medetomidine	-	67.5 66.3–68.7 (n = 1)	-	—	-	—
Ketamine/ Diazepam	-	48.5 not reported (n = 1)	-	—	-	—
Ketamine/ Midazolam	-	47 44–50 (n = 1)	-	—	-	—
Urethane	—	48.99 45.03– 52.95 (n = 9)	—	—	—	—
Isoflurane	—	48.05 46.52– 49.63 (n = 6)	—	—	—	—
Desflurane	—	41.6 40.08– 43.12 (n = 1)	—	—	—	—
Chloralose	—	—	—	—	—	—
Tribromethanol	—	52.6 50.4–54.8 (n = 2)	—	—	—	—
Ether	—	49.7 44.7–54.7 (n = 4)	—	—	—	—
Isolated Heart	—	44.5 41.8–47.2 (n = 2)	-	-	—	—

Data are presented as the average value of PR (PQ) interval duration (ms) (range); (n, number of baseline or control values from which heart rate was evaluated). Not specified - the methodology did not specify the lighted period when the experiments were performed.

Table 2.
Duration of PR (PQ) interval duration under individual types of anesthesia according to sex and light cycle (light [inactive]) versus dark [active]).

medetomidine [96], ketamine/diazepam [96], ketamine/midazolam, [97], anesthesia in isolated hearts [105, 115], and in tribromethal anesthesia [106, 116].

Duration of the PR (PQ) interval from telemetry studies [21, 23–25, 30, 117–119], inhalation (isoflurane) [72, 74, 75, 120, 121] pentobarbital [32, 34, 36, 37, 40, 43–47, 49, 122–126], thiopental [63–65, 68, 71], urethane [45, 52, 53, 56, 60, 128], and ether anesthesia [99–101, 104] did not differ significantly from one another. The shortened duration of the PR (PQ) interval was under ketamine/xylazine anesthesia [45, 78, 79, 84, 85, 89, 91, 92, 127–129]. The duration of the PQ (PR) interval in isolated hearts [105, 115] did not differ significantly from the duration with other types of anesthesia.

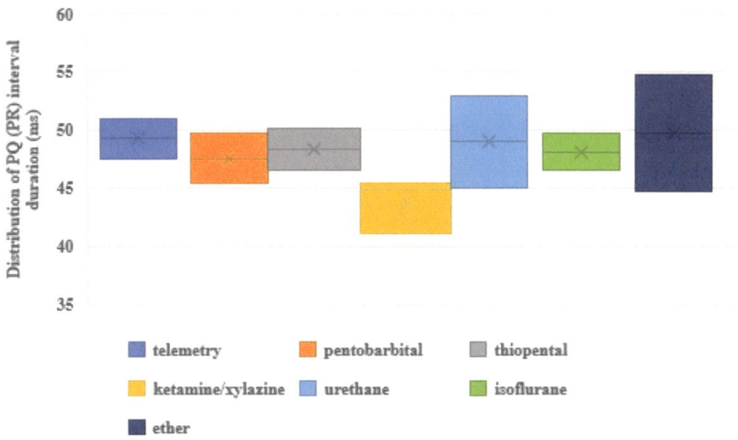

Figure 2.
Distribution of average values and ranges of PR (PQ) interval duration from telemetry studies and under different types of general anesthesia in male rats without taking into account the light periods of the rat regimen day when the experiments were performed. Only PR (PQ) interval ranges from at least three studies where PR (PQ) interval was evaluated and is shown in the figure. Telemetry studies (n = 10), pentobarbital anesthesia (n = 18), thiopental anesthesia (n = 6), ketamine/xylazine anesthesia (n = 13), isoflurane anesthesia (n = 6), ether anesthesia (n = 4), urethane anesthesia (n = 9). n, number of baseline or control values from which duration of PR (PQ) interval was evaluated.

For a given ECG parameter, it was difficult to determine sex differences, as well as differences dependent on the LD cycle because there was only one study (**Table 2**).

The P wave represents the depolarization of the atria. Atrial depolarization spreads from the SA node toward the AV node, and the right to the left atrium. In humans, but also in rats, the physiological sinus rhythm is characterized by the same P wave orientation as the R wave and its occurrence before each QRS complex in all cardiac cycles. P wave duration has been evaluated in Wistar rats, for which prolongation after myocardial infarction may be associated with increased sensitivity to supraventricular arrhythmias [130].

Other parameters of atrial complex evaluation include amplitude and polarity (either negative or positive, although it can also be so flat that it is indistinguishable from the isoelectric line). If the P wave is unusually high, it may reflect enlargement of the atria. Typically, an enlarged right atrium exhibits a high, spiked P wave, while an enlarged left atrium is reflected by a bifidic P wave on ECG. The absence of a P wave or its altered shape is present in various cardiac arrhythmias, the most common of which is atrial [131, 132]. Although the analysis of P wave duration and shape in humans provides clinically important information, there is a lack of experimental data from rats to draw definitive conclusions about sex-related changes and circadian rhythm in P wave amplitude and duration [45].

4.2 P wave duration and amplitude

The duration and amplitude of the P wave, despite their important prognostic significance, have only been sporadically evaluated in *in vivo* experiments involving rats. The average amplitudes of the P wave were essentially the same at all types of anesthesia (i.e., in studies where the given parameter was evaluated). Only one telemetry study [118] evaluated P wave duration, and if it is considered as a reference value, only in males, prolonged duration was under ketamine/xylazine anesthesia [84, 89]

Anesthesia	P wave amplitude (mV)	P wave duration (ms)
Telemetry studies	—	21.51 (19.84–23.18) n = 1
Pentobarbital	0.39 (0.34–0.44) n = 2	16.15 (15.65–16.65) n = 2
Thiopental	—	14 (12.8–15.2) n = 1
Phenobarbital	—	—
Nembutal	0.29 (0.27–0.32) n = 1	—
Ketamine/xylazine	0.05 (0.03–0.07) n = 4	26.25 (24.25–28.25) n = 2
Ketamine/medetomidine	0.08 (0.05–0.11) n = 1	32 (31–33) n = 1
Ketamine/diazepan	0.09 (0.06–0.13) n = 2	—
Ketamine/midazolam	0.04 (0.013–0.067) n = 1	15 (13.5–16.5) n = 1
Isoflurane	0.19 (0.17–0.21) n = 1	24.1 (23.1–25.1) n = 1
Desflurane	—	23.5 (22.6–24.4) n = 1
Chloralose	—	—
Tribromethanol	—	—
Ether	—	19.5 (17–22) n = 1
Urethane	0.077 (0.074–0.080) n = 1	22.1 (18.7–25.5) n = 2
Isolated heart	0.001 (0.00084–0.00116) n = 1	19.0 ± 0 n = 1

Data presented as average (range); (n, number of baseline or control values in which the amplitude and duration of the P wave were evaluated).

Table 3.
P wave amplitude and duration, regardless of synchronization of the male rats to the light and dark cycle under individual types of anesthesia.

and ketamine/medetomidine [96]. Shorter durations were under pentobarbital [46, 126] and thiopental [64] anesthesia. Approximately the same duration of the P wave was under the other types of anesthesia (**Table 3**). The amplitude of the P wave was the smallest in all combinations with ketamine (ketamine/xylazine) [82, 84, 89], ketamine/medetomidine [96], ketamine/diazepam [96, 98], ketamine/midazolam [97] and urethane [133], and isolated hearts [115].

The extent to which these values are valid cannot yet be assessed because there are an insufficient number of studies; this problem also affects sex and the LD effect on the amplitude and duration of the P wave. There is an indication, however, that there may be sex differences in the duration of the P wave under ketamine/xylazine anesthesia (21.99 ms [range 17.38 ms–26.62 ms]) for females and 20.37 ms (range 18.84 ms–26.49 ms) in males [19]. However, to date, this is not statistically demonstrable for other types of anesthesia.

5. Prognostic significance of changes in the ventricular complex in arrhythmogenesis

Evaluation of the parameters of the ventricular complex (QT interval, QTc interval, QRS complex, R, and T wave amplitudes) is undoubtedly important because it provides information about the course of depolarization and repolarization of the ventricles. The distance from the beginning of the QRS complex to the end of the T wave is measured, with the total length corresponding to the duration of depolarization and repolarization of the ventricular muscle.

5.1 QT interval

In rats, the determination of the QT interval is more complicated because the T wave is not clearly separated from the QRS complex. Therefore, it is necessary to develop a method for analyzing repolarization time in nonanesthetized rats. However, the importance of QT interval dispersion is a complex matter involving at least two different phenomena—namely, prolongation of the average action potential duration and myocardial heterogeneity [26]. Based on the evaluation of the QT, as well as the QTc interval in rat experimental models, cardioprotection was also assessed after stimulation of vitamin D receptors and the effect of isoprenaline [42], the effect of doxorubicin [134] and L-glutamine in diabetic rats [135], saffron on atrial and ventricular conduction velocity [64], or the effect of preconditioning at different doses of noradrenaline on ischemia-induced ventricular arrhythmias.

The mentioned examples confirm the informative value of changes in the duration of the QT interval in the evaluation of the severity of disorders in the dispersion of ventricular refractory periods and their impact on the onset and development of ventricular arrhythmias. If we consider the values from telemetry studies, in terms of reference value and range [21, 26, 117, 118], QT interval prolongation was measured with virtually every type of barbiturate anesthesia; as such, under pentobarbital [32, 34, 37, 38, 40, 41, 43–45, 47–50, 122, 124–126], thiopental [61–64, 66, 67, 69], and Nembutal anesthesia [114]. Ketamine/xylazine [45, 78, 85, 87, 89–92, 129, 136], ketamine/medetomidine [96], ketamine/diazepam [96, 98], and ketamine/midazolam [97], anesthesia had the greatest effect on QT interval prolongation. A moderate prolongation was also found under chloralose anesthesia [77] and similar prolongations under ether anesthesia [99–101, 103, 104]. The shorter QT interval duration was under urethane [45, 52, 55, 56, 60, 135, 137, 138] and tribromoethanol [106] anesthesia compared with telemetry studies. Isoflurane [72, 74, 75, 120, 121] and desflurane anesthesia [72] did not affect QT interval duration. There were virtually no significant changes in QT interval duration in working with isolated hearts [105, 115, 139, 140]. All experiments were performed on males without specifying the adaptation of the animals to the LD cycle and there were no studies investigating sex

Anesthesia.	Not specified		Light period		Dark period	
	Female	Male	Female	Male	Female	Male
Telemetry studies	—	58.02 51.7–64.34 (n = 4)	-	-	-	-
Pentobarbital	—	68.85 65.56–69.26 (n = 19)	73.5 58.1–88.9 (n = 1)	—	76.02 66.36–85.68 (n = 1)	—
Thiopental	—	64.75 54.03–67.52 (n = 8)	-	—	-	—
Phenobarbital	—	—	—	—	—	—

Anesthesia.	Not specified		Light period		Dark period	
	Female	Male	Female	Male	Female	Male
Nembutal	-	62 60–63 (n = 1)	-	—	-	—
Ketamine/xylazine	87 79–95 (n = 1)	74.97 70.88–79.23 (n = 11)	89.9 73–106.8 (n = 1)	—	91.7 82–101.4 (n = 1)	—
Ketamine/ medetomidine	-	65 63.1–66.9 (n = 1)	-	—	-	—
Ketamine/Diazepam	-	101.25 84.15–116.7 (n = 2)	-	—	-	—
Ketamine/midazolam	-	78 69–87 (n = 1)	-	—	-	—
Isoflurane	—	58.32 43.68–61.48 (n = 6)	—	—	—	—
Desflurane	-	69.0 67.72–0.28 (n = 1)	—	—	—	—
Chloralose	-	60.20 53.51–6.89 (n = 1)	—	—	—	—
Tribromethanol	-	36 33.5–38.5 (n = 1)	—	—	—	—
Ether	—	69.86 66.4–73.4 (n = 5)	—	—	—	—
Urethane	—	53.05 48.74–57.35 (n = 9)	—	—	—	—
Isolated heart	—	72.75 68,8–76.7 (n = 4)	—	—	—	—

Data presented as average (range); (n, number of baseline or control values from which QT interval was evaluated). Not specified—in the methodology does not specify the lighted period when the experiments were performed.

Table 4.
QT interval duration (ms) under individual types of anesthesia with regard to sex and the cycle of light (inactive) and dark (active).

differences. Similarly, it was not possible to determine the circadian fluctuation in the duration of the QT interval or the dependence on the LD cycle (**Table 4**, **Figure 3**).

5.2 QTc interval

In human cardiology, QTc interval assessment enables the comparison of QT values overtime at different HRs and improves the identification of patients at increased

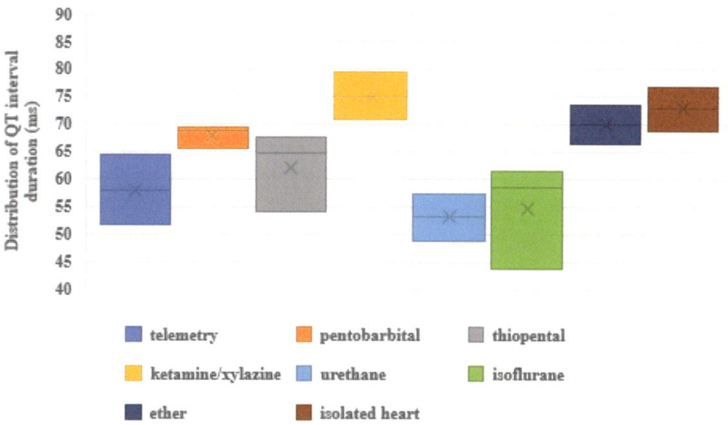

Figure 3.
Distribution of ranges of QT intervals from telemetry studies and under different types of general anesthesia in male rats without taking into account the light periods of the rat regimen day when the experiments were performed. Only QT interval ranges from at least three studies in which QT interval was evaluated are shown in the figure. Telemetry studies (n = 4), pentobarbital anesthesia (n = 19), thiopental anesthesia (n = 8), ketamine/xylazine anesthesia (n = 11), isoflurane anesthesia (n = 6), ether anesthesia (n = 5), urethane anesthesia (n = 9), isolated heart (n = 4). n, number of baseline or control values from which duration of the QT interval was evaluated.

risk for arrhythmias. Prolonged QTc is caused by premature action potentials during the late phases of depolarization. This increases the risk for ventricular arrhythmias, including fatal ventricular fibrillation [141]. These changes make it difficult to compare QT intervals measured at different HRs. To account for this and, thus, improve the reliability of QT measurements, the QT interval can be corrected for HR (QTc) using various mathematical formulae, a process that modern ECG recorders often perform automatically. The duration of the QTc interval is a key and critical factor in assessing changes in repolarization with regard to drug safety and cardiac disorders. There was only one study that reported changes in the duration of the QTc interval depending on commonly used drugs, especially when used in combination with other substances that affect their metabolism [142, 143]. Possible changes in QTc interval depending on sex and age have also been described in humans. Higher rates of prolonged QTc are observed in women, older patients, with high systolic blood pressure or HR, and low body height [144]. It was found that the rate of QT/RR hysteresis decreases with increasing age, while the duration of the individually corrected QTc interval increases with increasing age. In contrast to longer QTc intervals, the rate of QT/RR hysteresis was faster in women [145]. There are many causes of prolonged QT intervals, and acquired causes are more common than genetic causes [146].

Changes in the QTc interval have also been described in rats, where, for example, induction of ischemia shortened the QTc interval and led to ventricular arrhythmias. Administration of low doses of noradrenaline prevented shortening of the QTc interval during ischemia but could not significantly reduce the severity and incidence of arrhythmias [38]. However, in the experimental field, determination of QTc interval is somewhat more complicated because HR values are extremely variable among different species [147]. In rats, there is a lack of a validated approach to QT interval correction [143] and, despite some efforts [148, 149], there is no validated and widely used method for such QTc interval adjustment. Thus, most researchers in experimental cardiology, pharmacology, and toxicology must use formulas designed for other species, without commenting on their accuracy in rats [26, 150, 151], and its use should be considered carefully in case of very low HR [143] . This fact is reflected in the data reported in **Table 5** and **Figure 4** of the average values of the QTc interval, where relatively large deviations under different types of anesthesia are evident.

When comparing the duration of the QTc interval with the mean value from telemetry studies [26, 30, 31, 117, 118], significant prolongation occurred under pentobarbital [32, 38, 41–43, 47, 51] ketamine/xylazine [87, 90–92, 129, 136, 152, 153], and urethane [52, 57, 60] anesthesia, with moderate prolongation under thiopental [31, 62, 63, 66, 68, 71] anesthesia. The shortened QTc interval duration compared with the mean value from telemetry studies was under isoflurane anesthesia [72, 74, 75, 121].

Anesthesia	QTc interval (ms)	QRS complex (ms)	R wave amplitude (mV)	T wave amplitude (mV)
Telemetry studies	87.02 (81.79–92.31) n = 5	26.08 (25.68–29.52) n = 5	—	0.139 (0.118–0.16) n = 1
Pentobarbital	203.77 (196.2–211.5) n = 7	25.4 (23.68–27.13) n = 19	0.56 (0.54–0.58) n = 4	0.08 (0.07–0.9) n = 2
Thiopental	110.23 (100.5–120) n = 7	22.76 (21.12–24.47) n = 8	1.8 (1.76–1.84) n = 1	—
Phenobarbital	71.6 (69.36–73.84) n = 1	55 (45–65) n = 1	-	—
Nembutal	-	20 (19–21 n = 1	1.06 (0.99–1.12) n = 1	0.37 (0.34–0.41) n = 1
Ketamine/xylazine	143.76 (138.97–148.55) n = 8	23.9 (22.16–25.64) n = 12	0.49 (0.41–0.57) n = 5	0.09 (0.06–0.11) n = 5
Ketamine/ medetomidine	-	27.5 (22.5–32.5) n = 1	-	—
Ketamine/diazepam	-	18.5 (13.25–23.75) n = 2	-	—
Ketamine/ midazolam	-	18 (16.8–19.2) n = 1	-	0.07 (0.034–0.106) n = 1
Isoflurane	58.32 (43.68–61.48) n = 4	18.3 (16.75–19.85) n = 4	1.7 1.5–1.9 n = 1	0.11 (0.09–0.13) n = 1
Desflurane	184.7 (181.32–188.08) n = 1	28.8 (25.22–32.38) n = 1	—	—
Chloralose	-	66 (55.7–76.3) n = 1	—	—

Anesthesia	QTc interval (ms)	QRS complex (ms)	R wave amplitude (mV)	T wave amplitude (mV)
Tribromethanol	90.5 (85.5–95.5) n = 1	26.2 (25.3–27.1) n = 2	—	—
Ether	153 (151–155) n = 1	22.15 (18.8–25.5) n = 2	—	—
Urethane	165.5 (158.6–180.5) n = 3	18.41 (17.39–20.5) n = 15	0.65 (0.64–0.66) n = 2	0.337 (0.335–0.337) n = 1
Isolated heart	83.43 (52.65–114.2) n = 2	32.5 (31.4–33.6) n = 2	1.61 (not specified) n = 2	1.42 (0.95–1.89) n = 1

Data presented as average (range) n, number of experimental studies in which ventricular parameters were evaluated.

Table 5.
QTc interval, QRS complex duration, R and T wave amplitude, regardless of the synchronization of the animals to the light and dark cycle under individual types of anesthesia.

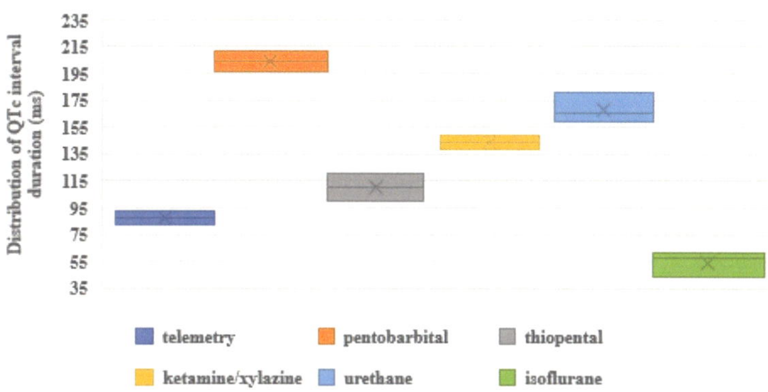

Figure 4.
Distribution of ranges of QTc interval from telemetry studies and under different types of general anesthesia in male rat males without taking into account the light periods of the rat regimen day when the experiments were performed. Only QTc interval ranges from at least three studies where QTc interval has been evaluated are shown in the figure. Telemetry studies (n = 5), pentobarbital anesthesia (n = 7), thiopental anesthesia (n = 7), ketamine/xylazine anesthesia (n = 8), urethane anesthesia (n = 3), isoflurane anesthesia (n = 4). n, number of baseline or control values from which duration of QTc interval was evaluated.

The problem is the comparison between the sexes and to evaluate the effect of the LD cycle, for which insufficient experimental data are available. LD differences were found in females under ketamine/xylazine anesthesia (light 174.5 ± 34.8 ms vs. dark 202.1 ms) [19], unlike pentobarbital anesthesia, where there were no significant differences (light 197.7 ± 40.9 ms vs. dark 190.7 ± 26.6 ms) [20]. Unfortunately, this dependence has not been tested with other types of general anesthesia. The age effect of rats was demonstrated under rather unconventional tribromoethanol anesthesia by da Silva et al. [106], where the duration of the QTc interval was two times longer in older rats (117 ± 4 ms vs. 64 ± 6 ms) than in young rats at relatively the same HR (young, 381 ± 1 beats/min. vs. old, 405 ± 11 beats/min).

5.3 QRS complex

In some cases, it is also important to evaluate other parameters related to the electrophysiology of the ventricles. For example, the QRS complex indicates depolarization of the right and left ventricles and the contraction of the large ventricular muscles. Any conduction abnormality lasts longer and causes "extended" QRS complexes. The duration, amplitude, and morphology of the QRS complex are useful in the diagnosis of cardiac arrhythmias, conduction abnormalities, ventricular hypertrophy, myocardial infarction, electrolyte disturbances, and other disease states. High-frequency analysis of the QRS complex may be useful for detecting coronary artery disease during a stress test. Evaluation of the amplitude of the R wave as well as the P wave in experimental work on rats also proved to be important. They are informative and changes can help to determine the tendency of the myocardium to arrhythmias.

When comparing the average value of QRS complex duration from telemetry studies [21, 31, 117–119] to barbiturate anesthesia—under pentobarbital [32, 34, 37, 40, 42, 44–49, 51, 122, 124–126, 154], thiopental [31, 61, 63, 64, 68, 69, 71], and Nembutal [114] anesthesia—the average value of the QRS complex duration was somewhat shorter and the ranges did not differ significantly.

Ketamine/xylazine [45, 78, 79, 84, 85, 89, 91, 92, 128, 129, 152], ketamine/diazepam [96, 98], and ketamine/midazolam [97] as well as ether [100, 101] and urethane anesthesia [45, 53, 55–58, 60, 135, 137, 138] shortened the duration of the QRS complex compared to the value(s) from telemetry studies. The longer duration was under phenobarbital [95], ketamine/medetomidine [96], desflurane [72], chloralose [77] anesthesia, and in isolated hearts [105, 115] (**Figure 5**). Of course, such comparisons can be misleading because the values were reported in only one study. Similar to previously described ECG parameters, all experiments were performed on males without specifying the adaptation of the animals to the LD cycle, and there was no study addressing sex differences. Similarly, it was not possible to determine the circadian fluctuation in the duration of the QT interval or the dependence on the LD cycle (**Table 5**, **Figure 5**).

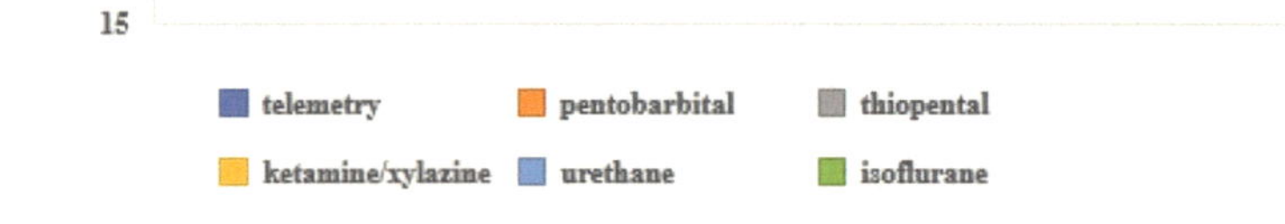

Figure 5.
Distribution of ranges of QRS complex from telemetry studies and under different types of general anesthesia in male rats without taking into account the light periods of the rat regimen day when the experiments were performed. Only QRS complex ranges from at least three studies where QRS complex has been evaluated are shown in the figure. Telemetry studies (n = 5), pentobarbital anesthesia (n = 19), thiopental anesthesia (n = 8), ketamine/xylazine anesthesia (n = 12), urethane anesthesia (n = 15), isoflurane anesthesia (n = 4). n, number of baseline or control values from which duration of QT interval was evaluated.

DOI: http://dx.doi.org/10.5772/intechopen.104928

6. Conclusions

In the discussion sections of many published *in vivo* studies, the results obtained are compared with previously published findings. Although changes in ECG parameters are often described, the type of anesthesia used in the experiments is not taken into account. Moreover, in acute *in vivo* experiments, the time of day the experiments are performed, and the adaptation of the animals to the LD cycle, and/or sex, are not taken into account whatsoever. This approach is self-evident and logical because the experiments are mostly performed only on males and during the workday, often without regard for chronobiological principles.

However, if changes in ECG parameters are considered to be important indicators of arrhythmogenesis, such comparisons may be misleading and must not be immediately regarded to indicate a difference in myocardial electrical stability. We should be more careful in interpreting results and, in discussing the mechanisms underlying a given type of arrhythmia, acknowledge that initial ECG parameters may already be affected to some extent by the anesthesia used and by regular daytime experimentation. The data presented in the tables clearly demonstrate the differences in baseline or control values with different types of anesthesia and whether the baseline or control value is "normal" or already altered by anesthesia should be taken into account. For example, a change in the evaluated ECG parameter after an intervention may not necessarily indicate a possible electrophysiological substrate for the development of an arrhythmia, it can only be "adjusted to a normal value" because we do not know the reference value.

Similarly, sex and time of day the experiments are performed can be a problem because it is not possible to determine sex differences as well as changes during the active and nonactive period of rat regimen day because there are no studies that have directly addressed this aspect. Telemetry studies that would reveal changes in ECG parameters in circadian dependence, to describe reference values and, possibly, sex differences, could help to facilitate interpretation of the results obtained. However, it is highly speculative to consider the values from the cited telemetry studies as reference values (although the ECG is measured from nonanesthetized rats) because the methodologies do not report whether the indicated baseline value is the 24 h average (mesor) or is the current value measured immediately before the intervention. Most likely, they are baseline values before the experimental intervention and this only applies to male rats, whereas the lighted (light or dark) period when the experiment is performed is not reported, although an adaptation of animals to the LD cycle is described.

Thus, the question "Which anesthetic is the most suitable anesthetic in *in vivo* rat cardiological experiments so that the initial electrophysiology of the heart is not significantly affected" is relatively difficult to address for several reasons. First, we do not currently have specified sex-related reference values for rats. Second, because there are circadian variations in the measurable parameters of the cardiovascular system, there are also changes in individual ECG parameters, depending on the light cycle (inactive period) and dark (active period). Finally, the effects of anesthetics at the level of ion channels are not described in detail because the entire electrophysiology of the myocardium depends on ionic currents and the overall metabolism of minerals.

As such, when evaluating changes in ECG parameters in rats, these possible variations should also be taken into account. The correct assessment of changes, in turn, depends on knowledge of the reference values according to sex and on the time of day the experiments or measurements are performed. Although rat ECG parameters are only analyzed in this study, these can be of basis to further researches and studies that may involve humans in the future.

Acknowledgements

This work was supported by a VEGA grant: 1/0008/20.

Conflict of interest statement

The authors declare that there is no conflict of interest.

Funding

This research received no specific grant from any funding agency in the public, commercial, or not-for-profit sectors.

Author details

Pavol Svorc Jr[1] and Pavol Svorc[1,2*]

1 Department of Physiology and Pathophysiology, Medical Faculty, Ostrava University, Ostrava, Czech Republic

2 Department of Physiology, Medical Faculty, Safarik University, Kosice, Slovak Republic

*Address all correspondence to: pavol.svorc@upjs.sk

References

[1] Fields RD. Vive la Différence. Scientific American. 2014;**311**(3):14

[2] Caetano J, Alves JD. Heart rate and cardiovascular protection. European Journal of Internal Medicine. 2015;**26**(4):217-222

[3] Zaza A, Ronchi C, Malfatto G. Arrhythmias and heart rate: Mechanisms and significance of a relationship. Arrhythmia & Electrophysiology Review. 2018;**7**(4):232-237

[4] Svorc P, Tomori Z, Bracokova I, Marossy A. Effect of pentobarbital and ketamine/xylazine anaesthesia on the electrical stability of the heart and heart rate in rat hypoventilation/reoxygenation model. Biologia. 2003;**58**(3):379-386

[5] Priori SG, Chen SR. Inherited dysfunction of sarcoplasmic reticulum Ca^{2+} handling and arrhythmogenesis. Circulation Research. 2011;**108**:871-883

[6] Haxxox JP. Effect of temperature on the heart rate, electrocardiogram and certain myocardial oxidations of the rat. Circulation Research. 1958;**6**: 771-778

[7] Baldwin A, Wagers C, Schwartz GE. Reiki improves heart rate homeostasis in laboratory rats. The Journal of Alternative and Complementary Medicine. 2008;**14**(4):417-422

[8] Heisser A. Effect of exercise and L-citrulline on heart rate in rats. Cantaurus. 2020;**28**:5-7

[9] James AF, Choisy SCM, Hancox JC. Recent advances in understanding sex differences in cardiac repolarization. Progress in Biophysics and Molecular Biology. 2007;**94**(3):265-319

[10] Harkness JE, Wagner JE. In Book: The Biology and Medicine of Rabbits and Rodents. Philadelphia: Lea & Febiger; 1977

[11] Leblanc N, Chartier D, Gosselin H, Rouleau JL. Age and gender differences in excitation-contraction coupling of the rat ventricle. Journal of Physiology (London). 1998;**511**(Pt 2):533-548

[12] Philp KL, Coker SJ, Hussain M, Hart G. Actions of 17b-oestradiol on the current-voltage relationship for the L-type calcium current (ICa) in ventricular myocytes isolated from male and female rats. Journal of Physiology (London). 2002;**544P**:57P-58P

[13] Hashimoto M, Kuwahara M, Tsubone H, Sugano S. Diurnal variation of autonomic nervous activity in the rat - investigation by power spectral analysis of heart rate variability. Journal of Electrocardiology. 1999;**32**(2): 167-171

[14] Hashimoto M, Harada T, Ishikawa T, Obata M, Shibutani Y. Investigation on diabetic autonomic neuropathy assessed by power spectral analysis of heart rate variability in WBN/Kob rats. Journal of Electrocardiology. 2001;**34**(3):243-250

[15] Koresh O, Kaplan Z, Zohar J, Matar MA, Geva AB, Cohen H. Distinctive cardiac autonomic dysfunction following stress exposure in both sexes in an animal model of PTSD. Behavioural Brain Research. 2016;**308**:128-142

[16] Molcan L, Teplan M, Vesela A, Zeman M. The long-term effects of phase advance shifts of photoperiod on cardiovascular parameters as measured by radiotelemetry in rats. Physiological Measurement. 2013;**34**:1623-1632

[17] Molcan L, Vesela A, Zeman M. Repeated phase shifts in the lighting regimen change the blood pressure response to norepinephrine stimulation in rats. Physiological Research. 2014;**63**(5):567-575

[18] Schlatter J, Zbinden G. Heart rate- and ECG-recording in the rat by biotelemetry. In: Chambers CM, Chambers PL, editors. New Toxicology for Old. Archives of Toxicology (Supplement) 5. Berlin: Heidelberg, Springer; 1982

[19] Svorc P, Svorc P Jr, Novakova M, Bacova I, Jurasova Z, Marossy A. Ketamine/xylazine anaesthesia in the chronobiological studies. Biological Rhythm Research. 2014;**45**(4):633-642

[20] SvorcJr. P, Svorc P, Bacova I, Gresova S. Pentobarbital anaesthesia in the chronobiological studies. Biological Rhythm Research 2015;46(3):445-452.

[21] Farmer JB, Levy GP. A simple method for recording the electrocardiogram and heart rate from conscious animals. British Journal of Pharmacology and Chemotherapy. 1968;**32**:193-200

[22] Sgoifo A, De Boer SF, Buwalda B, Korte-Bouws G, Tuma J, Bohus B, et al. Vulnerability to arrhythmias during social stress in rats with different sympathovagal balance. American Journal of Physiology. Heart and Circulatory Physiology. 1998;**275**(2):460-466

[23] Nijsen MJMA, Croiset G, Diamant M, Stam R, Delsing D, de Wied D, et al. Conditioned fear-induced tachycardia in the rat; vagal involvement. European Journal of Pharmacology. 1998;**350**(2-3):211-222

[24] Nijsen MJMA, Croiset G, Stam R, Bruijnzeel A, Diamant M, de Wied D. The role of the CRH type 1 receptor in autonomic responses to corticotropin-releasing hormone in the rat. Neuropsychopharmacology. 2000;**22**(4):388-399

[25] Nijsen MJMA, Croiset G, Diamant M, De Wied D, Wiegant VM. CRH signalling in the bed nucleus of the stria terminalis is involved in stress-induced cardiac vagal activation in conscious rats. Neuropsychopharmacology. 2001;**24**(1):1-10

[26] Baillard C, Mansier P, Ennezat PV, Mangin L, Medigue C, Swynghedauw B, et al. Converting enzyme inhibition normalizes QT interval in spontaneously hypertensive rats. Hypertension. 2000;**36**:350-354

[27] Towa S, Kuwahara M, Tsubone H. Characteristics of autonomic nervous function in Zucker-fatty rats: Investigation by power spectral analysis of heart rate variability. Experimental Animals. 2004;**53**(2):137-144

[28] Pereira-Junior PP, Marocolo M, Rodrigues FP, Medei E, Nascimento JHM. Noninvasive method for electrocardiogram recording in conscious rats: Feasibility for heart rate variability analysis. Anais Academia Brasileria de Ciências. 2010;**82**(2):431-437

[29] Koizumi S, Minamisawa S, Sasaguri K, Onozuka M, Sato S, Ono Y. Chewing reduces sympathetic nervous response to stress and prevents poststress arrhythmias in rats. American Journal of Physiology-Heart and Circulatory Physiology. 2011;**301**(4):H1551-H1558

[30] Carll AP, Hazari MS, Perez CM, Krantz QT, King CJ, Winsett DW, et al. Whole and particle-free diesel exhausts differentially affect cardiac electrophysiology, blood pressure, and autonomic balance in heart failure-prone rats. Toxicological Sciences. 2012;**128**(2):490-499

[31] Kumar P, Srivastava P, Gupta A, Bajpai M. Noninvasive recording of electrocardiogram in conscious rat: A new device. Indian Journal of Pharmacology. 2017;**49**(1):116-118

[32] Lessard Y, Vernhet L, Mainguy A. Relationships between transmembrane action potential changes and simultaneous changes in electrocardiograms of rats after a one-month aortic pressure overload. Physiological Research. 1997;**46**(4):257-269

[33] Miki K, Kosho A, Hayashida Y. Method for continuous measurements of renal sympathetic nerve activity and cardiovascular function during exercise in rats. Experimental Physiology. 2002;**87**(1):33-39

[34] Sugiyama A, Takahara A, Honsho S, Nakamura Y, Hashimoto K. A simple in vivo atrial fibrillation model of rat induced by transesophageal atrial burst pacing. Journal of Pharmacological Sciences. 2005;**98**:315-318

[35] Rivero DHRF, Sassaki C, Lorenzi-Filho G, Saldiva PHN. PM2.5 induces acute electrocardiographic alterations in healthy rats. Environmental Research. 2005;**99**(2):262-266

[36] Yokokawa M, Ohnishi S, Ishibashi-Ueda H, Obata H, Otani K, Miyahara Y, et al. Transplantation of mesenchymal stem cells improves atrioventricular conduction in a rat model of complete atrioventricular block. Cell Transplantation. 2008;**17**(10-11):1145-1155

[37] Kumar R, Kela A, Tayal G. Effect of acute stress on rat ECG. The Internet Journal of Pharmacology. 2009;**8**(1)

[38] Imani A, Faghihi M, Keshavarz DM, Karimian SM, Niaraki SS. Effect of different doses of noradrenaline against ischemia-induced ventricular arrhythmias in rat heart in vivo. Indian Pacing Electrophysiology Journal. 2009;**9**(1):35-44

[39] Chang YT, Wann SR, Wu PL, Hsieh KH, Lin CC, Huang MS, et al. Influence of age on heart rate variability during therapeutic hypothermia in a rat model. Resuscitation. 2011;**82**(10):1350-1354

[40] Howarth FC, Jacobson M, Shafiullah M, Ljubisavljevic M, Adeghate E. Heart rate, body temperature and physical activity are variously affected during insulin treatment in alloxan-induced type 1 diabetic rat. Physiological Research. 2011;**60**(1):65-73

[41] Liu B, Li S, Su Y, Xiong MT, Xu YW. Comparative study of the protective effects of terfenadine and amiodarone on barium chloride/aconitine-induced ventricular arrhythmias in rats: A potential role of terfenadine. Molecular Medicine Reports. 2014;**10**(6): 3217-3226

[42] Abbod AM, Elshal MF. VDR stimulation improves outcome of isoprenaline-induced myocardial infarction in rats via down-regulation of cardiac inos gene expression. Biomedical Research. 2015;**36**(4):755-764

[43] Ahmad A, Sattar MZ, Rathore HA, Khan SA, Lazhari MA, Hashmi F, et al. Impact of isoprenaline and caffeine on development of left ventricular hypertrophy and renal hemodynamic in Wistar Kyoto rats. Acta Poloniae Pharmaceutica. 2015;**72**(5): 1015-1026

[44] Pugsley MK, Hayes ES, Wang WQ, Walker MJA. Ventricular arrhythmia incidence in the rat is reduced by naloxone. Pharmacological Research. 2015;**97**:64-69

[45] Konopelski P, Ufnal M. Electrocardiography in rats: A comparison to human. Physiological Research. 2016;**65**(5):717-725

[46] Comerma-Steffensen SG, Carvacho I, Hedegaard ER, Simonsen U. Small and intermediate calcium-activated potassium channel openers improve rat endothelial and erectile function. Frontiers in Pharmacology. 2017;**8**:660

[47] Pezolato VA, Mascarin AL, Ferreira RB, Dias R, Silva CA. Acompanhamento eletrocardiográfico no desenvolvimento de ratos Wistar. Arquivo Brasileiro de Medicina Veterinaria e Zootecnia. 2017;**69**(01):39-47

[48] Wang S, Cheng ZY, Chen XJ, Xue HZ. Ulinastatin protects rats with myocardial infarction by activating Nrf2/NOS pathway. European Review for Medical and Pharmacological Sciences. 2018;**22**(24):8990-8998

[49] Chen XY, Guo HC, Li Q, Zhang Y, Liu HL, Zhang XF, et al. Protective effect of berberine on aconite-induced myocardial injury and the associated mechanisms. Molecular Medicine Reports. 2018;**18**(5):4468-4476

[50] Huang XW, Pan MD, Du PH, Wang LX. Arginase-2 protects myocardial ischemia-reperfusion injury via NF-kappa B/TNF-alpha pathway. European Review for Medical and Pharmacological Sciences. 2018;**22**(19):6529-6537

[51] Abdulsalam TM, Hasanin AH, Mohamed RH, Badawy AELS. Angiotensin receptor-neprilysin inhibitior (thiorphan/irbesartan) decreased ischemia-reperfusion induced ventricular arrhythmias in rat; in vivo study. European Journal of Pharmacology. 2020;**882**:173295

[52] Lin MT, Liu HH, Yang YL. Involvement of interleukin-1 receptor mechanisms in development of arterial hypotension in rat heatstroke. American Journal of Physiology. Heart and Circulatory Physiology. 1997;**273**(4):H2072-H2077

[53] Buschmann G, Schumacher W, Budden R, Kühl UG. Evaluation of the effect of dopamine and other catecholamines on the electrocardiogram and blood pressure of rats by means of on-line biosignal processing. Journal of Cardiovascular Pharmacology. 1980;**2**:777-795

[54] Chaswal M, Das S, Prasad J, Katyal A, Fahim M. Chemical sympathectomy restores baroreceptor-heart rate reflex and heart rate variability in rats with chronic nitric oxide deficiency. Physiological Research. 2015;**64**(4):459-466

[55] Aydin B, Hocaoglu N, Micili SC, Ergur BU, Kalkan S. Effects of 2-hydroxypropyl-beta-cyclodextrin on cardiovascular signs of amitriptyline poisoning in a rat model. Cardiovascular Toxicology. 2016;**16**(4):374-380

[56] Emeka PM, Al-Ahmed A. Effect of metformin on ECG, HR and BP of rats administered with cardiotoxic agent doxorubicin. International Journal of Basic & Clinical Pharmacology. 2017;**6**(5):1054-1059

[57] Younis NS, Al Ahmed A, Al Mulhim N, AlGarni AA, Madu EP. Exenatide attenuation of cardiac rhythm abnormalities and blood pressure changes induced by doxorubicin in rats. International Journal of Pharmacology. 2017;**13**(8):1098-1102

[58] Sharma S, Khan V, Najmi AK, Alam O, Haque SE. Prophylactic treatment with icariin prevents isoproterenol-induced myocardial oxidative stress via nuclear factor-like 2 activation. Pharmacognsy Magazine. 2018;**14**(suupl. S, 55): S227-S236

[59] Bozdogan O, Bozcaarmutlu A, Kaya ST, Sapmaz C, Ozarslan TO, Eksioglu D, et al. Decreasing myocardial estrogen receptors and antioxidant activity may be responsible for increasing ischemia- and reperfusion-induced ventricular arrhythmia in older female rats. Life Sciences. 2021;**271**:119190

[60] Lin C-C, Hsu K-H, Shih C-P, Chang G-J. Hemodynamic and electromechanical effects of paraquat in rat heart. PLoS One. 2021;**16**(4):e0234591

[61] Kralova E, Mokran T, Murin J, Stankovicova T. Electrocardiography in two models of isoproterenol-induced left ventricular remodeling. Physiological Research. 2008;**57**(suppl 2):583-589

[62] Kralova E, Racanska E, Vicenova A, Boselova I, Malik I, Stankovicova T. Pharmacological evaluation of the effects of phenylcarbamic acid derivatives on cardiovascular functions in rats. Acta Pharmaceutica. 2018;**68**(4):507-515

[63] Maciel NR, Reis PG, Kato KC, Vidal AT, Guimaraes HN, Frezard F, et al. Reduced cardiovascular alterations of tartar emetic administered in long-circulating liposomes in rats. Toxicology Letters. 2010;**199**(3):234-238

[64] Joukar S. Electrocardiogram alterations following one-week consumption of Crocus sativus L. (saffron). EXCLI Journal. 2012;**11**:480-486

[65] Joukar S, Ghorbani-Shahrbabaki S, Hajali V, Sheibani V, Naghsh N. Susceptibility to life-threatening ventricular arrhythmias in an animal model of paradoxical sleep deprivation. Sleep Medicine. 2013;**14**(12):1277-1282

[66] Klimas J, Vaja V, Vercinska M, Kyselovic J, Krenek P. Discrepant regulation of QT (QTc) interval duration by calcium channel blockade and angiotensin converting enzyme inhibition in experimental hypertension. Basic & Clinical Pharmacology & Toxicology. 2012;**111**(4):279-288

[67] Elsherbiny NM, Salama MF, Said E, El-Sherbiny M, Al-Gayyar MMH. Crocin protects against doxorubicin-induced myocardial toxicity in rats through down-regulation of inflammatory and apoptic pathways. Chemico-Biological Interactions. 2016;**247**:39-48

[68] Raji-Amirhasani A, Joukar S, Naderi-Boldaji V, Bejeshk MA. Mild exercise along with limb blood-flow restriction modulates the electrocardiogram, angiotensin, and apelin receptors of the heart in aging rats. Iranian Journal of Basic Medical Sciences. 2018;**21**(6):558-563

[69] Rahmanifard M, Vessal M, Noorafshan A, Karbalay-Doust S, Naseh M. The protective effects of coenzyme Q10 and lisinopril against doxorubicin-induced cardiotoxicity in rats: A stereological and electrocardiogram study. Cardiovascular Toxicology. 2021;**21**(11):936-946

[70] El-Marasy SA, El-Awdan SA, Hassan A, Abdallah HMI. Cardioprotective effect of thymol against adrenaline-induced myocardial injury in rats. Heliyon. 2020;**6**(7):e04431

[71] Haydari S, Nazari A, Moghimian M, Sedighi M, Ghaderpour S. Cardioprotective activity of ethanolic extract of Echinophora cinerea against aluminum phosphide poisoning in rats. Journal of Food Biochemistry. 2020;**44**:e13300

[72] Ozturk A, Altug ME. Effects of repeated application of isoflurane and desflurane on electrocardiogram, anaesthesia induction, and recovery characteristics in rats. Bulletin-Veterinary Institute in Pulawy. 2007;**51**(4):635-640

[73] Rey M, Weber E, Hess PD. Simultaneous pulmonary and systemic blood pressure and ECG interval measurement in conscious, freely moving rats. Journal of the American Association for Laboratory Animal Science. 2012;**51**(2):231-238

[74] Jiang M, Murias JM, Chrones T, Sims SM, Lui E, Noble EG. American ginseng acutely regulates contractile function of rat heart. Frontiers in Pharmacology. 2014;**5**:43

[75] Imoto K, Hirakawa M, Okada M, Yamawaki H. Canstatin modulates L-type calcium channel activity in rat ventricular cardiomyocytes. Biochemical and Biophysical Research Communications. 2018;**499**(4):954-959

[76] Kruger C, Landerer V, Zugck C, Ehmke H, Kubler W, Haass M. The bradycardic agent zatebradine enhances baroreflex sensitivity and heart rate variability in rats early after myocardial infarction. Cardiovascular Research. 2000;**45**(4):900-912

[77] Dai GF, Wang ZJY. Octreotide protects doxorubicin-induced cardiac toxicity via regulating oxidative stress. European Review for Medical and Pharmacological Sciences. 2018;**22**(18):6139-6148

[78] Mao PR, Jamali F. Methoxyflurane anesthesia augments the chronotropic and dromotropic effects of verapamil. Journal of Pharmacy & Pharmaceutical Sciences. 1999;**2**(1):30-35

[79] Regan CP, Cresswell HK, Zhang R, Lynch JJ. Novel method to assess cardiac electrophysiology in the rat: Characterization of standard ion channel blockers. Journal of Cardiovascular Pharmacology. 2005;**46**(1):68-75

[80] Trindade DC, Trindade RC, Marassi MP, Martins OPPR, Costa-E-Sousa RH, Mattos EC, et al. Role of renin-angiotensin system in development of heart failure induced by myocardial infarction in rats. Anais da Academia Brasileira de Ciências. 2007;**79**(2):251-259

[81] Yenisehirli A, Naseri E. Omeprazole, lansoprazole and pantoprazole had no effect on blood pressure and electrocardiogram of anesthetized rat. Pharmacological Research. 2008;**58**(1):65-71

[82] Parasuraman S, Raveendran R, Selvaraj RJ. Effects of cleistanthins a and B on blood pressure and electrocardiogram in Wistar rats. Zeitschrift für Naturforschung C. 2011;**66**(11-12):581-587

[83] Kannan M, Quine SD. Ellagic acid ameliorates isoproterenol induced oxidative stress: Evidence from electrocardiological, biochemical and histological study. European Journal of Pharmacology. 2011;**659**(1):45-52

[84] Mutiso SK, Rono DK, Bukachi F. Relationship between anthropometric measures and early electrocardiographic changes in obese rats. BMC Research Notes. 2014;**7**:931

[85] Selcuk EB, Sungu M, Parlakpinar H, Ermis N, Taslidere E, Vard N, et al. Evaluation of the cardiovascular effects of varenicline in rats. Drug Design, Development and Therapy. 2015;**9**:5705-5717

[86] Binu P, Priya N, Abhilash S, Vineetha RC, Nair RH. Studies on curative efficacy of monoterpene eugenol on anti- leukemic drug arsenic trioxide induced cardiotoxicity. Biomedicine & Pharmacotherapy. 2017;**91**:559-566

[87] Bora S, Erdogan MA, Yigitturk G, Erbas O, Parlak I. The effects of lipid emulsion, magnesium sulphate and metoprolol in amitriptyline-induced cardiovascular toxicity in rats. Cardiovascular Toxicology. 2018;**18**(6):547-556

[88] Pişkin Ö, Ayoğlu H. Effects of remifentanil pretreatment on bupivacaine cardiotoxicity in rats. Cardiovascular Toxicology. 2018;**18**(1):56-62

[89] Arini PD, Liberczuk S, Mendieta JG, Santa María M, Bertrán GC. Electrocardiogram delineation in a Wistar rat experimental model. Computational and Mathematical Methods in Medicine. 2018;**2018**(3):1-10

[90] Ramezani-Aliakbari F, Badavi M, Dianat M, Mard SA, Ahangarpour A. The effects of trimetazidine on QT-interval prolongation and cardiac hypertrophy in diabetic rats. Arquivos Brasileiros de Cardiologia. 2019;**112**(2):173-178

[91] Sohrabi F, Dianat M, Badavi M, Radan M, Mard SA. Does gallic acid improve cardiac function by attenuation of oxidative stress and inflammation in an elastase-induced lung injury? Iranian Journal of Basic Medical Sciences. 2020;**23**:1130-1138

[92] Boarescu PM, Boarescu I, Bulboacă AE, Bocsan IC, Pop RM, Gheban D, et al. Multi-organ protective effects of curcumin nanoparticles on drug-induced acute myocardial infarction in rats with type 1 diabetes mellitus. Applied Sciences. 2021;**11**:5497

[93] Miranda A, Costa-e-Sousa RH, Werneck-de-Castro JP, Mattos EC, Olivares EL, Ribeiro VP, et al. Time course of echocardiographic and electrocardiographic parameters in myocardial infarct in rats. Anais da Academia Brasileira de Ciências. 2007;**79**:639-648

[94] Ketabchi F, Sepehrinezhad A, Dehghanian A. The relationship between liver dysfunction, electrocardiographic abnormalities and metabolism in rat. Journal of Clinical and Experimental Cardiology. 2018;**9**(10):1000610

[95] Kumar P, Verma S, Singh S, Tiwari S, Khan MY. Effect of Aloe vera (Aloe barbadensis) gel extract on repolarization state of myocardium in albino rat. African Journal of Pharmacy and Pharmacology. 2010;**4**(12):885-889

[96] Barrasa JLM, Rodriguez NS, Rodriguez-Perez JC, Hidalgo AC, Garcia AT, Camarillo JAI, et al. Electrocardiographic changes in rats undergoing thoracic surgery under combined parenteral anesthesia. Lab Animal. 2008;**37**(10):469-174

[97] Sedmera D, Neckar J, Benes J Jr, Pospisilova J, Petrak J, Sedlacek K, et al. Changes in myocardial composition and conduction properties in rat heart failure model induced by chronic volume overload. Frontiers in Physiology. 2016;**7**:367

[98] Yadav RK, Rawat JK, Gautam S, Singh M, Kumar M, Ansari MN, Roy S, Saeedan AS, Kaithwas G. Antidiabetic activity of mefloquine via GLP-1 receptor modulation against STZ-NA-induced diabetes in albino wistar rats. 3 Biotech 2018;8(5), 1-10

[99] Normann SJ, Priest RE, Benditt EP. Electrocardiogram in the normal rat and its alteration with experimental coronary occlusion. Circulation Research. 1961;**9**:282-287

[100] Fraser RS, Harley C, Wiley T. Electrocardiogram in the normal rat.

Journal of Applied Physiology. 1967;**23**(3):401-402

[101] Kela AK, Reddy IP, Thombre DB. E.C.G. findings in normal rats and after administration isoproterenol. Indian Journal of Physiology and Pharmacology. 1980;**24**(2):84-90

[102] Krandycheva VV, Kharin SN, Shmakov DN. P-wave body surface potential distribution in rats. Journal of Electrocardiology. 2006;**39**(1): 88-92

[103] Upaganlawar AA, Balaraman R. Cardioprotective effects of co-administration of pomegranate extract and vitamin E on electrocardiographic, biochemical and apoptotic changes in isoproterenol induced myocardial infarction in rats. Pharmacologia. 2015;**6**(5):178-185

[104] Farag NE, El-Kherbetawy MK, Ismail HM, Abdelrady AM, Toraih EA, Abdelbasset WK, et al. Differential effect of three macrolide antibiotics on cardiac pathology and electrophysiology in a myocardial infarction rat model: Influence on sodium Nav1.5 channel expression. Pharmaceuticals. 2021;**14**:597-603

[105] Taskin E, Kindap EK, Ozdogan K, Aycan MBY, Dursun N. Acute adriamycin-induced cardiotoxicity is exacerbated by angiotension II. Cytotechnology. 2016;**68**(1):33-43

[106] Da Silva VJD, Neto EF, Salgado HC, Junior RF. Chronic converting enzyme inhibition normalizes QT interval in aging rats. Brazilian Journal of Medical and Biological Research. 2002;**35**(9):1025-1031

[107] Walsh EP, Alexander ME, Cecchin F. Chapter 12 - electrocardiography and introduction to electrophysiologic techniques. In: Nadas' Pediatric Cardiology. 2nd ed. Amsterdam: Elsevier Inc; 2006. pp. 145-181

[108] Surawicz B, Knilans TK. Normal electrocardiogram. PR interval. In: Chou's Electrocardiography in Clinical Practice. 6th ed. Amsterdam: Elsevier Inc; 2008

[109] Richig JW, Sleeper MM. PR (PQ), QRS, QT, and other issues. In: Electrocardiography of Laboratory Animals. 2nd ed. London, UK: Academic Press, Elsevier Inc; 2019

[110] Mauer DE, Naegeli B, Straumann E, Bertel O, Frielingsdorf J. Quality of life and exercise capacity in patients with prolonged PQ interval and dual chamber pacemakers: A randomized comparison of permanent ventricular stimulation vs intrinsic AV conduction. EP Europace. 2003;**5**(4):411-417

[111] Portnov A. PQ interval extension. Diseases of the heart and blood vessels (cardiology). PQ interval extension: symptoms, diagnosis, treatment (iliveok.com). 2021.

[112] Lown B, Ganong WF, Levine SA. The syndrome of short P-R interval normal QRS complex and paroxysmal rapid heart action. Circulation. 1952;**5**:693-706

[113] Zada M, Lo Q, Trivedi SJ, Harapoz M, Boyd AC, Devine K, et al. Electrocardiographic characteristics and their correlation with echocardiographic alterations in fabry disease. Journal of Cardiovascular Development and Disease. 2022;**9**(1):11

[114] Shumilova TE, Shereshkov VI, Yanvareva IN, Nozdrachev AD. Peculiarities of myocardial electrogenesis in laboratory rats under conditions of acute nitrite intoxication. Journal of Evolutionary Biochemistry and Phys. 2010;**46**(2):179-188

[115] Sadeghi N, Saadatfard S, Dianat M, Abedi H, Dehghani K. Combination effects of gallic acid and cyclosporine a during ischemia/ reperfusion on rat electrocardiogram parameters and arrhythmia. Physiology and Pharmacology. 2021;**25**:162-170

[116] Damasceno DD, Lima MP, Motta DF, Ferreira AJ, Quintão-Junior JF, Drummond-JuniorLR,etal.Cardiovascular and eletrocardiographic parameters after tonin administration in Wistar rats. Regulatory Peptides. 2013;**181**:30-36

[117] Gohma H, Kuramoto T, Kuwamura M, Okajima R, Tanimoto N, Yamasaki K, et al. WTC deafness Kyoto (dfk): A rat model for extensive investigations of Kcnq1 functions. Physiological Genomics. 2006;**24**:198-206

[118] Mamalyga ML. Heart rate regulation at different levels of convulsive readiness. Bulletin of Experimental Biology and Medicine. 2013;**155**(4):425-428

[119] Adeyemi O, Parker N, Pointon A, Rolf M. A pharmacological characterization of electrocardiogram PR and QRS intervals in conscious telemetered rats. Journal of Pharmacological and Toxicological Methods. 2020;**102**:106679

[120] Hamdy DA, Brocks DR. Experimental hyperlipidemia causes an increase in the electrocardiographic changes associated with amiodarone. Journal of Cardiovascular Pharmacology. 2009;**53**:1-8

[121] Patel JP, Brocks DR. Effect of experimental hyperlipidaemia on the electrocardiographic effects of repeated doses of halofantrine in rats. British Journal of Pharmacology. 2010;**161**(6):1427-1440

[122] Machidal K, Dol K, Kaburaki M, Sugano S. Electrocardiographical findings of WBN/Kob rats. Laboratory Animals. 1990;**24**(3):288-291

[123] Van Buren T, Schiereck P, De Ruiter GJW, Gispen WH, De Wildt DJ. Vagal efferent control of electrical properties of the heart in experimental diabetes. Acta Diabetologica. 1998;**35**(1): 19-25

[124] Lee JK, Nishiyama A, Kambe F, Seo H, Takeuchi S, Kamiya K, et al. Downregulation of voltage-gated K+ channels in rat heart with right ventricular hypertrophy. American Journal of Physiology. Heart and Circulatory Physiology. 1999;**277**(5):H1725-H1731

[125] Barrett TD, Hayes ES, Yong SL, Zolotoy AB, Abraham S, Walker MJA. Ischaemia selectivity confers efficacy for suppression of ischaemia-induced arrhythmias in rats. European Journal of Pharmacology. 2000;**398**(3):365-374

[126] Ghelfi E, Ramos-Rhoden C, Wellenius GA, Lawrence J, Gonzalez-Flecha B. Cardiac oxidative stress and electrophysiological changes in rats exposed to concentrated ambient particles are mediated by TRP-dependent pulmonary reflexes. Toxicological Sciences. 2008;**102**(2):328-336

[127] Regan CP, Stump GL, Wallace AA, Anderson KD, McIntyre CJ, Liverton NJ, et al. In vivo cardiac electrophysiologic and antiarrhythmic effects of an isoquinoline IKur blocker, ISQ-1, in rat, dog, and nonhuman primate. Journal of Cardiovascular Pharmacology. 2007;**49**(4):236-245

[128] Medeiros DM, Shiry LJ, McCune SA. Marginal copper intakes over a protracted period in genetically and nongenetically susceptible heart disease rats disturb electrocardiograms and enhance lipid deposition. Nutrition Research. 2005;**25**(7):663-372

[129] Medei E, Lima-Leopoldo AP, Pereira-Junior PP, Leopoldo AS, Campos DHS, Raimundo JM, et al. Could a high-fat diet rich in unsaturated fatty acids impair the cardiovascular system? The Canadian Journal of Cardiology. 2010;**26**(10):542-548

[130] Milliez P, Deangelis N, Rucker-Martin C, Leenhardt A, Vicaut E, Robidel E, et al. Spironolactone reduces fibrosis of dilated atria during heart failure in rats with myocardial infarction. European Heart Journal. 2005;**26**(20):2193-2199

[131] Haugan K, Lam HR, Knudsen CB, Petersen JS. Atrial fibrillation in rats induced by rapid transesophageal atrial pacing during brief episodes of asphyxia: A new *in vivo* model. Journal of Cardiovascular Pharmacology. 2004;**44**(1):125-135

[132] Nattel S, Shiroshita-Takeshita A, Brundel BJ, Rivard L. Mechanisms of atrial fibrillation: Lessons from animal models. Progress in Cardiovascular Diseases. 2005;**48**:9-28

[133] Gupta C, Omanwar S, Bubber P, Saidullah B. ECG alterations precedes cardiac hypertrophy in rat model of diabetes. Open Access Journal of Toxicology. 2018;**2**(5)

[134] Shamala S, Krishna KL. Cardioprotective activity of fruit extracts of momordica dioca roxb on doxorubicin induced toxicity on rats. Science International. 2013;**1**(12):392-400

[135] Badole SL, Jangam GB, Chaudhari SM, Ghule AE, Zanwar AA. L-glutamine supplementation prevents the development of experimental diabetic cardiomyopathy in streptozotocin-nicotinamide induced diabetic rats. PLoS One. 2014;**9**(3):e92697

[136] Cagiltay E, Pouwels S, Erbas O, Taskiran D, Tas SK, Aslan I. The prophylactic effects of metoprolol, diltiazem, and pilocarpine on hypoglycemia induced prolongation of QT interval. Cureus. 2021;**13**(3):e14058

[137] Jain PG, Mahajan UB, Shinde SD, Surana SJ. Cardioprotective role of FA against isoproterenol induced cardiac toxicity. Molecular Biology Reports. 2018;**45**(5):1357-1365

[138] Sultan F, Kaur R, Mir AH, Maqbool I, Lonare M, Singh D, et al. Rosuvastatin and retinoic acid may act as pleiotropic agents' against β-adrenergic agonist-induced acute myocardial injury through modulation of multiple signalling pathways. Chemico-Biological Interactions. 2020;**318**:108970

[139] Gogelein H, Ruetten H, Albus U, Englert HC, Busch AE. Effects of the cardioselective K-ATP channel blocker HMR 1098 on cardiac function in isolated perfused working rat hearts and in anesthetized rats during ischemia and reperfusion. Naunyn-Schmiedeberg's Archives of Pharmacology. 2001;**364**(1): 33-41

[140] Di Filippo C, D'Amico M, Marfella R, Berrino L, Giugliano D, Rossi F. Endothelin-1 receptor antagonists reduce cardiac electrical instability induced by high glucose in rats. Naunyn-Schmiedeberg's Archives of Pharmacology. 2002;**366**(3):193-197

[141] Panoulas VF, Toms TE, Douglas KMJ, Sandoo A, Metsios GS, Stavropoulos-Kalinoglou A, et al. Prolonged QTc interval predicts all-cause mortality in patients with rheumatoid arthritis: An association driven by high inflammatory burden. Rheumatology. 2014;**53**(1):131-137

[142] Jayasinghe R, Kovoor P. Drugs and the QTc interval. Australian Prescriber. 2002;**25**:63-65

[143] Kmecova J, Klimas J. Heart rate correction of the QT duration in rats. European Journal of Pharmacology. 2010;**641**(2-3):187-192

[144] Rossing P, Breum L, Major-Pedersen A, Sato A, Winding H, Pietersen A, et al. Prolonged QTc interval predicts mortality in patients with type 1 diabetes mellitus. Diabetic Medicine. 2001;**18**(3):199-205

[145] Andršová I, Hnatkova K, Šišáková M, Toman O, Smetana P, Huster KM, et al. Sex and rate change differences in QT/RR hysteresis in healthy subjects. Frontiers in Physiology. 2022;**12**:2473

[146] Van Noord C, Eijgelsjeim M, Stricker BHC. Drug- and non-drug-associated QT interval prolongation. British Journal of Clinical Pharmacology. 2010;**70**(1):16-23

[147] Hayes E, Pugsley MK, Penz WP, Adaikan G, Walker MJ. Relationship between QaT and RR intervals in rats, Guinea pigs, rabbits, and primates. Journal of Pharmacological and Toxicological Methods. 1994;**32**:201-207

[148] Tavakoli S, Hajrasouliha AR, Jabehdar-Maralani P, Ebrahimi F, Solhpour A, Sadeghipour H, et al. Reduced susceptibility to epinephrine-induced arrhythmias in cirrhotic rats: The roles of nitric oxide and endogenous opioid peptides. Journal of Hepatology. 2007;**46**:432-439

[149] Volk T, Nguyen TH, Schultz JH, Faulhaber J, Ehmke H. Regional alterations of repolarizing K^+ currents among the left ventricular free wall of rats with ascending aortic stenosis. The Journal of Physiology. 2001;**530**:443-455

[150] Allon N, Rabinovitz I, Manistersky E, Weissman BA, Grauer E. Acute and long-lasting cardiac changes following a single whole-body exposure to sarin vapor in rats. Toxicological Sciences. 2005;**87**:385-390

[151] Howden R, Hanlon PR, Petranka JG, Kleeberger S, Bucher J, Dunnick J, et al. Ephedrine plus caffeine causes age-dependent cardiovascular responses in Fischer 344 rats. American Journal of Physiology Heart and Circulatory Physiology. 2005;**288**:H2219-H2224

[152] Lamb CM, Hazari MS, Haykal-Coates N, Carll AP, Krantz QT, King C, et al. Divergent electrocardiographic responses to whole and particle-free diesel exhaust inhalation in spontaneously hypertensive rats. Toxicological Sciences. 2012;**125**(2):558-568

[153] Nwokocha C, Palacios J, Simirgiotis MJ, Thomas J, Nwokocha M, Young L, et al. Aqueous extract from leaf of *Artocarpus altilis* provides cardio-protection from isoproterenol induced myocardial damage in rats: Negative chronotropic and inotropic effects. Journal of Ethnopharmacology. 2017;**203**:163-170

[154] Mohammed HS, Hosny EN, Khadrawy YA, Magdy M, Attia YS, Sayed OA, et al. Protective effect of curcumin nanoparticles against cardiotoxicity induced by doxorubicin in rat. Biochimica et Biophysica Acta (BBA) - Molecular Basis of Disease. 1866;**2020**(5):165665

Chapter 3

G Protein-Coupled Receptor Regulation in Cardiovascular Disease: Role of G Protein-Coupled Receptor Kinases

Asma S. Alonazi, Anfal F. Bin Dayel, Tahani K. Alshammari and Nouf M. Alrasheed

Abstract

G protein-coupled receptor kinases (GRKs), the negative regulators of G protein-coupled receptors (GPCRs), have a key role in cardiovascular disease pathophysiology. Alteration in GRKs' expressions and/or kinase activity has been reported in preclinical animal models as well as in patients with cardiovascular diseases. This alteration might be a contributing factor to disease progression by a variety of mechanisms such as non-canonical transduction pathways. The current chapter is aimed to expand our knowledge and understanding of the function of GRKs in cardiovascular diseases, highlight their involvement, and illustrate the possible mechanistic role of GRKs in hypertensive vascular diseases and cardiac myopathy. The current chapter also is endeavoured to identify the potential molecular mechanisms by which GRKs participate in cardiovascular disease progression. Building the basics knowledge about GRKs in cardiovascular diseases will help to assess the potential utilization of GRKs as therapeutic targets and to examine the possible approaches to modulate their protein expression or to inhibit their kinase activity to prevent or attenuate cardiovascular disease progression.

Keywords: GRK2, GRK5, GPCR regulation, cardiovascular diseases, heart failure, hypertension, myocardial infarction

1. Introduction

Cardiovascular diseases consider as one of the major causes of death, contributing to approximately 30% of all deaths globally. In Kingdom of Saudi Arabia, approximately 37% deaths are caused by cardiovascular diseases [1]. Elevated cardiovascular disease-related morbidity and mortality result from a complex pathophysiological process including activation of many signaling transduction pathways, resulting in modification in cardiac/vascular structure, remodeling, and ultimately alteration in the functionality, which contributes to disease progression. Of importance, G protein-coupled receptors (GPCR) play a key fundamental role in various transductions signaling that participate in cardiovascular diseases pathophysiological progression. GPCRs are a superfamily of heptahelical integral membrane proteins, which respond to various stimuli. They are responsible for transduction of a plethora of signaling networks that involve in physiological and pathological actions in cardiovascular system [2, 3]. The activation of α-adrenergic, β-adrenergic, muscarinic, angiotensin II type 1 receptor (AT_1) and endothelin (ET_A) receptors are involved in cardiac contractility, vascular resistance, vascular and cardiac remodeling. In addition, the effect of neurohumoral systems on cardiac contractility and blood vessel tone mainly transmit their signals via corresponding GPCR. These types of receptors and their downstream transduction systems are targets of various drugs used in the treatment of cardiovascular diseases [4].

In case of hypertension, GPCRs play fundamental function in blood vessel diameter, which is mainly controlled by either contraction or relaxation of vascular smooth muscle cells. During contraction, GPCR mediated phosphorylation of contractile proteins [5]. Vasoactive peptides such as noradrenaline, angiotensin II, endothelin 1, and vasopressin activated their corresponding $G_{\alpha q}$ coupled GPCR, results in stimulation of phospholipase C-β, resulting in the formation of inositol-1,4,5-trisphosphate (IP_3) and diacylglycerol (DAG). IP_3 binds to their corresponding receptors which is inositol trisphosphate receptors (IP_3Rs) in the sarcoplasmic reticulum; the intracellular Ca^{2+} store. Activation of IP3Rs resulting in efflux of Ca^{2+} into the cytoplasm. On other hand, DAG activates protein kinase C (PKC), promoting Ca^{2+} influx via enhancing the vascular channels activity such as voltage-dependent L-type Ca^{2+} channels. Elevated intracellular Ca^{2+} concentration $[Ca^{2+}]_i$ binds to calmodulin, creating Ca^{2+}-calmodulin complex which activate MLC kinase (MLCK) followed by phosphorylation of contractile proteins that promote myosin-actin filament interactions and consequently smooth muscle contraction [6–11]. Contraction of vascular smooth muscle cells could persist via regulation of MLC phosphatase (MLCP). Vasoactive peptides also regulate the dephosphorylation of MLC phosphatase via different mechanisms. They utilize the PLC-DAG-PKC pathway, which in turn inhibits phosphatase activity and thus stimulates persistent contraction [12]. In addition, they activate RhoA-Rho kinase pathway, which phosphorylates MLCP and inhibits its activity [13, 14]. On the other hand, a low $[Ca^{2+}]_i$ concentration and increased activity of MLC phosphatase promoting vascular smooth muscle cell relaxation [15]. $G_{\alpha s}$-coupled GPCR mediated blood vessel relaxation. Adrenaline, as vasodilator, acts on corresponding receptors, recruiting $G_{\alpha s}$ to stimulate adenylyl cyclase (AC), leading to the formation of cAMP and then activation of protein kinase A (PKA). PKA plays important role in decreasing $[Ca^{2+}]_i$ concentrations via phosphorylation of MLCK. This results in activation of calcium pumps in the plasma membrane and sarcoplasmic reticulum. Furthermore, promotes cell hyperpolarization by opening K^+ channels promoting relaxation of vascular smooth muscle cells [8, 16, 17].

In case of heart failure, GPCR such as β-adrenergic receptors plays an essential role in cardiac function and in cardiac myocytes contractility. β1-adrenergic receptors couple to $G_{\alpha s}$ that activates adenylate cyclase (AC) and enhances cAMP mediate protein kinase A (PKA) activation which regulates different intracellular, sarcolemma, and myofibrillar substrates, mediating positive inotropic and chronotropic effects [18]. $G_{\beta\gamma}$ subunits also activate downstream effectors that participate in cardiac transduction pathways. Moreover, it has been reported that overexpression of β1-adrenergic receptors triggers early myocytes hypertrophy and interstitial fibrosis followed by marked cardiac dysfunction in mice [18]. In addition, β1-adrenergic receptors activate various downstream signaling participating in cardiac pathophysiological processes such as cardiac hypertrophy, which might progress to heart failure development [19–21]. β2-adrenergic receptors can couple to a dual $G_{\alpha s}/G_{\alpha i}$ subunits, it has been implicated in differential β2-adrenergic receptors mediated signaling such as in myocyte apoptosis [22]. Therefore, β-adrenoceptor blockers are one of the standard pharmacotherapeutics agents used in the treatment of heart failure patients [23]. β-blockers also have been shown to reduce disease progression, mortality, and morbidity in patients with heart failure with reduced ejection fraction (HFrEF) [24]. This effect appears primarily related to the ability of β-adrenoceptor blockers to protect the heart from the harmful effects of receptor over-stimulation [25].

As the effect of neurohumoral systems on cardiovascular system mainly transmits their signals via GPCRs, understanding of the GPCR regulation and their G-protein dependent/independent signaling reveals a novel therapeutic approach that could attenuate cardiovascular-related complications. In current chapter, we provide insight into the potential effect of GPCR negative regulators, focusing particularly on G protein-coupled receptor kinases (GRKs) and their possible effect on cardiovascular diseases.

2. GPCRs regulations

Repeated or prolonged/continues agonist stimulation of GPCRs resulted in loss of receptor response characterized as receptor desensitization. It can be described as physical uncoupling of G proteins from their associate receptors subsequent in diminish their ability to initiate intracellular signaling cascades [26]. As shown in **Figure 1**, receptor desensitization process is initiated by receptor phosphorylation. It can be mediated by G protein-coupled receptor kinases (GRKs), which phosphorylate agonist-bound active receptor inducing homologous type of receptor desensitization [27]. Receptor phosphorylation can be also mediated by second messenger kinases such as PKA and PKC, which can phosphorylate receptors regardless of whether the GPCR is occupied by agonist or not, thus producing heterologous type of receptor desensitization [27–29]. Receptor phosphorylation subsequently increases the affinity of the receptors for β-arrestins proteins binding, consequently prevents further receptors-G protein interactions and therefore termination of G protein-related signaling

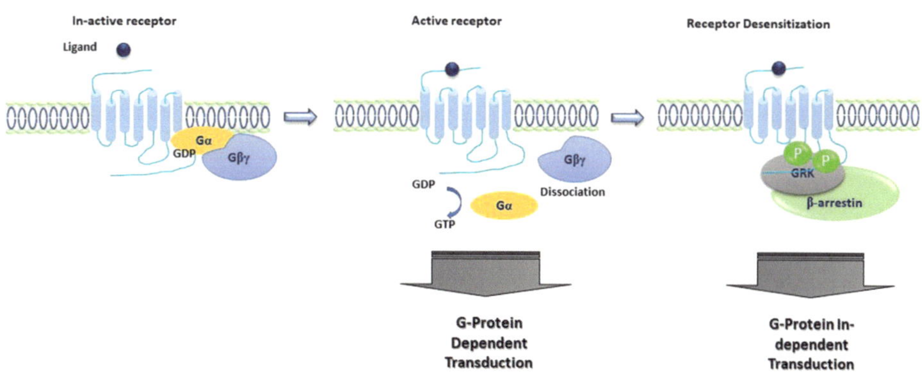

Figure 1.
GPCR desensitization and related signaling transductions pathways. GPCR desensitization by GRKs and β-arrestins process initiated with ligand binding, receptor activation and dissociation of G protein. Consequently, GRKs phosphorylate agonist-occupied GPCRs (activated receptors) at third intracellular loop or C-terminal. Receptor phosphorylation resulting in enhances the affinity for β-arrestin recruitment then binding to the receptors causing termination of G-protein dependent transduction signaling and receptor desensitization. After that, the receptors undergo internalization and initiation of G protein-independent transduction signaling.

[30]. Accordingly, the phosphorylated GPCR/β-arrestin complex is subjected for clathrin-mediated endocytosis, followed by either recycling, or degradation [31–33]. Importantly, β-arrestins function as ligand-regulated adaptor scaffolds that enable the transduction of signaling pathways in non-canonical manner [34].

3. G protein-coupled receptors kinases (GRKs)

G Protein-Coupled Receptors Kinases (GRKs) are family of seven members of serine/threonine kinases [35]. They are allocated into three subcategories: the first category is visual GRKs including GRK1 and GRK7; the second and third categories are non-visual GRKs including β-adrenergic receptor kinase subcategory, containing GRK2 (β-ARK1) and GRK3 (β-ARK2) and; the GRK4 subcategory, containing GRK4, GRK5, and GRK6 [27]. Regarding GRKs tissue distribution, GRK1 and GRK7 are primarily expressed in the retina mediating photoreceptor regulation. GRK2, GRK3, GRK5, and GRK6 are ubiquitously expressed in various tissues; however, GRK4 is limitedly distributed to testes, kidneys, and some areas of the brain. Hence, GRK2, GRK3, GRK5, or GRK6 is the potential regulator for the majority of GPCRs [36–38].

In cardiovascular system, the distribution pattern and expression levels of GRK are crucial factors contributing to their functionality in various cell types. Previous reports show that GRK2, GRK3, and GRK5 are highly expressed in the human heart [39]. GRK isoforms distribution is different among various heart cells. GRK2 and GRK5 are expressed in almost all cardiac cells, while GRK3 distribution is limited to cardiac myocytes [4, 40]. GRK2 is expressed in the vascular endothelium, arterial smooth muscle, and in the myocardium. GRK2 is also expressed in the kidney, especially in the renal proximal tubule [41].

The structure of GRKs comprises of three domains: N-terminal; an amino terminal domain, central serine/threonine protein kinase/catalytic domain, and C-terminal; a carboxyl terminal domain. The N-terminal domain is implicated in receptor recognition. It includes a region of a regulator of G protein signaling (RGS) homology domain (RH) [31, 35]. In GRK2, $G_{\beta\gamma}$ binding site has been mapped in the N-terminal region causing binding of GRK2 to cell membrane [42]. The central domain is a serine/threonine protein that exerts the kinase catalytic function in all GRKs. The C-terminal domain structure is different among GRKs subfamilies. It is implicated in GRK membrane localization. For instant, GRK5 is located at cell membrane level as the C-terminus of GRK5 contains lipid-binding sites that interact with the phospholipid in the cell membrane. On other hand, GRK2 and GRK3 are cytoplasmic proteins that are recruited to the plasma membrane upon agonist binding and receptor activation. Their C-terminal domains contain pleckstrin homology (PH) domain, which comprises binding sites for the cell membrane phospholipid (PIP_2) and $G_{\beta\gamma}$ subunits [26, 35, 43]. As a multi-domain protein, GRK acts as a negative GPCR signaling regulator, terminating G protein-dependent signaling and initiating other G protein-independent signaling pathways [30, 44]. For instance, reported evidence reported that GRK functions are expanded more than receptors phosphorylation. GRKs are able to interact with various cellular proteins mediating non-canonical GPCR signaling [31, 45]. Of importance, GRK expression and activity are changed in many cardiovascular diseases such as in case of hypertension or heart failure. Thus, better understanding of the diseases associated with alteration in GRKs' expression as well as their functional roles in cardiovascular system is fundamental to develop a new therapeutic target.

3.1 GRKs in hypertension

In hypertension, continuous activation of $G_{\alpha q}$ coupled receptors such as ET_A and AT_1 mediate vascular smooth muscle contraction and enhance peripheral vascular resistance [46]. Current evidence shows that GRK2 plays an important function in regulation of prolonged $G_{\alpha q}$-related signaling in vascular smooth muscle cells and consider as the main negative regulator of vasoactive peptide corresponding GPCRs. Moreover, previously published studies reported that GRK2 negatively regulate ET_A and $P2Y_2$ receptors in aortic smooth muscle cells [47, 48]. Reported evidence shows that inhibition of GRK2 kinase activity diminishes the desensitization process of AngII/AT_1 and UTP/$P2Y_2$ induced arterial smooth muscle contractions [49]. Indeed, published studies show that GRK2 expression is augmented in hypertension, in both hypertensive animal models and hypertensive patients [50–55]. Therefore, enhanced GRK2 expression may possibly participate in the pathophysiology of hypertension development. For instant, GRK2 has been reported to attenuate endothelial NO production [56]. Furthermore, GRK2 is reported to mediate the desensitization of β-adrenoceptors, which mediates vasodilation. Thus, enhanced GRK2 expressions may impair vasodilation in hypertension, which possibly contributes to enhancing vascular tone and elevation of blood pressure [53]. Additionally, it has been reported that GRK2 overexpression in vascular smooth muscle cells resulted in a 30% increase in vascular wall thickness [52], suggesting a possible link between GRK2 overexpression in hypertension and hypertension-induced vascular remodeling [57]. Recently published paper show that elevated GRK2 expression hypertension has a potential to promote vascular smooth muscle growth and proliferation possibly via PI3K-Akt signaling, followed by release the GSK3-mediated inhibition of cell cycling progression, therefore aggravate hypertensive induced pathophysiological vascular remodeling [58].

Still, it is not clear if the changes in GRK2 expression are a contributing factor for hypertension development or a consequence of hypertension, which needs further investigation. Moreover, further investigations are required to understand the molecular mechanisms underlying these changes and how the alterations in GRK expression implicated in triggering or progression of hypertension might contribute to the development of novel diagnostic and/or therapeutic strategies to control hypertension or prevent its complications.

3.2 GRKs in heart failure

Myocardial GRK2 and GRK5 have been shown to be involved in the pathophysiology of heart failure [40]. Indeed, several evidences highlight GRK2 as well as GRK5 as the key regulators of β-adrenoceptor [59, 60]. Of importance, recently published paper describes that GRK2 and GRK5 are new therapeutic targets for pathological cardiac hypertrophy and may attenuate morbidity and mortality rates [61]. Dysregulation of β-adrenoceptor is a pathological characteristic of heart failure; in particular, the receptors are considerably downregulated and desensitized as a result of the upregulated levels of GRK2 and GRK5 [16]. Enhanced expression and activity of GRK2 are associated with the loss of β-adrenoceptor functions that induces deleterious effects in the heart functionality contribute to progression of heart failure [62]. Overstimulation of β-adrenoceptor as a subsequent of continuous sympathetic activation, resulting in GRK and β-arrestins induced desensitization and downregulation of β-adrenoceptor [63]. Initially, this process is adaptive response to overcome receptor overactivation. However, prolonged excessive stimulation mediated receptor down-regulation has been reported inducing harmful effect to the heart and consequently heart failure development [63, 64]. Notably, alterations in GRKs have been observed in heart failure [39, 65, 66]. Indeed, several evidences highlight GRK2 as well as GRK5 as the key regulators of β-adrenoceptor [59, 60]. Several reported evidence have shown that GRK2 expression and activity are significantly increased in the failing heart [39, 67, 68]. Enhanced GRK2 expression and altered functionality have been found in heart failure status [39, 65, 66, 69]. Moreover, up-regulation of GRK2 level was detected in end-stage dilated heart failure patient [65]. Even though the mechanism of β-adrenoceptor overstimulation mediated GRK2 upregulation is not clearly understood, published reports show that GRK2 dysfunction plays an essential function in the pathophysiology of heart failure [70] suggesting that alteration in GRK2 function participates in heart failure pathology. Altered GRK2 expression or activity appears to contribute to disease progression through various molecular mechanisms. Therefore, targeting GRK2 expression or inhibition of its activity has been suggested as a therapeutics strategy for treatment of heart failure patients [71, 72].

Reported evidence shows that overexpression of a peptide inhibitor of GRK2; carboxy terminal domain (βARKct) which lacks to membrane translocation function inhibits GRK2 activity and prevents desensitization of the receptors resulting in restoring of β-adrenoceptor function and enhanced cardiac contractility in experimental animals of heart failure [73–75]. Moreover, $G_{\beta\gamma}$-GRK2 inhibition reduces pathological effect of myofibroblast activation. Thus, $G_{\beta\gamma}$-GRK2 inhibition might be a potential therapeutic strategy to attenuate pathological myofibroblast activation, interstitial fibrosis, cardiac remodeling, and progression of heart failure [76].

It has been reported that cardiac dysfunction could be attenuated by inhibition of GRK2 activity [62]. Interestingly, it has been reported that paroxetine, selective serotonin re-uptake inhibitor (SSRI) approved by FDA for treatment of depression, significantly inhibited GRK2 kinase activity [49, 77, 78]. Published studies showed capability paroxetine as GRK2 inhibitor in reversing cardiac remodeling in experimental models of acute myocardial infarction [79, 80]. Therefore, paroxetine may perhaps be used as a therapeutic approach for targeting GRK2 catalytic activity and potentially provide a protective role against cardiac hypertrophy development via its function as GRK2 inhibitor.

GRK5 another GRK member that mediates phosphorylation and desensitization of β-adrenoceptor is well known to regulate heart functions [72]. Several studies suggest that GRK5 plays a crucial role in various cardiovascular diseases. For instance, previous studies show that GRK5 overexpressing mice developed cardiac hypertrophy, which rapidly progressed to heart failure [81]. Moreover, GRK5 knockout mice showed attenuated hypertrophic responses [82]. Furthermore, GRK5 overexpressing mice showed an alteration in myocardial performance including attenuation of contractility, cardiac output, stroke work, and stroke volume [83]. Of note, GRK5 levels were shown to be markedly elevated in heart failure patients and patients with left ventricular volume overload disorders and dilated cardiomyopathic hearts [84–86].

GRK5 overexpressed transgenic mice exhibited enhanced susceptibility to pressure overload-induced cardiac hypertrophy and cardiac dysfunction [87]. Furthermore, cardiac-specific GRK5 transgenic mice demonstrated reduced cardiac function and increased adverse cardiac remodeling in a myocardial infarction-induced heart failure mice model [64]. On other hand, heart hypertrophic responses were attenuated in GRK5 knockout mice [88], these studies demonstrated the possible functions of GRK5 in pathological cardiac remodeling development. Interestingly, several lines of evidence show that GRK5 can translocate to the nucleus, exerting its non-canonical functions. For instance, it was shown that GRK5 in the cardiomyocyte nuclei acts as a class II histone deacetylase (HDAC) kinase, phosphorylating HDAC5 and leading to de-repression of myocyte enhancer factor 2 (MEF2)-mediated hypertrophic gene transcription [81, 89]. In addition, it was demonstrated that GRK5 interacts with hypertrophic transcription factors like nuclear factor of activated T cell (NFAT) and nuclear factor κ-B (NF-κB) [81, 87, 90, 91]. These studies indicate that GRK5 has a major role in the pathogenesis of the cardiovascular disorders and GRK5 might be a therapeutic target for heart failure. Recently, it has been demonstrated that KR-39038, a novel small molecule inhibitor of GRK5, significantly inhibited cellular hypertrophy and HDAC5 phosphorylation in neonatal rat ventricular myocytes. This inhibitor was able to minimize the left ventricular weight, improve cardiac function and ameliorate myocardial remodeling in animal model of heart failure [92]. Another important agent proposed as a GRK5 inhibitor is an anti-inflammatory and anti-allergic immunomodulator, named amlexanox [93]. This agent was able to inhibit GRK5 induced MEF2 activation in neonatal rat ventricular myocytes and inhibit GRK5 mediated HDAC5 phosphorylation in cellular model of cardiac hypertrophy [93, 94].

3.3 GRKs in myocardial infarction

It has been reported that GRK2 expressions upregulated in peripheral blood lymphocytes in patients with acute ST-segment elevation myocardial infarction. Enhanced lymphocyte GRK2 expressions are associated with worse cardiac functionality. These studies indicate that GRK2 could be predictive of myocardial remodeling after myocardial infarction [95, 96]. Enhanced GRK2 levels and activity are deleterious to post-ischemic myocardium in acute ischemia/reperfusion (I/R) injury animal model [97]. It has been reported that GRK2 peptide inhibitor; βARKct provides cardioprotective effect, which modulate GRK2-mediated PI3K-Akt-NOS signaling pathway in the ischemic heart which validates GRK2-related effect on survival and apoptotic signaling in the ischemic heart [97]. βARKct expression mediated GRK2 inhibition modulate Akt downstream pro-survival signaling such as reduced Caspase-3 activity, increased eNOS activation and NO production and then reduced apoptosis and cell death [97]. Furthermore, decreasing GRK2 expression in cardiomyocytes attenuate myocyte apoptosis possibly via Akt/Bcl-2 mediated mitochondrial protection and limits I/R- provoked injury and improves post-ischemia recovery in the heart [98]. Additionally, it has been reported that fibroblast specific GRK2 knockout has a protective effect after myocardial I/R injury in mice. GRK2 fibroblast knockout mice decreased the infarct size, increased ejection fraction, preserved cardiac function, and also reduced tumor necrosis factor-α expression, fibrotic gene expression, and fibrosis development [99].

4. Conclusions

Cardiovascular diseases are a leading cause of death worldwide. The pathophysiological mechanisms are regulated by a GPCR mediated complex network of transduction pathways. The functions of GRKs, negative regulators of GPCR, are not limited to receptors desensitization. It is expanded further to activations of many transductions in non-classical manner. As the expression and kinase activity of GRK2 and GRK5 are altered in cardiovascular diseases, Therefore, better knowledge of the transduction events which mediated by up-regulated GRK2 and/or GRK5 in terms of the expression, activity, and localization would help to develop a novel strategy for targeting their expressions or inhibiting activity. This will participate in building a knowledge-based platform identifying a new therapeutic target to prevent the progression of cardiovascular diseases. Many different approaches could be applied, including small molecule inhibitors, gene therapy, and the use of advanced drug delivery systems to potentially prevent the progression of cardiovascular disease. Overall, GRKs play an important role in cardiovascular diseases progression. Pharmacological intervention of GRK5 as well as GRK2 would provide a novel possible future target for cardiovascular disease progression prevention.

Acknowledgements

The authors extend their appreciation to the Deputyship for Research & Innovation, Ministry of Education in Saudi Arabia for funding this research work through project no. (IFKSUDR_H150).

Conflict of interest

The authors declare no conflict of interest.

Author details

Asma S. Alonazi*, Anfal F. Bin Dayel, Tahani K. Alshammari and Nouf M. Alrasheed
Department of Pharmacology and Toxicology, College of Pharmacy, King Saud University, Riyadh, Saudi Arabia

*Address all correspondence to: aaloneazi@ksu.edu.sa

References

[1] Organization WH. Noncommunicable Diseases Country Profiles 2018. 2018

[2] Fredriksson R, Lagerström MC, Lundin L-G, Schiöth HB. The G-protein-coupled receptors in the human genome form five main families. Phylogenetic analysis, paralogon groups, and fingerprints. Molecular Pharmacology. 2003;**63**(6):1256-1272

[3] Gether U. Uncovering molecular mechanisms involved in activation of G protein-coupled receptors. Endocrine Reviews. 2000;**21**(1):90-113

[4] Penela P, Murga C, Ribas C, Tutor AS, Peregrín S, Mayor F Jr. Mechanisms of regulation of G protein-coupled receptor kinases (GRKs) and cardiovascular disease. Cardiovascular Research. 2006;**69**(1):46-56

[5] Touyz RM, Alves-Lopes R, Rios FJ, Camargo LL, Anagnostopoulou A, Arner A, et al. Vascular smooth muscle contraction in hypertension. Cardiovascular Research. 2018;**114**(4):529-539

[6] Lymperopoulos A, Bathgate A. Arrestins in the cardiovascular system. Progress in Molecular Biology and Translational Science. 2013;**118**:297-334

[7] Hill-Eubanks DC, Werner ME, Heppner TJ, Nelson MT. Calcium signaling in smooth muscle. Cold Spring Harbor Perspectives in Biology. 2011;**3**(9):a004549

[8] Harris DM, Cohn HI, Pesant S, Eckhart AD. GPCR signalling in hypertension: Role of GRKs. Clinical Science (Lond). 2008;**115**(3):79-89

[9] Lozinskaya I, Matsuda K, Cox RH. Augmented contributions of voltage-Gated Ca2 channels to contractile responses in spontaneously hypertensive rat mesenteric arteries*. American Journal of Hypertension. 1997;**10**(11):1231-1239

[10] Allen BG, Walsh MP. The biochemical basis of the regulation of smooth-muscle contraction. Trends in Biochemical Sciences. 1994;**19**(9):362-368

[11] Ghosh D, Syed AU, Prada MP, Nystoriak MA, Santana LF, Nieves-Cintron M, et al. Calcium channels in vascular smooth muscle. Advances in Pharmacology. 2017;**78**:49-87

[12] Ringvold HC, Khalil RA. Protein kinase C as regulator of vascular smooth muscle function and potential target in vascular disorders. Advances in Pharmacology. 2017;**78**:203-301

[13] Loirand G, Pacaud P. The role of Rho protein signaling in hypertension. Nature Reviews Cardiology. 2010;**7**(11):637-647

[14] Puetz S, Lubomirov LT, Pfitzer G. Regulation of smooth muscle contraction by small GTPases. Physiology (Bethesda). 2009;**24**:342-356

[15] Webb RC. Smooth muscle contraction and relaxation. Advances in Physiology Education. 2003;**27**(1-4):201-206

[16] Fukunaga K, Kume H, Oguma T, Shigemori W, Tohda Y, Ogawa E, et al. Involvement of Ca(2+) signaling in the synergistic effects between muscarinic receptor antagonists and β2-adrenoceptor agonists in airway smooth muscle. International Journal of Molecular Sciences. 2016;**17**(9):1590

[17] Consigny PM. Vascular smooth muscle contraction and relaxation: Pathways and chemical modulation. Journal of Vascular and Interventional Radiology. 1991;**2**(3):309-317

[18] Engelhardt S, Hein L, Wiesmann F, Lohse MJ. Progressive hypertrophy and heart failure in beta1-adrenergic receptor transgenic mice. Proceedings of the National Academy of Sciences of the United States of America. 1999;**96**(12):7059-7064

[19] Xiang Y, Kobilka BK. Myocyte adrenoceptor signaling pathways. Science. 2003;**300**(5625):1530-1532

[20] Bernstein D, Fajardo G, Zhao M, Urashima T, Powers J, Berry G, et al. Differential cardioprotective/cardiotoxic effects mediated by β-adrenergic receptor subtypes. American Journal of Physiology-Heart and Circulatory Physiology. 2005;**289**(6):H2441-H24H9

[21] Khamssi M, Brodde O-E. The role of cardiac beta1-and beta2-adrenoceptor stimulation in heart failure. Journal of Cardiovascular Pharmacology. 1990;**16**:S133-S137

[22] Communal C, Singh K, Sawyer DB, Colucci WS. Opposing effects of beta(1)-and beta(2)-adrenergic receptors on cardiac myocyte apoptosis: Role of a pertussis toxin-sensitive G protein. Circulation. 1999;**100**(22):2210-2

[23] Chavey WE. The importance of beta blockers in the treatment of heart failure. American Family Physician. 2000;**62**(11):2453-2462

[24] Ponikowski P, Voors AA, Anker SD, Bueno H, Cleland JG, Coats AJ, et al. 2016 ESC Guidelines for the diagnosis and treatment of acute and chronic heart failure: The Task Force for the diagnosis and treatment of acute and chronic heart failure of the European Society of Cardiology (ESC). Developed with the special contribution of the Heart Failure Association (HFA) of the ESC. European Journal of Heart Failure. 2016;**18**(8):891-975

[25] Bristow MR. beta-adrenergic receptor blockade in chronic heart failure. Circulation. 2000;**101**(5):558-569

[26] Penela P, Ribas C, Mayor F. Mechanisms of regulation of the expression and function of G protein-coupled receptor kinases. Cellular Signalling. 2003;**15**(11):973-981

[27] Willets JM, Challiss RA, Nahorski SR. Non-visual GRKs: Are we seeing the whole picture? Trends in Pharmacological Sciences. 2003;**24**(12):626-633

[28] Hausdorff WP, Caron MG, Lefkowitz RJ. Turning off the signal: Desensitization of beta-adrenergic receptor function. FASEB Journal. 1990;**4**(11):2881-2889

[29] Stadel JM, Nambi P, Shorr RG, Sawyer DF, Caron MG, Lefkowitz RJ. Catecholamine-induced desensitization of turkey erythrocyte adenylate cyclase is associated with phosphorylation of the beta-adrenergic receptor. Proceedings of the National Academy of Sciences. 1983;**80**(11):3173-3177

[30] Brinks HL, Eckhart AD. Regulation of GPCR signaling in hypertension. Biochimica et Biophysica Acta. 2010;**1802**(12):1268-1275

[31] Penela P, Murga C, Ribas C, Lafarga V, Mayor F Jr. The complex G protein-coupled receptor kinase 2 (GRK2) interactome unveils new physiopathological targets. British Journal of Pharmacology. 2010;**160**(4):821-832

[32] Kelly E, Bailey CP, Henderson G. Agonist-selective mechanisms of GPCR desensitization. British Journal of Pharmacology. 2008;**153**(Suppl. 1): S379-SS88

[33] Oakley RH, Laporte SA, Holt JA, Caron MG, Barak LS. Differential affinities of visual arrestin, βArrestin1, and βArrestin2 for G protein-coupled receptors delineate two major classes of receptors. Journal of Biological Chemistry. 2000;**275**(22):17201-17210

[34] Luttrell LM, Miller WE. Arrestins as regulators of kinases and phosphatases. Progress in Molecular Biology and Translational Science. 2013;**118**:115-147

[35] Homan KT, Tesmer JJG. Structural insights into G protein-coupled receptor kinase function. Current Opinion in Cell Biology. 2014;**27**:25-31

[36] Premont RT, Gainetdinov RR. Physiological roles of G protein-coupled receptor kinases and arrestins. Annual Review of Physiology. 2007;**69**:511-534

[37] Pugh EN, Lamb TD. Chapter 5 Phototransduction in vertebrate rods and cones: Molecular mechanisms of amplification, recovery and light adaptation. In: Stavenga DG, DeGrip WJ, Pugh EN, editors. Handbook of Biological Physics. vol. 3. North-Holland; 2000. pp. 183-255. DOI: org/10.1016/S1383-8121(00)80008-1

[38] Premont RT, Macrae AD, Stoffel RH, Chung N, Pitcher JA, Ambrose C, et al. Characterization of the G protein-coupled receptor kinase GRK4. Identification of four splice variants. The Journal of Biological Chemistry. 1996;**271**(11):6403-6410

[39] Ungerer M, Böhm M, Elce J, Erdmann E, Lohse M. Altered expression of beta-adrenergic receptor kinase and beta 1-adrenergic receptors in the failing human heart. Circulation. 1993;**87**(2):454-463

[40] Vinge LE, Øie E, Andersson Y, Grøgaard HK, Andersen G, Attramadal H. Myocardial distribution and regulation of GRK and beta-arrestin isoforms in congestive heart failure in rats. The American Journal of Physiology-Heart and Circulatory Physiology. 2001;**281**(6):H2490-H2499

[41] Yang J, Villar VAM, Armando I, Jose PA, Zeng C. G protein-coupled receptor kinases: Crucial regulators of blood pressure. Journal of the American Heart Association. 2016;**5**(7):e003519

[42] Eichmann T, Lorenz K, Hoffmann M, Brockmann J, Krasel C, Lohse MJ, et al. The amino-terminal domain of G-protein-coupled receptor kinase 2 is a regulatory Gbeta gamma binding site. The Journal of Biological Chemistry. 2003;**278**(10):8052-8057

[43] Ribas C, Penela P, Murga C, Salcedo A, Garcia-Hoz C, Jurado-Pueyo M, et al. The G protein-coupled receptor kinase (GRK) interactome: Role of GRKs in GPCR regulation and signaling. Biochimica et Biophysica Acta. 2007;**1768**(4):913-922

[44] Reiter E, Lefkowitz RJ. GRKs and β-arrestins: Roles in receptor silencing, trafficking and signaling. Trends in Endocrinology & Metabolism. 2006;**17**(4):159-165

[45] Shenoy SK, Lefkowitz RJ. β-arrestin-mediated receptor trafficking and signal transduction. Trends in Pharmacological Sciences. 2011;**32**(9):521-533

[46] Harris DM, Cohn HI, Pesant S, Zhou RH, Eckhart AD. Vascular smooth muscle G(q) signaling is involved in high blood pressure in both induced

renal and genetic vascular smooth muscle-derived models of hypertension. The American Journal of Physiology-Heart and Circulatory Physiology. 2007;**293**(5):H3072-H3079

[47] Morris GE, Nelson CP, Everitt D, Brighton PJ, Standen NB, Challiss RA, et al. G protein-coupled receptor kinase 2 and arrestin2 regulate arterial smooth muscle P2Y-purinoceptor signalling. Cardiovascular Research. 2011;**89**(1):193-203

[48] Morris GE, Nelson CP, Standen NB, Challiss RA, Willets JM. Endothelin signalling in arterial smooth muscle is tightly regulated by G protein-coupled receptor kinase 2. Cardiovascular Research. 2010;**85**(3):424-433

[49] Rainbow RD, Brennan S, Jackson R, Beech AJ, Bengreed A, Waldschmidt HV, et al. Small-molecule G Protein-coupled receptor kinase inhibitors attenuate G protein-coupled Receptor Kinase 2-mediated desensitization of vasoconstrictor-induced arterial contractions. Molecular Pharmacology. 2018;**94**(3):1079-1091

[50] Willets JM, Nash CA, Rainbow RD, Nelson CP, Challiss RA. Defining the roles of arrestin2 and arrestin3 in vasoconstrictor receptor desensitization in hypertension. The American Journal of Physiology-Cell Physiology. 2015;**309**(3):C179-C189

[51] Cohn HI, Harris DM, Pesant S, Pfeiffer M, Zhou RH, Koch WJ, et al. Inhibition of vascular smooth muscle G protein-coupled receptor kinase 2 enhances alpha1D-adrenergic receptor constriction. The American Journal of Physiology-Cell Physiology. 2008;**295**(4):H1695-H1704

[52] Eckhart AD, Ozaki T, Tevaearai H, Rockman HA, Koch WJ. Vascular-targeted overexpression of G protein-coupled receptor kinase-2 in transgenic mice attenuates beta-adrenergic receptor signaling and increases resting blood pressure. Molecular Pharmacology. 2002;**61**(4):749-758

[53] Gros R, Chorazyczewski J, Meek MD, Benovic JL, Ferguson SS, Feldman RD. G-protein-coupled receptor kinase activity in hypertension: Increased vascular and lymphocyte G-protein receptor kinase-2 protein expression. Hypertension. 2000;**35**(1 Pt 1):38-42

[54] Cohn HI, Xi Y, Pesant S, Harris DM, Hyslop T, Falkner B, et al. G protein-coupled receptor kinase 2 expression and activity are associated with blood pressure in black Americans. Hypertension. 2009;**54**(1):71-76

[55] Gros Robert BJL, Tan Christopher M, Feldman Ross D. G-protein–coupled receptor kinase activity is increased in hypertension. Journal of Clinical Investigation. 1997;**99**:2087-2093

[56] Feldman RD. Deactivation of vasodilator responses by GRK2 overexpression: A mechanism or the mechanism for hypertension? Molecular Pharmacology. 2002;**61**(4):707-709

[57] Ramos-Ruiz R, Penela P, Penn RB, Mayor F Jr. Analysis of the human G protein-coupled receptor kinase 2 (GRK2) gene promoter: Regulation by signal transduction systems in aortic smooth muscle cells. Circulation. 2000;**101**(17):2083-2089

[58] Alonazi ASA, Willets JM. G protein-coupled receptor kinase 2 is essential to enable vasoconstrictor-mediated arterial smooth muscle proliferation. Cell Signal. 2021;**88**:110152

[59] Hu LA, Chen W, Premont RT, Cong M, Lefkowitz RJ. G protein-coupled

receptor kinase 5 regulates β1-adrenergic receptor association with PSD-95. Journal of Biological Chemistry. 2002;**277**(2):1607-1613

[60] Huang ZM, Gao E, Chuprun JK, Koch WJ. GRK2 in the heart: A GPCR kinase and beyond. Antioxidants & Redox Signaling. 2014;**21**(14):2032-2043

[61] Lieu M, Koch WJ. GRK2 and GRK5 as therapeutic targets and their role in maladaptive and pathological cardiac hypertrophy. Expert Opinion on Therapeutic Targets. 2019;**23**(3):201-214

[62] Petrofski JA, Koch WJ. The beta-adrenergic receptor kinase in heart failure. Journal of Molecular and Cellular Cardiology. 2003;**35**(10):1167-1174

[63] Lymperopoulos A, Rengo G, Koch WJ. Adrenergic nervous system in heart failure: Pathophysiology and therapy. Circulation Research. 2013;**113**(6):739-753

[64] de Lucia C, Eguchi A, Koch WJ. New insights in cardiac β-adrenergic signaling during heart failure and aging. Frontiers in Pharmacology. 2018;**9**:904

[65] Ungerer M, Parruti G, Böhm M, Puzicha M, DeBlasi A, Erdmann E, et al. Expression of beta-arrestins and beta-adrenergic receptor kinases in the failing human heart. Circulation Research. 1994;**74**(2):206-213

[66] Leineweber K, Rohe P, Beilfuß A, Wolf C, Sporkmann H, Bruck H, et al. G-protein-coupled receptor kinase activity in human heart failure: Effects of β-adrenoceptor blockade. Cardiovascular Research. 2005;**66**(3):512-519

[67] Harris CA, Chuang TT, Scorer CA. Expression of GRK2 is increased in the left ventricles of cardiomyopathic hamsters. Basic Research in Cardiology. 2001;**96**(4):364-368

[68] Sato PY, Chuprun JK, Schwartz M, Koch WJ. The evolving impact of G protein-coupled receptor kinases in cardiac health and disease. Physiological Reviews. 2015;**95**(2):377-404

[69] Bohm M, Lohse MJ. Quantification of beta-adrenoceptors and beta-adrenoceptor kinase on protein and mRNA levels in heart failure. European Heart Journal. 1994;**15**(Suppl. D):30-34

[70] Mangmool S, Parichatikanond W, Kurose H. Therapeutic targets for treatment of heart failure: Focus on GRKs and β-Arrestins affecting βAR signaling. Frontiers in Pharmacology. 2018;**9**:1336

[71] Williams ML, Hata JA, Schroder J, Rampersaud E, Petrofski J, Jakoi A, et al. Targeted beta-adrenergic receptor kinase (betaARK1) inhibition by gene transfer in failing human hearts. Circulation. 2004;**109**(13):1590-1593

[72] Cannavo A, Liccardo D, Koch WJ. Targeting cardiac β-adrenergic signaling via GRK2 inhibition for heart failure therapy. Frontiers in Physiology. 2013;**4**:264

[73] Koch WJ, Rockman HA, Samama P, Hamilton RA, Bond RA, Milano CA, et al. Cardiac function in mice overexpressing the beta-adrenergic receptor kinase or a beta ARK inhibitor. Science. 1995;**268**(5215):1350-1353

[74] Tachibana H, Naga Prasad SV, Lefkowitz RJ, Koch WJ, Rockman HA. Level of beta-adrenergic receptor kinase 1 inhibition determines degree of cardiac dysfunction after chronic pressure overload-induced heart failure. Circulation. 2005;**111**(5):591-597

[75] Rengo G, Lymperopoulos A, Leosco D, Koch WJ. GRK2 as a novel gene therapy target in heart failure. Journal of Molecular and Cellular Cardiology. 2011;**50**(5):785-792

[76] Travers JG, Kamal FA, Valiente-AlandiI,NiemanML,SargentMA, Lorenz JN, et al. Pharmacological and activated fibroblast targeting of Gβγ-GRK2 after myocardial ischemia attenuates heart failure progression. Journal of the American College of Cardiology. 2017;**70**(8):958-971

[77] Sugarman MA, Loree AM, Baltes BB, Grekin ER, Kirsch I. The efficacy of paroxetine and placebo in treating anxiety and depression: A meta-analysis of change on the Hamilton Rating Scales. PLoS One. 2014;**9**(8):e106337-e

[78] Thal DM, Yeow RY, Schoenau C, Huber J, Tesmer JJ. Molecular mechanism of selectivity among G protein-coupled receptor kinase 2 inhibitors. Molecular Pharmacology. 2011;**80**(2):294-303

[79] Tian X, Wang Q, Guo R, Xu L, Chen QM, Hou Y. Effects of paroxetine-mediated inhibition of GRK2 expression on depression and cardiovascular function in patients with myocardial infarction. Neuropsychiatric Disease and Treatment. 2016;**12**:2333-2341

[80] Schumacher SM, Gao E, Zhu W, Chen X, Chuprun JK, Feldman AM, et al. Paroxetine-mediated GRK2 inhibition reverses cardiac dysfunction and remodeling after myocardial infarction. Science Translational Medicine. 2015;**7**(277):277ra31

[81] Martini JS, Raake P, Vinge LE, DeGeorge BR, Chuprun JK, Harris DM, et al. Uncovering G protein-coupled receptor kinase-5 as a histone deacetylase kinase in the nucleus of cardiomyocytes. Proceedings of the National Academy of Sciences. 2008;**105**(34):12457-12462

[82] Gold JI, Gao E, Shang X, Premont RT, Koch WJ. Determining the absolute requirement of g protein–coupled receptor kinase 5 for pathological cardiac hypertrophy. Circulation Research. 2012;**111**(8):1048-1053

[83] Chen EP, Bittner HB, Akhter SA, Koch WJ, Davis RD. Myocardial function in hearts with transgenic overexpression of the G protein-coupled receptor kinase 5. The Annals of Thoracic Surgery. 2001;**71**(4):1320-1324

[84] Dzimiri N, Muiya P, Andres E, Al-Halees Z. Differential functional expression of human myocardial G protein receptor kinases in left ventricular cardiac diseases. European Journal of Pharmacology. 2004;**489**(3):167-177

[85] Yi XP, Zhou J, Baker J, Wang X, Gerdes AM, Li F. Myocardial expression and redistribution of GRKs in hypertensive hypertrophy and failure. The Anatomical Record Part A: Discoveries in Molecular, Cellular, and Evolutionary Biology: An Official Publication of the American Association of Anatomists. 2005;**282**(1):13-23

[86] Agüero J, Almenar L, D'Ocon P, Oliver E, Montó F, Moro J, et al. Correlation between beta-adrenoceptors and G-protein-coupled receptor kinases in pretransplantation heart failure. In: Transplantation Proceedings. Elsevier; 2008. The Journal of Heart and Lung Transplantation. DOI:10.1016/j.healun.2009.06.003. Epub 2009 Sep 26.

[87] Hullmann JE, Grisanti LA, Makarewich CA, Gao E, Gold JI, Chuprun JK, et al. GRK5-mediated exacerbation of pathological cardiac hypertrophy involves facilitation of

nuclear NFAT activity. Circulation Research. 2014;**115**(12):976-985

[88] Gold JI, Gao E, Shang X, Premont RT, Koch WJ. Determining the absolute requirement of G protein-coupled receptor kinase 5 for pathological cardiac hypertrophy: Short communication. Circulation Research. 2012;**111**(8):1048-1053

[89] Traynham CJ, Cannavo A, Zhou Y, Vouga AG, Woodall BP, Hullmann J, et al. Differential role of G protein-coupled receptor kinase 5 in physiological versus pathological cardiac hypertrophy. Circulation Research. 2015;**117**(12):1001-1012

[90] Islam KN, Bae J-W, Gao E, Koch WJ. Regulation of nuclear factor κB (NF-κB) in the nucleus of cardiomyocytes by G protein-coupled receptor kinase 5 (GRK5). Journal of Biological Chemistry. 2013;**288**(50):35683-35689

[91] Gold JI, Martini JS, Hullmann J, Gao E, Chuprun JK, Lee L, et al. Nuclear translocation of cardiac G protein-coupled receptor kinase 5 downstream of select Gq-activating hypertrophic ligands is a calmodulin-dependent process. PloS One. 2013;**8**(3):e57324

[92] Lee JH, Seo HW, Ryu JY, Lim CJ, Yi KY, Oh K-S, et al. KR-39038, a novel GRK5 inhibitor, attenuates cardiac hypertrophy and improves cardiac function in heart failure. Biomolecules & Therapeutics. 2020;**28**(5):482

[93] Homan KT, Wu E, Cannavo A, Koch WJ, Tesmer JJ. Identification and characterization of amlexanox as a G protein-coupled receptor kinase 5 inhibitor. Molecules. 2014;**19**(10):16937-16949

[94] Park CH, Lee JH, Lee MY, Lee JH, Lee BH, Oh K-S. A novel role of G protein-coupled receptor kinase 5 in urotensin II-stimulated cellular hypertrophy in H9c2 UT cells. Molecular and Cellular Biochemistry. 2016;**422**(1):151-160

[95] Gao WQ, Han CG, Lu XC, Liu YX, Hui HP, Wang H. GRK 2 level in peripheral blood lymphocytes of elderly patients with acute myocardial infarction. Journal of Geriatric Cardiology. 2013;**10**(3):281-285

[96] Santulli G, Campanile A, Spinelli L, Assante di Panzillo E, Ciccarelli M, Trimarco B, et al. G protein-coupled receptor kinase 2 in patients with acute myocardial infarction. The American Journal of Cardiology. 2011;**107**(8):1125-1130

[97] Brinks H, Das A, Koch WJ. A role for GRK2 in myocardial ischemic injury: Indicators of a potential future therapy and diagnostic. Future Cardiology. 2011;**7**(4):547-556

[98] Fan Q, Chen M, Zuo L, Shang X, Huang MZ, Ciccarelli M, et al. Myocardial ablation of G protein-coupled receptor kinase 2 (GRK2) decreases ischemia/reperfusion injury through an anti-intrinsic apoptotic pathway. PLoS One. 2013;**8**(6):e66234

[99] Woodall MC, Woodall BP, Gao E, Yuan A, Koch WJ. Cardiac fibroblast GRK2 deletion enhances contractility and remodeling following ischemia/reperfusion injury. Circulation Research. 2016;**119**(10):1116-1127

Chapter 4

Gut Microbial Metabolite Trimethylamine-N-Oxide and Its Role in Cardiovascular Diseases

Shubham Barik, Aritra Mukherjee, Angelina Job Kolady, Boda Karunakar and Tony Grace

Abstract

Atherosclerosis (AS) is the common pathological underpinning of numerous cardiovascular illnesses (CVDs), and it is the leading cause of death worldwide. In recent years, researchers have begun to recognize the importance of gut microbiota in AS. Gut microbial dysbiosis has been reported to be connected with various CVDs. Moreover, dietary choline, betaine, and L-carnitine produce trimethylamine N-oxide (TMAO), a key gut microbe-dependent metabolite. Multiple studies have found a link between plasma TMAO levels and the likelihood of developing AS. The mechanism underlying this link, however, is still unknown. In this chapter, we discuss the TMAO-mediated mechanisms of atherosclerotic CVD from the perspectives of dietary patterns and gut microbial metabolism. Finally, we explain how TMAO has emerged as a novel therapeutic target for CVDs, as well as many treatment options for lowering TMAO levels that are currently being investigated, such as medications, dietary changes, probiotics, and so on.

Keywords: cardiovascular disease, gut microbiota, trimethylamine (TMA), trimethylamine-N-oxide (TMAO), diet, metabolism

1. Introduction

Cardiovascular disease or *CVD* is a term for disorders affecting the heart or blood vessels. Except in Africa, cardiovascular illnesses are the main cause of mortality globally, resulting in 17.9 million deaths (32.1%) in 2015, an increase from 12.3 million (25.8%) in 1990 [1]. CVD deaths are more widespread and have been growing in most developing countries, whereas rates in most developed countries have declined since the 1970s [2]. Coronary artery disease and stroke account for 80% of CVD deaths in males and 75% in females. The majority of cardiovascular disease affects older people. In the United States, 11% of adults between the ages of 20 y and 40 y have CVD, 37% between the ages of 40 y and 60 y, 71% between the ages of 60 y and 80 y, and 85% above the age of 80 y have CVD. In developed countries, the average age of death from coronary artery disease is over 80 y, while it is roughly 68 y in the developing world [2]. Diagnosis of diseases typically occurs seven to ten years earlier in men than in women.

The underlying processes differ according to the illness. Dietary risk factors are responsible for 53% of CVD fatalities [3]. Atherosclerosis is a common factor in coronary artery disease, stroke, and peripheral artery disease [4]. High blood pressure, smoking, diabetes mellitus, lack of exercise, obesity, high blood cholesterol, poor food, excessive alcohol consumption, and poor sleep, among other factors, may contribute to this [5]. High blood pressure contributes around 13% of CVD fatalities, whereas tobacco accounts for 9%, diabetes accounts for 6%, lack of exercise factors for 6%, and obesity accounts for 5%. Untreated strep throat can potentially cause rheumatic heart disease. Up to 90% of cardiovascular disease is thought to be preventable [6]. Lowering risk factors through good food, exercise, avoiding cigarette smoke, and limiting alcohol use are all part of CVD prevention. It also treats risk factors such as high blood pressure, lipids, and diabetes. In those with strep throat, antibiotics can lower the risk of rheumatic heart disease [7].

The microbiome plays a beneficial role in the homeostatic regulation of different body tissues of the host [8]. The overall relationship between humans and their microbiota can be described as a mutualistic symbiosis, also known as eubiosis [9]. This healthy balance of gut bacteria can be disrupted, leading to the onset of a variety of chronic diseases with an underlying inflammatory condition [10]. A large population of microbiota, predominantly bacteria, that populate the human gut have a symbiotic connection with the host, and imbalances in host-microbial interaction (dysbiosis) hamper these homeostatic systems that govern health and activate numerous pathways that contribute to advancing CVD risk factors [11]. Dysbiosis is related to intestinal inflammation and decreased gut barrier integrity, which raises circulating levels of bacterial structural components and microbial metabolites such as trimethylamine-N-oxide and short-chain fatty acids, which may aid in the development of CVDs [11].

Trimethylamine-N- oxide (TMAO) is a type of osmolyte found in the tissues of marine crustaceans and fish, where it prevents protein distortion and, therefore, the animal's death [12]. The concentration of TMAO increases as the animal's depth in the seas increases [13]. It is a protein stabilizer that counteracts the protein-destabilizing effects of pressure. In general, the bodies of animals living at great depths are adapted to high-pressure environments by having pressure-resistant biomolecules and small organic molecules present in their cells, known as piezolytes, of which TMAO is the most abundant. These piezolytes give the proteins the flexibility to function properly under great pressure [13–15]. However, more importantly, TMAO has emerged not only as an important metabolite in the human diet but also as a major cardiometabolic risk factor. It has been associated with many cardiovascular complications including foam cell formation [16], endothelial dysfunction [17], acute heart failure [18], infracted coronary artery [19], inflammation [20] and vascular aging [21].

2. Role of gut microbes in regulating cardiovascular health and disease

The gut microbiome has emerged as a critical factor in human health and disease [22, 23] and cardio-metabolic diseases are no exception. Obesity and insulin resistance are serious cardiometabolic risk factors [24–27], and gut microbial composition is a major regulator of these conditions. Changes in fecal microbial community composition have been linked to the development of obesity and insulin resistance, and microbial transplantation has been shown to transmit increased adiposity in the host [28–30]. Disruptions to the microbiota early in life have since been identified to induce increased obesity [31]. Koren et al. [32] argued that microbiota could be associated with atherosclerosis since human atherosclerotic plaques were found to contain bacterial DNA, albeit it was unclear if the DNA came from live bacteria within the arterial wall. The initial research into a possible link between the gut microbiome and cardiovascular disease (CVD) focused on trimethylamine N-oxide (TMAO), a metaorganismal metabolite generated after ingestion of food substances plentiful in a Western diet (eg, carnitine, lecithin, choline) [16, 33, 34]. TMAO has swiftly established itself as a biomarker for human CVD risk as well as a promoter of atherothrombotic disease [35, 36]. In fact, a Western-style diet deficient in microbiota-accessible carbohydrates (MACs) may cause irreversible microbial diversity loss and the extinction of particular bacterial species in the digestive system [37]. As a result, the low intake of dietary fiber and increased levels of fat and sugar in our food, which are typical of a westernized lifestyle and diet, may contribute to the depletion of specific bacterial taxa, at least in part [38]. Fiber, fruit, legume and vegetable consumption is linked to an increased microbial richness in the gut microbiota [39, 40], and several recent epidemiological studies have found an inverse relationship between dietary fiber consumption and CVD risk variables [41–45]. Non -digestible carbohydrates present in dietary fiber are converted by intestinal bacteria into Short-Chain fatty acids(SCFAs) like acetate, propionate and butyrate [46, 47]. SCFAs have been shown to have a direct effect on renin release and vasomotor function, resulting in lower blood pressure [48–50]. Butyrate has been shown to have a potential adjuvant effect in the lowering of diastolic blood pressure by reducing inflammation in a recent controlled experiment [51]. Moreover, in early pregnancy, the presence of butyrate-producing bacteria was found to be inversely related to blood pressure and plasminogen activator inhibitor-1 levels [52].

2.1 Gut microbiota dysbiosis and implications in CVD risk

Most microbiome-related diseases have skyrocketed in the last century, implying that a change in lifestyle could disturb gut microbiota symbiosis by removing helpful, protective bacteria [53]. Patients with a variety of CVD risk factors, such as hypertension, dyslipidemia, insulin resistance, and other metabolic abnormalities, have been found to have variations in microbial composition [36, 37]. Dysbiosis of the gut microbiota can lead to chronic inflammation, which is a major contributor to obesity, cardiovascular disease, and notably atherosclerosis [38, 39]. In symptomatic atherosclerosis patients, metagenome research indicated a higher concentration of triglycerides and a lower level of high-density lipoprotein in the circulation, as well as an increased abundance of *Collinsella* and a decreased abundance of *Roseburia* and *Eubacterium* [54]. Jie et al. [55] discovered an elevated relative abundance of *Enterobacteriaceae* and *Streptococcus* spp. taxa in atherosclerotic CVD patients. In coronary artery disease patients, Emoto et al. discovered a distinct alteration in microbial composition, with a large increase in *Lactobacillales* (Firmicutes) and a decrease in Bacteroidetes [56]. In another study, patients with type 2 diabetes had a lower number of Firmicutes and a non-significant rise in Bacteroidetes and Proteobacteria [57]. Some cross-sectional studies have found evidence that high-protein and high-fat diets (associated with Western lifestyles) are linked to gut microbial populations characterized by the Bacteroides enterotype, while diets heavy in carbohydrates and simple sugars are linked to the Prevotella enterotype [58].

The metabolism-independent pathway and the metabolism-dependent pathway are two key pathways via which gut dysbiosis can contribute to the development and progression of atherosclerosis [59]. In the metabolism -independent pathways, bacterial components located on the outer membrane of Gram-negative bacteria, such as lipopolysaccharides (LPS), can encourage the production of foam cells, which are a primary component of atherosclerotic plaque [60]. To prevent the accumulation of excess cholesterol in peripheral tissues, the body has internal homeostatic systems in place, such as reverse cholesterol transport (RCT). Excess cholesterol is transported to the liver and transformed into bile acids through the RCT process [61–63]. By producing metabolic endotoxemia, gut dysbiosis can overload systems like RCT and encourage the development of foam cells [64–66]. Metabolic endotoxemia is a condition marked by a high level of LPS in the bloodstream [67]. The presence of *Bifidobacteria*, which typically enhance intestinal barrier function and inhibit bacterial translocation, is reduced in high-fat (HF) diet-induced dysbiosis [60].

3. Synthesis and metabolism of gut microbial metabolite TMA and TMAO

3.1 Production of trimethylamine by gut bacteria

Trimethylamine (TMA) is the source of TMAO in humans. TMA is derived either directly from meals high in TMA, such seafood, [68, 69] or indirectly from the bacterial metabolism of dietary choline and choline-containing substances in the colon, such as phosphatidylcholine [16], betaine [70], and dietary L-carnitine [33, 71]. The ability of different gut microbes to produce TMA from food precursors varies. This is because it is produced in the gut via a variety of microbial mechanisms (**Figure 1**). As a result, the composition of an individual's microbiota influences the magnitude of TMA production. It's worth noting that the genes essential for TMA formation are found in just a small percentage of the microorganisms in the intestine (less than 1%) [72]. TMA formation appears to be possible even at extremely low concentrations of these microorganisms, highlighting the importance of the gut microbiota in this context [73]. TMA and TMAO levels have been linked to increased activity in bacteria belonging to the phylum Firmicutes and Proteobacteria, which are known producers of this metabolite. Furthermore, because Bacteroidetes are unable to make TMA [74], TMA and TMAO levels have been connected to an enhanced Firmicutes/Bacteroidetes ratio, with higher levels of Firmicutes and lower levels of Bacteroidetes [57, 58]. The genes coding for the glycyl radical enzyme choline TMA-lyase (CutC) and its related radical S-adenosyl-L-methionine (SAM)(CutD) activating protein were discovered in the Choline Utilization (cut) gene cluster in gut bacteria, which is responsible for the anaerobic breakdown of choline into TMA [75]. A two-component CntA/CntB oxygenase/reductase system capable of cleaving L-carnitine into TMA and malic semialdehyde is another microbial metabolic route that generates TMA from L-carnitine [76]. The yeaW/X gene products (YeaW/X TMA lyase) are a closely similar bacterial lyase. Choline, betaine, L-carnitine, and -butyrobetaine can all be converted to TMA by this promiscuous lyase [74, 77]. Aside from these TMA-generating processes from dietary trimethylamines, some gut microbes like *E.coli* have also been found to have another pathway that converts TMAO to TMA via the activity of a torA-like gene product which acts as a reductase [78, 79].

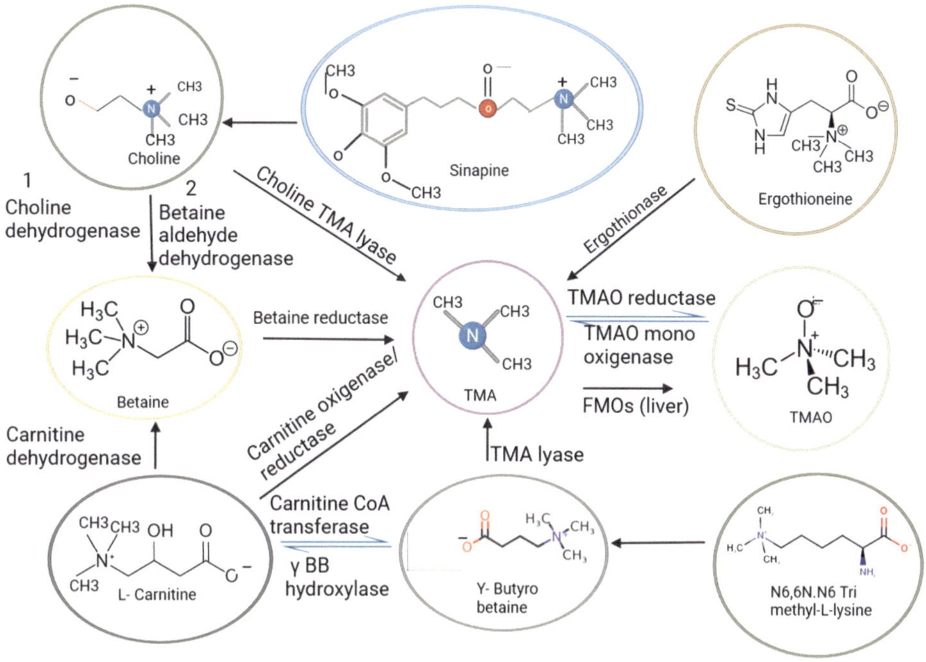

Figure 1.
Chemical formulae of TMA and TMAO's principal dietary precursors. The key metabolic pathways for the synthesis of TMA by the gut microbiota and endogenous enzymes, as well as the conversion of TMA to TMAO by hepatic FMOs, are depicted in this diagram.

3.2 Conversion of TMA into TMAO and its regulation

TMA generated from a choline -rich diet through various metabolic pathways is absorbed from the gut into the hepatic portal circulation and oxidized by the enzymes flavin-dependent monooxygenase isoforms 1 and 3 (FMO1 and FMO3) in the liver to create Trimethylamine-N-oxide(TMAO) (**Figure 2**) [80]. TMAO is excreted out of the body, usually through urine [81]. Sweat, feces (4%), exhaled air (less than 1%), and other body secretions are some of the other ways TMAO is excreted [82]. TMAO can be metabolized to DMA(Dimehtylamine), formaldehyde, ammonia, and methane by methanogenic bacteria that carry the TMAO demethylase enzyme [83]. Furthermore, it has been demonstrated that TMAO derived from food can be absorbed directly in the gut [84]. As a result, plasma TMAO levels are regulated by TMA synthesis and degradation, as well as the rate at which TMA, and TMAO are secreted [85].

3.3 Dietary precursors of TMAO and the relationship between TMAO levels and dietary habits

As discussed in Section 3.1, seafood is a rich source of dietary TMA/TMAO and various dietary precursors like L-carnitine, choline, ergothioneine and betaine (**Figure 1**) equally contribute to the generation of TMAO in the body. Free TMAO present in seafood is not metabolized by gut microbiota and is directly absorbed into the systemic circulation [86]. L-carnitine is present in high concentrations in meals derived from animals (meat and dairy products), and in smaller amounts in grains

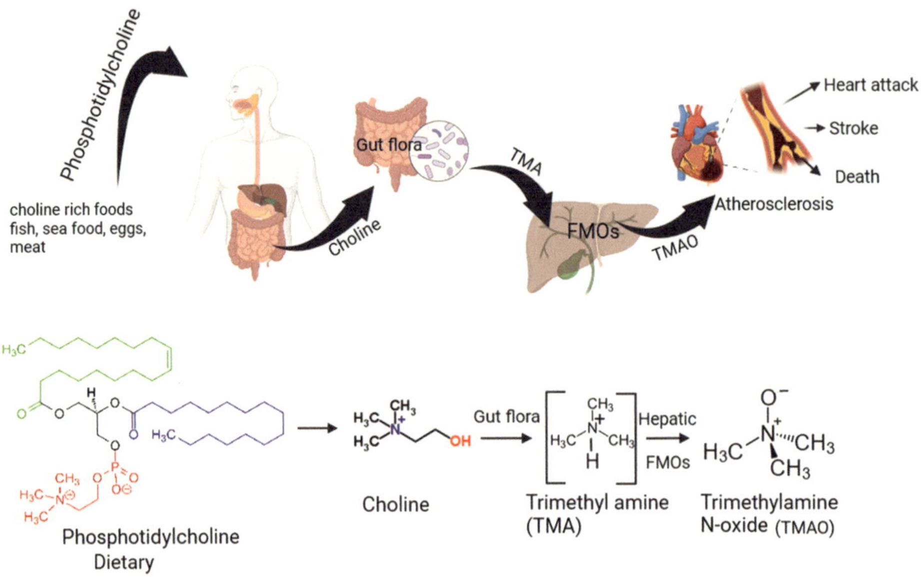

Figure 2.
Gut flora mediated synthesis of TMA and hepatic conversion to TMAO.

and vegetables [87]. The most common sources of choline in the diet are eggs and liver, followed by meats and fish, whole grain, cereal, vegetables, fruits, milk, fats, and oils [88]. One of the most important sources of betaine is cereal-based foods [89]. Betaine can also be found in spinach, beets, crabs, and finfish [90]. Dietary sources are the only way to get ergothioneine. Ergothioneine is found in only a few foods, with the largest quantities found in boletus and oyster mushrooms, as well as to a lesser level in chicken and pork liver and kidney, oat bran, and black and red beans [91]. As discussed in Section 2, a westernized lifestyle and diet full of junk fatty foods and refined sugar, devoid of fiber and important nutrients, predisposes one to increased CVD risk and other chronic diseases. Plasma TMAO levels have been observed to rise when people eat Western-style or high-fat diets [92–94]. However, conversely, epidemiological studies have linked the Mediterranean diet to a lower risk of cardiovascular disease (CVD) [95]. A typical Mediterranean diet is defined by plant based foods (vegetables, fruits, nuts,), olive oil based fats and moderate to low amounts of seafood, eggs and meats [96, 97]. This makes this type of diet high in fiber and low in choline -rich food. The importance of fiber- rich foods has already been mentioned in Section 2. High dietary fiber consumption, followed by gut microbiota-mediated fermentation, appears to reduce TMAO levels in experiments on animal models and clinical medicine [98].

4. Role of TMAO in increasing cardiovascular disease risk

A choline-rich diet puts a person at risk of increased TMAO levels [16], which is directly correlated to an increased CVD risk [99]. Angiographic markers of coronary artery atherosclerotic burden and cardiac risks have strong relationships with systemic TMAO levels, and higher levels of TMAO in the blood are linked to an increased risk of incident cardiovascular events such as myocardial infarction, recurrent stroke,

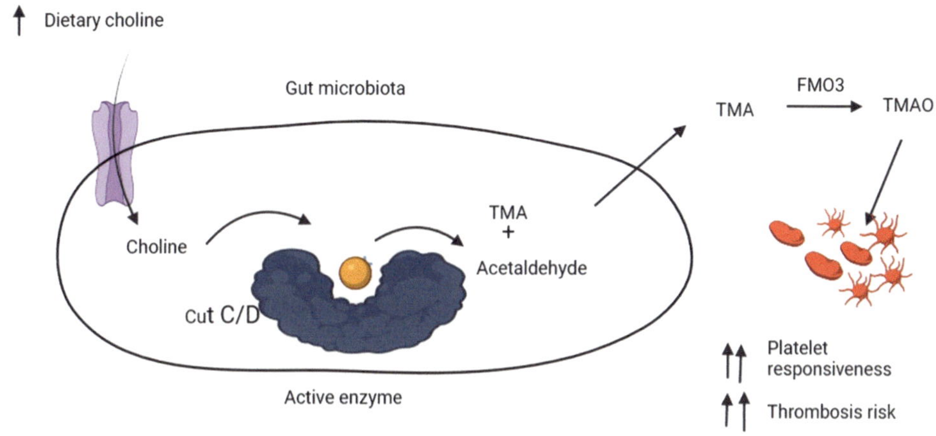

Figure 3.
TMAO- mediated platelet hyper-responsiveness and increased thrombosis risk.

and even cardiovascular death [55, 100]. Gut microbes play a role in modifying platelet reactivity and generating a pro-thrombotic phenotype in vivo by producing TMAO (**Figure 3**) [101]. Zhu *et al.,* has shown that direct exposure of platelets to TMAO, caused activation of the platelets by the release of intracellular calcium. This modulates the platelet hyper-responsiveness and the potential of thrombosis and causes thrombosis and atherosclerosis [101]. Rebecca *et al.*, states that knockdown of FMOs can protect mice from obesity, which is a major cause for cardiovascular diseases [102, 103]. Increased amount of TMAO, obtained from the diet, causes monocytes to enter the subendothelial space and differentiate into colony -stimulating factors when they encounter the growth factors. These form large cells known as dendritic cells and macrophages which possess high expression of SR-A1 and CD36 [104]. These cells take up oxidized, low- density lipid particles to create foam cells that are irregular in the uptake of cholesterol with fatty acids and ester bonds, thus stimulating atherosclerosis [105]. It is suggested that CD36/MAPK/JNK pathways play a vital role in the formation of foam cells [106]. Research studies show that apoe−/− mice fed with choline diet for 8 weeks, gradually exhibited an increase in TMAO, which further recruited macrophages and pro – inflammatory cytokines [107]. Another study by Boini et al. indicates the link between TMAO and inflammation, where TMAO induces NLRP3 inflammasome formation and causes other immune responses [108]. An imbalance of cholesterol transport is observed in individuals with high TMAO, and studies show that mice with administered TMAO inhibited the synthesis of hepatic bile acid by downregulating the expression of Cyp7a1, which promoted atherosclerosis [109]. The activation of oxidative stress pathways following exposure to TMAO, which triggers inflammatory cytokines, is the molecular basis for increasing cardiovascular illnesses. It can also activate the p38 MAPK and NF-kappa beta signaling pathways, which enhances NLRP3 production in the inflammasome and promotes vascular calcification and endothelial cell damage [110]. High administration of TMAO causes oxidative stress, inflammation and suppressed cellular functions, while low levels exhibit a contrary response [111]. A recent study proved that patients with aortic stenosis, had their TMAO levels as 5.5 μM, when the control was 3.6 μM. TMA is also associated with cardiovascular diseases as the levels of TMA in these patients were 59.5 μM and the control was 23.2 μM [112]. Thus, TMAO is considered to be an independent risk factor for cardiovascular diseases.

5. Targeting the TMA/TMAO pathway as a therapeutic strategy to combat CVD risk-current research and future directions

The gut microbiome is a growing area of research in metabolic health and its link to CVD risk. The development of high-throughput metagenomic tools has aided a new understanding of the gut microbiome's role in CVD risk [113]. The gut microbiome can be targeted to modify TMAO synthesis, according to recent fecal microbial transplant research [114] and as a result TMA/TMAO levels can be regulated. Based on research by Maisto et al., in healthy subjects, grape pomace polyphenolic extract has been found to lower serum levels of TMAO [115]. Resveratrol (RSV) reduces TMAO- induced atherosclerosis by lowering TMAO levels and enhancing hepatic bile acid synthesis through gut microbiota remodeling [116]. Antimicrobial phytochemicals, such as allicin, a dietary dosage derived from garlic, effectively neutralize the metabolic ability of gut microbiota to produce TMAO- induced by L-carnitine intake [117]. Luhong granules, a complex blend of herbs, flowers, animal parts, seeds, and roots, prolong ventricular remodeling after myocardial infarction by lowering TMAO and LPS levels in the bloodstream by increasing the gut microflora and intestinal barrier function [118]. A single oral dosage of a cutC/D inhibitor lowers plasma TMAO levels for up to three days and reverses diet-induced platelet reactivity and thrombus formation as studied in animal models, with no toxicity or increased bleeding risk [119]. In experiments with mice models, *Lactobacillus plantarum* ZDY04 significantly reduced serum TMAO and cecal TMA levels in mice by modulating the relative abundance of specific bacterial species, including *Bacteroids* and significantly inhibiting the development of TMAO-induced atherosclerosis in choline fed mice [120]. In high-fat diet-induced obese mice, capsanthin extract prevents obesity, lowers serum TMAO levels, and modifies the gut microbiota composition by decreasing serum triglycerides, total cholesterol, and TMAO levels and markedly increasing microbial diversity [121]. The ability of several oral probiotics to modify circulating TMAO levels in different cohorts, including healthy participants and patients with a CVD-related disease, has been investigated [122–125]. None of them, however, appeared to have a significant effect on TMAO levels in the treatment groups as compared to the placebo groups. In another study, TMA-degrading microorganisms were used by Qiu et al. (2017) to investigate another promising technique for lowering TMA levels in the gut where oral administration of a TMA-metabolizing strain (*Enterobacter aerogenes* ZDY01) reduced TMA in the cecum and TMAO in the serum, as well as changing the microbial community composition in mice, according to their findings [126]. In human studies, changes in urine TMAO levels have been discovered in untargeted metabolomics investigations following supplementation with *Origanum dictamus* tea and *Curcuma longa* extract [127, 128].

6. Conclusions

Diet has been shown to have an important role in the formation of TMAO because it offers the nutritional precursors needed to create TMA and TMAO. There is a positive correlation between circulating TMAO levels and the consumption of food rich in dietary precursors of TMAO like seafood, meat, eggs etc. Targeting the TMA/TMAO metabolism has emerged as a promising tool for cardiovascular disease prevention and treatment in recent years. Targeting the microbiota and host metabolic systems implicated in TMA and TMAO production shows potential for future intervention.

Animal models have largely established the capacity of specific diets, food ingredients, and phytochemicals found in herbs to reduce circulation of TMAO levels. The link between changes in TMAO levels and gut microbiota has only been shown in a few cases, and the exact processes behind the impacts of the dietary items under investigation are yet unknown. More importantly, there are few studies that suggest that lowering circulating TMAO levels has a favorable effect in humans. Because the majority of the studies have been conducted on animal models, the results are difficult to apply to humans. Future research in this area should address conventional microbial research obstacles as well as those more specific to the study of TMA/TMAO metabolism, such as the substantial intra-individual variability of plasma TMAO levels observed in some humans. With the advancement and availability of next-generation sequencing and other omics technologies, a change from studies focusing on defining microbial community composition to more function-oriented research on the gut microbiota is envisaged. Bioinformatic approaches, shotgun metagenomics, meta-transcriptomics, meta-proteomics, and metabolomics, are all expected to be crucial in unraveling the intricate relationships between nutrition, microbial metabolism, and host health.

Acknowledgements

All images in this manuscript were made using BioRender.

Conflict of interest

The authors declare no conflict of interest.

Author details

Shubham Barik, Aritra Mukherjee, Angelina Job Kolady, Boda Karunakar and Tony Grace*
Department of Genomic Science, Central University of Kerala, Kasaragod, Kerala, India

*Address all correspondence to: tonygrace@cukerala.ac.in

References

[1] GBD 2013 mortality and cause of death collaborators. Global, regional, and national age–sex specific all-cause and cause-specific mortality for 240 causes of death, 1990-2013: A systematic analysis for the global burden of disease study 2013. Lancet. 2015;**385**(9963):117-171

[2] Moran AE et al. Temporal trends in ischemic heart disease mortality in 21 world regions, 1980 to 2010: The global burden of disease 2010 study. Circulation. 2014;**129**(14):1483-1492

[3] Petersen KS, Kris-Etherton PM. Diet quality assessment and the relationship between diet quality and cardiovascular disease risk. Nutrients. 2021;**13**(12):4305

[4] Criqui MH, Denenberg JO. The generalized nature of atherosclerosis: How peripheral arterial disease may predict adverse events from coronary artery disease. Vascular Medicine. 1998;**3**(3):241-245

[5] deGoma EM, Knowles JW, Angeli F, Budoff MJ, Rader DJ. The evolution and refinement of traditional risk factors for cardiovascular disease. Cardiology in Review. 2012;**20**(3):118-129

[6] McGill HC, McMahan CA, Gidding SS. Preventing heart disease in the 21st century. Circulation. 2008;**117**(9):1216-1227

[7] Spinks A, Glasziou PP, Del Mar CB. Antibiotics for treatment of sore throat in children and adults. Cochrane Database of Systematic Reviews. 2021;**12, no. 12**:CD000023

[8] Schroeder BO, Bäckhed F. Signals from the gut microbiota to distant organs in physiology and disease. Nature Medicine. 2016;**22**(10):1079-1089

[9] Walter J, Britton RA, Roos S. Host-microbial symbiosis in the vertebrate gastrointestinal tract and the lactobacillus reuteri paradigm. Proceedings of the National Academy of Sciences. 2011;**108**(Supplement 1):4645-4652

[10] Hand TW, Vujkovic-Cvijin I, Ridaura VK, Belkaid Y. Linking the microbiota, chronic disease, and the immune system. Trends in Endocrinology and Metabolism. 2016;**27**(12):831-843

[11] Novakovic M et al. Role of gut microbiota in cardiovascular diseases. World Journal of Cardiology. 2020;**12**(4):110-122

[12] Yancey PH, Clark ME, Hand SC, Bowlus RD, Somero GN. Living with water stress: Evolution of Osmolyte systems. Science (80-.). 1982;**217**(4566):1214-1222

[13] Linley TD, Gerringer ME, Yancey PH, Drazen JC, Weinstock CL, Jamieson AJ. Fishes of the hadal zone including new species, in situ observations and depth records of Liparidae. Deep Sea Research part I: Oceanographic Research Papers. 2016;**114**:99-110

[14] Yancey PH. Organic osmolytes as compatible, metabolic and counteracting cytoprotectants in high osmolarity and other stresses. The Journal of Experimental Biology. 2005;**208**(15):2819-2830

[15] Velasquez MT, Ramezani A, Manal A, Raj DS. Trimethylamine N-oxide: The good, the bad and the unknown. Toxins (Basel). 8 Nov 2016;8(11):326. DOI: 10.3390/toxins8110326

[16] Wang Z et al. Gut flora metabolism of phosphatidylcholine promotes cardiovascular disease. Nature. 2011;**472**(7341):57-63

[17] Sun X et al. Trimethylamine N-oxide induces inflammation and endothelial dysfunction in human umbilical vein endothelial cells via activating ROS-TXNIP-NLRP3 inflammasome. Biochemical and Biophysical Research Communications. 2016;**481**(1-2):63-70

[18] Suzuki T, Heaney LM, Bhandari SS, Jones DJL, Ng LL. Trimethylamine N-oxide and prognosis in acute heart failure. Heart. 2016;**102**(11):841-848

[19] Mafune A et al. Associations among serum trimethylamine-N-oxide (TMAO) levels, kidney function and infarcted coronary artery number in patients undergoing cardiovascular surgery: A cross-sectional study. Clinical and Experimental Nephrology. 2016;**20**(5):731-739

[20] Chen ML, Zhu XH, Ran L, Lang HD, Yi L, Mi MT. Trimethylamine-N-oxide induces vascular inflammation by activating the NLRP3 Inflammasome through the SIRT3-SOD2-mtROS signaling pathway. Journal of the American Heart Association. 4 Sep 2017;**6**(9):e006347. DOI: 10.1161/JAHA.117.006347. Erratum in: J Am Heart Assoc.

[21] Li D et al. Trimethylamine-N-oxide promotes brain aging and cognitive impairment in mice. Aging Cell. 2018;**17**(4):e12768

[22] Clemente JC, Ursell LK, Parfrey LW, Knight R. The impact of the gut microbiota on human health: An integrative view. Cell. 2012;**148**(6):1258-1270

[23] Wang J, Jia H. Metagenome-wide association studies: Fine-mining the microbiome. Nature Reviews. Microbiology. 2016;**14**(8):508-522

[24] McFarlane SI, Banerji M, Sowers JR. Insulin resistance and cardiovascular disease. The Journal of Clinical Endocrinology and Metabolism. 2001;**86**(2):713-718

[25] Reaven G, Abbasi F, McLaughlin T. Obesity, insulin resistance, and cardiovascular disease. Recent Progress in Hormone Research. 2004;**59**:207-224

[26] Bonow RO, Eckel RH. Diet, obesity, and cardiovascular risk. The New England Journal of Medicine. 2003;**348**(21):2057-2133

[27] Sharma AM. Obesity and cardiovascular risk. Growth Hormone & IGF Research. 2003;**13**:S10-S17

[28] Ley RE, Bäckhed F, Turnbaugh P, Lozupone CA, Knight RD, Gordon JI. Obesity alters gut microbial ecology. Proceedings of the National Academy of Sciences. 2005;**102**(31):11070-11075

[29] Turnbaugh PJ, Ley RE, Mahowald MA, Magrini V, Mardis ER, Gordon JI. An obesity-associated gut microbiome with increased capacity for energy harvest. Nature. 2006;**444**(7122):1027-1031

[30] Bäckhed F et al. The gut microbiota as an environmental factor that regulates fat storage. Proceedings of the National Academy of Sciences. 2004;**101**(44):15718-15723

[31] Cho I et al. Antibiotics in early life alter the murine colonic microbiome and adiposity. Nature. 2012;**488**(7413):621-626

[32] Koren O et al. Human oral, gut, and plaque microbiota in patients with atherosclerosis. Proceedings of

the National Academy of Sciences. 2011;**108**(Supplement 1):4592-4598

[33] Koeth RA et al. Intestinal microbiota metabolism of L-carnitine, a nutrient in red meat, promotes atherosclerosis. Nature Medicine. 2013;**19**(5):576-585

[34] Tang WHW et al. Intestinal microbial metabolism of phosphatidylcholine and cardiovascular risk. The New England Journal of Medicine. 2013;**368**(17):1575-1584

[35] Guasti L et al. TMAO as a biomarker of cardiovascular events: A systematic review and meta-analysis. Internal and Emergency Medicine. 2021;**16**(1):201-207

[36] Randrianarisoa E et al. Relationship of serum trimethylamine N-oxide (TMAO) levels with early atherosclerosis in humans. Scientific Reports. 2016;**6**(1):1-9

[37] Sonnenburg ED, Smits SA, Tikhonov M, Higginbottom SK, Wingreen NS, Sonnenburg JL. Diet-induced extinctions in the gut microbiota compound over generations. Nature. 2016;**529**(7585):212-215

[38] Sonnenburg ED, Sonnenburg JL. Starving our microbial self: The deleterious consequences of a diet deficient in microbiota-accessible carbohydrates. Cell Metabolism. 2014;**20**(5):779-786

[39] Bourquin LD, Titgemeyer EC, Fahey GC Jr. Fermentation of various dietary fiber sources by human fecal bacteria. Nutrition Research. 1996;**16**(7):1119-1131

[40] Bourquin LD, Titgemeyer EC, Fahey GC Jr. Vegetable fiber fermentation by human fecal bacteria: Cell wall polysaccharide disappearance and short-chain fatty acid production during in vitro fermentation and water-holding capacity of unfermented residues. The Journal of Nutrition. 1993;**123**(5):860-869

[41] Liu L, Wang S, Liu J. Fiber consumption and all-cause, cardiovascular, and cancer mortalities: A systematic review and meta-analysis of cohort studies. Molecular Nutrition & Food Research. 2015;**59**(1):139-146

[42] Micha R et al. Etiologic effects and optimal intakes of foods and nutrients for risk of cardiovascular diseases and diabetes: Systematic reviews and meta-analyses from the nutrition and chronic diseases expert group (NutriCoDE). PLoS One. 2017;**12**(4):e0175149

[43] McRae MP. Dietary fiber is beneficial for the prevention of cardiovascular disease: An umbrella review of meta-analyses. Journal of Chiropractic Medicine. 2017;**16**(4):289-299

[44] Kim Y, Je Y. Dietary fibre intake and mortality from cardiovascular disease and all cancers: A meta-analysis of prospective cohort studies. Archives of Cardiovascular Diseases. 2016;**109**(1):39-54

[45] Hajishafiee M, Saneei P, Benisi-Kohansal S, Esmaillzadeh A. Cereal fibre intake and risk of mortality from all causes, CVD, cancer and inflammatory diseases: A systematic review and meta-analysis of prospective cohort studies. The British Journal of Nutrition. 2016;**116**(2):343-352

[46] Duncan SH, Belenguer A, Holtrop G, Johnstone AM, Flint HJ, Lobley GE. Reduced dietary intake of carbohydrates by obese subjects results in decreased concentrations of butyrate and butyrate-producing bacteria in feces. Applied and Environmental Microbiology. 2007;**73**(4):1073-1078

[47] Cummings J, Pomare EW, Branch WJ, Naylor CP, MacFarlane G. Short chain fatty acids in human large intestine, portal, hepatic and venous blood. Gut. 1987;**28**(10):1221-1227

[48] Pluznick JL et al. Olfactory receptor responding to gut microbiota-derived signals plays a role in renin secretion and blood pressure regulation. Proceedings of the National Academy of Sciences. 2013;**110**(11):4410-4415

[49] Marques FZ et al. High-fiber diet and acetate supplementation change the gut microbiota and prevent the development of hypertension and heart failure in hypertensive mice. Circulation. 2017;**135**(10):964-977

[50] Natarajan N et al. Microbial short chain fatty acid metabolites lower blood pressure via endothelial G protein-coupled receptor 41. Physiological Genomics. 2016;**48**(11):826-834

[51] Roshanravan N et al. Effect of butyrate and inulin supplementation on glycemic status, lipid profile and glucagon-like peptide 1 level in patients with type 2 diabetes: A randomized double-blind, placebo-controlled trial. Hormone and Metabolic Research. 2017;**49**(11):886-891

[52] Gomez-Arango LF, Barrett HL, McIntyre HD, Callaway LK, Morrison M, Dekker Nitert M. Increased systolic and diastolic blood pressure is associated with altered gut microbiota composition and butyrate production in early pregnancy. Hypertension. 2016;**68**(4):974-981

[53] Logan AC, Jacka FN, Prescott SL. Immune-microbiota interactions: Dysbiosis as a global health issue. Current Allergy and Asthma Reports. 2016;**16**(2):1-9

[54] Karlsson FH et al. Symptomatic atherosclerosis is associated with an altered gut metagenome. Nature Communications. 2012;**3**(1):1-8

[55] Jie Z et al. The gut microbiome in atherosclerotic cardiovascular disease. Nature Communications. 2017;**8**(1):845

[56] Emoto T, Yamashita T, Sasaki N, Hirota Y, Hayashi T, So A, et al. Analysis of Gut Microbiota in Coronary Artery Disease Patients: a Possible Link between Gut Microbiota and Coronary Artery Disease. Journal of Atherosclerosis and Thrombosis. 1 Aug 2016;**23**(8):908-921. DOI: 10.5551/jat.32672

[57] Wong JMW. Gut microbiota and cardiometabolic outcomes: Influence of dietary patterns and their associated components. The American Journal of Clinical Nutrition. 2014;**100**(suppl_1):369S-377S

[58] Wu GD et al. Linking long-term dietary patterns with gut microbial Enterotypes. Science (80-.). 2011;**334**(6052):105-108

[59] Brown JM, Hazen SL. The gut microbial endocrine organ: Bacterially derived signals driving cardiometabolic diseases. Annual Review of Medicine. 2015;**66**:343-359

[60] Manco M, Putignani L, Bottazzo GF. Gut microbiota, lipopolysaccharides, and innate immunity in the pathogenesis of obesity and cardiovascular risk. Endocrine Reviews. 2010;**31**(6):817-844

[61] Ohashi R, Mu H, Wang X, Yao Q, Chen C. Reverse cholesterol transport and cholesterol efflux in atherosclerosis. QJM. 2005;**98**(12):845-856

[62] Spady DK. Reverse cholesterol transport and atherosclerosis regression. Circulation. 1999;**100**(6) Am Heart Assoc:576-578

[63] Annema W, Tietge UJF. Regulation of reverse cholesterol transport-a

comprehensive appraisal of available animal studies. Nutrition & Metabolism (London). 2012;**9**(1):1-18

[64] Cuchel M, Rader DJ. Macrophage reverse cholesterol transport: Key to the regression of atherosclerosis? Circulation. 2006;**113**(21):2548-2555

[65] Lo Sasso G et al. Intestinal specific LXR activation stimulates reverse cholesterol transport and protects from atherosclerosis. Cell Metabolism. 2010;**12**(2):187-193

[66] Castrillo A et al. Crosstalk between LXR and toll-like receptor signaling mediates bacterial and viral antagonism of cholesterol metabolism. Molecular Cell. 2003;**12**(4):805-816

[67] Mohammad S, Thiemermann C. Role of metabolic endotoxemia in systemic inflammation and potential interventions. Frontiers in Immunology. 11 Jan 2021;**11**:594150. DOI: 10.3389/fimmu.2020.594150

[68] Seibel BA, Walsh PJ. Trimethylamine oxide accumulation in marine animals: Relationship to acylglycerol storagej. The Journal of Experimental Biology. 2002;**205**(3):297-306

[69] Zeisel SH, DaCosta K-A. Increase in human exposure to methylamine precursors of N-nitrosamines after eating fish. Cancer Research. 1986;**46**(12 Part 1):6136-6138

[70] Day-Walsh P et al. The use of an in-vitro batch fermentation (human colon) model for investigating mechanisms of TMA production from choline, l-carnitine and related precursors by the human gut microbiota. European Journal of Nutrition. 2021;**60**(7):3987-3999

[71] Rajakovich LJ, Fu B, Bollenbach M, Balskus EP. Elucidation of an anaerobic pathway for metabolism of l-carnitine–derived γ-butyrobetaine to trimethylamine in human gut bacteria. Proceedings of the National Academy of Sciences. 2021;**118**(32):e2101498118

[72] Rath S, Heidrich B, Pieper DH, Vital M. Uncovering the trimethylamine-producing bacteria of the human gut microbiota. Microbiome. 2017;**5**(1):1-14

[73] Romano KA, Vivas EI, Amador-Noguez D, Rey FE. Intestinal microbiota composition modulates choline bioavailability from diet and accumulation of the proatherogenic metabolite trimethylamine-N-oxide. MBio. 2015;**6**(2):e02481-e02414

[74] Falony G, Vieira-Silva S, Raes J. Microbiology meets big data: The case of gut microbiota–derived trimethylamine. Annual Review of Microbiology. 2015;**69**:305-321

[75] Smaranda C, Balskus EP. Microbial conversion of choline to trimethylamine requires a glycyl radical enzyme. Proceedings of the National Academy of Sciences. 2012;**109**(52):21307-21312

[76] Yijun Z et al. Carnitine metabolism to trimethylamine by an unusual Rieske-type oxygenase from human microbiota. Proceedings of the National Academy of Sciences. 2014;**111**(11):4268-4273

[77] Wang Z et al. Non-lethal inhibition of gut microbial trimethylamine production for the treatment of atherosclerosis. Cell. 2015;**163**(7):1585-1595

[78] McCrindle SL, Kappler U, McEwan AG. Microbial dimethylsulfoxide and trimethylamine-N-oxide respiration. Advances in Microbial Physiology. 2005;**50**:147-198. DOI: 10.1016/S0065-2911(05)50004-3

[79] Méjean V, Lobbi-Nivol C, Lepelletier M, Giordano G, Chippaux M, Pascal M. TMAO anaerobic respiration in Escherichia coli: Involvement of the tor operon. Molecular Microbiology. 1994;**11**(6):1169-1179

[80] Bennett BJ et al. Trimethylamine-N-oxide, a metabolite associated with atherosclerosis, exhibits complex genetic and dietary regulation. Cell Metabolism. 2013;**17**(1):49-60

[81] Yu D et al. Urinary levels of trimethylamine-N-oxide and incident coronary heart disease: A prospective investigation among urban Chinese adults. Journal of the American Heart Association. 2019;**8**(1):e010606

[82] Papandreou C, Moré M, Bellamine A. Trimethylamine N-oxide in relation to cardiometabolic health—Cause or effect? Nutrients. 2020;**12**(5):1330

[83] Chhibber-Goel J, Gaur A, Singhal V, Parakh N, Bhargava B, Sharma A. The complex metabolism of trimethylamine in humans: Endogenous and exogenous sources. Expert Reviews in Molecular Medicine. 29 Apr 2016;**18**:e8. DOI: 10.1017/erm.2016.6. Erratum in: Expert Rev Mol Med. 2016 Nov 23;**18**:e19.

[84] Zhang AQ, Mitchell SC, Smith RL. Dietary precursors of trimethylamine in man: A pilot study. Food and Chemical Toxicology. 1999;**37**(5):515-520

[85] Gessner A, di Giuseppe R, Koch M, Fromm MF, Lieb W, Maas R. Trimethylamine-N-oxide (TMAO) determined by LC-MS/MS: Distribution and correlates in the population-based PopGen cohort. Clinical Chemistry and Laboratory Medicine. 2020;**58**(5):733-740

[86] Canyelles M, Tondo M, Cedó L, Farràs M, Escolà-Gil JC, Blanco-Vaca F. Trimethylamine N-oxide: A link among diet, gut microbiota, gene regulation of liver and intestine cholesterol homeostasis and HDL function. International Journal of Molecular Sciences. 2018;**19**(10):3228

[87] Steiber A, Kerner J, Hoppel CL. Carnitine: A nutritional, biosynthetic, and functional perspective. Molecular Aspects of Medicine. 2004;**25**(5):455-473

[88] Patterson KY et al. USDA Database for the Choline Content of Common Foods, Release Two. Center, ARS, USDA: Nutr. Data Lab. Beltsv. Hum. Nutr. Res; 2008

[89] Filipčev B, Kojić J, Krulj J, Bodroža-Solarov M, Ilić N. Betaine in cereal grains and grain-based products. Foods. 2018 Mar 29;**7**(4):49. DOI: 10.3390/foods7040049

[90] Zeisel SH, Mar M-H, Howe JC, Holden JM. Concentrations of choline-containing compounds and betaine in common foods. The Journal of Nutrition. 2003;**133**(5):1302-1307

[91] Ey J, Schömig E, Taubert D. Dietary sources and antioxidant effects of Ergothioneine. Journal of Agricultural and Food Chemistry. 2007;**55**(16):6466-6474

[92] Malinowska AM, Szwengiel A, Chmurzynska A. Dietary, anthropometric, and biochemical factors influencing plasma choline, carnitine, trimethylamine, and trimethylamine-N-oxide concentrations. International Journal of Food Sciences and Nutrition. 2017;**68**(4):488-495

[93] Chen K, Zheng X, Feng M, Li D, Zhang H. Gut microbiota-dependent metabolite trimethylamine N-oxide contributes to cardiac dysfunction in Western diet-induced obese mice. Frontiers in Physiology. 21 Mar 2017;8:139. DOI: 10.3389/fphys.2017.00139

[94] Boutagy NE et al. Short-term high-fat diet increases postprandial trimethylamine-N-oxide in humans. Nutrition Research. 2015;**35**(10):858-864

[95] Serra-Majem L, Román-Viñas B, Sanchez-Villegas A, Guasch-Ferré M, Corella D, La Vecchia C. Benefits of the Mediterranean diet: Epidemiological and molecular aspects. Molecular Aspects of Medicine. 2019;**67**:1-55

[96] Willett WC et al. Mediterranean diet pyramid: A cultural model for healthy eating. The American Journal of Clinical Nutrition. 1995;**61**(6):1402S-1406S

[97] Bach-Faig A et al. Mediterranean diet pyramid today. Science and cultural updates. Public Health Nutrition. 2011;**14**(12A):2274-2284

[98] Li Q, Wu T, Liu R, Zhang M, Wang R. Soluble dietary fiber reduces trimethylamine metabolism via gut microbiota and Co-regulates host AMPK pathways. Molecular Nutrition & Food Research. Dec 2017;**61**(12). DOI: 10.1002/mnfr.201700473

[99] Haghikia A et al. Gut microbiota–dependent trimethylamine N-oxide predicts risk of cardiovascular events in patients with stroke and is related to proinflammatory monocytes. Arteriosclerosis, Thrombosis, and Vascular Biology. 2018;**38**(9):2225-2235

[100] Hoyles L et al. Metabolic retroconversion of trimethylamine N-oxide and the gut microbiota. Microbiome. 2018;**6**(1):1-14

[101] Zhu W et al. Gut microbial metabolite TMAO enhances platelet hyperreactivity and thrombosis risk. Cell. 2016;**165**(1):111-124

[102] Schugar RC et al. The TMAO-producing enzyme flavin-containing monooxygenase 3 regulates obesity and the beiging of white adipose tissue. Cell Reports. 2017;**19**(12):2451-2461

[103] Liu Y, Dai M. Trimethylamine N-oxide generated by the gut microbiota is associated with vascular inflammation: New insights into atherosclerosis. Mediators of Inflammation. 17 Feb 2020;**2020**:4634172. DOI: 10.1155/2020/4634172

[104] Yang S et al. Gut microbiota-dependent marker TMAO in promoting cardiovascular disease: Inflammation mechanism, clinical prognostic, and potential as a therapeutic target. Frontiers in Pharmacology. 2019;**10**:1360

[105] Wu K et al. The gut microbial metabolite trimethylamine N-oxide aggravates GVHD by inducing M1 macrophage polarization in mice. Blood. 2020;**136**(4):501-515

[106] Geng J et al. Trimethylamine N-oxide promotes atherosclerosis via CD36-dependent MAPK/JNK pathway. Biomedicine & Pharmacotherapy. 2018;**97**:941-947

[107] Lindskog Jonsson A et al. Impact of gut microbiota and diet on the development of atherosclerosis in Apoe−/− mice. Arteriosclerosis, Thrombosis, and Vascular Biology. 2018;**38**(10):2318-2326

[108] Boini KM, Hussain T, Li P-L, Koka SS. Trimethylamine-N-oxide instigates NLRP3 inflammasome activation and endothelial dysfunction. Cellular Physiology and Biochemistry. 2017;**44**(1):152-162

[109] Ding L et al. Trimethylamine-N-oxide (TMAO)-induced atherosclerosis is associated with bile acid metabolism. Lipids in Health and Disease. 2018;**17**(1):1-8

[110] Wang B, Qiu J, Lian J, Yang X, Zhou J. Gut Metabolite Trimethylamine-N-Oxide in Atherosclerosis: From Mechanism to Therapy. Frontiers in Cardiovascular Medicine. 23 Nov 2021;**8**:723886. DOI: 10.3389/fcvm.2021.723886

[111] Chou R-H et al. Trimethylamine N-oxide, circulating endothelial progenitor cells, and endothelial function in patients with stable angina. Scientific Reports. 2019;**9**(1):1-10

[112] Jaworska K et al. TMA, a forgotten uremic toxin, but not TMAO, is involved in cardiovascular pathology. Toxins (Basel). 2019;**11**(9):490

[113] Kelly TN et al. Gut microbiome associates with lifetime cardiovascular disease risk profile among Bogalusa heart study participants. Circulation Research. 2016;**119**(8):956-964

[114] Gregory JC et al. Transmission of atherosclerosis susceptibility with gut microbial transplantation. The Journal of Biological Chemistry. 2015;**290**(9):5647-5660

[115] Annunziata G et al. Effects of grape pomace polyphenolic extract (Taurisolo®) in reducing TMAO serum levels in humans: Preliminary results from a randomized, placebo-controlled, cross-over study. Nutrients. 2019;**11**(1):139

[116] Chen M et al. Atherosclerosis by regulating TMAO synthesis and bile acid metabolism via remodeling of the gut microbiota. MBio. 2016;7:E02210-E02215

[117] Wu W-K, Panyod S, Ho C-T, Kuo C-H, Wu M-S, Sheen L-Y. Dietary allicin reduces transformation of L-carnitine to TMAO through impact on gut microbiota. Journal of Functional Foods. 2015;**15**:408-417

[118] Yang T, Qu H, Song X, Liu Q, Yang X, Xu J, et al. Luhong granules prevent ventricular remodelling after myocardial infarction by reducing the metabolites TMAO and LPS of the intestinal flora. Evidence-Based Complementary and Alternative Medicine. 16 Nov 2019;**2019**:8937427. DOI: 10.1155/2019/8937427. PMID: 31827566; PMCID: PMC6885292

[119] Roberts AB et al. Development of a gut microbe–targeted nonlethal therapeutic to inhibit thrombosis potential. Nature Medicine. 2018;**24**(9):1407-1417

[120] Qiu L, Tao X, Xiong H, Yu J, Wei H. Lactobacillus plantarum ZDY04 exhibits a strain-specific property of lowering TMAO via the modulation of gut microbiota in mice. Food & Function. 2018;**9**(8):4299-4309

[121] Wu T et al. Capsanthin extract prevents obesity, reduces serum TMAO levels and modulates the gut microbiota composition in high-fat-diet induced obese C57BL/6J mice. Food Research International. 2020;**128**:108774

[122] Montrucchio C et al. Serum trimethylamine-N-oxide concentrations in people living with HIV and the effect of probiotic supplementation. International Journal of Antimicrobial Agents. 2020;**55**(4):105908

[123] Borges NA et al. Effects of probiotic supplementation on trimethylamine-N-oxide plasma levels in hemodialysis patients: A pilot study. Probiotics Antimicrobial Proteins. 2019;**11**(2):648-654

[124] Tripolt NJ, Leber B, Triebl A, Köfeler H, Stadlbauer V, Sourij H. Effect of lactobacillus casei Shirota supplementation on trimethylamine-N-oxide levels in patients with metabolic syndrome: An open-label,

randomized study. Atherosclerosis. 2015;**242**(1):141-144

[125] Boutagy NE et al. Probiotic supplementation and trimethylamine-N-oxide production following a high-fat diet. Obesity. 2015;**23**(12):2357-2363

[126] Qiu L, Yang D, Tao X, Yu J, Xiong H, Wei H. Enterobacter aerogenes ZDY01 attenuates choline-induced trimethylamine N-oxide levels by remodeling gut microbiota in mice. Journal of Microbiology and Biotechnology. 2017;**27**(8):1491-1499

[127] Takis PG, Oraiopoulou M-E, Konidaris C, Troganis AN. 1H-NMR based metabolomics study for the detection of the human urine metabolic profile effects of Origanum dictamnus tea ingestion. Food & Function. 2016;**7**(9):4104-4115

[128] Dall'Acqua S et al. New findings on the in vivo antioxidant activity of Curcuma longa extract by an integrated 1H NMR and HPLC–MS metabolomic approach. Fitoterapia. 2016;**109**:125-131

Chapter 5

Obesity and Cardiovascular Risk

Pedro Felipe Parra Velasco

Abstract

Obesity is considered a pandemic of the present century and is associated with severe noncommunicable chronic diseases, especially cardiovascular diseases, which remain the leading cause of death in the world. Visceral adiposity is a usual localization for ectopic fat depots and increases the risk of cardiovascular diseases. Endothelial dysfunction in obesity explains atherosclerosis and higher risk of incident coronary artery disease. Further microvascular disease caused by chronic inflammatory state increases cytokines and reduces the nitric oxide, and chronic inflammation has been characterized by the imbalance between proinflammatory and procoagulant and anti-inflammatory and anticoagulant activities of the endothelium to generate a procoagulant state. An important topic is the gut microbiota that influences the progression of atherosclerosis. Some studies have shown the influence of gut dysbiosis and progression of atherosclerosis and cardiovascular disease. Additionally studies talking about overweight and obesity with coronary artery disease are explained by levels of blood pressure, cholesterol, and glucose; however, another important causative factor is the ectopic fat deposition, especially pericardial and epicardial spaces, which may further contribute to the burden of coronary atherosclerosis. So, diagnosis of cardiovascular diseases in obesity requires a lot of knowledge to suspect, diagnose, and to treat.

Keywords: obesity, cardiovascular risk, fatty tissue, atherosclerosis, coronary artery disease (CAD)

1. Introduction

Obesity is a disorder characterized by a disproportionate increase in body weight in relation to height, mainly due to the accumulation of fat, is considered a pandemic of the present century. It is associated with several noncommunicable chronic diseases, namely metabolic syndrome, type 2 diabetes mellitus (T2DM), cardiovascular diseases (CVD), obstructive sleeping apnea, osteoarthropathies, and cancer [1].

It is estimated that 39–49% of the world's population (2.8–3.5 billon people) are overweight. Among adult men, the prevalence of obesity in the Hispanic, black, and white is higher than in Asians, respectively. In women, the prevalence of obesity behavior is almost the same as the men. The black women have the most prevalence following the Hispanic, white, and Asian. In addition, children and adolescents are also affected; between 2 and 19-year-olds, 17% are obese and the males and females are equally [2, 3].

Knowing that the obesity is a complex disease, the prevalence is based on racial/ethnic and sex factors. For example, among adult men, the prevalence of obesity in the Hispanic, black, and white is higher than in Asians, respectively. In women, the prevalence is almost the same as the men. The black women have the most prevalence following the Hispanic, white, and Asian showing there is a socioeconomic inequality structure as well. In addition, children and adolescents are also affected; between 2 and 19-year-olds 17% are obese and the males and females are equally [2].

In general terms, the trends in obesity prevalence around the world are getting up constantly, which means it highlights the significant impact that the obesity will continue to have on CVD the incidence, prevalence, and deaths globally.

At this time, obesity is linked to numerous diseases of the cardiovascular system: stroke, venous thromboembolic disease and pulmonary hypertension, cardiovascular disease, heart failure, arrhythmias such as atrial fibrillation, and sudden cardiac death [4].

2. Visceral adiposity, liver fat, and cardiovascular risk

There is a strongly correlation between overall obesity and abdominal obesity; although, there are two kinds of patients: either the ones with overall obesity but not abdominal obesity.

Abdominal obesity is linked to increased cardiovascular diseases. Along these lines, there still exists underdiagnosis to classify the CVD risk among obese patients. Trying to unmask and making a good clinical patient evaluation, organizations, expert panels, and a lot of evidence support have shown and recommended the waist circumference (WC) measurements with body mass index (BMI) applied in the clinical practice may add critical information and successful prediction of cardiovascular risk and mortality focusing on visceral adiposity.

Fortunately imaging techniques can be used to quantify adipose tissue and ectopic fat depots volumes. The National Library of Medicine described the adipose tissue as a storage of energy in the form of triacylglycerols and ectopic fat depots and is defined by excess adipose tissue in locations not classically associated with adipose tissue storage, some fat depots are more linked to risk factors for disease than others. Techniques such as computed tomography (CT) and magnetic resonance imaging (MRI) are extraordinary and the most advanced in the study of human body composition and of its relationship with CVD risk. However, other techniques such as bio-impedance body composition are more available in the practice [5].

The abdominal adiposity can be divided into: obesity, subcutaneous, and visceral obesity. Overweight or obese patients with low levels of visceral adipose tissue (VAT) have been identified as having a more favorable cardiovascular risk profile, commonly known as metabolically healthy obese patients. Some recent data suggest that metabolically healthy obesity may be a transitory phenotype, the time of which may be variable by race, ethnicity, and gender. The relationship between visceral adipose tissue and cardiovascular risk is known, the first one being a clear accelerator for the development of cardiovascular diseases.

The concept called adipose tissue expandability refers to the ability of the adipocyte to be contained in the places where it normally lives. When this expansion capacity of adipose tissue is exceeded, it begins to be located in organs abnormally, developing diseases such as hepatic steatosis, which is directly related to a higher risk of developing cardiovascular events. Thus, it is important to identify that patients with increased visceral adiposity are the ones with the highest risk independent of weight.

3. Ectopic fat depots and CVD risk

3.1 Ectopic fat depots

Although the major known ectopic fat depot is the hepatic depot, there are other abnormal fat depots that contribute to the development of cardiovascular diseases. Some of these are: pericardial and epicardial depots despite being used many times in an undifferentiated way, they have a different anatomical locations and their relationship with cardiovascular diseases is different. The pericardial depot is located at the level of the pericardial sac and has been related to a high BMI, traditional cardiovascular risk (CVR) risk factors, and elevated atherogenic cholesterol. Additionally, the amount of pericardial fat has been associated with an increased risk of coronary heart disease, atherosclerosis, and heart failure adjusting for age, sex, BMI, and abdominal circumference; but not adjusting for traditional CVR factor and either when adjusting for levels of more atherogenic cholesterol particles [6].

VAT on the other hand represents the visceral fat contained between the external myocardium wall and the visceral lamina of the pericardium. It has been associated with a general CVR score and arterial stiffness in patients with CVD and DM2 [7].

Reports from multiple studies presented a high association between the pericardial depots and CVD. For example, a study of atherosclerosis showed the pericardial fat and a higher risk of all CVD causes, hard atherosclerotic CVD, and HF but not intrathoracic fat [8]. Another study that analyzed all-cause mortality risk after adjustment for age, sex, lifestyle variables, lipids, glucose, and adipocytokines was higher by increment in pericardial fat, but it did not proof enough information to predict the events of CVD beyond traditional risk factors [9].

Epicardial adipose tissue (EAT) is the visceral fat layer located around the heart and is believed to be important for the buffering of the coronary arteries and in providing fatty acids as a source of energy for the cardiac muscle. Reviews have shown that this deposit may be considered highly insulin resistant and also indicator of cardiovascular risk because of the secretion of pro-inflammatory cytokines and carotid artery stiffness. In addition, this can produce sleep apnea severity in woman independently of BMI, and this last one is associated with higher CVD risk [10, 11].

Currently, the way to reduce the announced ectopic fat (adipose tissue depots) has been investigated. There are a lot of nonpharmacological strategies to be applied based on lifestyle interventions, some authors dare to say could be more effective than pharmacological therapies. One of those strategies are exercises such as aerobic in nature, which may reduce VAT unchanged on weight loss; and reports of losing VAT by only resistance and high-intensity raining are equivocal [12, 13]. Thus, exercise interventions not just can decrease the VAT, apparently have impact in reducing hepatic, epicardial, and pericardial fat. However, there is not enough information to support a significant reduction in epicardial fat with exercise as the caloric restriction strategy to reduce it [14].

The recommendation for physical activity of 150 min per week may be sufficient to reduce VAT with no further reduction with additional activity. It is very important to highlight that exercise can reduce VAT even in the absence of weight loss [15].

According to data from the National Health and Nutrition Examination Survey, central obesity has higher risk of cardiovascular mortality compared with patients with the same BMI but without central adiposity. This has been called normal weight central obesity and expected survival estimates were consistently lower for those with central obesity when controlled for age and BMI [16, 17].

4. Endotelial disfunction

4.1 Atherosclerosis in obesity

The process to atherosclerosis begins with fatty streaks resulting in thickening of the intima arterial layer. Obesity is considered a storm, which accelerates this process by several mechanisms such as insulin resistance through adipocytokines, endothelial dysfunction, hypercoagulability, and inflammation. The VAT makes systemic and vascular inflammation that promotes atherogenesis. Further, insulin resistance has been associated to metabolic syndrome, proinflammatory, and prothrombotic states.

Endothelial dysfunction in obesity has two principal causes: diminished bioavailability of nitric oxide and increased oxidative stress. A good marker of early atherosclerosis is carotid intima media thickness [18].

Several prospective epidemiological studies demonstrate that obesity and higher risk of incident coronary artery disease (CAD) are strongly linked. Excess visceral fat rather than body weight has been linked to increased risk of cardiovascular events. BMI, higher measures of central adiposity, including WC and waist-to-hip ratio (WHR), were aligned with a higher risk of CAD and cardiovascular mortality independently of BMI [19, 20].

Another important concept is the duration of obesity and abdominal adiposity, expressed as excess BMI-years and WC-years, which are stronger predictors of CAD, highlighting these measurements must be evaluated together [21].

4.2 Microvascular disease and obesity

The chronic inflammatory conditions developed from the obesity are linked to abnormalities in the coronary microvasculature. Coronary microvascular disease is pathophysiologically associated with endothelial dysfunction and possibly to small vessel remodeling and also disturbing coronary blood flow; this microvascular disease is independently associated with higher BMI [22].

Obesity has implications in macrophages and adipocytes that generate a proinflammatory state that increases the cytokines and reduces the nitric oxide. All this cascade promotes endothelial dysfunction (**Figure 1**).

Proinflamatory state: ↑IL1β, IL 6, Leptin, TNFα, PCR, ↓NO.
Endothelial Dysfunction: ↑ROS, angiotensinogen, calprotectin ↓NO, Ghrelin.
Metabolic disorders: Changes in glucose and lipid metabolism, insulin resistance, hypertension, atherosclerosis.

IL1 β: Interleukin 1 β, IL6: Interleukin 6, TNF Tumor Necrosis Factor, Nitric Oxide, ROS: Reactive Oxygen Species.

Normally the endothelium regulates vascular homeostasis; it is the natural inner lining of the vessels. Its layers are: tunica intima, tunica media, and the vascular smooth muscle cell (VSMC). But there is a combination-coordination of multiple factors such as blood flow, distribution of nutrients, hormones, and other macronutrients, and migration and proliferation of VSMC. The VSMC is an important

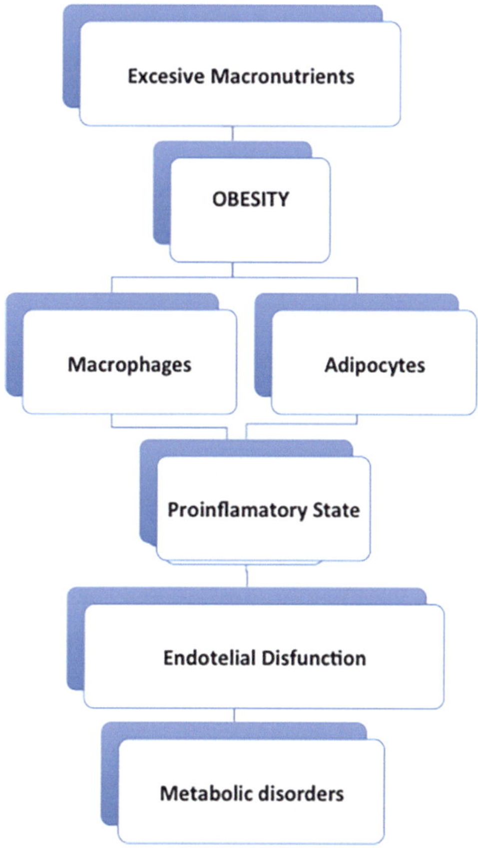

Figure 1.
OBESTITY and PROINFLAMATORY STATE.

component of vessel wall remodeling in response to injury, which controls coagulation and fibrinolysis activities, reduces vascular tone and regulates cellular and vascular adhesions, inhibits leukocyte adhesions, and modulates inflammatory activities and angiogenesis (**Figure 2**).

Vasodilators: Apelin, H2S, NO, PGI2, IgF1.
Permeability: NO, VEGF, ROS, PGI2, PAI1, FGF, Leptin.
Anticoagulant factors: Anti thrombin III, Thrombomodulin.
Angiogenic factors: FGF, TGFβ, VEGF.
Vasoconstrictors: ROS, VCAM, PgH2, Ang II, Resistin.
Inflammatory mediators: Leucotriens, integrins Inmunoglobulins.
Procoagulant factors: TF, PAF, vWF, TXA2, PAI.
Proliferation: NO, TxA2, ROS, PgH2.

H2S: Hydrogen Sulfide, NO: Nitric Oxide, PGI2*: Proctaciclin, IgF1: Insulin Like growth factor 1, VEGF: vascular endothelial growth factor, PAI1: Plaminogen Activator Inhibitor, FGF: Fibroblast Growth Factor, TGFβ: Transforming Growth Factor β, ROS: Reactive Oxygen Species, VCAM: Vascular Cell Adhesion Molecule1, PgH2: Prostaglandin H2, Ang II: Angiotensin II, TF: Tissue Factor; vWF: Von Willebrand Factor, PAF: Platelet Activating Factor, TXA2: thromboxane A2, PAI: Plasminogen Activator Inhibitor1.*

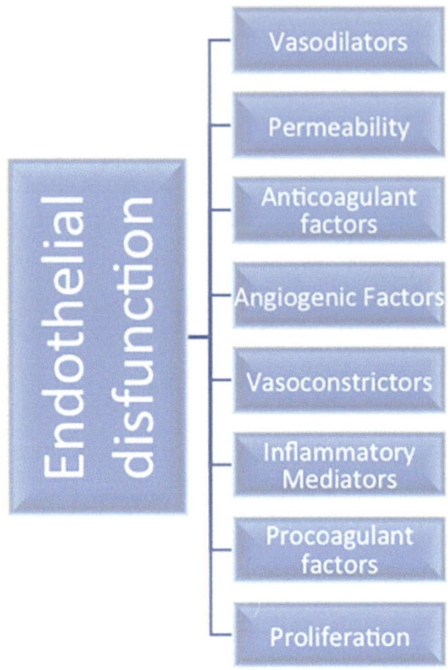

Figure 2.
Endothelial dysfunction and obesity.

Nevertheless, the endothelial dysfunction is usually characterized by the disrupt between secretion and release of vasoconstriction and vasodilation agents, pushing the vascular endothelial toward prothrombotic and proatherogenic effects [23].

Secondly, the distorted provokes that the leukocyte adhesion, activation of platelets, pro-oxidation of mitogens, impaired PGI2, coagulation, and nitric oxide (NO) productions are the features or ¨faulty physiological properties¨ resulted from a dysfunction of endothelium, as well decreased synthesis of EDHF, and vasoconstriction factors including Ang II and prostaglandin (PGH2), atherosclerosis, and thrombosis (**Figure 3**) [23].

The major participating agents of endothelial dysfunction in obesity include: insulin resistance, oxidized form of low-density lipoprotein (oxLDL), adipose tissues related inflammation, and decreased NO bioavailability. Others such as elevated production of ROS and arginase, advanced glycation end products (RAGE), and phenotypic alterations in perivascular adipose tissue result in mild inflammation and elevated leptin with subsequent reduction of adiponectin secretions [24].

Further obesity generates a procoagulant state, which is explained by several mechanisms:

1. Adipose tissue in obesity secretes decreased levels of adiponectin, thereby facilitating the susceptibility of platelets aggregation with the subsequent increased PAI-1 production, which further inhibits fibrinolysis.

2. Macrophages found in adipose tissue also produce TF, which combines with the elevated liver secretion of FVII and FVIII to promote the possibility of coagulation abnormalities.

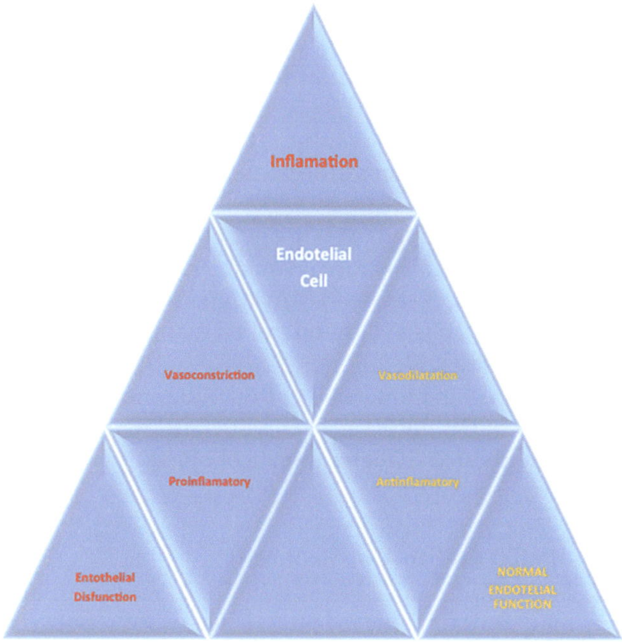

Figure 3.
Proinflamatory and anti-inflammatory state in obesity.

3. Inflammation has been characterized by the imbalance between proinflammatory and procoagulant, and anti-inflammatory and anticoagulant activities of the endothelium, leading to disturbance of the hemostatic system.

4.3 Endothelial dysfunction, epigenetic modifications, and vascular calcification

Epigenetic modifications such as DNA methylation and histone acetylation are described. Previous studies have recognized changes in expression of methyltransferase linked with hypomethylation of hypermethylated genomic regions. These findings are linked between epigenetic modifications and atherosclerosis.

Vascular calcification (VC) is one of the mechanisms that influences vascular remodeling due to the differentiation of vascular smooth muscle cells (VSMCs), alterations in elastin, collagen, and endothelial dysfunction. VC increases the chances of cardiovascular mortality and morbidity, especially in individuals with obesity, type 2 diabetes mellitus (T2DM), and chronic kidney disease [25]. Several studies have identified the correlation between ROS generation, particularly H2 O2 (hydrogen peroxide), and the progression of vascular calcification. An elevated level of ROS triggers MMP (matrix metalloproteinase) activity and alteration in collagen and elastin deposition [26].

4.4 How the gut microbiota affects on vascular endothelium

Gut microbiota is the collection of bacteria that inhabitat gastrointestinal tract and have many repercussions in health. Several studies have indicated that gut microbiota plays a contributing role in atherosclerosis through modulating inflammation and the secretion of microbial metabolites. Recent studies have shown the influence of gut disbiosis and progression of atherosclerosis and cardiovascular disease. Bacteria such as *Akkermansia muciniphila* promote barrier function and have attenuating effect against atherosclerosis [27].

Scientists have found that the relative abundance of Roseburia and Eubacterium was lower, while Collinsella was higher in atherosclerosis patients compared with healthy controls [28].

Variety of metabolites are derived from the gut microbiota, as well as co-metabolism of gut microbiota such as amines methylamines, polyamines, short-chain fatty acids (SCFAs), trimethylamine N-oxide (TMAO), and secondary bile acids (BAs). SCFAs are a group of well-established gut microbial metabolites that are critically involved in metabolic diseases [27].

Diet has an important role in biodiversity of microbiome and hemostasis for maintaining human health. Disbiosis has been associated with progression of various diseases including CVD, obesity, diabetes, nonalcoholic fatty liver disease, and some types of cancer.

4.5 Molecular endothelial dysfunction in obesity

There are many bioquimical makers of endothelial dysfunction: first MCP1 (monocyte chemotactic and activating factor). This protein is synthesized by several types of cells, including inflammatory and inflammation-mediated cells, monocytic cells, human tubular epithelial cells (TECs), and renal-mediated cells in response to various stimuli and when joint to chemokine receptor 2 (CCR2) initiates various monocyte-mediated proinflammatory signals and monocyte chemoattractant activities, facilitating monocytes migration to the subendothelium and combines with ox-LDL to form foam cells, forming a fatty streak and eventual atherosclerotic plaque (**Figure 4**) [29].

5. Obesity and atherosclerosis

Obesity increases morbidity and mortality especially when associated to hypertension and CAD [30].

Obesity is associated with overt atherosclerotic lesions even after accounting for the impact of these metabolic cardiovascular risk factors. The association of obesity with raised atherosclerotic lesions among men in the Pathobiological Determinants of Atherosclerosis in Youth study was present only for those with a thick abdominal panniculus, indicating the fundamental role of central adiposity in the development of atherosclerotic disease [31]. Chronic inflammation induced by obesity increases the likelihood of low-density lipoprotein oxidation, which promotes atherogenesis [32]. Other factors together increase atherosclerosis are insulin resistance and metabolic syndrome.

Endothelial dysfunction in obesity is principally caused by diminished bioavailability of nitric oxide in the setting of inflammation and oxidative stress [33].

A prospective study published by Whintlock et al. describes an increase of probability of mortality stroke in a range of 25–50 kg/m2, each 5 kg/m2 is associated with 40% higher stroke mortality. A prospective cohort study with 3.2 million person-year by follow-up from 1964 to 2015 concluded that overweight and obesity shortened longevity and increased lifetime risk [34].

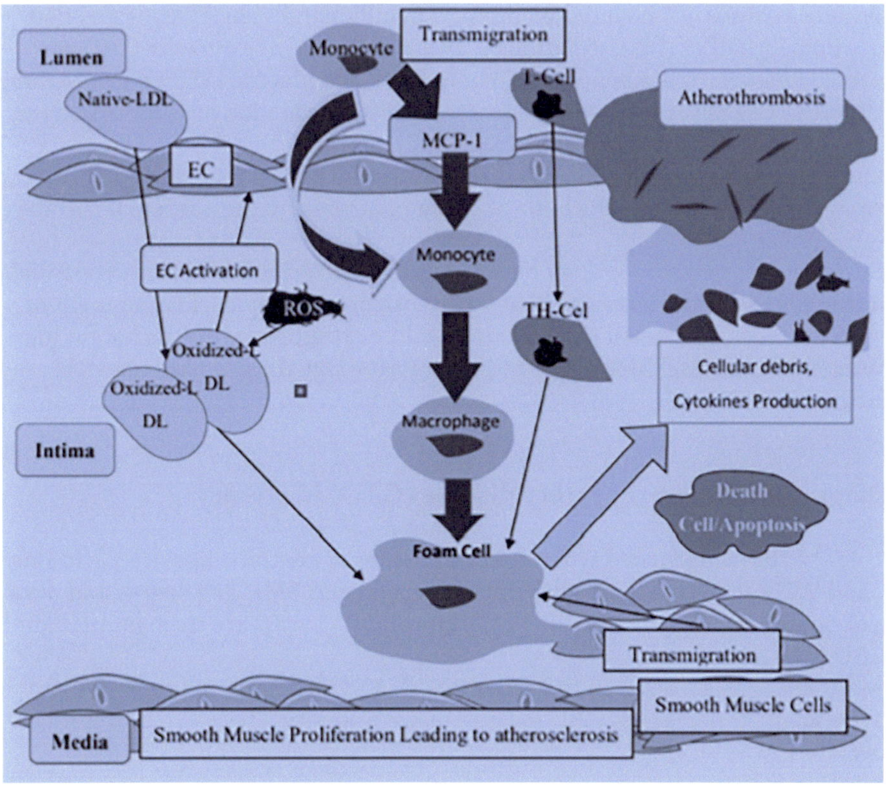

Figure 4.
Bioquimical markers of endothelial dysfunction.

There are important differences in obesity according to gender that must be taken into account, such as the impact of hormones in women against the development of atherosclerosis.

Before menopause, women generally have greater vagal than sympathetic tone, and lower levels of total cholesterol and LDL-C than men. Additionally, differences in glucose and lipid metabolism, sex hormones, and cytokine production are thought to explain why men are at an increased risk of CVD [35, 36]. This recalls the protective effect of estrogens in maintaining health and distribution of body fat. This is likely explained by the aforementioned differences in hormone-driven patterns of fat distribution, with men more likely to deposit visceral fat, compared with subcutaneous fat in women, considering that visceral fat has been associated with greater cardiometabolic risk [37, 38].

Obesity is characterized by an increased risk of diabetes, hypertension, and dyslipidemia, and independently associated with CVD. Several prospective epidemiological studies demonstrate that obesity is associated with higher risk of incident coronary artery disease [39]. There are controversies if obesity causes high risk of CVD or the complications of obesity are the cause of them. Some large prospective analyses have indicated that the link between obesity and CAD is mediated largely by hypertension, dyslipidemia, diabetes, and other comorbidities, whereas other prospective studies suggest a significant residual CAD risk in obesity even after accounting for these risk factors [40].

A meta-analysis of 21 studies including 1.8 million individuals suggested that approximately half of the associations of overweight and obesity with CAD are explained by levels of blood pressure, cholesterol, and glucose [41]. There are three mechanisms linked to metabolic syndrome, that is, production of adipocytokines, oxidative stress, and a prothrombotic state [42].

Other important causative factor is the ectopic fat deposition, especially pericardial and epicardial spaces, which may further contribute to the burden of coronary atherosclerosis [43].

Some studies of pathobiology have shown that arteries with intramyocardial course in perfect condition could have atherosclerosis in epicardial segment of the same artery. Thus, local production of adipocytokines by epicardial fat may modulates blood vessel biology through paracrine signaling or through vasa vasorum [44].

6. Diagnosis of coronary artery disease (CAD) in obesity

CAD has been associated with higher measures of central adiposity, including WC and WHR inclusive those with normal weight and BMI. The degree and duration of obesity expressed as excess BMI years and WC years are stronger predictors of CAD [21].

Many changes can occur in the patients with CAD. There are noninvasive and invasive modalities to assess CAD in patients with obesity. These will be described below.

6.1 Noninvasive CAD assessment

6.1.1 Electrocadiography

Obesity has the potential to affect the ECG in several ways: displacing the heart by elevating the diaphragm in the supine position, increasing the cardiac workload, and increasing the distance between the heart and the recording electrodes.

Several electrocardiographic changes are associated with obesity (**Table 1**).

More frequent ST-segment depression is seen in patients with overweight and CAD, and insulin concentration may be related to the development of the ST-segment depression over time [21].

↑Hear rate
↑QRS interval
↑QT interval
False-positive criteria for inferior myocardial infraction
↑PR interval
ST-T abnormalities
Left axis deviation

Table 1.
Electrocardiographic changes in importance order.

6.1.2 Treadmill stress test

Many patients with obesity fail to achieve 80–85% of the age-predicted heart rate needed for diagnostically valid results.

Chronotropic competence can be reduced in obesity, with a prior study showing that peak heart rate, heart rate recovery, and chronotropic index are lower in patients with obesity, regardless of fitness level [45].

6.1.3 Stress ecocardiography

Stress echocardiography is highly feasible in most cases for patients with obesity through either physiological stress (treadmill exercise) or pharmacological stress (dobutamine).

However, stress echocardiography is highly operator-dependent and can be limited in the presence of poor acoustic windows related to pulmonary disease, breast size, obesity, and respiratory motion. Contrast study in obesity patients is suggested because the sensitivity is better than without contrast. Contrasted images improved sensitivity and specificity (82% vs 70% and 78% vs. 67%, respectively) [46].

6.1.4 PET (positron emission tomography) rubidium

PET rubidium has a 91% sensitivity and 89% specificity and produces less irradiation exposure, better quality of images, a greater degree of diagnosis, reduces invasive examination, and low cardiac death rates in obesity [47].

Therefore, PET rubidium is the nuclear imaging technique of choice for patients with obesity.

6.1.5 Stress cardiac MRI (magnetic resonance imaging)

Stress cardiac MRI and PET are likely the diagnostic techniques least affected by obesity.

The presence of ischemia predicted adverse events at 5 years of follow-up, regardless of whether scar was present. Lack of inducible ischemia is associated with a low annual major adverse coronary events (MACEs) rate of 0.3% at 2 years in patients with obesity [48].

6.1.6 CT calcium score

CAC (coronary artery calcium) is a marker of atherosclerosis that is predictive of cardiovascular events. This technique offers the possibility of determining the presence and extent of calcified coronary artery plaque. Some studies suggest that waist circumference (WC) and waist-to-hip ratio (WHR) provide more useful prognostic information than BMI on the likelihood of elevated CAC. This concept emphasizes the importance of abdominal obesity and pathophysiology of atherosclerosis [49].

6.1.7 Cardiac CT coronary angiography

CT coronary angiography is an alternative for the quantification of calcified or noncalcified plaque. This approach is useful in specific subset of symptomatic patients with obesity or when stress test is equivocal, uninterpretable stress test, or in cases when a discrepancy exists between clinical presentation and stress test results. This technique allows evaluation of luminal stenosis and plaque characterization and quantification [50].

One major challenge with CT coronary angiography is that image quality degrades as BMI increases; this degradation increases in background noise. In patients with overweight can reduce signal-to-noise ratio, and low vessel opacification may occur when contrast is inspected.

6.2 Invasive evaluation of CAD in obesity

6.2.1 Coronary angiography

Patients undergoing catheterization have potential difficulties: suboptimal radiographic visualization, vascular access laborious, bleeding, radial access is preferred in obesity patients because it has been associated with three times lower rate of complications than transfemoral access and higher radiation exposure to both patients with obesity and staff [51].

6.2.2 PCI and obesity

In the Cath PCI Registry after multivariable adjustment obesity was independently associated with a greater mortality rate and lower bleeding rate. Adequate anticoagulation is important in this subpopulation [52, 53]. Another study reported that patients with severe obesity have major risk of contrast-induced nephropathy. Dialysis and vascular complications, gastrointestinal bleeding, and MACE (Major Adverse Cardiovascular Events) are not statistically different [54].

6.2.3 Intravascular ultrasound

Several intravascular imaging techniques such as intravascular ultrasound, virtual histology intravascular ultrasound, and optical coherence tomography allow in vivo assessment of plaque burden, plaque morphology, and response to therapy.

Abdominal visceral adiposity independently predicted the presence and extent of noncalcified coronary plaque that also contained multiple features of plaque vulnerability [55].

The appropriate choice of test to assess CVD depends on local expertise, the relative strengths and weaknesses of each modality, and individual patient characteristics that contribute to the pretest likelihood of CVD and the risk/benefit ratio of using a given modality.

7. Clinical management, treatment, and secondary cardiac disease

Obesity paradox refers to the fact that although obesity increases the risk of CVD for those who had already an CVD, excess weight is not a risk factor to develop adverse outcomes including death [56].

Although weight loss would be believed to significantly benefit cardiovascular outcomes, this benefit has only been shown in weight loss performed through bariatric surgery in which more than 10–15% of body weight is lost; therefore, that modest weight loss has not been shown to impact cardiovascular outcomes [57, 58].

To treat obesity requires a multidisciplinary management in which the eating pattern, amount of exercise, stress, sleep pattern are evaluated. So, it is not enough exercise and nutrition to evaluate all the factors related to weight gain together.

Some clinical trials demonstrate the cardiovascular impact of Mediterranean diet in reducing MACE in patients with high cardiovascular risk. However, lifestyle changes in diabetes patients have failed to show a significant reduction in MACE, only those with weight loss greater than 10% had significant results [59, 60].

Pharmacological treatment has impact on weight reduction as well. For example, liraglutide has been shown to reduce death by 13% and 22% from cardiovascular causes in patients with type 2 diabetes in LEADER trial [61].

Recently semaglutide at 2.4 mg dose in obese patients without diabetes has demonstrated a significant body weight reduction (14.9% vs. 2.4% with placebo). In total, 69% of body weight reduction ≥10% at 68 weeks and 50% body weight reduction ≥15% .

Further reduction in waist circumference, systolic blood pressure, and improvement of physical function [62].

Orlistat was approver in 1998 for the treatment of obesity and demonstrated 37% reduction in progression from prediabetes to diabetes and significant reduction of associated disease such as hypertension and blood lipid levels [63].

Naltrexone SR/Bupropion SR is another drug approved in the United States for the treatment of obesity and has cardiovascular security trial (LIGHT trial – Cardiovascular Outcomes Study of Naltrexone SR/Bupropion SR in Overweight and obese subjects with cardiovascular risk factors). Bupropion suppresses appetite transiently due to an endorphin-mediated mechanism of action. Naltrexone blocks the endorphin, which allows a long-term appetite suppression effect [64]. However, because of the early unanticipated termination of the trial, it is not possible to assess non-inferiority to the prespecified upper limit of 1.4. Consequently, the cardiovascular safety of this treatment remains uncertain and will require evaluation in a new adequately powered outcome trial.

Lorcaserine was approved in the obesity treatment but recently was removed for the Food and Drug Administration (FDA), due to a possible increased risk of cancer [65].

Finally, patients with body mass index greater than 35 kg/m^2 with comorbidities or greater than 40 kg/m^2 without them get benefit from bariatric surgery. Non-randomized prospective studies desmonstrated a reduction of cardiovascular death in this group of patients [66].

8. Conclusions

In conclusion, obesity patients have an important difference than patients with normal weight. First, the chronic inflammation is the principal cause of molecular and cellular changes that have been linked to development of chronic diseases and manifestations due to decreased expansibility of adipose tissue. Endothelial dysfunction is an important factor that contributes to vascular calcification and atherosclerosis. In addition, the intestinal microbiota plays an important role in the development and inflammation of atherosclerotic plaque. Obesity is linked to major risk of CVD and is directly proportional to the amount of excess weight, it can be explained by blood pressure, cholesterol, and glucose levels. Diagnosis must be evaluated according to the risk and the clinical probability of suffering an event, evaluating the expected changes at the electrocardiographic level that can lead to overdiagnosis. Finally, remember that there are currently multiple noninvasive studies for the early diagnosis of cardiovascular disease, which have allowed more timely diagnoses to be made in obese patients.

Conflict of interest

The authors declare no conflict of interest.

Author details

Pedro Felipe Parra Velasco
Luz Karina Rojas Cañaveral, (s), Popayan, Colombia

*Address all correspondence to: doctorpedroparra@gmail.com

References

[1] Rangel-Huerta OD, Pastor-Villaescusa B, Gil A. Are we close to defining a metabolomic signature of human obesity? A systematic review of metabolomics studies. Metabolomics. 13 Jun 2019;**15**(6):93. DOI: 10.1007/s11306-019-1553-y. PMID: 31197497; PMCID: PMC6565659

[2] Flegal KM, Kruszon-Moran D, Carroll MD, Fryar CD, Ogden CL. Trends in obesity among adults in theunited states, 2005 to 2014. Journal of the American Medical Association. 2016;**315**(21):2284-2291

[3] Bray GA, Heisel WE, Afshin A, Jensen MD, Dietz WH, Long M, et al. The science of obesity management: An endocrine society scientific statement. Endocrine Reviews. 2018;**39**(2):79-71

[4] Heit JA, Spencer FA, White RH. The epidemiology of venous thromboembolism. Journal of Thrombosis and Thrombolysis. 2016;**41**:3-14. DOI: 10.1007// s11239-015-1311-6

[5] Sahakyan KR, Somers VK, Rodriguez-Escudero JP, Hodge DO, Carter RE, Sochor O, et al. Normal-weight central obesity: Imlications for total and cardiovascular mortality. Annals of Internal Medicine. 2015;**163**:827-835. DOI: 10.7326/M14-2525

[6] Larsen BA, Laughlin GA, Saad SD, Barrett-Connor E, Allison MA, Wassel CL. Pericardial fat is associated with all casus mortality but not incidente CVD: The rancho Bernardo study. Atherosclerosis. 2015;**239**:470-475. DOI: 10.1016/j.atherosclerosis.2015.02.022

[7] Al-Talabany S, Mordi I, Graeme Houston J, Colhoun HM, Weir-McCall JR, Matthew SZ, et al. Epicardial adipose tissue is related to arterial stiffness and inflammation in patients with cardiovascular disease and type 2 diabetes. BMC Cardiovascular Disorders. 2018;**18**:31. DOI: 10.1186/ s12872-018-0770-z

[8] Shah RV, Anderson A, Ding JZ, Budoff M, Rider O, Petersen SE, et al. Pericardial, but not hepatic, fat by CT is associated with cv outcomes and structure: The multi-ethnic study of atherosclerosis. JACC Cardiovascular Imaging. 2017;**10**:1016-1027. DOI: 10.1016/j.jcmg.2016.10.024

[9] Larsen BA, Laughlin GA, Saad SD, Barrett-Connor E, Allison MA, Wassel CL. Pericardial fat is associated with all-cause mortality but not incident CVD: The rancho Bernardo. Study. Atherosclerosis. 2015;**239**:470-475. DOI: 10.10.1016/j. atherosclerosis.2015.02.022

[10] Iacobellis G. Local and systemic effects of the multifaceted epicardial adipose tissue depot. Nature Reviews Endocrinology. Jun 2015;**11**(6):363-371. DOI: 10.1038/nrendo.2015.58. Epub 2015 Apr 7. PMID: 25850659

[11] St-Onge MP, Grandner MA, Brown D, Conroy MB, Jean-Louis G, Coons M, et al. On behalf of the American Heart Association obesity, behavior change, diabetes, and nutrition committees of the council on lifestyle and Cardiometabolic health; council on cardiovascular disease in the young; council on clinical cardiology; and stroke council. Sleep duration and quality: Impact. Association. Circulation. 2016;**134**:e367-e386

[12] Verheggen RJ, Maessen MF, Green DJ, Hermus AR, Hopman MT, Thijssen DH.

A systematic review and meta-analysis on the effects of exercise training versus hypocaloric diet: Distinct effects on body weight and visceral adipose tissue. Obesity Reviews. 2016;**17**:664-690. DOI: 10.1111/obr.12406

[13] Hintze LJ, Messier V, Lavoie MÉ, Brochu M, Lavoie JM, Prud'homme D, et al. A one-year resistance training program following weight loss has no significant impact on body composition and energy expenditure in postmenopausal women living with overweight and obesity. Phyisiology Behaviour. 15 May 2018;**189**:99-106. DOI: 10.1016/j.physbeh.2018.03.014. Epub 2018 Mar 13. PMID: 29549030

[14] Rabkin SW, Campbell H. Comparison of reducing epicardial fat by exercise, diet or bariatric surgery weight loss strategies: A systematic review and meta-analysis. Obesity Reviews. 2015;**2015**(16):406-415. DOI: 10.1111/obr.12270

[15] Friedenreich CM, Neilson HK, O'Reilly R, Duha A, Yasui Y, Morielli AR, et al. Effects of a high vs moderate volume of aerobic exercise on adiposity outcomes in postmenopausal women: A randomized clinical trial. JAMA Oncology. 2015;**1**:766-776. DOI: 10.1001/jamaoncol.2015.2239

[16] Sahakyan KR, Somers VK, Rodriguez-Escudero JP, Hodge DO, Carter RE, Sochor O, et al. Normal-weight central obesity: Implications for total and cardiovascula mortality. Annals of Internal Medicine. 2015;**163**:827-835

[17] Coutinho T, Goel K, de Sa DC, Carter RE, Hodge DO, Kragelund C, et al. Combining body mass index with measures of central obesity in the assessment of mortality in subjects with coronary disease: Role of normal weight central obesity. Journal of the American College of Cardiology. 2013;**61**:553-560. DOI: 10.1016/j.jacc.2012.10.035

[18] De Michele M, Panico S, Iannuzzi A, Celentano E, Ciardullo AV, Galasso R, et al. Association of obesity and central fat distribution with carotid artery wall thickening in middle-aged women. Stroke. 2002;**33**:2923-2928. DOI: 10.1161/01.str.0000038989.90931.be

[19] Romero-Corral A, Somers VK, Sierra-Johnson J, Korenfeld Y, Boarin S, Korinek J, et al. Normal weight obesity: A risk factor for cardiometabolic dysregulution and cardiovascular mortality. European Heart Journal. 2010;**31**:737-746. DOI: 10.1093/eurheartj/ehp487

[20] Sahakyan KR, Somers VK, Rodriguez-Escudero JP, Hodge DO, Carter RE, Sochor O, et al. Normal-weight central obesity: Implications for total and cardiovascular mortality. Annals of Internal Medicine. 2015;**163**:827-835. DOI: 10.7326/M14-2525

[21] Reis JP, Allen N, Gunderson EP, Lee JM, Lewis CE, Loria CM, et al. Excess body mass index- and waist circumference-years and incident cardiovascular disease: The CARDIA study. Obesity. 2015;**23**:879-885. DOI: 10.1002/oby.21023

[22] Kwaifa IK, Bahari H, Yong YK, Md NS. Endothelial dysfunction in obesity-induced inflammation: Molecular mechanisms and clinical implications. Biomolecules. 2020;**10**(2):291

[23] Sena CM, Pereira AM, Seica R. The endothelial dysfunction-a major mediator of diabetic vascular disease. Biochimica et Biophysica Acta. 2013;**1832**:2216-2231

[24] Olive M, Harten I, Mitchell R, Beers JK, Djabali K, Cao K, et al.

Cardiovascular pathology in Hutchinson-Gilford progeria: Correlation with the vascular pathology of ageing. Arteriosclerosis, Thrombosis, and Vascular Biology. 2010;**30**:2301-2309

[25] Omar A, Chatterjee TK, Tang Y, Hui DY, Weintraub NL. The proinflammatory phenotype of perivascular adipocytes. Atherosclerosis Thrombosis and Vascular Biology. 2014;**34**:1631-1636

[26] Gerhard M, Roddy MA, Creager SJ, Creager MA. Aging progressively impairs endothelium-dependent vasodilation in forearm resistance vessels of humans. Hypertension. 1996;**27**:849-853ç

[27] Li X, Shimizu Y, Kimura I. Gut microbial metabolite short-chain fatty acids and obesity. Bioscience, Microbiota Food Health. 2017;**36**:135-140

[28] Karlsson FH, Fak F, Nookaew I, Tremaroli V, Fagerberg B, Petranovic D, et al. Symptomatic atherosclerosis is associated with an altered gut metagenome. Nature Communications. 2012;**3**:1245. DOI: 10.1038/ncomms2266

[29] Zhang X, Liu X, Shang H, Xu Y, Qian M. Monocyte chemoattractant protein-1 induces endothelial cell apoptosis in vitro through a p53-dependent mitochondrial pathway. Acta Biochimica et Biophysica Sinica. 2011;**43**:787-795

[30] Rocha VZ, Libby P. Obesity, inflammation, and atherosclerosis. Nature Reviews. Cardiology. 2009;**6**(6):399-409. DOI: 10.1038/nrcardio.2009.55

[31] Zieske AW, Malcom GT, Strong JP. Natural history and risk factors of atherosclerosis in children and youth: The PDAY study. Pediatric Pathology & Molecular Medicine. 2002;**21**:213-237. DOI: 10.1080/15227950252852104

[32] Romero-Corral A, Somers VK, Sierra-Johnson J, Korenfeld Y, Boarin S, Korinek J, et al. Normal weight obesity: A risk factor for cardiometabolic dysregulation and cardiovascular mortality. European Heart Journal. 2010;**31**:737-746. DOI: 10.1093/eurheartj/ehp487

[33] Engin A. Endothelial dysfunction in obesity. Advances in Experimental Medicine and Biology. 2017;**960**:345-379. DOI: 10.1007/978-3-319-48382-5_15

[34] Prospective Studies C, Whitlock G, Lewington S, Sherliker P, Clarke R, Emberson J, et al. Body-mass index and cause-specific mortality in 900 000 adults: Collaborative analyses of 57 prospective studies. Lancet. 2009;**373**(9669):1083-1096. DOI: 10.1016/S0140-6736(09)60318-4

[35] Khan SS, Ning H, Wilkins JT, Allen N, Carnethon M, Berry JD, et al. Association of body mass index with lifetime risk of cardiovascular disease and compression of morbidity. JAMA Cardiology. 2018;**3**(4):280-287. DOI: 10.1001/jamacardio.2018.0022

[36] Song X, Tabak AG, Zethelius B, Yudkin JS, Soderberg S, Laatikainen T, et al. Obesity attenuates gender differences in cardiovascular mortality. Cardiovascular Diabetology. 2014;**13**(1):144. DOI: 10.1186/s12933-014-0144-5

[37] Varlamov O, Bethea CL, Roberts CT Jr. Sex-specific differences in lipid and glucose metabolism. Frontiers in Endocrinology. 2014;**5**:241

[38] Sironi AM, Petz R, De Marchi D, Buzzigoli E, Ciociaro D, Positano V, et al. Impact of increased visceral and cardiac

fat on cardiometabolic risk and disease. Diabetic Medicine. 2012;**29**(5):622-627. DOI: 10.1111/j.1464-5491.2011.03503.x

[39] Calle EE, Thun MJ, Petrelli JM, Rodriguez C, Heath CW Jr. Body-mass index and mortality in a prospective cohort of U.S. adults. betwen multiple cardiovascular risk factors and atherosclerosis in children and young adults. N Engl J Med. 198;**338**:1650-1656. DOI: 10.1056/NEJM199806043382302

[40] Hubert HB, Feinleib M, McNamara PM, Castelli WP. Obesity as an independent risk factor for cardiovascular disease: A 26-year follow-up of participants in the Framingham heart study. Circulation. 1983;**67**:968-977. DOI: 10.1161/01.cir.67.5.968

[41] Lu Y, Hajifathalian K, Ezzati M, Woodward M, Rimm EB, Danaei G. Global burden of metabolic risk factors for chronic diseases collaboration (BMI mediated effects). Metabolic mediators of the effects of body-mass index, overweight, and obesity on coronary heart disease and stroke: A pooled analysis of 97 prospective cohorts with 1·8 million participants. Lancet. 2014;**383**(9921):970-983. DOI: 10.1016/S0140-6736(13)61836-X

[42] Grundy SM. Metabolic syndrome update. Trends in Cardiovascular Medicine. 2016;**26**:364-373. DOI: 10.1016/j.tcm.2015.10.004

[43] Shimabukuro M, Hirata Y, Tabata M, Dagvasumberel M, Sato H, Kurobe H, et al. Epicardial adipose tissue volume and adipocytokine imbalance are strongly linked to human coronary atherosclerosis. Arteriosclerosis, Thrombosis, and Vascular Biology. 2013;**33**:1077-1084. DOI: 10.1161/ATVBAHA.112.300829

[44] Ishii T, Asuwa N, Masuda S, Ishikawa Y. The effects of a myocardial bridge on coronary atherosclerosis and ischaemia. J Pathol. 1998;**185**:4-9

[45] Adachi H, Hashimoto R, Tsuruta M, Jacobs DR Jr, Crow RS, Imaizumi T. Hyperinsulinemia and the development of ST-T electrocardiographic abnormalities: An 11-year follow-up study. Diabetes Care. 1997;**20**:1688-1692. DOI: 10.2337/diacare.20.11.1688

[46] Gondoni LA, Titon AM, Nibbio F, Augello G, Caetani G, Liuzzi A. Heart rate behavior during an exercise stress test in obese patients. Nutrition, Metabolism, and Cardiovascular Diseases. 2009;**19**:170-176. DOI: 10.1016j.numecd.2008.07.001

[47] Hu SJ, Liu SX, Katus HA, Luedde M. The value of contrast dobutamine stress echocardiography on detecting coronary artery disease in overweight and obese patients. The Canadian Journal of Cardiology. 2007;**23**:885-889. DOI: 10.1016/s0828-282x(07)70844-9

[48] Chow BJ, Dorbala S, Di Carli MF, Merhige ME, Williams BA, Veledar E, et al. Prognostic value of PET myocardial perfusion imaging in obese patients. JACC: Cardiovascular Imaging. 2014;**7**:278-287. DOI: 10.1016/jjcmg.2013.12.008

[49] Shah RV, Heydari B, Coelho-Filho O, Abbasi SA, Feng JH, Neilan TG, et al. Vasodilator stress perfusion CMR imaging is feasible and prognostic in obese patients. JACC: Cardiovascular Imaging. 2014;**7**:462-472. DOI: 10.1016/j.jcmg.2013.11.011

[50] See R, Abdullah SM, McGuire DK, Khera A, Patel MJ, Lindsey JB, et al. The association of differing measures of overweight and obesity with prevalent atherosclerosis: The Dallas

heart study. Journal of the American College of Cardiology. 2007;**50**:752-759. DOI: 10.1016/j.jacc.2007.04.066

[51] Labounty TM, Gomez MJ, Achenbach S, Al-Mallah M, Berman DS, Budoff MJ, et al. Body mass index and the prevalence, severity, and risk of coronary artery disease: An international multicentre study of 13 874 patients. European Heart Journal Cardiovascular Imaging. 2013;**14**:456-463. DOI: 10.1093/ehjci/jes179

[52] Hibbert B, Simard T, Wilson KR, Hawken S, Wells GA, Ramirez FD, et al. Transradial versus transfemoral artery approach for coronary angiography and percutaneous coronary intervention in the extremely obese. JACC. Cardiovascular Interventions. 2012;**5**:819-826. DOI: 10.1016/j.jcin.2012.04.009

[53] Ohashi N, Yamamoto H, Horiguchi J, Kitagawa T, Kunita E, Utsunomiya H, et al. Association between visceral adipose tissue area and coronary plaque morphology assessed by CT angiography. JACC: Cardiovascular Imaging. 2010;**3**:908-917. DOI: 10.1016/j.jcmg.2010.06.014

[54] Payvar S, Kim S, Rao SV, Krone R, Neely M, Paladugu N, et al. In hospital outcomes of percutaneous coronary interventions in extremely obese and normal-weight patients: Findings from the NCDR (National Cardiovascular Data Registry). Journal of American College of Cardiology. 2013;**62**:692-696. DOI: 10.1016/j.jacc.2013.05.058

[55] Buschur ME, Smith D, Share D, Campbell W, Mattichak S, Sharma M, et al. The burgeoning epidemic of morbid obesity in patients undergoing percutaneous coronary intervention: Insight from the blue cross blue shield of Michigan cardiovascular consortium. Journal of the American College of Cardiology. 2013;**62**:688-689. DOI: 10.1016/j.jacc.2013.06.004 [PubMed: 23948512]

[56] Lavie CJ, Laddu D, Arena R, Ortega FB, Alpert MA, Kushner RF. Healthy weight and obesity prevention: JACC health promotion series. Journal of the American College of Cardiology. 25 Sep 2018;**72**(13):1514-1515. DOI: 10.1016/j.jacc.2018.08.1037. PMID: 30236314

[57] Ma C, Avenell A, Bolland M, Hudson J, Stewart F, Robertson C, et al. Effects of weight loss interventions for adults who are obese on mortality, cardiovascular disease, and cancer: Systematic review and meta-analysis. BMJ. 2017;**359**:j4849. DOI: 10.1136/bmj.j4849

[58] Sjöström L, Peltonen M, Jacobson P, Sjöström CD, Karason K, Wedel H, et al. Bariatric surgery and long-term cardiovascular events. JAMA. 2012;**307**:56-65. DOI: 10.1001/jama.2011.1914

[59] Estruch R, Ros E, Salas-Salvadó J, Covas M-I, Corella D, Arós F, et al. Primary prevention of cardiovascular disease with a Mediterranean diet supplemented with extra-virgin Olive oil or nuts. The New England Journal of Medicine. 2018;**378**(25):e34

[60] Gregg EW, Jakicic JM, Lewis CE, Regensteiner JG, Pi-Sunyer X, Wing RR, et al. Look AHEAD research group. Association of the magnitude of weight loss and changes in physical fitness with long-term cardiovascular disease outcomes in overweight or obese people with type 2 diabetes: A post-hoc analysis of the look AHEAD randomised clinical trial. The Lancet Diabetes and Endocrinology. 2016;**4**:913-921. DOI: 10.1016/S2213-8587(16)30162-0

[61] Mann JFE, Nauck MA, Nissen SE, Pocock S, Ph D, Zinman B, et al. Liraglutide and cardiovascular outcomes in type 2 diabetes. Drug and Therapeutics Bulletin. 2016;**54**(9):101

[62] Wilding JPH, Batterham RL, Calanna S, Davies M, Van Gaal LF, Lingvay I, et al. Once-weekly Semaglutide in adults with overweight or obesity. The New England Journal of Medicine. 2021;**384**(11):989-1002

[63] Js T, J H, Mn B, L S. Xenical in the prevention of diabetes in obese subjects (XENDOS) study. Diabetes Care. 2004;**27**(1):155-161

[64] Nissen SE, Wolski KE, Prcela L, Wadden T, Buse JB, Bakris G, et al. Effect of naltrexone-bupropion on major adverse cardiovascular events in overweight and obese patients with cardiovascular risk factors: A randomized clinical trial. JAMA. 2016;**315**(10):990-1004

[65] FDA. El ensayo clínico de seguridad demuestra un posible aumento del riesgo de cáncer con el medicamento para la perdida de peso Beviq, Belviq R (lorcaserina). Estados Unidos: Food and Drug administration; 14 de Enero de 2020, 24 de Julio de 2022

[66] English WJ, Spann MD, Aher CV, Williams DB. Cardiovascular risk reduction following metabolic and bariatric surgery. Annals of Translation Medicine. 2020;**8**(S1):S12-S12

Chapter 6

Thrombotic Events in Cancer Patients

Azin Alizadehasl and Haniye Hajiali Fini

Abstract

Cancer poses the highest clinical and social burden throughout the world and is the second cause of death after is chemic heart disease, although will be predicted the first in 2060. Cancer patients are high risk for thrombotic events that are characterized as the second cause of death after cancer itself. Thrombotic events seem to be increasing over recent years according to improved patients survival, novel thrombogenic cancer treatment and central catheter using. As we know thromboprophylaxis reduces the risk of VTE and primary prevention seems to be more effective way to reduce morbidity and mortality in these patients several criteria was designed to reduce this risk. Khorana risk score is the most important of them which designed for ambulatory cancer patients. Some other risk factors for thrombotic events consist of major abdominal surgery and prolonged immobility after surgery, use of thrombogenic medications (chemotherapy agents), old age, obesity, distant metastasis or advanced stage at the time of diagnosis, hyperthermic intraperitoneal chemotherapy (HIPEC) as a new surgery technique, anemia that requires blood transfusion that recommend special attention should be paid to them.

Keywords: cancer, cancer-associated thrombosis, thromboprophylaxis, Khorana score, venous thromboembolism, arterial thromboembolism, cardiotoxicity, cardiooncology

1. Introduction

Cancer poses the highest clinical and social burden throughout the world which is nonsignificantly higher in men than women. The risk of developing cancer is 20.2% for lifelong (22.4% in men and 18.2% in women). Cancer is the second cause of death after ischemic heart disease, although it will be predicted the first in 2060 [1]. The Studies demonstrated 19.3 million new cancer patients and about 10 million cancer deaths occurred in 2020 [2].

Breast cancer has recognized as the most common malignancy followed by lung, liver, colorectal, prostate, and stomach cancers [1, 2]. Despite breast cancer prevalence outstrip lung cancer over the time, the most common causes of death include lung, liver, and stomach cancers, respectively [2, 3].

Thrombus can involve either veins or arteries and is associated with substantial morbidity and mortality as the third most common cardiovascular disease [4]. Acute vein and artery thrombosis is computed as the most common causes of death in developed country. The epidemiology of thrombus depends on if it is venous versus arterial, provoked versus unprovoked, or first episode versus subsequent episode. Thrombus etiology is multifactorial [5]. Main components of thrombus consist of fibrin, platelets, red blood cells (RBCs), leukocytes [6]. Thrombosis occurs with low shear flow and intact endothelial wall in veins and is associated with severe shear, damaged endothelial wall, and platelet-rich clot formation in arteries [4]. Vein thrombosis is more common due to low velocity of venous blood flow. Sedentary lifestyle, immobilization, contraception agents, pregnancy, surgery, coagulation disorders, high haematocrit level and increased blood viscosity, varicose veins, obesity, infectious disease, and using intravenous drug can contribute to it [4].

Vein or artery thrombus can break away and be transferred to lung or cerebral and peripheral vessels, respectively. Thus, it is important to protect thrombus formation or be diagnosed and start adequate treatment as soon as possible [4].

Cancer patients are high risk for both venous and arterial thromboembolism that are characterized as the second cause of death after cancer itself. Malignancies are responsible for about 18% of all cases with venous thromboembolism (VTE) [7, 8]. Venous thrombosis prevalence in patients with cancer is four- to sevenfold higher compared to healthy individuals [8], and some research reported this risk may be increased up to 28-fold in certain malignancies [7]. A study showed that arterial thrombosis assigns about 5.6% of death in cancer patients. Thrombotic events seem to be increasing over recent years according to improved patients survival, novel thrombogenic cancer treatment, and using central catheter. Venous thromboembolism (VTE) in cancer patients is not limited to deep veins and pulmonary embolism, unusual sites of thrombosis are reported such as upper extremities and cerebral or splanchnic veins. Arterial thromboembolism (ATE) also manifests as myocardial infarction (MI) or cerebrovascular accident (CVA) predominantly [8].

2. Risk factors of thrombosis in cancer patients

2.1 Patient-related risk factors include as follows

- Age of 70 years or older—aging is accompanied by increased immobility and systemic activation of coagulation.

- Black ethnic—some studies suggested higher rate of thrombosis in black patients with cancer, although data show conflicting too.

- Immobility—bed rest of greater than 3 days is related to higher rate of thrombotic events.

- Poor functional status.

- Inherited coagulation disorders such as antithrombin (AT), protein C and protein S deficiency, or factor V leiden and factor II G20210A are related to thrombotic events at younger age.

- Medical comorbidities such as heart disease, obesity, infection, respiratory disease, renal disease, and anemia lead to 1.5-fold and higher risk for thrombus formation in cancer patients.

- Prior history of thromboembolism—risk of venous thromoembolism (VTE) recurrence is about six- to sevenfold in patients with malignancy and history of VTE [8, 9].

2.2 Cancer-related risk factors are delineated based on malignancy site, stage, histopathology, and time after diagnosis

- Malignancy site—the highest risk for thrombotic events is for pancreatic cancer and then primary brain tumor, stomach, esophagus, uterus and ovarian, lung cancers, and hematologic malignancies such as non-hodgkin lymphoma and multiple myeloma.

- Malignancy stage—researches show that almost half of cancer patients with thromboembolism at time of cancer diagnose have advanced stage or metastasis. A study reported fourfold increased risk of venous thromboembolism (VTE) in cancer patients without metastasis compared to increased 58-fold in patients who had distant metastasis.

Peritoneal surface malignancy (PSM) can be a manifestation of cancer metastasis from colorectal or ovarian malignant sites. Although, new methods of treatment such as cytoreductive surgery (CRS) and hyperthermic intraperitoneal chemotherapy (HIPECH) can improve survival, these procedures are related to activating of coagulation cascade. Postoperative venous thromboembolism risk in PSM patients is as high as 30-50% without thrombo prophylaxis.

- Tumor histopathology—the studies have shown that histological subtypes of some cancers may have different risk for thrombotic events.

- Time after cancer diagnosis: 3–6 months after cancer diagnosis is highest risk full time for thrombotic events. Although, some other research suggest that greatest risk of thromboembolism is within the first year following diagnosis [8–10]. Eventually, this risk decreases within 10 years after cancer diagnosis [11].

2.3 Treatment-related factors—thrombotic events can increase with surgery, anticancer therapies, and supportive care in cancer patients

- Chemotherapy agents—using some chemotherapeutic agents lead to increase two- to sixfold risk of thrombosis. Cisplatin regimen has a known effect in this way and increases risk for both vein and arterial thrombosis events. Immunomodulatory agents like thalidomide and lenalidomide can increase risk for venous and arterial thromboembolism, about 1.98% for myocardial infarction (MI) and 3.4% for cerebrovascular accident (CVA). Bevacizumab, a monoclonal antibody against vascular endothelial growth factor receptor (VEGFR), increases the risk of arterial rather than the vein thromboembolism events.

- Hospital admission for acute medical illness or surgery (especially pelvic and abdominal cancer surgery) is associated with increasing risk of thrombosis formation. The reports demonstrated two- to threefold risk of thrombotic events in these cases.

- Supportive care—supportive treatment including erythropoiesis-stimulating agents, red blood cell, and platelet transfusion lead to venous thromboembolism in cancer patients [8, 9].

Central venous catheters are important access to delivery of intravenous drugs in cancer patients. The incidence of catheter-related thrombosis is estimated about 5–30% and can interrupt chemotherapy treatment or cause substantial morbidity including pulmonary emboli and post-phlebitic syndrome [9].

Recent studies reported that high leukocyte and platelet counts and low hemoglobin level are associated with higher risk of venous thromboembolism in patients with malignancy [8].

3. Cancer-associated thrombosis mechanisms

Patients with malignancy often have several predisposing factors for thrombus formation. Traditionally, Virchow's triad including stasis, thrombophilia, and endothelial damage have a critical role in pathophysiology of thromboembolism in these patients. Tumor compression and bed rest condition can lead to blood stasis. Homeostasis disturbance, hypercoagulable state, and inflammation have a key role in pathogenesis of thrombosis. Endothelial dysfunction can be the result of abnormal tumor vascularity as a mechanism for thrombosis formation [4, 12–14]. Cancer can conduce to the presence of antiphospholipid antibody, decrease in hepatic anticoagulant synthesis, and reduced hepatic clearance of coagulation factors, too [14]. Finally, imbalance between procoagulative factors and fibrinolytic system lead to cancer-associated thrombosis [12].

3.1 Directed mechanism of cancer-associated thrombosis: several factors expressed on or released from cancer cells

- Tissue factor (TF) is the most important tumor-derived procoagulant protein that expresses on tumoral cells as an initiator of extrinsic pathway in coagulation cascade and results in the activation of factor II and fibrin synthesis and platelet activation. Although, the relation between tumor TF expression and risk of thrombotic events has been observed only in pancreatic and ovarian cancers.

- Microparticle (MP) is membrane vesicle that is released from cancer cells, and its procoagulative effect is associated with the expression of active tissue factor on it which cause platelet activation and thrombus formation. Although, this relation between microparticles and thrombotic events has only been in pancreatic cancer.

- Podoplanin (PDPN) is expressed by cancer-associated fibroblasts and causes platelets activation and aggregation. It has been reported in pancreatic cancer cells.

- Plasminogen activator inhibitor- (PAI-1) has been shown to be expressed on pancreatic cancer cells and is an inhibitor of fibrinolysis, thus increasing the risk of thrombosis formation.

- Cancer cells can secrete and generate platelets agonists such as adenosine diphosphate (ADP) and thrombin that cause platelets activation and aggregation [9, 12, 15].

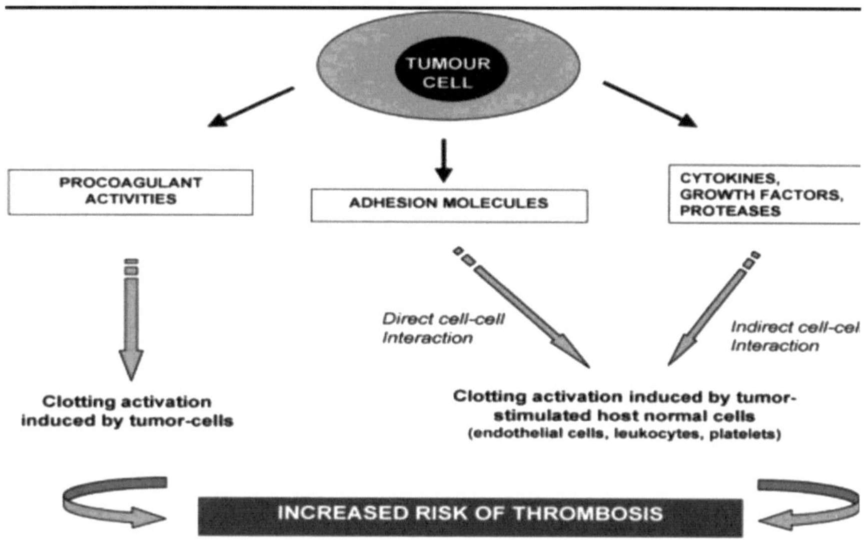

Figure 1.
Hemeostatic system activation by tumor cells [16].

3.2 Indirect mechanism of cancer-associated thrombosis

Indirect mechanism also promotes thrombosis events in cancer patients. Tumoral cells can synthesis and secrete numerous thrombogenic inflammatory cytokines which lead to the expression of specific adhesion molecules on surface of endothelial cells and monocytes, so cause activation of endothelial cells and procoagulant properties [9, 13, 14] (**Figure 1**).

4. Prophylaxis of vein thrombotic events in cancer patients

Venous thromboembolism in cancer patients is accompanied with poor prognosis due to complications such as pulmonary embolism or reflecting the advanced stages of cancer as the more important factor. Cancer patients are prone to failure of anticoagulation therapy. Receiving anticoagulant agents can lead to major bleeding two to six times. In contrast, venous thromboembolism (VTE) recurrences occur two to three times in these patients. Thus, primary prevention seems to be more effective way to reduce morbidity and mortality related with thrombotic events in patients with malignancy [17]. However, about 75% of patients do not receive appropriate prophylaxis treatment [18].

4.1 Hospitalized cancer patients

Risk of thrombotic events in cancer patients undergoing surgery is as high as 50% which can reduce about 50–80% by thromboprophylaxis agents [17]. Since recent decades, multiples guidelines support the using of venous thromboembolism (VTE) prophylactic drugs in hospitalized active cancer patients unless contraindications which intermittent pneumatic compression or graduated compression stockings are recommended in these cases **Table 1** [14, 19]. Although, it is uncertain if hospital

1. Active uncontrollable bleeding*	10. Heparin-induced thrombocytopenia (HIT)
2. Active or recent cerebrovascular hemorrhage	11. Epidural catheter placement
3. Intracranial or intraspinal lesions at high risk for bleeding	12. Platelet count <50,000/mm^{3}***
4. Dissection or aneurysm of cerebral vessels	13. Severe platelet dysfunction
5. Endocarditis, pericarditis	14. Recent operation at high risk for bleeding
6. Active peptic ulceration	15. Severe coagulopathy
7. Severe uncontrolled or malignant hypertention	16. High risk for falling
8. Severe head trauma	17. Renal impairment
9. Pregnancy**	

**Active bleeding that requires at least two units of blood products within 24 h.*
***Pregnancy is relative contraindication for warfarin.*
****International Society of Thrombosis and Homeostasis 2014 (ISTH) recommended thromboprophylaxis agents for patients with platelets more than 50,000/mm^{3}, individualize approach in cases with platelets 25,000–49,000/mm^{3}, and against pharmacologic therapy for platelet lesser than 25,000/mm^{3}, [14, 19, 20].*

Table 1.
Relative contraindications for thromboprophylaxis drug in hospitalized cancer patients.

admission for chemotherapy or bone marrow transplantation displays a risk for venous thromboembolism [20].

American Society of Clinical Oncology 2020 (ASCO) recommended pharmacological thromboprophylaxis for hospitalized cancer patients with acute medical illness, reduced mobility, or undergoing major surgery. However, it should not be advised thromboprophylaxis to patients admitted for minor procedures, chemotherapy infusion, or stem cell/bone marrow transplantation.

Low-molecular-weight heparin (LMWH), fondaparinux, unfractionated heparin (UFH) are proposed prophylaxis drugs by International Society of Thrombosis and Homeostasis 2014 (ISTH), International Initiative on Thrombosis and Cancer 2019 (IITC), and National Comprehensive Cancer Network 2020 [20]. American Society of Hematology 2021 (ASH) guideline recommended low molecular heparin weight (LMHW) over unfractionated heparin (UFH) in hospitalized cancer patients and LMWH or fondaparinux rather than UFH for cancer patients undergoing surgery [21]. They against use of direct oral anticoagulants (DOACs) as prophylactic drugs in these patients [20]. Trials showed the rate of thrombosis has been significantly lower with low-molecular-weight heparin (LMWH) than unfractionated heparin (UFH) without noticeable increase in major bleeding [19].

According to American Society of Clinical Oncology 2020 (ASCO), prophylactic drugs should be commenced preoperatively (one dose 12 hours prior or evening before procedure rather than one dose on the operating table) and continued for at least 7–10 days. Extended prophylaxis with low-molecular-weight heparin (LMWH) is advised up to 4 weeks postoperatively, for high-risk patients undergoing major open or laparascopic abdominal or pelvic cancer surgery [20, 21]. American Society of Hematology 2021 recommended discontinuing thromboprophylaxis at the time of discharge rather than continuing beyond it in hospitalized cancer patients due to medical illness [21].

Non-pharmacological prophylaxis should not be recommended for cancer patients undergoing cancer surgery unless contraindication for using of pharmacological prophylaxis. Combined prophylaxis (pharmacological and mechanical) may be effective for high-risk patients for thrombotic events [20]. American Society of Hematology

2021 (ASH) also suggested pharmacological thromboprophylaxis over combination or mechanical prophylaxis. Although, it recommended mechanical thromboprophylaxis over pharmacological for cancer inpatient undergoing surgery with high bleeding risk. In contrast, early ambulation is over mechanical thromboprophylaxis in post-surgery cancer patients to the opinion of American Society of Hematology Guideline 2021 [21]. International Initiative on Thrombosis and Cancer 2019 (IITC) did not recommend inferior vena cava (IVC) filter for prophylaxis, routinely [20].

4.2 Ambulatory cancer patients

Ambulatory cancer patients receiving chemotherapy have increased risk for thromboembolism [20]. Primary prophylaxis decreases the risk of thromboembolism events in these patients, but the related bleeding risk and frequent daily injection have increased [22] and absolute event rate is low in cancer outpatients, too. Thus, thromboprophylaxis is not recommended by guidelines for all ambulatory cancer patients, routinely [20].

Risk stratification can guide selection of ambulatory cancer patient at high risk of venous thromboembolism [23]. Khorana score (KRS) is used as an ideal, simple, and validated risk stratification tool since 2008, to identify patients at risk of venous thromboembolism (VTE) based on clinical and laboratory variables before starting new systematic therapy. It uses platelet and leukocyte counts, hemoglobin level, body mass index, and site of cancer as the predictor for thromboembolism events **Table 2**, [23, 24]. Two randomized trials evaluated the role of anticoagulant agents for primary prevention of venous thromboembolism based on Khorana scoring in outpatients with cancer and demonstrated reduction in incidence of venous thromboembolism [22]. Khorana score seems to be the best known risk stratification tool in recent years which is endorsed by the latest guidelines [23]. Based on Khorana score, score of 0 displays that the patients are at low risk of venous thromboembolism, a score of 1–2 associates with intermediate risk, and a score of ≥3 (maximum score is 6) indicates high-risk patients. This scoring classification relates to symptomatic venous thromboembolism risk of 0.3–1.5%, 1.8–4.8%, and 6.7–12.9% in ambulatory cancer patients under chemotherapy, respectively [25].

Some guidelines suggest Khorana score 3 points or higher as potential indication for anticoagulation but most recommend a threshold of equal and more than 2 points for anticoagulant agent using [22]. Floris T.M. Bosch et al. evaluated thromboprophylaxis effects in ambulatory cancer patients with intermediate risk (2 points) Khorana

	Score
1. Site of cancer:	
Very high risk (stomach and pancreatic)	2
High risk (lung, lymphoma, gynecological, bladder, and testicular)	1
2. Pre-chemotherapy platelet count $\geq 350 \times 10^9$/L	1
3. Pre-chemotherapy hemoglobin level < 100 g/l or use of red cell growth factors	1
4. Pre-chemotherapy leukocyte count $>11 \times 10^9$/L	1
5. Body mass index (BMI) ≥ 35 kg/m^2	1
Score 0: low risk, score 1–2: intermediate risk, ≥3: high risk.	

Table 2.
Khorana score for risk stratification in ambulatory cancer patients [24].

score, intermediate to high risk (≥2 points) and high risk score (≥3 points) separately, as a systemic review and meta-analysis involving 4626 cancer patients in 2020. They showed significant reduction in venous thromboembolism in intermediate-, intermediate-to-high-, and high-risk patients with no important difference in major bleeding or all-cause mortality. These results explained the indication of thromboprophylaxis for ambulatory cancer patients with intermediate-to-high-risk Khorana score (≥2 points) to reducing the risk of venous thromboembolism [26].

American Society of Clinical Oncology 2020 (ASCO) recommended thromboprophylaxis with apixaban, rivaroxaban, or low-molecular-weight heparin (LMWH) for high-risk outpatients with cancer with Khorana score 2 points and higher, prior to starting a systemic chemotherapy regimen (strength of recommendation: moderate) [20]. Outpatients with multiple myeloma undergoing treatment with immonomodulatory drugs such as thalidomide or linalidomide-based regimens in combination with steroids or systemic chemotherapy drugs are at risk for venous thromboembolism. So, guidelines such as American Society of Clinical Oncology 2020 (ASCO) and International Initiative on Thrombosis and Cancer 2019 (IITC)) recommended low-dose aspirin or low-molecular-weight heparin (LMWH) for these patients as thromboprophylaxis [20]. American Society of Hematology 2021 (ASH) recommended fixed low-dose vitamin K antagonists (VKAs) in these patients, too [21].

5. Anticoagulant agents in cancer patients thromboprophylaxis

5.1 Aspirin

Platelets activation is a part of coagulation process and venous thrombosis. Aspirin is an inhibitor of platelet-derived cyclooxygenaze1 (COX1) and thromboxane A and is the most common used antiplatelet agents through the world. Studies showed that aspirin can decrease thrombotic events in older patients with cancer without evidence of increased major bleeding [27, 28].

5.2 Unfractionated heparin

It is an anticoagulant which activate antithrombin to inhibit clotting enzymes, especially thrombin and factor Xa. Research showed that unfractionated heparin is effective to prevent thromboembolism events in cancer patients. Although, the use of low-molecular-weight heparin (LMWH) is associated with higher reduction in thrombotic events compared to unfractionated heparin in patients with malignancy, especially solid tumor due to increasing of inflammatory component on solid tumor rather than others [27, 29].

5.3 Low-molecular-weight heparin (LMHW)

It includes smaller fragments of heparin which activate antithrombin to inhibit thrombin and factor Xa. Inhibition of factor X is more than thrombin compared to unfractionated heparin. Studies demonstrated effectiveness of low-molecular-weight heparin in thrombotic events treatment with low mortality risk in cancer patients. Benefit of it on patient's survival is ambiguous. Although, it is characterized to be associated with reduction in venous thromboembolism as a thromboprophylaxis agent in these patients [27, 30].

Unfractionated heparin is preferred over low-molecular-weight heparin for cancer patients with severe renal impairment (clearance of creatinine less than 30 ml/min) [21].

5.4 Funadparinux

It is indirect synthetic analog that binds to antithrombin, thus inhibiting factor Xa and thrombin activation. Fondaparinux is used as anticoagulation agent for venous thrombus or pulmonary emboli. Although, it is mostly used as thromoprophylaxis agent compared to other anticoagulant agents. Megan Taguay et al. evaluated the role of fondaparinux in high-risk patients and demonstrated fondaparinux potential for cancer-associated thrombus refractory to low-molecular-weight heparin and unfractionated heparin. It has bioavailability of 100%, too, and its specificity for antithrombin results in more predictable anticoagulation effects. It is contraindication in patients with clearance of creatinine less than 30 ml/min and should be used with caution in clearance of creatinine between 30 and 50 ml/min [27, 31].

5.5 Direct oral anticoagulants (DOACs)

DOACs target thrombin and factor Xa and are more convenient to descript than warfarin [27]. Rivaroxaban and apixaban are the only DOACs using as the primary thromboprophylaxis for ambulatory cancer patients receiving chemotherapy [21]. Studies showed low-dose direct oral anticoagulants (including 2.5 mg twice a day for apixaban and 10 mg once a day for rivaroxaban) can reduce incidence of thrombotic events in high-risk patients with cancer receiving systemic therapy. Rivaroxaban dosage should be reduced in clearance of creatinine more than 15 and less than 50 ml/min. Apixaban dosage should be reduced if age is more than 80 years old and body weight is less than 60 kg and creatinine more than 1.5 g/l [27, 32].

6. Conclusion and future horizons

The world's population has been growing, and life expectancy is increasing. The growth of population aging also occurs in parallel with increase in life expectancy [33]. The incidence of most cancers rises with age due to some same mechanisms [34], and old age is a risk factor for cancer-associated thrombosis too, as has been discussed above [8]. Fortunately, early diagnosis and adequate treatment of malignancies result in the improvement of these patients outcome [35]. Although, these therapeutic methods such as some chemotherapy agents or surgery can increase the risk of thrombosis in cancer patients [8, 9]. Despite the life expectancy of cancer survivors has been increased, other illnesses such as cardiovascular disease have developed in these patients [35]. Cancer patients who presented with atrial fibrillation (AF) rhythm or coronary arteries disease have worse outcome including increased thrombotic risk [36]. Thus, thrombotic events risk is a vast issue in cancer patients. It is associated with patients prognosis. Malignancies nature patients-related factors, new therapeutic agents, even improved patients survival, and developing other illnesses or complications in cancer survivors can affect thromboemboli risk in cancer patients. Risk stratification tools and prevention methods are used to evaluate this risk and reduce thrombotic events. Albeit, thromboemboli is still one of the most common causes of death in patients with cancer. Awareness of thromboemboli risk is important for both patients and physicians, and all cancer patients should be educated about symptoms and signs of thrombotic events. More studies are needed to assess tumor nature and identify new molecular markers as predictor of thrombotic events and help to develop accuracy and specificity of traditional risk stratification tools.

Abbreviations

ADP	adenosine diphosphate
AF	atrial fibrillation
ASCO	American Society of Clinical Oncology
ASH	American Society of Hematology
AT	antithrombin
ATE	arterial thrombotic event
CRS	cytoreductive surgery
CVA	cerebrovascular accident
DOACs	direct acting dual anticoagulants
HIPECH	hyperthermic intraperitoneal chemotherapy
HIT	heparin-induced thrombocytopenia
IITC	international initiative on thrombosis and cancer
ISTH	international society of thrombosis and homeostasis
IVC	inferior vena cava
KSR	Khorana score
LMWH	low-molecular-weight heparin
MI	myocardial infarction
PAI-1	plasminogen activator inhibitor-1
PDPN	podoplanin
PSM	peritoneal surface malignancy
TF	tissue factor
UFH	unfractionated heparin
VEGFR	vascular endothelial growth factor receptor
VKA	vitamin K antagonist
VTE	venous thromboembolism

Author details

Azin Alizadehasl[1*] and Haniye Hajiali Fini[2]

1 Cardio-Oncology Research Center, Rajaie Cardiovascular Medical and Research Center, Iran University of Medical Sciences, Tehran, Iran

2 Department of Adult Echocardiography, Rajaie Cardiovascular Medical and Research Center, Iran University of Medical Sciences, Tehran, Iran

*Address all correspondence to: alizadeasl@gmail.com

References

[1] Mattiuzzi C, Lippi G. Current cancer epidemiology. Journal of Epidemiology and Global Health. 2019;**9**(4):217-222. DOI: 10.2991/jegh.k.191008.001

[2] Sung H, Ferlay J, Siegel RL, Laversanne M, Soerjomataram I, Jemal A, et al. Global cancer statistics 2020: GLOBOCAN estimates of incidence and mortality worldwide for 36 cancers in 185 countries. CA: A Cancer Journal for Clinicians. 2021;**71**:209-249. DOI: 10.3322/caac.21660

[3] Ferlay J, Colombet M, Soerjomataram I, Parkin DM, Piñeros M, Znaor A, et al. Cancer statistics for the year 2020: An overview. International Journal of Cancer. 2021;**149**:778-789. DOI: 10.1002/ijc.33588

[4] Lichota A, Szewczyk EM, Gwozdzinski K. Factors affecting the formation and treatment of thrombosis by natural and synthetic compounds. International Journal of Molecular Sciences. 2020;**21**(21):7975. DOI: 10.3390/ijms21217975

[5] Ashorobi D, Ameer MA, Fernandez R. Thrombosis. In: StatPearls. Treasure Island (FL): StatPearls Publishing; 2022. Available from: https://www.ncbi.nlm.nih.gov/books/NBK538430

[6] Chernysh IN, Nagaswami C, Kosolapova S, Peshkova AD, Cuker A, Cines DB, et al. The distinctive structure and composition of arterial and venous thrombi and pulmonary emboli. Scientific Reports. 2020;**10**(1):5112. DOI: 10.1038/s41598-020-59526-x

[7] Noble S, Pasi J. Epidemiology and pathophysiology of cancer-associated thrombosis. British Journal of Cancer. 2010;**102**(Suppl. 1):S2-S9. DOI: 10.1038/sj.bjc.6605599

[8] Gervaso L, Dave H, Khorana A, et al. Venous and arterial thromboembolism in patients with cancer. JACC: CardioOncology. 2021;**3**(2):173-190. DOI: 10.1016/j.jaccao.2021.03.001

[9] Abdol Razak NB, Jones G, Bhandari M, Berndt MC, Metharom P. Cancer-associated thrombosis: An overview of mechanisms, risk factors, and treatment. Cancers (Basel). 2018;**10**(10):380. DOI: 10.3390/cancers10100380

[10] Dranichnikov P, Mahteme H, Cashin PH, Graf W. Coagulopathy and venous thromboembolic events following cytoreductive surgery and hyperthermic intraperitoneal chemotherapy. Annals of Surgical Oncology. 2021;**28**(12):7772-7782. DOI: 10.1245/s10434-021-09941-9

[11] Hamza MS, Mousa SA. Cancer-associated thrombosis: Risk factors, molecular mechanisms, future management. Clinical and Applied Thrombosis/Hemostasis. 2020;**26**:1076029620954282. DOI: 10.1177/1076029620954282

[12] Fernandes Caio J, Morinaga LTK, Alves José L, Castro Marcela A, Jardim CD, Carlos VP, et al. Cancer-associated thrombosis: The when, how and why. European Respiratory Review. 2019;**28**(151):180119. DOI: 10.1183/16000617.0119-201. Available from: http://err.ersjournals.com/content/28/151/180119

[13] Piazza G. Venous thromboembolism and cancer. Circulation. 2013;**128**(24):2614-2618. DOI: 10.1161/CIRCULATIONAHA.113.002702

[14] Sheth RA, Niekamp A, Quencer KB, Shamoun F, Knuttinen MG, Naidu S,

et al. Thrombosis in cancer patients: Etiology, incidence, and management. Cardiovascular Diagnosis and Therapy. 2017;**7**(Suppl. 3):S178-S185. DOI: 10.21037/cdt.2017.11.02

[15] Mukai M, Oka T. Mechanism and management of cancer-associated thrombosis. Journal of Cardiology. 2018;**72**(2):89-93. DOI: 10.1016/j.jjcc.2018.02.011

[16] Falanga A, Zacharski L. Deep vein thrombosis in cancer: The scale of the problem and approaches to management. Annals of Oncology. 2005;**16**(5):696-701. DOI: 10.1093/annonc/mdi165 Epub 2005 Mar 31

[17] Brose KM, Lee AY. Cancer-associated thrombosis: Prevention and treatment. Current Oncology. 2008;**15**(Suppl 1):S58-S67. DOI: 10.3747/co.2008.177

[18] Elyamany G, Alzahrani AM, Bukhary E. Cancer-associated thrombosis: An overview. Clinical Medicine Insights. Oncology. 2014;**8**: 129-137. DOI: 10.4137/CMO.S18991

[19] Khorana AA. Cancer and thrombosis: Implications of published guidelines for clinical practice. Annals of Oncology. 2009;**20**(10):1619-1630. DOI: 10.1093/annonc/mdp068

[20] Streiff MB, Abutalib SA, Farge D, Murphy M, Connors JM, Piazza G. Update on guidelines for the management of cancer-associated thrombosis. The Oncologist. 2021;**26**(1):e24-e40. DOI: 10.1002/onco.13596

[21] Lyman GH, Carrier M, Ay C, Di Nisio M, Hicks LK, Khorana AA, et al. American Society of Hematology 2021 guidelines for management of venous thromboembolism: Prevention and treatment in patients with cancer. Blood Advances. 2021;**5**(4):927-974. DOI: 10.1182/bloodadvances.2020003442

[22] Overvad TF, Ording AG, Nielsen PB, Skjøth F, Albertsen IE, Noble S, et al. Validation of the Khorana score for predicting venous thromboembolism in 40 218 patients with cancer initiating chemotherapy. Blood Advances. 2022;**6**(10):2967-2976. DOI: 10.1182/bloodadvances.2021006484

[23] Mulder FI, Candeloro M, Kamphuisen PW, Di Nisio M, Bossuyt PM, Guman N, et al. CAT-prediction collaborators. The Khorana score for prediction of venous thromboembolism in cancer patients: A systematic review and meta-analysis. Haematologica. 2019;**104**(6):1277-1287. DOI: 10.3324/haematol.2018.209114

[24] Khorana A, et al. Risk Assessment for Cancer-Associated VTE. JACC: Asia. 2021; 1 (2): 271-273. doi:10.1016/j.jacasi.2021.07.007

[25] Khorana AA, Cohen AT, CarrierM, Meyer G, Pabinger I, Kavan P, et al. Prevention of venous thromboembolism in ambulatory patients with cancer. ESMO Open. 2020;**5**(6);e000948. DOI: 10.1136/esmoopen-2020-000948

[26] Bosch FTM, Mulder FI, Kamphuisen PW, Middeldorp S, Bossuyt PM, Büller HR, et al. Primary thromboprophylaxis in ambulatory cancer patients with a high Khorana score: A systematic review and meta-analysis. Blood Advances. 2020;**4**(20):5215-5225. DOI: 10.1182/bloodadvances.2020003115

[27] Libby P, Bonow R, Mann D, Tomaselli G, Bhatt D, Solomon SD, et al. Braunwald 's Heart Disease. Philadelphia: Elsevier; 2021

[28] Li P, Ning Y, Li M, Li M, Cai P, Siddigui AD, et al. Aspirin is associated with reduced rates of venous thromboembolism in older

patients with cancer. Journal of Cardiovascular Pharmacology and Therapeutics. 2020;**25**(5):456-465. DOI: 10.1177/1074248420925021

[29] Van Matre ET, Reynolds PM, MacLaren R, Mueller SW, Wright GC, Moss B, et al. Evaluation of unfractionated heparin versus low-molecular-weight heparin and fondaparinux for pharmacologic venous thromboembolic prophylaxis in critically ill patients with cancer. Journal of Thrombosis and Haemostasis. 2018;**16**(12):2492-2500. DOI: 10.1111/jth.14317

[30] Zhang N, Lou W, Ji FL, Qiu B, Tsang K, et al. Low molecular weight heparin and cancer survival: Clinical trials and experimental mechanisms. Journal of Cancer Research and Clinical Oncology. 2016;**142**:1807-1816. DOI: 10.1007/s00432-016-2131-6

[31] Tanguay M, Séguin C. Recurrent thrombosis rescued by fondaparinux in high-risk patients: A case series. Research and Practice in Thrombosis and Haemostasis. 2022;**6**:e12773. DOI: 10.1002/rth2.12773

[32] Li A, Kuderer NM, Garcia DA, et al. Direct oral anticoagulant for the prevention of thrombosis in ambulatory patients with cancer: A systematic review and meta-analysis. Journal of Thrombosis and Haemostasis. 2019;**17**:2141-2151. DOI: 10.1111/jth.14613

[33] Gu D, Andreev K, Dupre ME. Major trends in population growth around the world. China CDC Weekly. 2021;**3**(28):604-613. DOI: 10.46234/ccdcw2021.160

[34] White MC, Holman DM, Boehm JE, Peipins LA, Grossman M, Henley SJ. Age and cancer risk: A potentially modifiable relationship. American Journal of Preventive Medicine. 2014;**46**(3 Suppl 1):S7-S15. DOI: 10.1016/j.amepre.2013.10.029

[35] Paterson D, Wiebe N, Cheung W, et al. Incident cardiovascular disease among adults with cancer. JACC: CardioOncology. 2022;**4**(1):85-94. DOI: 10.1016/j.jaccao.2022.01.100

[36] Leiva O, AbdelHameid D, Connors J, et al. Common pathophysiology in cancer, atrial fibrillation, atherosclerosis, and thrombosis. JACC: CardioOncology. 2021;**3**(5):619-634. DOI: 10.1016/j.jaccao.2021.08.011

Chapter 7

Cardio-Oncology and the COVID-19 Pandemic

Zahra Mortezaei and Narges Hosseini

Abstract

As one of the novel interesting fields of cardiology, cardio-oncology focuses on monitoring, detecting, and treating cardiovascular diseases caused due to chemotherapy or radiotherapy side effects. It has been observed that cardiovascular patients have a higher risk of viral infections and poorer treatment outcomes. COVID-19 is a disease caused by the new coronavirus, SARS-CoV-2, which emerged in Wuhan, China, in 2019 and then distributed worldwide. Recent evidence showed that the risk of COVID-19 and its mortality rate is higher in patients suffering from cardiovascular side effects of cancer therapies. Additional diagnosis complexity in cardio-oncology is another problem due to overlapping with COVID-19. Therefore, the cardio-oncology community had to re-evaluate the best clinical care in the COVID-19 pandemic. The present study aims to review previous studies focusing on the interaction between COVID-19 and cardio-oncology, which will pave the way for studying human diseases overlapping with COVID-19.

Keywords: cardio-oncology, COVID-19, cancer, cardiovascular, SARS-CoV-2, signaling pathway

1. Introduction

At the end of 2019, a novel corona virus called severe acute respiratory syndrome coronavirus 2 (SARS-CoV-2) was identified, which was caused respiratory-related diseases in China, and the disease caused by this virus was named COVID-19 by the World Health Organization and then in 12 March 2020 has been notified as a pandemic [1, 2]. Although COVID-19 mostly manifests in the lung, this virus invades to all part of the body such as heart, eyes, kidneys, the central nervous system (CNS), and other physiological systems (**Figure 1**) [3–7]. The virus directly affects the CNS or the peripheral nervous system (PNS), or other organs which ultimately causes disease in the CNS/PNS [3].

One of the crises in public health which emerged as a global pandemic is related to the coronavirus disease 2019 (COVID-19) increasing infectious outbreaks among broad population. During that pandemic, an unprecedented upheaval in the field of medicine has been observed. Cancer patients are vulnerable to adverse cardiac events, and therefore healthcare interactions have to be increased for them. Increasing cardiovascular disease due to cancer treatment led to the development of cardio-oncology field of research with the aim of monitoring, detecting, and

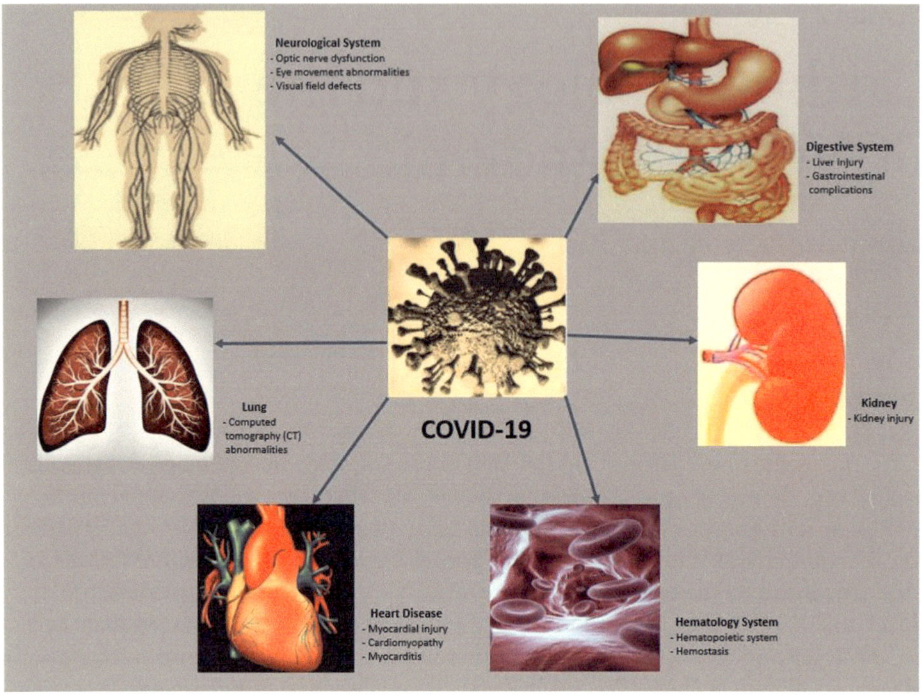

Figure 1.
COVID-19 invades most part of the body.

treating cardiovascular diseases caused due to chemotherapy or radiotherapy side effects. The aim of this research is to study the effects of cardio-oncology and COVID-19 on each other in different perspectives which can suggest strategies for future similar phases [8–11].

Cancer and cardiovascular diseases are vulnerable to COVID-19 because of an increased amount of infection risks and healthcare exposure. For example, one study among 426 hospitalized patients in Wuhan indicated that about 20% of patients have cardiac injury. Also, it has been reported that more unfavorable courses and severe outcomes of COVID-19 have been increased in cancer and cardiovascular diseases. In addition, that study indicated that irrespective of the COVID-19 pandemic, frequent use of healthcare system and anticancer therapies are required for cancer patients [12].

Due to the mentioned infection vulnerability for cancer and cardiovascular diseases, some publications focused on COVID-19 susceptibility for cancer and cardiovascular patients. Previous studies reported COVID-19 patients with cancer history and the statistics indicated that the amount of cancer patients with COVID-19 is higher than the amount of reported cancer patients before the pandemic. For example, one study reported that 6% of patients have both cancer and COVID-19. One case–control COVID-19 study among patients with cancer and those without cancer indicated that lung cancer, malignancies, or metastatic cancer are more in a risk of severe events than others. It has been shown in subsequent meta-analysis results that COVID-19 patients have an increase amount of cancer prevalence and risk of death. Some governments categorized cancer and cardiovascular patients having high risk of virus infection and severe clinical course in COVID-19 pandemic [13, 14].

There is evidences of increased mortality and morbidity rates in COVID-19 patients with comorbid cancer and cardiovascular. Cardiovascular complications such as myocarditis, arrhythmia, heart failure, and myocardial infarction have been observed due to the severe host immune response and cytokine release syndrome. In addition, there is a lot of evidence that shows cancer patients under immunosuppressive treatment have an increased risk of COVID-19 infection [15].

2. Global health system in COVID-19 pandemic

Beyond COVID-19 direct consequences, global health system has enormously been impacted by the pandemic. Since COVID-19 pandemic may affect and disturb access to clinical care, it is important to establish a clinical guideline and pathway. One of the essential and critical part of patient management is cardiac imaging. Because cardio-oncology patients are highly at both delayed care complications and COVID-19 infections risks, some countries developed strategies for cardiac imaging during oncology care in COVID-19 pandemic. In addition, for high-risk patients and to prevent an asymptomatic spread of COVID-19, some instruments have been proposed through regular COVID-19 testing and full personal protective equipment. The assessment of ST elevation myocardial infarction has been impacted during the COVID-19 affecting mortality rates. Therefore, the healthcare system must prepare for rebound effect that can increase disease incidence like heart failure [16, 17].

In COVID-19 pandemic, to assess cardio-oncology care pathways, the success of cardiotoxicity monitoring and COVID-19 mitigation effects, big data analysis is essential. For developing new strategies to overcome ongoing research barriers and to address patient risks in COVID-19 pandemic, some innovations should be inspired. Cardio-oncology in the COVID-19 pandemic has implemented clinical cares and monitoring protocols such as telemedicine systems, teleconsultation, cardiac imaging, limited clinical visits, and biomarker reliance [17].

For the purpose of better understanding similarities and relations between cardio-oncology and COVID-19, some common biological pathways between them will be discussed below [18].

3. Common signaling pathways and their effects

Considering that the virus survival depends on its host cell, cellular functions including signaling pathways can be important to discuss [2]. In coronavirus disease, viruses bind to host proteins and use different cellular pathways as their targets. Corona infection effects on multiple signal transduction pathways with important roles such as mitogen-activated protein kinase (MAPK) pathway, phosphatidylinositol-3-kinase (PI3K)/protein kinase B (AKT)/mammalian target of rapamycin (mTOR) pathway, janus kinase (JAK)–signal transducer and activator of transcription (STAT) signaling pathway, toll-like receptor (TLRI) signaling, and nuclear factor kappa-B (NF-κB) pathway cascades. Also, the virus can cause a series of hypercytokinemia [19].

3.1 MAPK pathway

Controlling several cell functions (proliferation, apoptosis, and differentiation) are done by MAPK signaling pathways. The MAPK pathways have three pathways in mammals that are Jun amino-terminal kinases/stress-activated protein kinases (JNK/SAPK), p38 MAPK, and MAPK/extracellular signal-regulated kinase (ERK). Environmental stimuli initially activate the p38 MAPK pathway, which has a significant impact on the inflammatory processes and immune response [19]. The host activates the immune system during viral infections to fight pathogenic microorganisms. As a result, if one of the immune responses is out of control, it can lead to significant damage during an infection such as COVID-19 [20]. It has been shown that Raf/MEK/ERK pathway inhibitors can be used as antiviral candidates for COVID-19 treatment [20].

Among severe infected COVID-19 patients, increased amount of cardiac injury has been observed. Clear mechanism of cardiac injury is not completely identified, but it is suggested to be involved in a combination of immune-mediated and viral damages by cytotoxic and cytokines/chemokines immune responses. In SARS-CoV-2 infection, cytokine storm contributors and the host immune responses are complex. In immune hyperactivity and dysregulation, T lymphocytes depletion may contribute [21].

Activation of the p38 pathway cause increases the level of pro-inflammatory cytokines such as IL-1, IL-1, and tumor necrosis factor (TNF), which play an important role in the cytokine storm stimulated by COVID-19 infection. Maybe shift balance toward harmful p38 signaling with angiotensin II if ACE2 is lost during viral infection. ACE2 activity was found in both the heart and lung. Excessive activation of p38 MAPK in infected cardiomyocytes, which causes promote fibrosis and apoptosis, can be one of the causes of cardiac dysfunction in patients with coronavirus. The cells can reduce p38 signaling which expands the viral lifespan and also causes inflammation. As a result, if p38 is suppressed, the infection of COVID-19 is reduced. Losmapimod is the most important p38 inhibitor that can be useful for patients with COVID-19 [19].

Another pathway that is effective in this infection is the c-jun NH2-terminal kinase (JNK) pathway, which may lead to an increase in lung damage and an increase in pro-inflammatory factors. This pathway is involved in tissue cytokine production, apoptotic pathway, metabolism, and inflammation [19].

3.2 Notch signaling pathway

Notch signaling pathway has a main role in development and controlling cell fate. This signaling pathway plays a role in maintaining the homeostasis of the cardiovascular system, and it can be a new target to reduce the progression of atherosclerosis and also is a main regulator of cardiovascular function and as well as involved in biological processes with viral infections. This article reported than may be able to use this signaling pathway to combat heart and lung disease caused by SARS-CoV-2 infection [22].

3.3 WNT/B-catenin pathway

This signaling pathway is activated in response to cardiac injury and has important roles in cardiac remodeling and hypertrophy [23]. It has been shown that WNT/b-catenin pathway upregulation can be associated with COVID-19, acute respire distress syndrome [24], and cytokine storm [25].

As a result, it can be said that this virus can effect on the functioning of heart cell by disrupting the signaling pathways.

As mentioned before, COVID-19 affects different organs, including lungs and most probably also the heart. Increase in COVID-19 mortality rates has been seen in cardiovascular diseases. It has been shown in studies that various organ systems to express the primary SARS-CoV-2 entry receptor, angiotensin-converting enzyme 2 (ACE2) [26]. ACE2 plays a major role in the regulation of cardiovascular and renal functions, and also in SARS-CoV-2 infection [27].

In one previous study, single-cell nuclei RNA sequencing in 40 failing explanted hearts and 15 healthy donor hearts has been used. As a result, low expression of ACE2 in cardiomyocytes and high pericytes expression have been observed. Therefore, SARS-CoV-2 infection in human heart can attack primarily pericytes and cause capillary endothelial cell dysfunction. The results of that can be microcirculation disorders and expanding cardiac damages' observed markers [26].

Expression of ACE2 in human hearts has been published in the European Heart Journal and by Nicin et al. used single-nuclei RNA sequencing for analyzing the expression of ACE2 and ACE in two patients with heart failure with reduced ejection fraction (HFrEF), five patients with aortic stenosis (AS), and two samples from one healthy donor heart with different cell types of the human heart. Finally, they reported an increased amount of ACE2 expression in cardiomyocytes of patients with heart disease compared with healthy controls [26, 28].

It has been shown that monitoring of SARS-CoV-2-infected patients for cardiovascular complications can be important because of ARB (angiotensin II receptor blocker)/ACE inhibitor therapy (driver of cardiovascular pathologies) [28]. One study showed that increase in level of ACE2 was related with cardiovascular male patients, and this can be a major risk factor for COVID-19 infection and complications [29]. Many cases of heart complications have been reported due to COVID-19 infection, and chemotherapy and cancer appear to be risk factors for COVID-19 [24].

In one study, cardiac complications were investigated in a cancer patient who was undergoing chemotherapy with anthracyclines and had corona disease. This patient was a 49-year-old woman with breast cancer who did not have any other medical history. The patient was admitted for coronavirus disease, and she had received chemotherapy 10 days before being admitted. At the time of admission, she had a normal electrocardiogram (normal QTc interval and narrow QRS complex), but on the second day, she had bad respiratory function, and abnormal electrocardiogram (QRS widening and QTc interval lengthening) was also reported from the patient, and finally the patient she died due to cardiorespiratory arrest [30].

In a series of recent studies, it has been reported that cancer patients with COVID-19 had a higher prevalence of severe events compared to the general population and showed a death rate more than 10 times higher than all patients in China [30].

4. Conclusions

In COVID-19 pandemic, in the field of medicine, an unprecedented upheaval has been observed. For example, it has been observed that cancer and cardiovascular diseases are vulnerable to COVID-19. Also, unfavorable courses and severe outcomes of COVID-19 have been observed in cancer and cardiovascular diseases. In addition, COVID-19 patients have an increased risk of cancer prevalence and death. Establishing clinical guidelines in COVID-19 pandemic is essential for high-risk patients. For example, monitoring protocols and clinical cares have been implemented for cardio-oncology care during COVID-19 pandemic. In order to better understand the effects of cardio-oncology and COVID-19 on each other, some common biological pathways like mitogen-activated protein kinase (MAPK) pathway, PI3K/AKT/mTOR pathway, JAK–STAT signaling pathway, TLRI signaling, and NF-κB pathway have been explained.

Author details

Zahra Mortezaei[1*] and Narges Hosseini[2]

1 Human Genetic Research Center, Baqiyatallah University of Medical Sciences, Tehran, Iran

2 Faculty of Basic Sciences and Advanced Technologies in Biology, Department of Molecular Genetics, University of Science and Culture, Tehran, Iran

*Address all correspondence to: zmortezaie@gmail.com

References

[1] Ciotti M, Ciccozzi M, Terrinoni A, Jiang WC, Wang CB, Bernardini S. The COVID-19 pandemic. Critical Reviews in Clinical Laboratory Sciences. 2020;**57**(6):365-388

[2] Ghasemnejad-Berenji M, Pashapour S. SARS-CoV-2 and the possible role of Raf/MEK/ERK pathway in viral survival: is this a potential therapeutic strategy for COVID-19? Pharmacology. 2021;**106**(1-2):119-122

[3] Finsterer J, Stollberger C. Update on the neurology of COVID-19. Journal of Medical Virology. Nov 2020;**92**(11):2316-2318

[4] Yende S, Parikh CR. Long COVID and kidney disease. Nature Reviews Nephrology. 2021;**17**(12):792-793

[5] Zhou F, Xia J, Yuan HX, Sun Y, Zhang Y. Liver injury in COVID-19: Known and unknown. World Journal of Clinical Cases. 2021;**9**(19):4980

[6] Zhong P, Xu J, Yang D, Shen Y, Wang L, Feng Y, et al. COVID-19-associated gastrointestinal and liver injury: Clinical features and potential mechanisms. Signal Transduction and Targeted Therapy. 2 Nov 2020;**5**(1):256

[7] Terpos E, Ntanasis-Stathopoulos I, Elalamy I, Kastritis E, Sergentanis TN, Politou M, et al. Hematological findings and complications of COVID-19. American Journal of Hematology. 2020;**95**(7):834-847

[8] Kostakou PM, Kouris NT, Kostopoulos VS, Damaskos DS, Olympios CD. Cardio-oncology: A new and developing sector of research and therapy in the field of cardiology. Heart Failure Reviews. 2019;**24**(1):91-100

[9] Bisceglia I, Canale ML, Gallucci G, Turazza FM, Lestuzzi C, Parrini I, et al. Cardio-oncology in the COVID era (Co & Co): The never ending story. Frontiers in Cardiovascular Medicine. 2022;**9**:821193. DOI: 10.3389/fcvm.2022.821193

[10] Bisceglia I, Gabrielli D, Canale ML, Gallucci G, Parrini I, Turazza FM, et al. ANMCO position paper: Cardio-oncology in the COVID era (CO and CO). European Heart Journal Supplements. 2021;**23**(Supplement_C):C128-C153

[11] Addison D, Campbell CM, Guha A, Ghosh AK, Dent SF, Jneid H. Cardio-oncology in the era of the COVID-19 pandemic and beyond. Journal of the American Heart Association. 2020;**9**(19):e017787

[12] Lenihan D, Carver J, Porter C, Liu JE, Dent S, Thavendiranathan P, et al. Cardio-oncology care in the era of the coronavirus disease 2019 (COVID-19) pandemic: An International Cardio-Oncology Society (ICOS) statement. CA: A Cancer Journal for Clinicians. 2020;**70**(6):480-504

[13] Sadler D, DeCara JM, Herrmann J, Arnold A, Ghosh AK, Abdel-Qadir H, et al. Perspectives on the COVID-19 pandemic impact on cardio-oncology: Results from the COVID-19 International collaborative network survey. Cardio-oncology. 2020;**6**(1):1-3

[14] Brown SA. Cardio-oncology and COVID 19: Lessons learned, past reflections and future deliberations. American Heart Journal Plus: Cardiology Research and Practice; 2022. p. 100137

[15] Abraham S, Manohar SA, Patel R, Saji AM, Dani SS, Ganatra S. Strategies

for cardio-oncology care during the COVID-19 pandemic. Current Treatment Options in Cardiovascular Medicine. 2022;**24**(8):137-153

[16] Brown SA, Rhee JW, Guha A, Rao VU. Innovation in precision cardio-oncology during the coronavirus pandemic and into a post-pandemic world. Frontiers in Cardiovascular Medicine. 2020;**7**:145

[17] Bisceglia I, Gabrielli D, Canale ML, Gallucci G, Parrini I, Turazza FM, et al. ANMCO position paper: Cardio-oncology in the COVID-19 era. Giornale Italiano di Cardiologia. 2021;**22**(10):800-825

[18] Martinez DS, Noseworthy PA, Akbilgic O, Herrmann J, Ruddy KJ, Hamid A, et al. Artificial intelligence opportunities in cardio-oncology: Overview with spotlight on electrocardiography. American Heart Journal Plus. 1 Apr 2022:100129

[19] Peyvandi AA, Niknazar S, Zare Mehrjerdi F, Abbaszadeh HA, Khoshsirat S, Peyvandi M. Molecular mechanisms and signaling pathways involved in immunopathological events of COVID-19. Physiology and Pharmacology. 2021;**25**(3):193-205

[20] Scudiero O, Lombardo B, Brancaccio M, Mennitti C, Cesaro A, Fimiani F, et al. Exercise, immune system, nutrition, respiratory and cardiovascular diseases during COVID-19: A complex combination. International Journal of Environmental Research and Public Health. 2021;**18**(3):904

[21] Zhu H, Rhee JW, Cheng P, Waliany S, Chang A, Witteles RM, et al. Cardiovascular complications in patients with COVID-19: Consequences of viral toxicities and host immune response. Current Cardiology Reports. 2020;**22**(5):1-9

[22] Rizzo P, Vieceli Dalla Sega F, Fortini F, Marracino L, Rapezzi C, Ferrari R. COVID-19 in the heart and the lungs: Could we "Notch" the inflammatory storm? Basic Research in Cardiology. 2020;**115**(3):1-8

[23] Ozhan G, Weidinger G. Wnt/β-catenin signaling in heart regeneration. Cell Regeneration. 2015;**4**(1):4-3

[24] Villar J, Zhang H, Slutsky AS. Lung repair and regeneration in ARDS: Role of PECAM1 and Wnt signaling. Chest. 2019;**155**:587-594. DOI: 10.1016/j.chest.2018.10.022

[25] Choi EY, Park HH, Kim H, Kim HN, Kim I, Jeon S, et al. Wnt5a and Wnt11 as acute respiratory distress syndrome biomarkers for severe acute respiratory syndrome coronavirus 2 patients. The European Respiratory Journal. 2020;**56**:2001531. DOI: 10.1183/13993003.01531-2020

[26] Thum T. SARS-CoV-2 receptor ACE2 expression in the human heart: Cause of a post-pandemic wave of heart failure? European Heart Journal. 2020;**41**(19):1807-1809

[27] Vallee A, Lecarpentier Y, Vallee JN. Interplay of opposing effects of the WNT/β-catenin pathway and PPARγ and implications for SARS-CoV2 treatment. Frontiers in immunology. 2021;**12**:666693

[28] Nicin L, Abplanalp WT, Mellentin H, Kattih B, Tombor L, John D, et al. Cell type-specific expression of the putative SARS-CoV-2 receptor ACE2 in human hearts. European Heart Journal. 2020;**41**(19):1804-1806

[29] Wallentin L, Lindbäck J, Eriksson N, Hijazi Z, Eikelboom JW, Ezekowitz MD, et al. Angiotensin-converting enzyme 2 (ACE2) levels in relation to risk factors for COVID-19 in two large cohorts of patients with atrial fibrillation. European Heart Journal. 2020;**41**(41):4037-4046

[30] Mechal H, Benmalek R, Choukrallah H, Maaroufi A, Habbal R, Mounir A, et al. Cardiac involvement in cancer patients under chemotherapy and diagnosed with COVID-19: Case report and literature review. The Pan African Medical Journal. 2022:41

Chapter 8

Cardiovascular Complications Related to Lower Limb Revascularization and Drug-Delivering Technology in Peripheral Arterial Disease

Saritphat Orrapin

Abstract

The cardiovascular complication related to lower limb revascularization is the common cause of mortality in patients with peripheral arterial disease (PAD). The coexisting multisite atherosclerotic vascular disease is increasing risk of major adverse cardiovascular events (MACE). The minimally invasive approach for revascularization, namely, endovascular-first strategy for decreasing risk of intervention is the modern approach. The novel technology of the drug delivering device by paclitaxel, sirolimus, and other antiproliferative drug coated balloon (DCB) and drug eluting stent (DES) to increase the patency of the target artery are trending to use in patients with CLTI. However, the long-term result and safety of a drug delivering device are still controversial. The paclitaxel related to MACE and major adverse limb events (MALE) need to be investigated. The new drug coating balloon, sirolimus demonstrated the excellent short-term result. However, there are some limitations of previous randomized studies and meta-analyses to conclude the best strategy and device to perform the best result for revascularization without increasing risk of MACE and MALE in CLTI patients who candidate for revascularization. This article is summarized the pathophysiology of MACE and MALE in the patients with PAD during revascularization, paclitaxel related cardiovascular complications and sirolimus coated balloon.

Keywords: major adverse cardiovascular events, MACE, peripheral arterial disease, PAD, chronic limb-threatening ischemia, CLTI, drug delivering technology, drug coated balloon, DCB, drug eluting stent, DES, paclitaxel, sirolimus coated balloon

1. Introduction

Peripheral arterial disease (PAD) is a chronic condition in which stenosis or occlusion of the peripheral arteries [1–3]. The scopes range from the arteries that feed the brain are the carotid artery and the vertebral artery, the upper extremity arteries, the mesenteric arteries, the renal arteries, and the lower extremity arteries [1, 2, 4]. The PAD is primarily caused by the systemic atherosclerosis [5, 6]. There are other causes of PAD, such as thromboangiitis obliterans (TAO) or Buerger's disease, chronic arterial embolism, arterial entrapment, fungal arteritis, Takayasu's disease, inflammatory arterial disease from other causes such as polyarteritis nodosa (PAN) or other uncommon arteriopathies such as drug-induced arteriopathy [7], exercise-related external Iliac arteriopathy, radiation arteritis, fibromuscular dysplasia (FMD), vasculitis secondary to connective tissue diseases), such as rheumatoid arthritis, systemic lupus erythematosus (SLE), etc. [1, 8, 9].

The PAD of the lower extremity or lower extremity arterial disease (LEAD) due to atherosclerosis is a common disease in patients over the age of 60 years [2, 10, 11]. Males having a 1–2 times higher risk of developing PAD than females [1]. There have been 200 million cases of PAD worldwide, with a prevalence in 13–28%. The prevalence rate is expected to be underestimate due to a lack of screening system, which makes it impossible to document the exact number of patients in the group who have no symptoms or have minor symptoms [1–3]. In addition, a half of patients presenting with gangrene and ischemic ulcer of lower limb have no prior document of PAD [3]. According to previous publications data, the presentation of PAD is not typical. 50% of PAD patients are asymptomatic, In addition, among diabetics mellitus (DM) with PAD, have no symptoms of up to 80%. 15% of PAD patients are intermittent claudication. Only 1–3% of PAD patients are chronic limb-threatening ischemia (CLTI) which is a clinical syndrome of the PAD in combination with rest pain, gangrene or lower limb ulceration [3, 12, 13].

The major cause of death in patients with PAD is a cardiovascular disease. A cerebrovascular disease (CVD) and coronary artery disease (CAD) lead to high mortality rates for LEAD patients [14, 15]. The 5-year mortality rate of diagnosed PAD patients is 10–15%. Three-quarters of mortality group are fatal stroke and myocardial infarction (MI). For CLTI patients, the mortality rate is increasing to 25% with 4.5% of fatal stroke and 6.5% acute MI [16]. Thus, the four-point major adverse cardiovascular events (MACE) including acute MI, stroke, cardiovascular mortality, hospitalization for unstable angina or revascularization procedures is an increasingly primary outcome of interest in PAD. Recently, five-point MACE further expands on this with the inclusion of heart failure (HF) [3, 17, 18].

The PAD patients who need to revascularization of lower extremity artery include (1) CLTI which associated with increased mortality, risk of amputation, and impaired quality of life. (2) Disabling claudication patients who have limitation of daily activity and impaired quality of life due to their symptom [3, 13, 17]. All of them are risk of MACE during hospitalization for lower limb procedure such as revascularization, debridement, and amputation. MACE is rapid increasingly during perioperative period due to the stress from the foot infection or active comorbid disease and risk of the anesthesia and operation including revascularization (open vascular bypass, endovascular treatment) as well as amputation. Moreover, the poor performance status which occurred in patients who loss of ambulatory state due to non-functional limb, amputation, limb ulceration, gangrene, rest pain or disabling claudication are increased risk of MACE (**Figure 1**). The Society for Vascular Surgery (SVS) Objective Performance Goals (OPGs) established standardized tools for report benchmark of perioperative outcome including MACE and major adverse limb events (MALE) after revascularization procedures in patients with CLTI. The major adverse limb events (MALE) include major amputation of the revascularized limb and reintervention [19, 20].

Over the past decade, revascularization procedure for treating both simple and complex lower extremity arterial occlusive disease in a minimally invasive fashion

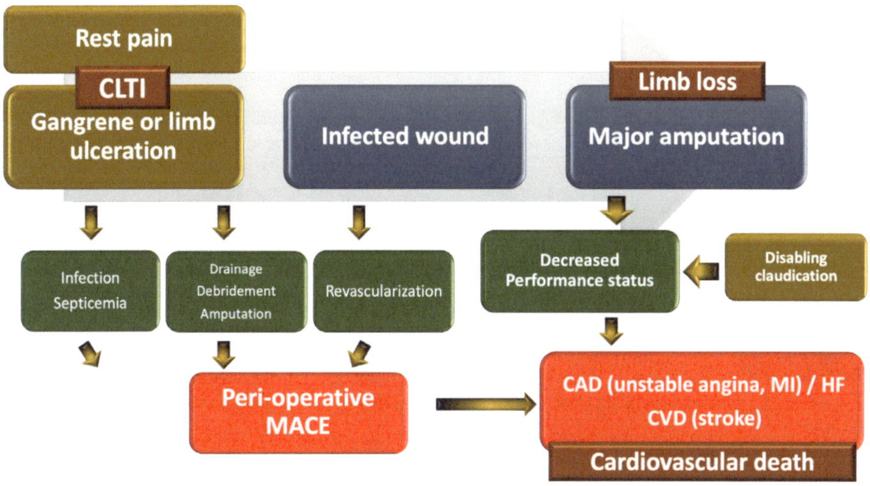

Figure 1.
The pathologic process of amputation and MACE during hospitalization in patients with PAD. CAD, coronary artery disease; CLTI, chronic limb-threatening ischemia; CVD, cerebrovascular disease; HF, heart failure; MACE, major cardiovascular events; MI, myocardial infarction; PAD, peripheral arterial disease.

have increased significantly and induce some to support an "endovascular-first strategy" for most patients with PAD who candidate for revascularization [3, 13]. Most of the endovascular treatment (ET) in CLTI is a minimally invasive intervention which can perform under local anesthesia, which decreased the risk of general anesthesia, especially in multiple co-morbidities patients who cannot tolerate the major operation. In addition, ET can avoid the surgical wound complication and adjacent tissue injury. The length of hospital stay is also decreased in CLTI patients who performed ET when compare with open vascular bypass procedures.

Recently, the novel technology developed the antiproliferative agent -coated and -eluting device which can deliver the drugs to the vessel wall to limit the neointimal growth within de novo vascular system and stent [21–26]. However, some literatures report the MACE, aneurysmal degeneration, vascular fibrinoid necrosis, small vessel inflammation, and budget impact after drug technology device including drug coated balloon (DCB) and drug eluting stent (DES) in patients with ET [27–31]. The long-term MACE after DCB and DES device usage in patients with CLTI is still controversy [30, 32, 33]. This chapter describes the fundamental pathophysiology of MACE related to revascularization in patients with PAD and summarizes the most current data to guide an appropriate strategic treatment with drug-delivering technology under the risk and benefit assessment for ET in CLTI patients.

2. Pathophysiology of MACE related to PAD and atherosclerotic risk factors

In patients with diagnosed PAD, the risk of MACE appears to be greater than patients without PAD [3, 14]. The major atherosclerotic risk factors including DM, hypertension, dyslipidemia, and smoking are increased the MACE due to the atherosclerotic involvement of arterial system in vascular beds that affect blood supply to the target organs (**Figure 2**).

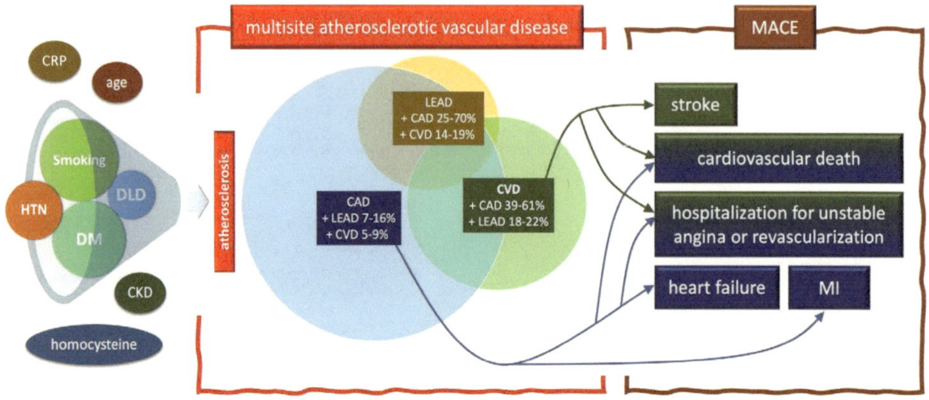

Figure 2.
The relationship between atherosclerotic risk factors and major adverse cardiovascular events with overlap in multisite atherosclerotic vascular disease. HTN, hypertension; DM, diabetes mellitus; DLD, dyslipidemia; CKD, chronic kidney disease; CRP, C-reactive protein; CAD, coronary artery disease; LEAD, lower extremity arterial disease; CVD, cerebrovascular disease; MACE, major cardiovascular events; MI, myocardial infarction.

The metabolic abnormality in patients with DM lead to hyperglycemia, insulin resistance, and increasing of free fatty acid. Three fundamental dysmetabolism process led to endothelial dysfunction and atherosclerosis [34]. Hyperglycemia increases the oxidative stress by increasing of reactive oxygen species (ROS). In addition, the cellular mitogenic pathway activation through the mitochondrial generation of the superoxide anion including advanced glycation end products (AGEs), protein kinase C (PKC) activation, and nuclear factor kappa B (NF-κB) are induced by high blood glucose level. In patients with long duration DM, insulin resistance cause endothelial dysfunction, decreasing of nitric oxide (NO) synthase, expression of adhesion molecules, and atherosclerotic lesions [34]. In addition, a thrombosis risk in DM is increasing though the hypercoagulation and platelet aggregation. The elevation of plasminogen activator inhibitor 1 (PAI-1), tissue factors and decreasing of NO are promoting coagulation cascade and platelet activation. Finally, insulin resistance is also promoted atherosclerotic process due to lipid metabolism disturbance such as high triglycerides (TG), high apolipoprotein B (ApoB), small and dense low-density lipoprotein (LDL), low high-density lipoprotein (HDL) cholesterol [35–37].

In early atherosclerotic process, the endothelial dysfunction is associate with hypertensive patients. A reduction in NO result in a reduced vasodilatory response, and result in an inflammation, thrombosis, and activate coagulation cascade [34, 38, 39]. The repetitive blood pressure alterations in patients with hypertension cause ongoing renin-angiotensin system activation. Angiotensin II, the product of renin-angiotensin system is a potent vasoconstrictor has an impact on the atherosclerotic lesions [35–37]. In the setting of dyslipidemia, a foam cell which is an intracellular droplets of cholesterol ester are occurred under the high LDL and low HDL in peripheral blood. The damaged endothelial of vessel wall cause the foam cells adhere and migrate into the intima layer and developed macrophages. The ongoing thickening of the intima by foam cell is developed after the vascular smooth muscle cell (VSMC) proliferates above the endothelial damaged area until the fibrous cap formation to create the atherosclerotic plaque [40].

Smoking causes an inflammation of vessel wall which related to atherosclerotic plaque formation through interleukin-6, tissue necrosis factor-α, interleukin-1-β, leukocyte, C-reactive protein (CRP), and other inflammatory markers [34, 38, 39]. The endothelial dysfunction by the increasing of ROS productions through the reduction of NO, and activation of enzymes are present in smoker patients. In addition, the prothrombotic state of platelet activation and aggregation are create by increasing of thromboxane A2 (TXA2), von Willebrand factor (vWF), thrombin, fibrin and decreasing of prostacyclin, antithrombotic, and fibrinolytic substances (PAI-1) [35–37].

The atherosclerosis of lower extremity artery is systemic disease which involved other vascular beds that affect blood supply to the cardiac and brain (**Figure 2**). So, it is usually that the LEAD, CAD, and CVD commonly occur together (**Figure 2**). So, the presence of lower extremity stenosis/occlusion is associated with an increased risk of stenosis/occlusion of coronary artery, carotid and vertebrobasilar arterial system which is clinically presented by MI and stroke [3, 14]. 25–70% and 14–19% of patients who present with LEAD often coexists with CAD and CVD, respectively. Conversely, only 7–16% and 18–22% of patients with CAD and severe carotid stenosis are coexists with LEAD, respectively [35]. Patients with severe LEAD which indicate by ankle brachial index (ABI) <0.4 or severe atherosclerosis on anatomic distribution by Trans-Atlantic Inter-Society Consensus for the management of PAD (TASC II) exhibit more extensive calcified and progressive coronary atherosclerosis [14, 35]. Therefore, the MACE is categorized into two fundamental parts including CAD and CVD based on vascular bed involvement which focus on the morbidity (stroke, MI, HF) and mortality (fatal stroke and fatal MI) (**Figure 2**). Currently, updated MACE is expanded to five-point including acute MI, stroke, hospitalization for unstable angina or revascularization procedures, HF, and cardiovascular mortality [3, 4, 14, 35, 36].

The risk of ongoing development to CLTI appears to be greater in patients who have a pre-existing CAD and CVD such as history of stroke, MI or HF. Comparing with PAD, patients with CLTI have a higher risk of MACE and premature death due to cardiovascular disease. In patients with developed CLTI, the risk of amputation and mortality rate is extremely increased to 30% and 25%, respectively [3, 14, 35]. For this reason, treatment of patients with CLTI is not only revascularization to salvage a functional limb but also aggressive best medical treatment to reduce MACE. The medical management of patients with PAD including atherosclerotic risk factors modification, statin therapy and antiplatelet therapy for symptomatic PAD can decreased risk of development of CLTI and overall prognosis for patients with PAD [3, 13].

3. Pathophysiology of MACE related to revascularization procedure in patients with CLTI

Almost CLTI patients need to be revascularization to salvage a functional limb and improve the quality of life [14, 35, 39]. Because the risk of perioperative MACE and other coexisting co-morbidities, some patients who indicate for limb revascularization are not candidate to perform the operation. Although, the novel medical technology including ET, medical risk optimization, the intensive care knowledge is significantly developed during the last century. The poor functional capacity and multiple co-morbidities patients are still very high risk of perioperative MACE during revascularization [3, 18, 37]. Active cardiac condition (including acute coronary syndrome including unstable angina (UA), non-ST elevation MI (NSTEMI) and

ST-elevation MI (STEMI) as well as symptomatic carotid stenosis are usually need for coronary and carotid revascularization before lower limb revascularization [3, 4, 14, 18, 35, 37, 39].

In healthy people, the systemic organs are functioning in parallel and simultaneously. The consequences of the organ functioning including (1) the stroke volume which is ejected from the heart and feeding to the various organs before entering the capillaries and venous system of the organ, (2) the arterial blood feeding each organ has the same composition, (3) the blood pressure at the entrance to each organ is the same, and (4) the blood flow to each organ can be controlled independently (local regulation of blood flow, namely, "autoregulation") [3, 41, 42]. The autoregulation is the human body physiologic response of functional hyperemia to maintain the blood flow to the vascular bed of the vital end-organ such as brain, kidney. The responsibility of the human body physiologic alteration and autoregulation after revascularization are impact to the incidence of perioperative MACE in patients with CLTI.

Physiologic changes and the autoregulation process after revascularization procedure by decreasing afterload (peripheral vascular resistance) are the burden to cardiovascular system. The cardiac reserve and response after lower limb revascularization, the anatomic distribution and severity of lower limb arterial occlusive disease as well as the type of revascularization are determining the risk of perioperative MACE [14, 37, 43].

3.1 Cardiac reserve and response after lower limb revascularization related to MACE

The blood flow rate which feed to the end organs are determined by the cardiovascular system. Each organ can adjust their vascular resistance or afterload which maintaining the blood flow and pressure to their vascular bed by the autoregulation mechanisms. Therefore, revascularization procedures which result in the reduction of afterload rapidly are significantly increased blood flow to the lower

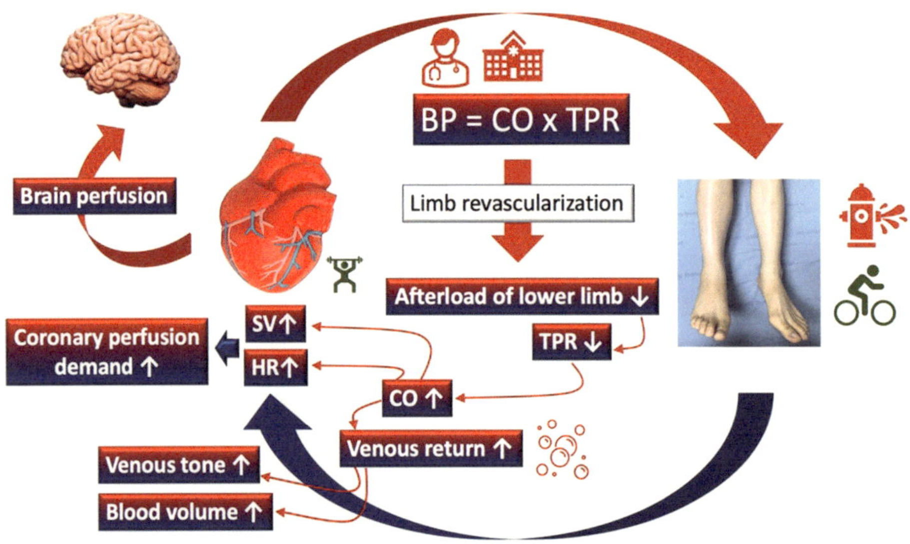

Figure 3.
The normal physiologic changes of cardiovascular system and cardiac response after lower limb revascularization. BP, blood pressure; CO, cardiac output; TPR, total peripheral resistant; SV, stroke volume; HR, heart rate.

extremities [39, 42, 43]. The preoperative cardiac reserve and cardiac response after lower limb revascularization are the important risk factors of perioperative MACE [14, 37, 43]. The rapidly increasing of the lower limb perfusion after revascularized procedures causes the alteration of cardiac physiology and activation of autoregulation process [3, 41, 42]. The cardiac responsibility is dependent on the increasing of blood flow rate to the revascularized limb which is determined by the degree of revascularization. If the revascularization is successful, almost stenotic, or occlusive lesions are well recanalization by endovascular therapy or open vascular bypass procedure which is cross all vascular lesions from the good inflow to the good run-off vessel, the after load of the lower limb are decreasing rapidly. The decreasing afterload leads to the reduction of total peripheral resistance (TPR) (**Figure 3**).

In the normal cardiac reserve patients, the immediate cardiac response to maintain the mean arterial blood pressure (MAP) is increasing of the cardiac output (CO) by the mechanoreceptors, known as baroreceptor reflex which are in the aortic arch and carotid sinus. The baroreceptors activity is decreasing lead to the reduction of impulse toward to the cardiovascular center. The increasing of sympathetic activity and the reduction of parasympathetic activity cause the increasing of CO (Eq. (1)). The increasing of CO is performed by the increasing of stroke volume (SV) and heart rate (HR) which are regulated by an autonomic nervous system (ANS) and a hormonal system though the positive chronotropic substances in human body. (Eq. (2)) (**Figure 3**).

$$\text{MAP} = \text{CO} \times \text{TPR} \tag{1}$$

$$\text{MAP} = (\text{SV} \times \text{HR}) \times \text{TPR} \tag{2}$$

The good cardiac reserve patients with good ejection fraction (EF) are regulated the SV by increasing of cardiac contractility and venous return (Eq. (3)). The increasing of cardiac contractility is activated by the neurohormonal system through the positive inotropic substances. The venous return which is regulated by the blood volume and venous tone are increased by the renin-angiotensin-aldosterone system (RAAS) activation, antidiuretic hormone (ADH) releasing, sympathetic nervous system, and central nervous system (Eq. (4)) (**Figure 3**).

$$\text{MAP} = (\text{cardiac contraction} \times \text{venous return}) \times \text{HR} \times \text{TPR} \tag{3}$$

$$\text{MAP} = \text{cardiac contraction} \times (\text{blood volume} \times \text{venous tone}) \times \text{HR} \times \text{TPR} \tag{4}$$

During the lower limb revascularization in patients with CLTI, the cardiac response by the increasing of SV through the cardiac contractility and increasing of HR are requiring the adequate perfusion of a myocardium which is more than resting cardiac metabolic requirement in non-revascularization of lower limb patients. So, the good functional status and cardiac reserve by the coronary artery perfusion which feeding to the myocardium is very important to prevent perioperative MI. In addition, the normal cardiac response and autoregulation process are controlling the MAP to keep a constant blood flow to the other vital organ including the brain and renal to prevent perioperative stroke and acute kidney injury (AKI), respectively (**Figure 3**) [37, 41, 42].

For poor functional status and poor cardiac reserve patients, the cardiac response after revascularization though the increasing of heart rate and cardiac contractility to maintain MAP which increase the perfusion demand of myocardium are risk of acute

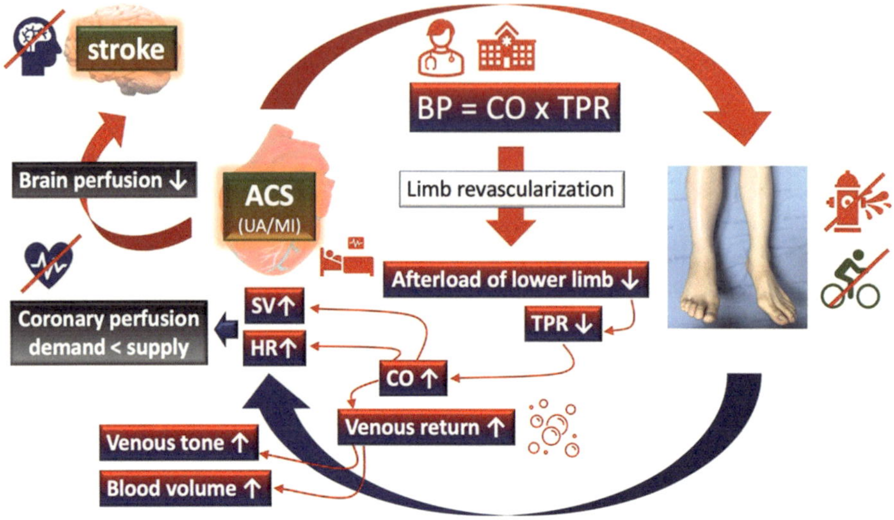

Figure 4.
The physiologic disturbance of cardiovascular system after lower limb revascularization in patients with coexisting coronary artery disease. BP, blood pressure; CO, cardiac output; TPR, total peripheral resistant; SV, stroke volume; HR, heart rate; ACS, acute coronary syndrome; UA, unstable angina; MI, myocardial infarction.

coronary syndrome (ACS) (Eq. (3)). The coexisting CAD or HF causes the limitation of blood supply to the myocardium and poor ejection fraction (EF) cause the insufficient perfusion to the heart and other organ. Therefore, the MI and acute HF are usually precipitated during revascularization procedure in CLTI patients with cardiac comorbidities. The ACS including UA, STEMI, and NSTEMI. After the mismatch of cardiac demand–supply, the severity of myocardial ischemia can present from the UA without myocardial necrosis to the myocardial infarction (MI) which there is myocardial ischemia with detectable myonecrosis by the releasing of cardiac biomarkers such as creatine kinase, troponin, myoglobin in the systemic circulation (**Figure 4**) [41, 42].

The consequence of MI or acute HF are systemic poor perfusion and cardiogenic shock. The autoregulation process to keep the adequate perfusion to the brain is the vital role to prevent stroke for this situation. The concomitant significant arterial occlusive disease of the carotid and vertebral arterial system can precipitate the perioperative stroke after revascularization because the decompensate in cardiac responsibility and autoregulation process which lead to the failure to maintain the constant blood flow to the brain. For this reason, the concomitant CAD, HF or CVD in patient with CLTI are high risk of MACE during lower limb revascularization. The early detection, optimization of the functional status, aggressive medical treatment in the preoperative phase before lower limb revascularization should be performed intensively to decrease the risk of perioperative MACE and to increase the chance of a functional limb salvage and long-term ambulatory status which effect on quality of life and cardiovascular mortality in patients with CLTI [19, 20].

3.2 The anatomic distribution and severity of lower limb arterial occlusive disease related to perioperative MACE

A reduction in arterial lumen more than 75% of cross-sectional area or 50% of luminal diameter causes the significant stenosis which are limiting blood flow to

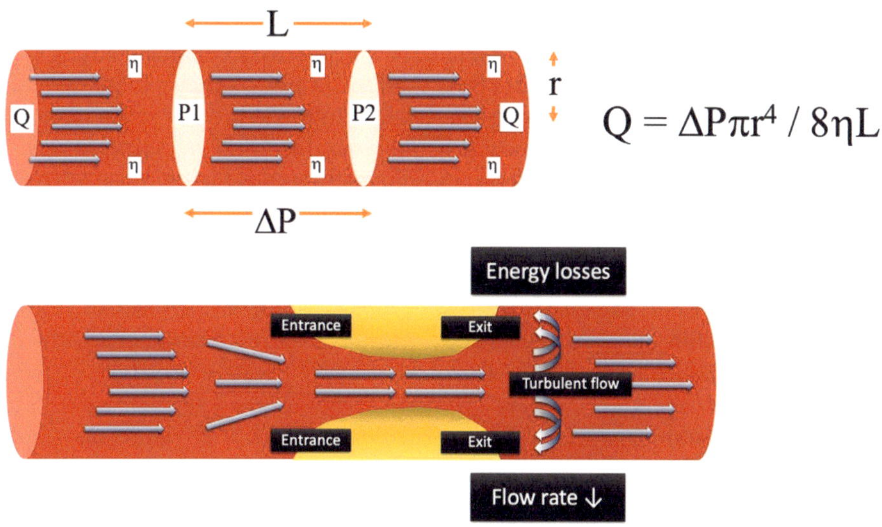

Figure 5.
The energy losses in the arterial stenotic lesion according to Poiseuille's law and the reduction in blood flow across an arterial stenosis due to the inertial energy losses by the turbulent flow in entrance and exit effects. Q, flow rate; ΔP, pressure gradient (P1-P2); r, radius; L, length; η, fluid viscosity.

lower limbs [3, 35]. From the Poiseuille's law [44, 45], the flow rate (Q) of the fluid in a hollow cylindrical shape tube is a direct variation of the fluid pressure (ΔP) and tube's radius (r) whereas the tube's length (L) and fluid viscosity (η) is indirect variation of the flow rate (Eq. (5)) (**Figure 5**).

$$Q = \Delta P \pi r^4 / 8\eta L \tag{5}$$

Therefore, the stenotic or occlusive arterial lesions are affecting to the decreasing of blood flow rate in the PAD of lower extremity. A severe stenosis and long length of the arterial lesions, meaning a greater decrease in blood flow and perfusion to lower limb when compare with a mild stenosis and short lesions. For the geographic pattern of stenosis. The irregular and abrupt change of arterial lumen results in more reduction of blood flow rate than a gradual tapering of the lumen (**Figure 5**) [37, 44, 45].

In addition, the blood flow rate is also affected by the anatomic distribution of a stenosis or occlusion. The inertial losses, an entry and exit of blood in a stenosis area which are resulting in the reduction of blood flow rate is important factors to the lower limb perfusion. The abrupt change of luminal stenosis of the entry site and expansion of the flow stream of the exit site has created the dissipation of kinetic energy in a zone of turbulence flow (**Figure 3**). Thus, the multiple short stenotic lesions result in more energy losses than single long stenotic lesion [37, 44, 45]. Commonly, the anatomic distribution of atherosclerosis in CLTI patients usually presents in multilevel occlusive disease [3]. The concomitant FP occlusive disease and IP arterial occlusive lesions usually occurred. The pattern of disease often presents the long occlusion or multiple severe stenosis lesions in CLTI [3, 35, 39].

In mild to moderate severity of LEAD, a stenosis vascular lesions are not influenced to lower limb perfusion at resting blood flow rates but become critical when flow rates are increased by reactive hyperemia through the vasodilatation which produce the intermittent claudication symptom during walking or exercise [12, 37, 43].

So, the revascularization strategy in patients with intermittent claudication have only increased flow rate to prevent the insufficiency perfusion during walking or exercise. In CLTI patients, the goal of lower limb revascularization is to increase the blood flow rate which is ensuring adequate straight inline to the wound or maintain resting metabolic requirement of lower limb for tissue loss and rest pain, respectively [3, 35, 43]. Therefore, the alterations of physiologic flow rate during revascularization in intermittent claudication is lower than CLTI which more extensive calcified and severe atherosclerotic stenotic or occlusive lesions. Moreover, the associated coronary and cerebrovascular disease are usually occurred and more severity in patients with extensive anatomic distribution of atherosclerotic CLTI [14, 35]. Altogether, the perioperative MACE is frequently present during revascularization in CLTI which is severe, multilevel atherosclerotic disease.

3.3 Type of lower limb revascularization related to MACE

The best choice for lower limb revascularization is dependent on multiple factors which determine, by the characteristic of patients, disease, and expertise of physicians. The patient's co-morbidities, anatomic distribution and severity of disease, patient's clinical presentation or degree of tissue loss, availability of venous conduit for below the knee lesion as well as doctor's preference, and experience (doctors included vascular surgeons, interventionist, cardiologist, and angiologist) are established to the important factors to determine the type of revascularization [14, 37, 43, 46–48].

Currently, the "endovascular-first strategy" or "endovascular-first approach" for lower limb revascularization in patients with LEAD have increased significantly [46]. This minimally invasive approach is aimed to decrease the morbidity and mortality of the open vascular bypass procedure. There are a lot of publications report the ET in CLTI patients with suprainguinal disease (aortoiliac disease, AIOD) and infrainguinal disease such as FP, IP, and inframalleolar arteries segment (IM) [3, 35, 46, 47]. Complex, severe, multilevel atherosclerotic occlusive can performed revascularization by ET which is associated with amputation free survival improvement over the long-term with modest relative increased risk of reintervention [47]. CLTI patients with multiple co-morbidities, the initial surgical bypass is associated with poorer amputation-free survival compare with an endovascular-first approach due to increased severity of wounds at the time of presentation [46]. The study of CLTI in the Vascular Quality Initiative (VQI) reports the ET procedures are more offered to older and more co-morbidities patients. The patients who performed ET demonstrated the lower perioperative mortality when compare with open vascular bypass. However, the benefit of ET is not demonstrated when treating patients with few comorbidities or less advanced disease [48]. Finally, the CLTI which is the advance form of atherosclerosis of LEAD are usually involved to other vascular bed. The coexisting multiple co-morbidities due to systemic atherosclerotic disease including CAD and CVA are usually present in CLTI patients who plan for revascularization [34, 43]. Therefore, the endovascular-first strategy is still the preferred approach for the majority of CLTI patients. The open vascular bypass procedures are more likely to perform for reintervention procedures, young patients, and few comorbidities [48].

However, long term patency and freedom from reintervention rate of open vascular bypass procedures are better than ET. The selection of CLTI patients to performed open vascular bypass or ET should be considered carefully. The patient's based individual approach and risk–benefit consideration including the risk of perioperative

MACE, MALE, quality of life, morbidity, and mortality of each procedure are very important [3, 35, 43].

3.3.1 MACE related to open vascular bypass

The open vascular bypass procedures are significant impact of the physiological changes of the cardiovascular system by decreasing afterload which is loaded to the cardiac function [41–43]. The degree of revascularization and increasing of blood flow rate of open vascular bypass procedures are determined by the level of inflow artery, quality of distal runoff and unimpaired of foot arch arteries as well as the total length of the bypass which cross to the atherosclerotic lesion. Higher or larger arterial inflow, better quality of distal runoff and foot arch arteries, longer length of bypass are more increasing of blood flow and pressure to lower limb [37, 41–43, 49]. Example: The CLTI patients with multisegmented AIOD, FP, and IP disease who performed common iliac artery to tibial artery bypass which allow inline flow to the complete foot arch artery is a higher physiologic alteration of the cardiovascular system during revascularization than the CLTI patients who performed distal superficial femoral artery to tibial artery short bypass with incomplete foot arch artery to treat the isolated IP disease [37, 41]. The in-situ anatomical bypass procedures such as aortobifemoral bypass is a higher risk of perioperative MACE than extra-anatomical bypass such as axillobifemoral bypass due to more rapid increasing of blood flow rate, third space loss from abdominal exploration of the in-situ anatomical bypass procedures. Therefore, a complexity and planning of open vascular bypass are related to risk of perioperative MACE. Comparing with ET, the open vascular bypass procedure is a higher risk of perioperative MACE because more rapid increasing of blood flow and more alteration of the cardiovascular system (**Figure 6**).

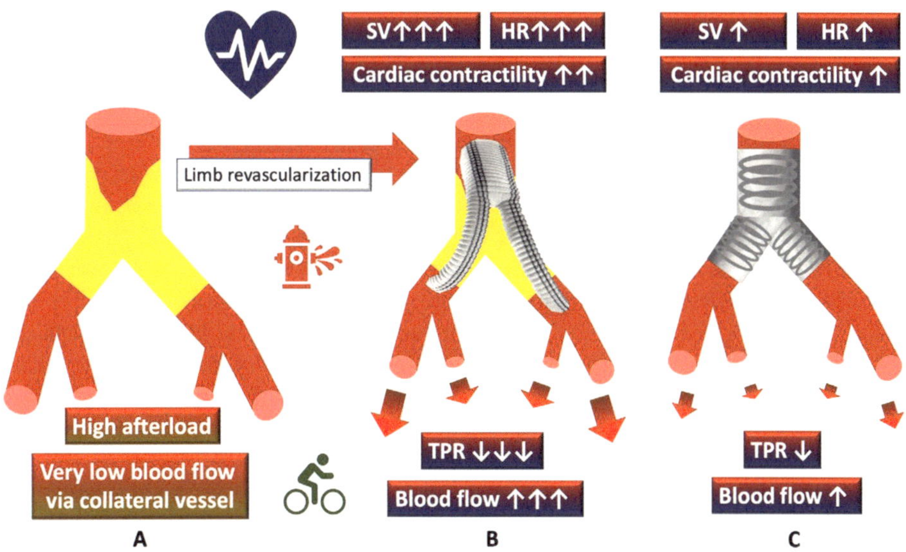

Figure 6.
The impact of revascularization in CLTI patients with TASC-D AIOD (A) open vascular bypass by vascular bifurcate graft (B) and endovascular treatment by stent graft (C) on the blood flow of lower limb and cardiovascular system. TASC, trans-Atlantic inter-society consensus; AIOD, aortoiliac occlusive disease; CLTI, chronic limb-threatening ischemia.

The risk of open vascular bypass also includes the risk of anesthesia which related to perioperative MACE. Most of the open bypass procedure needs to perform under general or spinal anesthesia which impact on the cardiovascular system [37]. Most anesthetic agent and muscle relaxant during anesthesia are negative impact on the cardiovascular system. The potential complications and morbidities of open vascular bypass procedures include surgical wound infection, bleeding, adjacent tissue/organ injury (such as nerve injury) due to the vessel dissection, and manipulation in open vascular bypass operation [37]. The surgical infection is usually present in CLTI with a history of wound infection, major tissue loss, diabetic foot ulcer, below the knee vascular bypass, redo-open vascular bypass in the previous surgical area [3, 13, 37]. All perioperative non-cardiovascular complication led to reintervention or the stress and inflammation which are precipitate the perioperative MACE.

The risk of bleeding and perianastomotic pseudoaneurysm or hematoma are a significant increase in patient who take multiple antiplatelets or anticoagulants [35]. Most of perianastomotic pseudoaneurysm requires the surgical treatment which increases the perioperative MACE due to anesthesia and bleeding during the redo operation. The CLTI patients with coexisting ACS or CVD usually take dual antiplatelet such as aspirin and clopidogrel especially in CAD patients with recent percutaneous coronary intervention (PCI) with stent [35, 37]. The cardiac arrhythmic patients need to take the oral anticoagulants to prevent intracardiac clot formation. The patients who had a history of CVD usually take an anticoagulant or antiplatelet to prevent recurrent stroke. So, the open vascular bypass procedures in CLTI patients with coexisting CAD and CVD are higher risk of bleeding and wound complications than ET. On the other hand, the discontinuation of antiplatelets or anticoagulants in high-risk MACE patients preoperatively are prohibited and increasing of the incidence of recurrent MACE during lower limb revascularization [14, 35, 37]. The appropriate post-operative care of CLTI patients who underwent open vascular bypass including wound care, ambulation training, rehabilitation, and atherosclerotic risk factors modification are decreased risk of perioperative complications, perioperative MACE, and long-term MACE [37, 42, 50].

3.3.2 MACE related to endovascular treatment

The ET can decrease the risk of perioperative MACE through the two main mechanisms. (1) The risk of anesthesia, proper anesthesia is allowing safe, less complication, comfortable, and well operated of the interventions. Most of CLTI patients are classified in class III and class IV of the American Society of Anesthesiologists (ASA) physical status due to severe systemic disease such as poorly controlled DM, hypertension, HF, history of ACS or CVD, chronic kidney disease, etc. High ASA physical status is associated with perioperative morbidity and mortality, namely, perioperative MACE [37]. Most of the ET procedures are preferred under local anesthesia with adequate sedation or analgesia which decreased the risk of general and spinal anesthesia. Anesthetic agents in general and spinal anesthesia usually impacts on the cardiovascular system [37]. (2) The risk of the operation, ET procedures reported less bleeding, less surgical wound complications, and less adjacent tissue/organ injury when compare with open vascular bypass procedures. The incidence of the surgical infection such as groin wound infection, vascular graft infection is very low in CLTI patients who underwent ET. In addition, less post-operative pain due to minimally invasive procedure allow early ambulation in patients with CLTI when compare with open vascular bypass. Thus, the risk of post-operative complications due to non-ambulatory status including deep vein thrombosis (DVT), lung atelectasis, aspiration pneumonia, urinary tract infection, and bowel ileus are decreased [37, 42, 50]. Especially in suprainguinal lesion or AIOD, the in-situ open vascular bypass procedure is needed for abdominal exploration which is significantly higher morbidity and mortality when compare with ET or hybrid operation. Because of the development of a new generation of aortoiliac stent and endograft, ET was associated with high initial technical success with equal short- to mid-term patency rate and fewer in-hospital systemic complications when compare with open vascular bypass for simple and complex AIOD [35, 37, 49].

To avoid the major operation of open vascular bypass procedures, the advance age and multiple co-morbidities usually undergo revascularized procedure by ET [48]. So, the risk of perioperative MACE during ET due to revascularization process are still present in the real-world practice because of poor cardiac reserve and multiple comorbidities such as CAD, HF and CVD. The burden to cardiovascular system depends on the degree of physiologic changes after ET because of the increasing of blood flow to the lower extremity after successful revascularization [41, 42, 48]. The high level of occlusion (such as suprainguinal disease) and single stage multisegmented revascularization are high risk of perioperative MACE due to rapidly decreasing of afterload and rapid increasing of blood flow to lower limbs (**Figure 6**) [41, 42]. In addition, the new technology of the antiproliferative agent embeds endovascular device which has increased the patency of the target arterial lesion are increasing to use in CLTI patients who undergo ET [21–26]. Some cohort study and meta-analysis report the high incidence of MACE in CLTI patients after revascularization by DCB and DES. The complication such as aneurysmal degeneration in patients with ET are reported [27–31]. Therefore, the MACE related to DCB, and DES is still debatable [30, 32]. The mechanism of drug-delivering technology and pathophysiology of MACE which may precipitated by DCB and DES, and latest evidence of the relationship between drug-delivering technology and MACE and potential complications are described under the Section 4 of this Chapter.

4. Drug-delivering technology concept and their effect on the perioperative MACE

The drug delivering technology of the paclitaxel, sirolimus, everolimus and other antiproliferative agent coated balloon and eluting stent to increase the patency of native artery and in-stent restenosis (ISR) through the aggressively inhibition of arterial damage induced neointimal hyperplasia are trending to increase for ET in patient with CLTI [21–26]. Due to the controversy of the MACE and potential complications related to DCB, and DES, the pharmacologic effect of drug-delivering technology and pathophysiology of MACE are very important to guide the individual patients-based approach and determine the strategies to offer the drug delivering technology in CLTI patients who undergo ET [30, 32, 33].

4.1 Strategies for drug-delivering technology and concept in endovascular treatment

The management of LEAD included (1) the risk modification and medical treatment to prevent MACE and MALE, (2) Revascularization procedures to improve the quality of life and salvage a functional limb with maintaining ambulatory status for disabling intermittent claudication and CLTI, respectively [3, 13, 35, 39]. The ET is usually the first-line option in CLTI patients who are high risk for perioperative MACE [3, 46]. The fundamental steps of revascularization in ET include (1) percutaneous vascular access, (2) guidewire and catheter passage, (3) vessel preparation and, (4) definitive therapy of arterial occlusive lesion [37, 50–52]. After the vascular access approach and intraluminal passage of the wire across the stenotic or occlusive arterial lesion, the vessel preparation is the most important step to determine the definitive therapy of de novo arterial lesion which effect to the patency of the target arterial lesion in short- and long-term [51–53]. The aim of vessel preparation is modified local environment of the vessel prior to leaving something behind including stent or a non-stent anti-proliferative agent. The concept of vessel preparation included the altering residual mechanical forces in the vessel, improving luminal gain to deliver an implant and, debulking calcium or barriers to diffused of anti-proliferative agent. Thus, the vessel preparation allows an intraluminal maximal lumen diameter without thrombosis, early recoil, plaque-burden and, flow-limiting dissection is the ideal treatment for the best patency of target arterial lesion and limit the mechanism of late target vessel failure after intervention, namely, restenosis including negative vascular remodeling and intimal hyperplasia by definitive therapy [37, 50–55].

Plain balloon angioplasty (POBA) is used to dilate significant arterial stenotic or occlusive lesions with variable results. POBA can increase the luminal diameter of a target vessel by several mechanism including stretching or rupture of plaque and connective fibers in the intima and media, compression of plaque and thrombus, compression of the medial layers, redistribution of plaque or thrombus at the inner surface of an artery, and overstretching of the artery [51, 53]. The drug delivering technology which offer the best long-term patency and prevent restenosis in de novo arterial lesion which does not indicate to scaffolding or stenting after the vessel preparation process is DCB [22–25, 32, 55].

DCB is a balloon-mounted surround by an antiproliferative chemotherapeutic agent for delivering biologically active materials into the vessel wall. The paclitaxel is a majority of chemotherapeutic agent which is effects by binding to the beta subunit of tubulin, resulting in the cessation of microtubular function and the inhibition of cellular division [37, 55]. The technique of DCB in ET include (1) adequate vessel preparation by predilatation and gradually increasing diameter of the POBA to the optimal size of the target vessel diameter are achievable without the dissection or recoil, (2) transfer phase of DCB which needs to touch and press the vessel wall for agent release. The size of DCB need to be equal the last uncoated balloon or one by one ratio of the POBA:DCB diameter and, (3) The action phase of DCB, the agent should stay as long as possible as a reservoir for long-term antiproliferative effect on the vessel wall after the drug transfer [37, 55, 56]. The long-term effect on the vessel wall is needed the lipophilicity properties of the agent without any toxicity to the target arterial lesion and other vascular bed when the drug is released in the systemic circulation in minimal level. The paclitaxel is a highly lipophilic property which limits the ability to transfer into the vessel wall but long-term embedded in the vessel wall. So, the excipient co-drug is needed to facilitate absorption in transfer phase. The stable configuration during kept on the shelf, during transport and handling with minimal loss of the agents on the delivering device are very important factors which effect on the efficacy of the DCB. Several DCB for use in the peripheral vascular intervention on the market are developed currently. The main differences in each manufacturer including excipient molecules bound to the drug, nature of coating, and the concentration of drug lead to difference in the efficacy, effectiveness, and safety of DCB in real-world practice and their studies [53, 55, 56].

For FP disease, there are a lot of the studies which are reporting the results in a common theme of a significantly better patency and freedom from CD-TLR when comparing DCB to POBA [24]. Therefore, the conclusion of DCB in FP arterial occlusive disease confirm the safety and effectiveness of in both simple and complex FP lesions [25, 53–55]. On the other hand, the IP arterial occlusive disease which are significant restenosis and progression of disease after POBA are still lack of the high evidence base and long-term data to conclude the result of DCB in IP disease. Currently, DCBs are ongoing evaluation for the treatment of IP target arterial lesions. Because of the downstream risk of embolization due to the increased paclitaxel dose and crystalline conferred by the early generation of DCB, the early study result of DCB in the IP patients who undergo ET is a trend toward higher 1-year major amputation rate as compared with POBA [57]. However, the next generation stage of DCB demonstrated the favorable result of freedom from CD-TLR and major amputations at 12 months. Thus, the long-term outcome data are needed to investigate in DCB of CLTI patients with IP arterial occlusive disease before implementation with the trend to early benefit in treatment of IP arterial occlusive disease by DCB [58, 59].

If flow-limiting dissection or recoil are present after POBA, the scaffolds are necessary to maintain the luminal diameter and prevent thrombosis by the closure of the dissection area [50, 51, 53]. Over recent years, the self-expanding nitinol stents has achieved the treatment of recoil, flow-limiting dissection. In addition, there are a lot of publications reported the significantly improved clinical results after nitinol stenting for the long arterial occlusive disease. However, the very long lesions are higher risk of ISR after bare metal stenting. Drug-eluting technology including DES has also limit ISR and increase freedom from clinical driven target lesion revascularization (CD-TLR) [51].

Drug delivering technology of the stents, namely, DES has demonstrated an aggressively inhibition the neointimal hyperplasia and improve patency rates. Initial clinical practice, paclitaxel, sirolimus, and everolimus have been attached to balloon-expandable stents (BES) for coronary arteries stenting in patients who undergo PCI which has a high technical success rate and reduction in restenosis rate [37, 53, 59]. Currently, DES loaded with chemotherapeutic agents such as paclitaxel, sirolimus, and everolimus usually using polymers. However, the chemotherapeutic agents which are inhibit the intimal response cause delay stent thrombosis as high as 4% after 1 year [37]. The stent thrombosis mechanism is the exposed raw surface of the stent to the blood circulation due to a minimal incorporation and a lack of endothelialization of the DES into the arterial wall. The latest generation of DES demonstrated the better patency freedom from CD-TLR when compare with bare metal stent in both FP and IP occlusive diseases [24, 26, 37, 60–62].

The FP disease which indicates for the stent deployment due to flow-limiting dissection or recoil, the first generation of DES, including sirolimus and everolimus coated self-expanding stent (SES) does not demonstrate the benefit for long-term patency and restenosis between DES and bare metal stents [63]. The next generation of DES which is a polymer-free paclitaxel coated SES demonstrates a sustained 2-year benefit for decreased target lesion revascularization and improve patency with 2% of stent thrombosis and less than 2% of stent fracture in FP occlusive disease. A polymer-free DESs release 95% of the antiproliferative within the first 24 hours. For long-term follow up, the relative risk reduction of 5-year reintervention or restenosis are greater than 40% in DES when compare with POBA and bare metal stent in FP occlusive disease [64–66]. The latest generation of DES in FP disease are elute the paclitaxel using a fluoropolymer coating which release 40% of the paclitaxel within the first 30 days and continue to release a drug over time with an estimated 90% eluted at 12 months. So, the sustaining of paclitaxel levels in the arterial wall of the fluoropolymer coating DES are longer periods than the previous version polymer-free DES [26, 37, 53, 67, 68]. The latest ongoing clinical trial demonstrate the better initial 1-year outcome of the primary patency of latest DES when compare with bare metal stent [60]. In addition, the ongoing trial demonstrate the comparable result of the all-cause death and target-limb major amputation between the DES and bare metal stent at 12 months [60].

For IP disease, the POBA with bailout stenting is still the standard treatment for revascularization. Because of the similarity in size between the coronary and IP arteries, the IP arterial occlusive disease which needs to be stenting due to the significant dissection or recoil are treated by the coronary stent. The off-label use of fluoropolymer with everolimus eluting BES which use in the coronary artery system are reported in RCTs and the real-world practice studies [61, 62]. The DES in focal IP disease significantly inhibit vascular restenosis and improve primary patency, decrease reintervention, and improve wound healing in patients with CLTI [61]. In addition, DES of IP disease may decrease risk of CD-TLR, restenosis rate and, amputation rate without any impact on mortality [62].

Heavy calcifications of the vessel wall which are usually present in CLTI patients with DM, advance age and chronic kidney disease remain the risk of early restenosis, thrombosis, and high CD-TLR [51]. The mechanism of the poor patency of target arterial lesion in calcification of the vessel wall includes (1) The mechanical effect of the vessel wall calcification act as the barrier to optimal dilatation of POBA and stenting. The calcific arterial lesions are increased risk of flow limiting dissection, recoil, and other angiographic complications [51, 53]. In addition, an inadequate vessel preparation due to retain plaque burden lesion and calcified lesion are still limiting the maximal luminal gain, stent apposition and stent expansion which effect to the long-term patency and increased risk of ISR in both bare metal stent and DES. (2) The pharmacological effect, the drug absorption of drug delivering device including DCB and DES are decrease in high calcific lesions [53, 54]. So, the plaque modifying device such as focal pressure balloon, cutting balloon, scoring balloon, serranator balloon, and lithoplasty device are developed for achieving of the vessel preparation in plaque burden and calcified arterial lesion. For heavy and circumferential severe atherosclerotic plaque and calcification, there are several atherectomy devices on the market currently which can debulking the calcification to increase the drug uptake to the vessel wall by the DCB and DES [53, 55, 69, 70]. The atherectomy include directional atherectomy, rotational atherectomy, orbital atherectomy, and laser atherectomy. The best choice for plaque modifying device and atherectomy are still debate and beyond the scope of this article. The result of DCB combined techniques with the atherectomy trend toward better outcomes in severely calcified long segment lesions and chronic total occlusion (CTO). However, the recent randomized control trial (RCT) and real-world practice study result are a debate in the risk of dissection and bailout stenting result with limited 1-year patency benefit in the combination of DCB with atherectomy as compared to DCB alone [69, 70].

For the ISR lesion, the characteristic of the restenosis lesion is different from the de novo arterial lesion. The "sandwich" structure including (1) a cell-dense neointimal hyperplasia within the stent struts which has ingrain and elastic consistency and (2) a cell-poor layer with a fibrous matrix which is embedded in the intimal layer at the outer margin of the stent struts results in a rubbery consistency of the lesions which poor response to POBA. Therefore, the significant recurrent stenosis of the ISR lesions usually presents after POBA without any specialty device [51, 53]. The DCB appears to be a significant benefit to treating ISR as opposed to POBA [21, 56, 71]. The combination of DCB with atherectomy devices is offered to increase the patency in patients with ISR. However, the results of these combinations for ISR have a little benefit when compare with DCB alone [53, 72].

4.2 Pharmacologic effect and pathophysiology of drug-delivering technology related to MACE

The healing response of vascular endothelium after POBA and stent placement which induce vascular endothelial injury is the activation of a local inflammatory response and the proliferation of smooth muscle cells (SMC) as well as migration of SMC into the neointima leading to significant restenosis [73, 74]. Paclitaxel and sirolimus coating devices directly inhibit the proliferation and migration of SMC which cause neointimal hyperplasia inhibition [31].

The paclitaxel is a diterpenoid antineoplastic agent which inhibits the cell proliferation. The oncologist used the paclitaxel as the chemotherapy to treat cancers, including gastric, ovarian, endometrial, breast, non-small cell lung cancer, and other cancers. The antiproliferative effect of paclitaxel can prevent the restenosis of the LEAD by the inhibition of the intimal hyperplasia [31, 75]. In normal human body physiology, microtubules are maintained cell shape and intracellular transport function, signaling, protein secretion, and motility function. The antimicrotubule effect of paclitaxel causes the formation of stable dysfunctional microtubules by binding to intracellular tubulin and interfering with spindle formation. The mitotic cell division is inhibited by the prevention of tubulin depolymerization through the irreversible of paclitaxel-tubulin binding. The prevention of tubulin depolymerization led to a microtubular dynamics disruption and cell death. The inhibition of cytokine response, migration, and secretion of matrix metalloproteinases (MMP) are the main mechanism to prevent the intimal hyperplasia after ET [31]. Consequently, the SMC proliferation and migration are inhibited which prevent neointimal hyperplasia of the vessel wall [31, 73, 74]. After DCB treatment, the paclitaxel particles are localized in fibroblast and SMC layers to inhibit the neointimal hyperplasia [73, 74]. Following DCB inflation in post-vessel preparation artery, the tissue absorption of the paclitaxel is occurring. Because of the low solubility and solid state of the paclitaxel is lower than tissue metabolic clearance rate, the paclitaxel accumulated in the target arterial lesion and cause durable effect on intimal hyperplasia [30, 55]. Overall, the pharmacokinetics of paclitaxel which is multiphasic and non-linear cause long lasting tissue accumulation of paclitaxel. The prevention of intimal hyperplasia is effective in long-term period with unknown long-term biological side effects [76, 77].

The pathophysiology and mechanism of the cardiac side effect of paclitaxel is not well established. The current studies concluded that the paclitaxel is one of cardiotoxicity chemotherapeutic agents. Some studies report the severe reduction in EF and cardiac arrhythmia [77, 78]. Theoretically, paclitaxel-induced cardiotoxicity can be occurred by the two main mechanisms: (1) direct effect of the myocardial damage which reduce in EF and precipitate HF through a subcellular organelle disturbance, (2) indirect effect of the releasing of histamine and QT interval prolongation which disturbed the cardiac electrical conduction led to cardiac arrhythmia such as atrial fibrillation (AF) and bradycardia (**Figure 7**). There are a lot of literatures report the cardiac side effects which is the most serious adverse effects of chemotherapy in malignancy patients. The early cardiac side effect of paclitaxel in chemotherapeutic

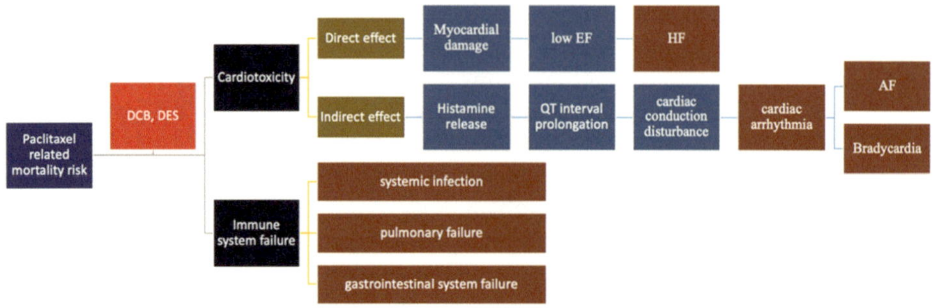

Figure 7.
Pathophysiology of paclitaxel-induced cardiotoxicity related to mortality risk. DCB, drug coated balloon; drug eluting balloon. DES; EF, ejection fraction; HF, heart failure; AF, atrial fibrillation.

dose can occur in first month including ACS, myocardial dysfunction, reversible cardiac arrhythmias, ventricular repolarization abnormality, QT interval prolongation on electrocardiogram, and pericardial reaction. Long-term cardiac adverse events include cardiac dysfunction, which lead to HF and other MACE [77, 78]. However, most malignancy patients who have a paclitaxel-induced cardiotoxicity usually to be asymptomatic or mild severity. Under carefully monitoring of cardiac function, the safely use of paclitaxel as a chemotherapy in malignancy patients with cardiac co-morbidities including the UA, HF, and AF have been reported [76].

For the paclitaxel in ET, the dosage of paclitaxel in drug delivering technology including DCB and DES is less than 1% of chemotherapy in malignancy patients. Only asymptomatic bradycardia is seen in CLTI patients who perform ET with paclitaxel agent use [31, 55]. The other early cardiotoxicity of paclitaxel is unlikely to be from the direct effect of myocardial damage [77, 78]. However, the sustained retention of the drug in the vessel wall due to the crystalline form with a paclitaxel spacer may create the ongoing distal embolization of the paclitaxel in the systemic circulation which may relate to the increasing risk of MACE and MALE including the increasing of amputation rate [25, 27, 30]. In addition, the anti-neoplastic effect of paclitaxel causes the toxicity to the immune system (**Figure 7**). The human body immune system is inhibited by the paclitaxel which increased risk of non-cardiac deaths including systemic infection, pulmonary and gastrointestinal system failure.

The potential complications due to local toxicity of the paclitaxel which report in the literatures include aneurysmal degeneration, vascular fibrinoid necrosis, small vessel inflammation, and downstream muscle necrosis. The inhibition of intimal hyperplasia after balloon angioplasty causes the post-angioplasty injured artery dilatation and aneurysmal formation in long-term period. The paclitaxel particles which insoluble cause downstream embolization led to ischemia and repetitive inflammation of the small vessel. The primary hypothesis of downstream paclitaxel particulate showers is concordant to the higher amputation rate and MALE of the DCB when compare with POBA in CLTI patients with IP arterial occlusive disease [25, 27, 30, 62]. However, there are some studies report no significant adverse effects related to distal paclitaxel crystalline embolization. The early result of recent study demonstrated the promising safety and efficacy of paclitaxel coated balloon in CLTI patients with IP arterial occlusive disease [58, 62]. Thus, large well RCT and real-world registry are needed to investigate the long-term safety and efficacy of DCB for treatment of PAD.

For the DES, the total dose of the paclitaxel is lower than DCB. The release kinetic of DCB via the transfer and action (releasing) phase of paclitaxel after balloon angioplasty are use the concept "the greater injury, the greater penetration of the drug" in injured vessel after balloon angioplasty. The large amount of paclitaxel on DCB which delivery to the vessel wall has a high rate of distal embolization. On the other hand, the release kinetic of DES is a polymer controlled sustained release process. Thus, the downstream paclitaxel showers are not occurred when the DES is used in CLTI patients with IP arterial occlusive disease. Previous studies report the non-significant distal embolization in coronary polymer coated paclitaxel eluting stents of IP arteries. Therefore, the DES is significant reducing of CD-TLR, MALE and major amputations in 5-year and 10-year period when compare with POBA and DCB. The DCB has no obvious advantage in the treatment of IP arterial occlusive disease [23, 57, 62].

Because of the pathophysiology of cardiotoxicity associated with paclitaxel used to not be well understood, the pathophysiology of the MACE related to drug delivering technology is not well determined [33, 77, 78]. However, previous study report high-risk features which associated with paclitaxel-induced cardiotoxicity including age >60 years, DM, hypertension, Eastern Cooperative Oncology Group (ECOG) Performance Status (PS) scale 2, and chest radiotherapy [76, 77]. The patients with CLTI usually have multiple co-morbidities including DM, hypertension, old age and poor ECOG PS scale [3, 35, 39]. Thus, closed monitoring of cardiac function after paclitaxel treatment is still required in CLTI patients who have high-risk features. Therefore, long-term result of paclitaxel related MACE and MALE needs to be more investigated [3, 22].

Because of the hypothesis of the paclitaxel delivering device related MACE in CLTI patients and some evidence of the paclitaxel related MALE through the particulate embolization induced slow flow or no-flow phenomenon especially in CLTI patients with the IP arterial occlusive disease [25, 27, 30, 62]. The sirolimus coated balloons to prevent the intimal hyperplasia are investigated. The sirolimus, also known as rapamycin, is a macrocyclic lactone antibiotic which produced by bacteria *Streptomyces hygroscopicus.* The sirolimus is isolated from the Easter Island soil which use as an antifungal medication especially in Candidiasis. The potent anti-neoplastic effect through the inhibition of the mammalian target of rapamycin (mTOR) of the sirolimus is investigated. Currently, the sirolimus is an immunosuppressive agent for prevention of organ transplant rejections and antineoplastic agent for treatment of lymphangioleiomyomatosis, and perivascular epithelioid cell tumors. The pathophysiology of the inhibition of neointimal hyperplasia has been less well studied. There are a lot of recent publications suggested excellent 6-month primary patency and encouraging 12-month freedom from CD-TLR, amputation-free survival rate, and limb salvage rates without early safety concerns [79]. In addition, particulate embolization due to downstream showers of drug particle and less found in the sirolimus coated balloon when compare with paclitaxel coated balloons. Comparing with paclitaxel coated balloon, the slow flow or no-flow phenomenon induced CD-TLR and MALE are less present in sirolimus coated balloon in patients with CLTI patients [80]. Thus, the sirolimus coated balloon may have a benefit to prevent restenosis of the target artery without significant MACE and MALE in ET in CLTI patients who candidate for revascularization. The further large randomized and real-world registry study in both short-term and long-term safety and efficacy is required to establish the result of sirolimus coated balloon in CLTI patients [81].

5. Summary and update of the best evidence of drug-delivering technology related to MACE in PAD

The drug delivering device have been extensively investigated to inhibit arterial restenosis and ISR to improve clinical outcomes, patency, CD-TLR, amputation free survival rate after revascularization by ET. Because the positive results of drug delivering technology from several industry-sponsored studies which demonstrated the improvement in the primary patency and reduction of CD-TLR in CLTI patients FP arterial occlusive disease, the DCB and DES are widely used for ET in CLTI patients who indicate for revascularization [25, 58, 60, 65, 68]. Both FP and IP arterial occlusive disease are investigated the limb, morbidity and mortality outcome including MALE and MACE [3, 23–25, 27, 30, 31, 33, 54, 56, 57, 59, 61, 62, 74, 75]. Concerns about a long-term mortality in PAD patients who use the paclitaxel delivering device are first reported by a meta-analysis in 2018 that described the increasing of mortality rate in comparison to POBA or bare metal stent beginning at 2 years after ET [33]. In addition, the concerning of paclitaxel related MALE including major amputation rate and CD-TLR is raised after recent studies report the higher amputation rate in the paclitaxel coated balloon when compare with POBA under the particulate embolization hypothesis [27, 30, 61].

However, there are a lot of recent publication between 2020 and 2022 report the comparable result of MACE, mortality and amputation between paclitaxel delivering devices and non-drug device [82–86]. The 5-year follow-up of RCT for the safety and effectiveness of IP arterial occlusive disease report comparable risk of amputation and all-cause mortality rate between paclitaxel coated balloon and POBA in patients with CLTI [25, 85]. The independent patient-level meta-analysis revealed the safety of paclitaxel coated balloon without the relationship between level of paclitaxel exposure and mortality [84]. The recent study report no dose–response relationship between paclitaxel and mortality in drug delivering device [83]. In addition, the ET with drug delivering technology in patients with claudication are safety and effectiveness without increasing of mortality rate or MACE [86].

For the paclitaxel eluting stent, no difference in mortality between a DES and bare metal stent. Currently, ongoing study of polymer-coated DES had demonstrated the 1-year safety and efficacy with better patency when compare with bare metal stent [60]. As the United States Food and Drug Administration (FDA) and others have recommended follow patients to 5 years to collect safety and efficacy data, the result of long-term safety of DES is not completely concluded. The systematic review and meta-analysis report no significant difference in 12-month all-cause mortality between DES and DCB. Primary patency and freedom from CD-TLR are also comparable between the two groups [23].

For the local complications of drug delivering device, there are only few reports about aneurysmal degeneration, vascular fibrinoid necrosis, small vessel inflammation, and downstream skeletal muscle necrosis after paclitaxel agent device in ET. The risk of local complication for drug delivering technology in CLTI patients are not well identified. The further study is required to concluded about the local complication of DCB and DES in PAD [28–30, 78].

The limitation of meta-analysis and RCTs about the DCB and DES include: (1) most RCTs did not report the mortality rate, MACE or major amputations as the primary outcome or main outcome. So, the imprecision due to inadequate power of study can occurred and indued the error of the study result, (2) The heterogeneity of patient's characteristic and demographic data such as ratio of CLTI and claudicants, (3) The different of the paclitaxel dose, paclitaxel crystallinity, balloon platforms and coating of agent technology. Low dose balloons may demonstrate the better outcome in safety with same efficacy due to the small number of events and lack of adequate statistical power to detect a true effect, (4) Lack of actual cause of death and the clinical indications to major amputation, (5) The chronology bias due to the long period to published of all RCTs. The improvements in MACE and co-morbidities management and the different in the design of newer paclitaxel coated balloon platforms over time, (6) Some RCT report the mortality outcome and analyzed under subgroup analysis and post-hoc analysis. The patient level time to event data should be extracted and analyzed with a one stage model to increase power and precision and there was also consistent size and direction of the summary effect in the various subgroups and sensitivity tests.

Due to the controversy result of the paclitaxel coated balloon related MACE and limitation of the previous studies, the additional patient-level, adequately powered meta-analyses with larger RCT data sets will be needed to confirm the correlation between paclitaxel and MACE. For the new drug coating balloon to avoid the possible adverse event and paclitaxel related MACE, sirolimus is promising the safety and efficacy of short-term period. However, to conclude the outcome of sirolimus coated device, the large RCT with long-term follow up is necessary.

6. Conclusion

Cardiovascular disease is the life-threatening condition with high morbidity and mortality rate. The PAD is the vascular disease which has a strong relationship with the MACE. The revascularization is usually indicated in CLTI patients who have a high risk of perioperative MACE. The revascularization procedure in patients with CLTI to salvage a functional limb with aggressive best medical treatment can reduce MACE during the revascularization. Because of the physiologic changes and the autoregulation process after revascularization procedure by decreasing of the peripheral vascular resistance are the burden to the cardiovascular system. The cardiac reserve and response after lower limb revascularization, the anatomic distribution and severity of lower limb arterial occlusive disease as well as the type of revascularization are the important predictive factors of perioperative MACE.

The minimally invasive fashion of revascularization by endovascular-first strategy can reduce perioperative MACE by decreasing risk of anesthesia and operative risk. The drug-delivering technology including DCB, and DES can improve the long-term patency of ET in CLTI patients. However, the paclitaxel effect on the MACE and MALE are still debatable. The decision making of physicians under the individual patients-based approach and determine the strategies to offer the drug delivering technology in CLTI patients who undergo ET is a key to success in both short-term and long-term safety and efficacy of revascularization in PAD.

Acknowledgements

We would like to thank the Research group in surgery, Faculty of Medicine, Thammasat University.

Conflict of interest

The authors declare no conflict of interest. All industry-sponsored of endovascular device and drug delivering technology are not involved to contribute this chapter.

Author details

Saritphat Orrapin
Faculty of Medicine, Vascular Surgery Division, Department of Surgery, Thammasat University Hospital, Thammasat University, Pathum Thani, Thailand

*Address all correspondence to: sam3_orra@hotmail.com

References

[1] Dosluoglu HH. Chapter 108 Lower Extremity Arterial Disease: General Considerations. In: Cronenwett JL, Johnston KW, editors. Rutherford's vascular surgery. 8th ed. Philadelphia: Elsevier; 2014. p 1660-1674

[2] Tendera M, Aboyans V, Bartelink ML, Baumgartner I, Clement D, Collet JP, et al. ESC guidelines on the diagnosis and treatment of peripheral artery diseases: Document covering atherosclerotic disease of extracranial carotid and vertebral, mesenteric, renal, upper and lower extremity arteries: The task force on the diagnosis and treatment of peripheral artery diseases of the European Society of Cardiology (ESC). European Heart Journal. 2011;**32**:2851-2906

[3] Conte MS, Bradbury AW, Kolh P, White JV, Dick F, Fitridge R, et al. Global vascular guidelines on the management of chronic limb-threatening ischemia. European Journal of Vascular and Endovascular Surgery. 2019;**58**:S1-S109

[4] Orrapin S, Rerkasem K. Carotid endarterectomy for symptomatic carotid stenosis. Cochrane Database of Systematic Reviews. 2017;**6**:CD001081

[5] Gallino A, Aboyans V, Diehm C, Cosentino F, Stricker H, Falk E, et al. Non-coronary atherosclerosis. European Heart Journal. 2014;**35**:1112-1119

[6] Owens CD. Chapter 5: Atherosclerosis. In: Cronenwett JL, Johnston KW, editors. Rutherford's vascular surgery. 8th ed. Philadelphia: Elsevier; 2014. p. 66-77

[7] Orrapin S, Reanpang T, Orrapin S, Arwon S, Kattipathanapong T, Lekwanavijit S, et al. Case series of HIV infection-associated arteriopathy: Diagnosis, management, and outcome over a 5-year period at Maharaj Nakorn Chiang Mai hospital, Chiang Mai University. The International Journal of Lower Extremity Wounds. 2015;**14**:251-261

[8] Kullo IJ, Rooke TW. Clinical practice. Peripheral artery disease. The New England Journal of Medicine. 2016;**374**:861-871

[9] Brunicardi FC. Schwartz's Principle of Surgery. 10th ed. New York: The McGraw-Hill Companies Inc.; 2015

[10] Kroger K, Stang A, Kondratieva J, Moebus S, Beck E, Schmermund A, et al. Prevalence of peripheral arterial disease—Results of the Heinz Nixdorf recall study. European Journal of Epidemiology. 2006;**21**:279-285

[11] Crawford F, Welch K, Andras A, Chappell FM. Ankle brachial index for the diagnosis of lower limb peripheral arterial disease. The Cochrane Database of Systematic Reviews. 2016;**9**:Cd010680

[12] Mutirangura P, Ruangsetakit C, Wongwanit C, Sermsathanasawadi N, Chinsakchai K. Atherosclerosis obliterans of the lower extremities in Thai patients. Journal of the Medical Association of Thailand. 2006;**89**:1612-1620

[13] Mills JL Sr, Conte MS, Armstrong DG, Pomposelli FB, Schanzer A, Sidawy AN, et al. The society for vascular surgery lower extremity threatened limb classification system: Risk stratification based on wound, ischemia, and foot infection (WIfI). Journal of Vascular Surgery. 2014;**59**:220-234

[14] Norgren L, Hiatt WR, Dormandy JA, Nehler MR, Harris KA, Fowkes FG. Inter-society consensus for the management

of peripheral arterial disease (TASC II). Journal of Vascular Surgery. 2007;**45**(Suppl. S):S5-S67

[15] Carmo GA, Calderaro D, Gualandro DM, Pastana AF, Yu PC, Marques AC, et al. The ankle-brachial index is associated with cardiovascular complications after noncardiac surgery. Angiology. 2016;**67**:187-192

[16] Alberts MJ, Bhatt DL, Mas JL, Ohman EM, Hirsch AT, Rother J, et al. Three-year follow-up and event rates in the international REduction of atherothrombosis for continued health registry. European Heart Journal. 2009;**30**:2318-2326

[17] Aboyans V, Criqui MH, Abraham P, Allison MA, Creager MA, Diehm C, et al. Measurement and interpretation of the ankle-brachial index: A scientific statement from the American Heart Association. Circulation. 2012;**126**:2890-2909

[18] Bosco E, Hsueh L, McConeghy KW, Gravenstein S, Saade E. Major adverse cardiovascular event definitions used in observational analysis of administrative databases: A systematic review. BMC Medical Research Methodology. 2021;**21**:241

[19] Conte MS, Geraghty PJ, Bradbury AW, Hevelone ND, Lipsitz SR, Moneta GL, et al. Suggested objective performance goals and clinical trial design for evaluating catheter-based treatment of critical limb ischemia. Journal of Vascular Surgery. 2009;**50**:1462-1473

[20] Saraidaridis JT, Patel VI, Lancaster RT, Cambria RP, Conrad MF. Applicability of the Society for Vascular Surgery's objective performance goals for critical limb ischemia to current practice of lower-extremity bypass. Annals of Vascular Surgery. 2016;**30**:59-65

[21] Zhen Y, Ren H, Chen J, Chang Z, Wang C, Zheng J. Systematic review and Meta-analysis of drug-coated balloon angioplasty for In-stent restenosis in femoropopliteal artery disease. Journal of Vascular and Interventional Radiology. 2022;**33**:368-374.e366

[22] Dominguez Yulanka C, Pichert M, Alabi O, Huang J, Arham A, Brice A, et al. Predictros of drug-coated balloon and drug-eluting stent use in femoropopliteal endovascular interventions. Insights from the vascular quality initiative. Journal of the American College of Cardiology. 2021;**77**:1005-1005

[23] Wang J, Chen X, Zhao J, Zhang WW. Systematic review and meta-analysis of the outcomes of drug eluting stent versus drug coated balloon angioplasty for lower extremity peripheral artery diseases. Annals of Vascular Surgery. 11 May 2022;**S0890-S5096**(22):00225-00224

[24] Zeller T, Rastan A, Macharzina R, Tepe G, Kaspar M, Chavarria J, et al. Drug-coated balloons vs. drug-eluting stents for treatment of long femoropopliteal lesions. Journal of Endovascular Therapy. 2014;**21**:359-368

[25] Shishehbor MH, Schneider PA, Zeller T, Razavi MK, Laird JR, Wang H, et al. Total IN.PACT drug-coated balloon initiative reporting pooled imaging and propensity-matched cohorts. Journal of Vascular Surgery. 2019;**70**:1177-1191.e1179

[26] Iida O, Fujihara M, Kawasaki D, Mori S, Yokoi H, Miyamoto A, et al. 24-month efficacy and safety results from Japanese patients in the IMPERIAL randomized study of the eluvia drug-eluting stent and the Zilver PTX drug-coated stent. Cardiovascular and Interventional Radiology. 2021;**44**:1367-1374

[27] Katsanos K, Spiliopoulos S, Teichgräber U, Kitrou P, Del Giudice C, Björkman P, et al. Risk of major amputation following application of paclitaxel coated balloons in the lower limb arteries: A systematic review and meta-analysis of randomised controlled trials. European Journal of Vascular and Endovascular Surgery. 2022;**63**:60-71

[28] Tsujimura T, Iida O, Asai M, Masuda M, Okamoto S, Ishihara T, et al. Aneurysmal degeneration of fluoropolymer-coated paclitaxel-eluting stent in the superficial femoral artery: A rising concern. CVIR Endovascular. 2021;**4**:56-56

[29] Altaf N, Ariyaratne TV, Peacock A, Deltetto I, El-Hoss J, Thomas S, et al. A budget impact model for the use of drug-eluting stents in patients with symptomatic lower-limb peripheral arterial disease: An Australian perspective. Cardiovascular and Interventional Radiology. 2021;**44**:1375-1383

[30] Katsanos K, Spiliopoulos S, Kitrou P, Krokidis M, Paraskevopoulos I, Karnabatidis D. Risk of death and amputation with use of paclitaxel-coated balloons in the Infrapopliteal arteries for treatment of critical limb ischemia: A systematic review and Meta-analysis of randomized controlled trials. Journal of Vascular and Interventional Radiology. 2020;**31**:202-212

[31] Beckman JA, White CJ. Paclitaxel-coated balloons and eluting stents: Is there a mortality risk in patients with peripheral artery disease? Circulation. 2019;**140**:1342-1351

[32] Siablis D, Kitrou PM, Spiliopoulos S, Katsanos K, Karnabatidis D. Paclitaxel-coated balloon angioplasty versus drug-eluting stenting for the treatment of Infrapopliteal long-segment arterial occlusive disease: The IDEAS randomized controlled trial. JACC. Cardiovascular Interventions. 2014;7:1048-1056

[33] Katsanos K, Spiliopoulos S, Kitrou P, Krokidis M, Karnabatidis D. Risk of death following application of paclitaxel-coated balloons and stents in the femoropopliteal artery of the leg: A systematic review and Meta-analysis of randomized controlled trials. Journal of the American Heart Association. 2018;**7**:e011245

[34] Ross R. The pathogenesis of atherosclerosis: A perspective for the 1990s. Nature. 1993;**362**:801-809

[35] Aboyans V, Ricco JB, Bartelink ML, Björck M, Brodmann M, Cohnert T, et al. 2017 ESC guidelines on the diagnosis and treatment of peripheral arterial diseases, in collaboration with the European Society for Vascular Surgery (ESVS). European Journal of Vascular and Endovascular Surgery. 2018;**55**:305-368

[36] Naylor AR, Ricco JB, de Borst GJ, Debus S, de Haro J, Halliday A, et al. Management of atherosclerotic carotid and vertebral artery disease: 2017 clinical practice guidelines of the European Society for Vascular Surgery (ESVS). European Journal of Vascular and Endovascular Surgery. 2018;**55**:3-81

[37] Sidawy AN, Perler BA. Rutherford's Vascular Surgery and Endovascular Therapy. 9th ed. Philadelphia: Elsevier; 2019

[38] Pearson TA, Mensah GA, Alexander RW, Anderson JL, Cannon RO, Criqui M, et al. Markers of inflammation and cardiovascular disease. Circulation. 2003;**107**:499

[39] Gerhard-Herman MD, Gornik HL, Barrett C, Barshes NR, Corriere MA, Drachman DE, et al. 2016 AHA/ACC guideline on the management of patients

with lower extremity peripheral artery disease: Executive summary: A report of the American College of Cardiology/ American Heart Association task force on clinical practice guidelines. Circulation. 2017;**135**:e686-e725

[40] Steinberg D. Thematic review series: The pathogenesis of atherosclerosis. An interpretive history of the cholesterol controversy: Part I. Journal of Lipid Research. 2004;**45**:1583-1593

[41] Pittman RN. Chapter 2: The circulatory system and oxygen transport. In: Regulation of Tissue Oxygenation [Internet]. San Rafael, CA: Morgan & Claypool Life Sciences; 2011 Available from: https://www.ncbi.nlm.nih.gov/books/NBK54112/

[42] Fashandi AZ, Mehaffey JH, Hawkins RB, Kron IL, Upchurch GR Jr, Robinson WP. Major adverse limb events and major adverse cardiac events after contemporary lower extremity bypass and infrainguinal endovascular intervention in patients with claudication. Journal of Vascular Surgery. 2018;**68**:1817-1823

[43] Farber A, Rosenfield K, Menard M. The BEST-CLI trial: A multidisciplinary effort to assess which therapy is best for patients with critical limb ischemia. Techniques in Vascular and Interventional Radiology. 2014;**17**:221-224

[44] Yokokawa K, Hamashima S, Shibata M. In vivo evaluation of peripheral vascular resistance based on Poiseuille's law. Transactions of Japanese Society for Medical and Biological Engineering. 2014;**52**:O-432-O-433

[45] Sutera SP, Skalak R. The history of Poiseuille's law. Annual Review of Fluid Mechanics. 1993;**25**:1-20

[46] Lin JH, Brunson A, Romano PS, Mell MW, Humphries MD. Endovascular-first treatment is associated with improved amputation-free survival in patients with critical limb ischemia. Circulation. Cardiovascular Quality and Outcomes. 2019;**12**:e005273

[47] Wiseman JT, Fernandes-Taylor S, Saha S, Havlena J, Rathouz PJ, Smith MA, et al. Endovascular versus open revascularization for peripheral arterial disease. Annals of Surgery. 2017;**265**:424-430

[48] Abu Dabrh AM, Steffen MW, Asi N, Undavalli C, Wang Z, Elamin MB, et al. Bypass surgery versus endovascular interventions in severe or critical limb ischemia. Journal of Vascular Surgery. 2016;**63**:244-253

[49] Mayor J, Branco BC, Chung J, Montero-Baker MF, Kougias P, Mills JL Sr, et al. Outcome comparison between open and endovascular management of TASC II D aortoiliac occlusive disease. Annals of Vascular Surgery. 2019;**61**:65-71

[50] Shishehbor MH, Jaff MR. Percutaneous therapies for peripheral artery disease. Circulation. 2016;**134**:2008-2027

[51] Schneider P. Endovascular Skills: Guidewire and Catheter Skills for Endovascular Surgery. 4th ed. Boca Raton: CRC Press; 2019

[52] Thukkani AK, Kinlay S. Endovascular intervention for peripheral artery disease. Circulation Research. 2015;**116**:1599-1613

[53] Lindquist J, Schramm K. Drug-eluting balloons and drug-eluting stents in the treatment of peripheral vascular disease. Seminars in Interventional Radiology. 2018;**35**:443-452

[54] Mills JL, Conte MS, Murad MH. Critical review and evidence implications

of paclitaxel drug-eluting balloons and stents in peripheral artery disease. Journal of Vascular Surgery. 2019;**70**:3-7

[55] Ang H, Koppara TR, Cassese S, Ng J, Joner M, Foin N. Drug-coated balloons: Technical and clinical progress. Vascular Medicine. 2020;**25**:577-587

[56] Brodmann M, Keirse K, Scheinert D, Spak L, Jaff MR, Schmahl R, et al. Drug-coated balloon treatment for femoropopliteal artery disease: The IN.PACT global study De novo In-stent restenosis imaging cohort. JACC: Cardiovascular Interventions. 2017;**10**:2113-2123

[57] Zeller T, Baumgartner I, Scheinert D, Brodmann M, Bosiers M, Micari A, et al. Drug-eluting balloon versus standard balloon angioplasty for infrapopliteal arterial revascularization in critical limb ischemia: 12-month results from the IN.PACT DEEP randomized trial. Journal of the American College of Cardiology. 2014;**64**:1568-1576

[58] Thieme M, Lichtenberg M, Brodmann M, Cioppa A, Scheinert D. Lutonix® 014 DCB global below the knee registry study: Interim 6-month outcomes. The Journal of Cardiovascular Surgery. 2018;**59**:232-236

[59] Spiliopoulos S, Vasiniotis Kamarinos N, Brountzos E. Current evidence of drug-elution therapy for infrapopliteal arterial disease. World Journal of Cardiology. 2019;**11**:13-23

[60] Goueffic Y. Editor the EMINENT study: Primary results of the randomized trial of eluvia DES vs bare metal stents. In: Vascular InterVentional advances (VIVA). Las Vegas, NV: TCT MD; 2021

[61] Katsanos K, Spiliopoulos S, Diamantopoulos A, Karnabatidis D, Sabharwal T, Siablis D. Systematic review of Infrapopliteal drug-eluting stents: A meta-analysis of randomized controlled trials. Cardiovascular and Interventional Radiology. 2013;**36**:645-658

[62] Zhang J, Xu X, Kong J, Xu R, Fan X, Chen J, et al. Systematic review and meta-analysis of drug-eluting balloon and stent for infrapopliteal artery revascularization. Vascular and Endovascular Surgery. 2017;**51**:72-83

[63] Duda SH, Bosiers M, Lammer J, Scheinert D, Zeller T, Tielbeek A, et al. Sirolimus-eluting versus bare nitinol stent for obstructive superficial femoral artery disease: The SIROCCO II trial. Journal of Vascular and Interventional Radiology. 2005;**16**:331-338

[64] Dake MD, Ansel GM, Jaff MR, Ohki T, Saxon RR, Smouse HB, et al. Durable clinical effectiveness with paclitaxel-eluting stents in the femoropopliteal artery. Circulation. 2016;**133**:1472-1483

[65] Iida O, Takahara M, Soga Y, Nakano M, Yamauchi Y, Zen K, et al. 1-year results of the ZEPHYR registry (Zilver PTX for the femoral artery and proximal popliteal artery): Predictors of restenosis. JACC: Cardiovascular Interventions. 2015;**8**:1105-1112

[66] Kichikawa K, Ichihashi S, Yokoi H, Ohki T, Nakamura M, Komori K, et al. Zilver PTX post-market surveillance study of paclitaxel-eluting stents for treating femoropopliteal artery disease in Japan: 2-year results. Cardiovascular and Interventional Radiology. 2019;**42**:358-364

[67] Müller-Hülsbeck S, Benko A, Soga Y, Fujihara M, Iida O, Babaev A, et al. Two-year efficacy and safety results from the IMPERIAL randomized study of the eluvia polymer-coated drug-eluting stent and the Zilver PTX polymer-free drug-coated stent. Cardiovascular and Interventional Radiology. 2021;**44**:368-375

[68] Gray WA, Keirse K, Soga Y, Benko A, Babaev A, Yokoi Y, et al. A polymer-coated, paclitaxel-eluting stent (eluvia) versus a polymer-free, paclitaxel-coated stent (Zilver PTX) for endovascular femoropopliteal intervention (IMPERIAL): A randomised, non-inferiority trial. Lancet. 2018;**392**:1541-1551

[69] Feng Z, Yang S, Sang H, Xue G, Ni Q, Zhang L, et al. One-year clinical outcome and risk factor analysis of directional atherectomy followed with drug-coated balloon for femoropopliteal artery disease. Journal of Endovascular Therapy. 2021;**28**:927-937

[70] Zeller T, Langhoff R, Rocha-Singh KJ, Jaff MR, Blessing E, Amann-Vesti B, et al. Directional atherectomy followed by a paclitaxel-coated balloon to inhibit restenosis and maintain vessel patency: Twelve-month results of the DEFINITIVE AR study. Circulation. Cardiovascular Interventions. 2017;**10**:e004848

[71] Grotti S, Liistro F, Angioli P, Ducci K, Falsini G, Porto I, et al. Paclitaxel-eluting balloon vs standard angioplasty to reduce restenosis in diabetic patients with In-stent restenosis of the superficial femoral and proximal popliteal arteries: Three-year results of the DEBATE-ISR study. Journal of Endovascular Therapy. 2015;**23**:52-57

[72] van den Berg JC, Pedrotti M, Canevascini R, Chevili SC, Giovannacci L, Rosso R. In-stent restenosis: Mid-term results of debulking using excimer laser and drug-eluting balloons: Sustained benefit? The Journal of Invasive Cardiology. 2014;**26**:333-337

[73] Vallabhajosyula S, Greenberg-Worisek AJ, Gulati R, Vallabhajosyula S, Windebank AJ, Misra S, et al. Paclitaxel-coated balloons and stents for lower extremity peripheral arterial disease interventions: A regulatory perspective for the practicing clinician. Mayo Clinic Proceedings. 2020;**95**:1569-1573

[74] Krawisz AK, Secemsky EA. The safety of paclitaxel-coated devices for patients with peripheral artery disease. Current Cardiology Reports. 2021;**23**:48

[75] Klumb C, Lehmann T, Aschenbach R, Eckardt N, Teichgräber U. Benefit and risk from paclitaxel-coated balloon angioplasty for the treatment of femoropopliteal artery disease: A systematic review and meta-analysis of randomised controlled trials. eClinicalMedicine. 2019;**16**:42-50

[76] Han X, Zhou Y, Liu W. Precision cardio-oncology: Understanding the cardiotoxicity of cancer therapy. NPJ Precision Oncology. 2017;**1**:31

[77] Osman M, Elkady M. A prospective study to evaluate the effect of paclitaxel on cardiac ejection fraction. Breast Care (Basel). 2017;**12**:255-259

[78] Farb A, Malone M, Maisel WH. Drug-coated devices for peripheral arterial disease. The New England Journal of Medicine. 2021;**384**:99-101

[79] Choke E, Tang TY, Peh E, Damodharan K, Cheng SC, Tay JS, et al. MagicTouch PTA sirolimus coated balloon for femoropopliteal and below the knee disease: Results from XTOSI pilot study up to 12 months. Journal of Endovascular Therapy. Oct 2022;**29**(5):780-789

[80] Tang TY, Sulaiman MSB, Soon SXY, Yap CJQ, Patel A, Chong TT. Slow-flow phenomena following lower limb paclitaxel- and sirolimus-coated balloon angioplasty in the setting of chronic limb threatening ischaemia—A case series. Quantitative Imaging in Medicine and Surgery. 2022;**12**:2058-2065

[81] Teichgräber U, Ingwersen M, Platzer S, Lehmann T, Zeller T, Aschenbach R, et al. Head-to-head comparison of sirolimus- versus paclitaxel-coated balloon angioplasty in the femoropopliteal artery: Study protocol for the randomized controlled SIRONA trial. Trials. 2021;**22**:665

[82] Gray WA, Jaff MR, Parikh SA, Ansel GM, Brodmann M, Krishnan P, et al. Mortality assessment of paclitaxel-coated balloons: Patient-level meta-analysis of the ILLUMENATE clinical program at 3 years. Circulation. 2019;**140**:1145-1155

[83] Schahab N, Prengel A-K, Mahn T, Schaefer C, Fimmers R, Nickenig G, et al. Long-term clinical outcome and mortality risks after paclitaxel-coated balloon angioplasty in patients with peripheral artery disease: An observational clinical study. Health Science Reports. 2021;**4**:e236-e236

[84] Schneider PA, Laird JR, Doros G, Gao Q, Ansel G, Brodmann M, et al. Mortality not correlated with paclitaxel exposure: An independent patient-level Meta-analysis of a drug-coated balloon. Journal of the American College of Cardiology. 2019;**73**:2550-2563

[85] Zeller T, Micari A, Scheinert D, Baumgartner I, Bosiers M, Vermassen Frank EG, et al. The IN.PACT DEEP clinical drug-coated balloon trial. JACC. Cardiovascular Interventions. 2020;**13**:431-443

[86] Schneider PA, Brodmann M, Mauri L, Laird J, Soga Y, Micari A, et al. Paclitaxel exposure: Long-term safety and effectiveness of a drug-coated balloon for claudication in pooled randomized trials. Catheterization and Cardiovascular Interventions. 2020;**96**:1087-1099

Chapter 9

Diabetes Mellitus Type 2, Prediabetes, and Chronic Heart Failure

Valeh Mirzazada, Sadagat Sultanova, Natavan Ismayilova, Aygun Huseynova, Gulnara Nurmammadova, Sevil Ismayilova and Aygun Aliyeva

Abstract

Impaired glucose metabolism and its consequence diabetes mellitus is still challenging the health care system worldwide. According to the International Diabetes Federation in 2021, the number of adult people living with diabetes was approximately 537 million and 860 million adults had prediabetes. It is predicted that numbers will rise in the future. Numerous researches have shown that prediabetes and diabetes mellitus are serious risk factors for cardiovascular diseases. Lots of epidemiological evidence figured out that diabetes mellitus is associated with the risk of developing heart failure. Diabetes mellitus is highly prevalent among patients with heart failure. Moreover, several anti-diabetics (anti-prediabetic) medications are contributing their share into developing heart failure by increasing risk of mortality and hospitalization for heart failure. This chapter will discuss the connection between prediabetes, diabetes mellitus, and chronic heart failure.

Keywords: diabetes mellitus type 2, prediabetes, chronic heart failure, diabetes risk factors, diabetes management

1. Introduction

Diabetes mellitus (DM) is one of the major healthcare problems worldwide. According to the International Diabetes Federation (IDF) 2021 Atlas, 537 million adults (20–79 years) are living with diabetes. This number is predicted to rise to 783 million by 2045 [1]. Of persons with diabetes, 21.4% were not aware of or did not report having diabetes, and only 15.3% of persons with prediabetes reported being told by a health professional that they had this condition [2]. The prevalence of DM type 2 (T2D) is overwhelming. It is accounted for more than 90% of diabetes cases all over the world [1]. High incidence of T2D is thought to be because of population aging, lack of physical activity, urbanization, and obesity [3].

DM is diagnosed by using following criteria: fasting plasma glucose level of ≥126 mg/dl, glycated hemoglobin (HbA1c) level of ≥48 mmol/mol, and 2-hour plasma glucose after 75 g oral glucose load (oral glucose tolerance test-OGTT) level of ≥11.1 mmol/l.

Diabetes should be diagnosed if one or more diagnostic criteria are met [1]. Symptoms of diabetes include thirst, fatigue, polyuria, hunger, weight loss, blurred vision, etc.

The classification of DM is not unified and there are some differences between proposed classification by the American Diabetes Association (ADA) [4], IDF [1], and the World Health Organization (WHO) [3]. Precise classification is important for identifying the individual treatment approach since sometimes it is quite difficult to distinguish types of DM [4].

Variety of genetic and environmental factors can lead to the progressive loss of ß-cell mass and/or function that manifest as hyperglycemia which result in DM. Deficient ß-cell insulin secretion, often on the background of insulin resistance, appears to be the common pathophysiological factor for T2D. T2D is associated with insulin secretory defects related to genetics, inflammation, and metabolic stress [4].

2. Risk factors for diabetes mellitus

Risk factors for DM include adults, with a history of cardiovascular disease (CVD), hypertension (≥140/90 mmHg or on therapy for hypertension), HDL cholesterol level < 35 mg/dL (0.90 mmol/L) and/or a triglyceride level > 250 mg/dL (2.82 mmol/L), physical inactivity, and other clinical conditions associated with insulin resistance (e.g., severe obesity, acanthosis nigricans) and etc. Also, patients with prediabetes and women who were diagnosed with gestational diabetes mellitus are at risk of diabetes [4]. People living with diabetes are at risk of macrovascular complications such as CVD and microvascular complications (such as diabetic kidney disease, diabetic retinopathy, and neuropathy). These complications lead to increased mortality, blindness, kidney failure, and decreased quality of life in individuals with diabetes [5]. T2D is a common metabolic disease leading to diabetic myocardiopathy and atherosclerotic cardiovascular disorder. These conditions may induce heart failure through a range of mechanisms along with myocardial infarction (MI) and chronic pressure overload [6].

Atherosclerotic cardiovascular diseases are determined as coronary artery disease, cerebrovascular disease, and peripheral artery diseases. Among patients with DM atherosclerotic CVD remains the main cause of death and disability [7]. This results in $37.3 billion in cardiovascular-related spending in patients with diabetes per year [8]. CVD and T2D share several common pathophysiological features such as insulin resistance, inflammation, oxidative stress, hypercoagulability, high blood pressure (BP), dyslipidemia, and obesity. Classical cardiovascular risk factors, such as dyslipidemia, hypertension, and obesity can also raise the risk of T2D [6].

Although T2D and heart failure (HF) are each individually associated with morbidity and mortality, they often occur together, which further worsens adverse patient outcomes, quality of life, and costs of care [9].

Observational studies of patients with DM (predominantly type 2) have identified an approximately two to fourfold risk of HF compared to individuals without DM [10]. While the relative risk of HF in patients with DM compared with patients without DM is higher in younger individuals [11], the frequency of HF is higher in older adults with DM who were ≥ 65 years of age [12].

Although studies have shown an association between poor glycemic control and risk of HF, improved glucose control has not been shown to reduce incident HF. A meta-analysis including 27,049 patients with T2D found that more intensive glucose control, compared with less intensive control, did not decrease incident HF or mortality, although major cardiovascular events (primarily MI) were decreased [13].

Glycemic control is assessed by HbA1c level measurement, continuous glucose monitoring (CGM) using either time in range and/or blood glucose monitoring. In a clinical scenario HbA1c measurement is used more often. The HbA1c measurement should be performed in all diabetes patients at initial assessment and once in every 3 months. Measurement of HbA1c every 3 months determines whether patients' glycemic targets have been achieved and maintained. The HbA1c checking may have limitations in patients with medical conditions that can affect red blood cell turnover (hemodialysis, erythropoietin therapy, etc.). In such cases plasma blood glucose measurements are conducted by using BGM by fingerstick and CGM. Glycemic targets should be determined individually in each diabetes patient. There is evidence that more intensive glycemic control in newly diagnosed diabetes patients can be beneficial in reducing long-term CVD [14]. However, available data show that strict glycemic control in patients with established DM does not eliminate the risk of developing HF [15]. Overall, there is obscurity on choosing glycemic targets in diabetes mellitus with HF.

Prognosis in patients with HF and DM having DM led to worse outcomes in comparison with those who did not have DM among patients with HF. This was also demonstrated by randomized trial data in patients with HF with reduced ejection fraction (HFrEF; LVEF ≤40%) or HF with preserved ejection fraction (HFpEF) [9, 16–22].

A study of data from the Candesartan in Heart Failure-Assessment of Reduction in Mortality and morbidity (CHARM) program on outcomes in patients with HF found that concurrent DM was associated with a greater increased risk of cardiovascular death or HF hospitalization in patients with LVEF >40% than in patients with LVEF ≤40% [21]. The risk by DM was similar in the two groups for all-cause mortality.

In the Prospective Comparison of ARNI with ACEI to Determine Impact on Global Mortality and Morbidity in Heart Failure (PARADIGM-HF) trial with patients with HFrEF, there was an increased risk of the primary outcome of HF hospitalization or cardiovascular mortality in patients with previously undiagnosed DM or known DM [19].

It has been shown that, there is disturbingly high prevalence, incidence, and mortality for HF in individuals with diabetes [12]. DM patients who developed HF had poor prognosis.

It has been shown that, there is disturbingly high prevalence, incidence, and mortality for heart failure in individuals with diabetes [12]. DM patients who developed HF had poor prognosis.

3. Management of DM type in patients with HF

The initial management of blood glucose as well as the general medical care in adults with T2D or type 1 DM and HF is similar to that for other adults. In selecting initial therapy, patient presentation should be considered (e.g., presence or absence of symptoms of hyperglycemia, comorbidities, baseline HbA1c level). Treatment plans should include individualized treatment goals and preferences. The glucose-lowering efficacy of individual drugs, their adverse effect profile, tolerability, and cost should be considered individually for each patient. In the absence of specific contraindications, metformin should be suggested as initial therapy for patients with newly diagnosed T2D who are asymptomatic. Metformin is the preferred initial therapy because of glycemic efficacy, absence of weight gain and hypoglycemia, general tolerability, and favorable cost. Metformin does not have adverse cardiovascular effects, and it appears to decrease cardiovascular events [23–25]. The cost of metformin is more affordable and practically it has more experience than glucagon-like peptide 1 (GLP-1) receptor agonists and sodium-glucose co-transporter 2 (SGLT2i) inhibitors. Metformin usage instigates less episodes of hypoglycemia compared with sulfonylureas, and less edema, congestive HF, and weight gain compared with thiazolidinediones. The benefit of metformin in HFpEF has been studied. It has been shown that, metformin was beneficial in reduction of mortality in both preserved and reduced EF after adjustment with HF therapies such as angiotensin converting enzyme inhibitors (ACEi) and beta-blockers. Metformin treatment along with insulin, ACEi, and beta-blocker therapy were also shown to have a reduction in mortality, whereas female gender was associated with worse outcomes [26].

Sulfonylurea medications are commonly used in DM as second- or third-line treatment if needed, especially when the cost is the issue for a patient [27]. They are the oldest class of antidiabetic medications [28]. Sulfonylureas are classified as first and second generation, as second generation of sulfonylureas are the most prescribed (glibenclamide, glimepiride, gliclazide, etc.) [29]. The pharmacokinetic and pharmacodynamic features of sulfonylureas differ [30]. Not all sulfonylureas are selective for pancreas, they can also bind to cardiac myocytes and vascular smooth muscle. This can lead to ischemia and deterioration of the cardiovascular outcome. It has been suggested that gliclazide is selective for pancreas, while glimepiride and glibenclamide are non-selective [31]. Usage of sulfonylurea is complicated with hypoglycemia [32]. Hypoglycemia is associated with a higher risk of CVD [33]. One of the meta-analyses demonstrated significant associations between hypoglycemia and death, dementia, macrovascular and microvascular complications, and CVD [34]. Therefore, there is clinical uncertainty on the usage of sulfonylurea medications in diabetic patients with CVD. It also has been shown that the use of sulfonylureas in T2D increases mortality and risk of stroke, although the overall incidence of major adverse cardiovascular events (MACE) seems to be unchanged [35]. In another cardiovascular outcomes trial assessing linagliptin with glimepiride in patients with T2D and increased cardiovascular risk, the nonfatal MI and nonfatal stroke outcome was similar in both groups. It was demonstrated that hospitalization for HF was the same in patients who received glimepiride in comparison with linagliptin. Episodes of hypoglycemia events occurred in both groups and the rate was low, although it was higher in the glimepiride group [36]. Widely used sulfonylurea, gliclazide was associated with a lower risk of all-cause and cardiovascular mortality [37]. Although the data regarding long-acting sulfonylureas may be conflicting [38]. There are no randomized control trials assessing their effects on outcomes.

Thiazolidinediones are insulin sensitizing glucose-lowering medication which shows their effect by activating PPAR-gamma (peroxisome proliferator–activated receptor γ) [39]. Their effects regulate glucose, lipids, and protein metabolism. They are hugely effective in insulin resistance [39]. The commonly used thiazolidinediones are rosiglitazone and pioglitazone, which are indicated as FDA black box warning [27]. In diabetic patients their use is moderated by concerns over cardiovascular safety, weigh gain, edema, fracture risk, and bladder cancer [27]. The randomized clinical trials demonstrated that rosiglitazone and pioglitazone increase the risk of HF [40–42].

GLP-1 are efficient glucose-lowering medications used for the treatment of T2D. GLP-1 RA include liraglutide once daily, semaglutide once weekly, dulaglutide once weekly, exenatide twice daily, exenatide once weekly, lixisenatide once daily, which are injectable medications. Recently semaglutide has been introduced also in oral form which can be taken once daily.

GLP-1 have a reliable safety and tolerability profile in the management of the T2D [43]. As it has been shown in numerous studies and trials, this class of glucose-lowering medication proved itself as an effective tool in blood glucose and weight management [44–46]. The class effect is based on glucose-dependent insulin secretion. They also delay gastric emptying and increase satiety [47]. GLP-1 improve lipid levels with decreased triglyceride levels and increase high-density lipoprotein levels and provide low risk of hypoglycemia [9]. They significantly reduce HbA1c levels and systolic BP [48]. GLP-1 usage is proved to be beneficial in T2D and established atherosclerotic CVD and is recommended as part of the cardiovascular risk reduction and/or glucose-lowering medication [49]. Semaglutide demonstrated decrease in the rate of cardiovascular death, MI, and stroke by 26% [50]. Overall GLP-1 have no effect on HF hospitalization [9] and are not recommended for the prevention of HF events in patients with T2D.

Dipeptidyl peptidase-4 inhibitors (DPP4) are oral glucose-lowering medications that inhibit native enzyme dipeptidyl peptidase [51]. This enzyme is expressed on the surface of the most cell types that affects native gastrointestinal peptides and GLP-1. DPP4 inhibit the degradation of native GLP1 and enhance the incretin effect [52]. The commonly used DPP4 are sitagliptin, vildagliptin, linagliptin, alogliptin, and saxagliptin. It should be noted that, saxagliptin demonstrated the increased risk of hospitalization in patients with DM and HF [53]. Sitagliptin, linagliptin, and alogliptin showed no effect on HF events. However, in another trial vildagliptin increased the left ventricular volumes [54]. Overall, DPP4 are not recommended to reduce cardiovascular events in T2D with HF [55].

SGLT2i are one of the effective glucose-lowering drugs used in the treatment of DM. Their effect is based on reducing renal tubular glucose reabsorption [56]. They decrease blood glucose levels without stimulation of insulin secretion which makes them very useful in patients with a long duration of diabetes [56]. SGLT2i include canagliflozin, dapagliflozin, empagliflozin, ertugliflozin, and sotagliflozin. The usage of dapagliflozin and canagliflozin has been associated with reduced incidence of HF [57, 58]. Those T2D patients with a high risk of cardiovascular events who received empagliflozin demonstrated reduction of the primary composite cardiovascular outcome and of death from any cause [59]. Empagliflozin and canagliflozin reduced the primary composite endpoint of major CV adverse events, including CV death or non-fatal MI or non-fatal stroke, and HF hospitalizations [59, 60]. Dapagliflozin demonstrated a lower rate of cardiovascular death or hospitalization for HF in T2D in the DECLARE-TIMI 58 trial [57]. The other SGLT2i, ertugliflozin, showed statistically significant reduction in HF hospitalization and repeated hospitalizations, although it did not reduce the primary major CV event endpoint and key secondary outcome of cardiovascular death or HF hospitalization [61, 62]. Meta-analysis of Empagliflozin, Cardiovascular Outcomes, and Mortality in Type 2 Diabetes (EMPA-REG OUTCOME), Canagliflozin Cardiovascular Assessment Study (CANVAS), Dapagliflozin Effect on CardiovasculAR Events (DECLARE-TIMI 58), and Canagliflozin and Renal Events in Diabetes with Established Nephropathy Clinical Evaluation (CREDENCE) trial demonstrated the significant reduction in HF and cardiovascular hospitalization [49, 55].

Therefore, it is recommended to use SGLT2i as first-line therapy in diabetes as well as add on to patients with T2D with or at high risk of HF or chronic kidney disease (CKD) and ASCVD [49]. Additionally, the SGLT2i canagliflozin, dapagliflozin, empagliflozin, ertugliflozin, and sotagliflozin are recommended to prevent HF and CV death and worsening kidney function in patients with T2D and CV disease and/or

CV risk factors, or CKD. Dapagliflozin and empagliflozin are also indicated for the treatment of patients with T2D and HFrEF [55].

Insulin is one of the effective and oldest glucose-lowering medications in the management of DM. In cases when glycemic treatment goals are not achieved, adding of insulin therapy should not be delayed. Insulin treatment can be added to oral and injectable anti-diabetic medications. Insulin usage is associated with high efficacy and improved glycemic control [27]. Despite the high efficacy insulin treatment can lead to hypoglycemia and weight gain [27]. Both acute and chronic hypoglycemia increase CVD risk [63, 64]. Moreover, severe hypoglycemia was shown to be an independent risk factor for heart failure incidence [65]. Another trial also demonstrated that insulin usage is associated with deterioration in patients with HFpEF [64]. Therefore, patients with HF should be monitored thoroughly after starting insulin treatment [55].

4. Prediabetes and chronic heart failure

4.1 Definition, prevalence, diagnostics, and types of prediabetes

Prediabetes (PD) is a serious health condition where blood sugar levels are higher than normal, but not enough yet to be diagnosed as T2D [66]. IDF estimates that, worldwide, 541 million individuals aged 20–79 years have impaired glucose tolerance (IGT) and 319 million have impaired fasting glucose. These numbers are projected to increase to 730 million and 440 million, respectively by 2045 [1].

According to the 2022 National Diabetes Statistics Report, in 2019, 96 million (38.0%) adults age 18 and older in the United States were diagnosed with PD. This means that 1 in 3 people have PD, but 8 in 10 are unaware of their carbohydrate metabolism disorder. Meanwhile, 26.4 million (48.8%) people age 65 and older have PD. 10.8% of American adults had PD based on both elevated fasting plasma glucose and A1C levels. Based on fasting glucose or A1C levels, PD was more common in men (41.0%) than in women (32.0%). For example, in the United States, 1 in 3 people have PD and 1 in 10 people have DM, i.e., the prevalence of PD is several times higher than that of DM [67].

DM does not appear suddenly. Every person diagnosed with diabetes first goes through a PD stage [68]. PD not only is associated with high risk of progression to T2D; it also confers an increased risk of cardiovascular morbidity and mortality [69], microangiopathy [70], and neuropathy [71]. An essential difference between PD and DM is the possibility of early detection, proper diagnosis, and an optimal management; PD can be returned to normal glucose metabolism (NGM) or its progression to diabetes may be slowed [72]. The medical and social significance of PD and DM requires the earliest detection of these conditions. The diagnostic criteria for diabetes are generally accepted [73–79], but the community of experts has not yet been able to fully agree on diagnostic criteria for PD.**Table 1** presents the diagnostic criteria for PD in accordance with international and national recommendations [73–79].

A range of risk scores are used for screening diabetes and PD [80, 81]. The relationship between PD and types of PD as IGT, IFG, elevated HbA1c (or their various combinations) with heart failure (HF) has been studied [82–85]. In one of the studies, it was demonstrated that, for all-cause mortality risk, the association was stronger for IGT- than for IFG- or HbA1c-defined prediabetes, suggesting that OGTT is more useful for identifying high-risk individuals [82].

Source of recommendations	Diagnostic criteria		
	FG	**OGTT**	**HbA1c**
ADA	100–125 (mg/dl) 5.6–6.9 (mmol/l)	140–199 (mg/dl) 7.8–11.0 (mmol/l)	5.7–6.4 (%) 39–47 (mmol/mol)
WHO/IDF	110–125 (mg/dl) 6.1–6.9 (mmol/l)	140–199 (mg/dl) 7.8–11.0 (mmol/l)	Not recommended
Canada/UK/Australia	110–125 (mg/dl) 6.1–6.9 (mmol/l)	140–199 (mg/dl) 7.8–11.0 (mmol/l)	6.0–6.4 (%) 42–47 (mmol/mol)
AAEDTE	110–125 (mg/dl) 6.1–6.9 (mmol/l)	140–199 (mg/dl) 7.8–11.0 (mmol/l)	5.7–6.4 (%) 39–47 (mmol/mol)

Note: ADA—American Diabetes Association, WHO—World Health Organization, IDF—International Diabetes Federation, Canada—The Canadian Diabetes Association, UK—The British Diabetic Association, Australia—Diabetes Australia, AAEDTE—Azerbaijan Association of Endocrinology, Diabetology and Therapeutic Education, FG—fasting glucose, OGTT—oral glucose tolerance test, HbA1c—glycohemoglobin.

Table 1.
Comparative characteristics of diagnostic criteria for prediabetes based on the recommendations of different societies.

In a recently published article in the journal Cardiovascular Diabetology, Sinha et al. analyzed 40,117 participants from 6 population-based cohorts in the United States. They found that PD (defined as an FPG concentration of 100–125 mg/dL) was associated with a higher lifetime risk of HF in middle-aged white adults and black women, while the association was less pronounced in older black women. It was observed that middle-aged adults with prediabetes had a higher lifetime risk of HF and, on average, lived fewer years without HF than adults with normoglycemia. This difference was seen in all racial-gender groups except for middle-aged black men with PD, where the difference was not consistently significant, but the trend was similar. The results can probably be explained by two mechanisms that are not mutually exclusive. First, cumulative effects on glucose levels in the PD range in middle-aged and older men may contribute to cardiac dysfunction and the development of chronic HF. This explanation is supported by mechanistic and clinical studies demonstrating direct and indirect effects of insulin resistance and hyperglycemia on myocardial energetics, fibrosis, and subclinical cardiac dysfunction. Second, middle-aged adults with PD are more likely to develop diabetes later in life, leading to a greater lifetime risk of HF [83].

In the study about glucose abnormalities and heart failure among participants with normal glucose metabolism, HF was diagnosed in 3.2% compared with IGT and IFG in 6.0%, respectively. Also, IGT and IFG and HF were in 0.7% of men and in 0.6% of women. In this study, it is proved once again that there is a relationship between impaired glucose metabolism (IGM) and HF [84]. In one of the studies it was demonstrated that, PD with high levels of HbA1c is associated with an increased risk of HF [85].

4.2 HF as a risk factor for PD

The 5-year risk of HF was assessed among participants with diabetes and PD by biomarker assessment groups (0–4). The primary outcomes included 6799 patients with dysglycemia (diabetes: 33.2%; PD: 66.8%). The 5-year risk of HF increased stepwise with a rising biomarker score, with the highest risk seen in patients with scores ≥3 (diabetes: 12.0%; PD: 7.8%). Therefore, the study demonstrated that among adults with IGM (DM + PD), a biomarker score would stratify HF [86].

4.3 Management of PD in heart failure

Until now there is no information on the usage of Metformin and DPP4 inhibitors in the treatment of PD and HF. Thiazolidinediones are contraindicated with HF. One of the studies had showed, orlistat which is used for the treatment of PD had lower rates of first-time HF [87].

SGLT2i are recommended in HF; however, there are no effective data on the reversing PD to NGM by using SGLT2i. Various studies have examined the effects of GLP1 in the treatment of PD on HF. Based on the results of trials as Functional Impact of GLP-1 for Heart Failure Treatment (FIGHT) [88] and LIVE [89], the effect of the glucagon-like peptide-1 analogue in HF patients without diabetes was demonstrated. The effect of Liraglutide on left ventricular function in chronic heart failure patients with and without type 2 diabetes (LIVE) study has noticed that, Liraglutide had no effect on left ventricular systolic function compared with placebo in patients with stable HF with and without diabetes. Liraglutide resulted in weight loss, improved glycemic control, and improved physical performance [89].

5. Chronic heart failure and diabetes mellitus

5.1 Classification and epidemiology of heart failure

LVEF is the criterion that is taken into consideration when diagnosing HF in groups. Based on the 'Report on the Universal Definition and Classification of HF' [90] and the last 2021 European Society of Cardiology (ESC) guidelines [91], there are three major categories of HF proposed: HF where EF is preserved (HFpEF, LVEF ≥50%), HF where EF is mildly reduced (HFmrEF, LVEF between 41 and 49%), and HF where EF is reduced (HFrEF, LVEF ≤40%). Improved LVEF is used to describe patients who have been previously diagnosed with HFrEF whose LVEF is now >40%.

Approximately 50% of all HF instances are caused by HFpEF, and its prevalence is rising—making this category of HF the most common one in the future [92, 93]. HFrEF has distinct risk factors including male gender and CVD history (for example, MI) [94]. In comparison with HFpEF, patients with HFrEF have a greater mortality rate [92, 95]. HF with mildly reduced EF, previously named "HF with mid-range EF" since similar therapies work for both patients with HFmrEF and HFrEF, is the latest type of HF (introduced by ACCF/AHA in 2013 [96] and by the ESC in 2016 [91, 94]).

Hypertension, CKD, obesity, and diabetes are all important predictors of HF [97, 98]. The etiological relationship between DM and HF is mutually directed. Prolonged diabetes contributes to the development of myocardial dysfunction and HF [99]. This is due to potentiation of endothelial dysfunction, dyslipidemia, and hypercoagulability, and is also the result of a direct effect of hyperglycemia on myocardial function and morphology. On the other hand, HF can be complicated by the development of DM as a result of organ hypoperfusion and hyperactivation of neurohumoral systems, which contribute to an increase in blood glucose concentration as a result of a decrease in glucose consumption by muscle tissue, increased gluconeogenesis in the liver, and the contra-insular effect of catecholaminemia [100]. Also, HF in patients with DM is considered direct damage to the heart muscle as a result of prolonged hyperglycemia. Myocardial damage against the background of hyperglycemia is mediated by microangiopathy, impaired calcium transport, and fatty acid metabolism [101]. A classic example of the myocardial effect of hyperglycemia is diabetic cardiomyopathy.

Diabetic cardiomyopathy describes impaired cardiac function as a result of decreased glucose metabolism and increased fatty acid (FA) metabolism [102]. It also includes myocardial structural and performance anomalies in people with diabetes not diagnosed with coronary artery disease, valvular disease, or other CV risk factors such as hypertension and dyslipidemia [103]. Irregularities that are usually seen in diabetes, such as hyperglycemia, hyperinsulinemia, systemic insulin resistance, and inflammation, are the factors that directly lead to the development of cardiomyopathy in people with diabetes (CMiPD) [103]. Regardless of LVEF or HF etiology, insulin therapy may be linked with higher mortality compared to oral hypoglycemic agents [104].

Insulin therapy in type 1 diabetes improves hyperglycemia and increases myocardial ischemia and death of cardiomyocytes, thereby inducing HF. There is evidence of a direct relationship between myocardial tissue perfusion, oxygen supply, energy substrate availability, and myocardial function in patients with DM, suggesting microcirculatory damage as a cause of diabetic cardiomyopathy [105]. Thus, the prevalence of CMiPD is increasing at the same rate as T2D [103].

As CMiPD advances from the first stage through the last, muscle contraction is impaired and fibrosis develops [102]. Stage I is characterized by abnormal myocardial relaxation, however normal EF [102]. During stage IV, HF is developed due to overt ischemia and infarct [102]. Hyperglycemia, hyperinsulinemia, inflammation, and hyperlipidemia due to diabetes can lead to cardiac dysfunction along with changes in the structure of the heart [106]. In the case of CMiPD, insulin resistance causes glucose metabolism in the cardiac myocyte to be altered; more specifically, glucose uptake, glycolytic activity, and oxidation of pyruvates are decreased [102]. In CMiPD while glucose is available in small amounts, there is an accumulation of circulating FAs that act as an energy source for the cardiomyocytes [102]. As a result of overactive FA oxidation and metabolic inflexibility, the heart is exposed to a variety of secondary pathways making it less capable of dealing with increased workloads [102].

An increase in free FA and hyperglycemia leads to an undesirable accumulation of lipids in the heart. Cardiomyocytes are not adapted to the accumulation of large amounts of lipids that have a direct cytopathic effect on them, and lipid fragments lead to the activation of inflammatory signaling pathways, including protein kinase C, which interfere with insulin signaling. As a result, insulin resistance develops, which limits the consumption of glucose by cells and a shift happens toward fatty acid oxidation [107].

Particularly, as FA-rich cardiomyocytes produce ATP less effectively and accumulate diverse toxic intermediates and lipids, pro-inflammatory and profibrotic responses are induced [102]. These processes ultimately lead to CMiPD through cardiac hypertrophy and diastolic dysfunction [102].

The accumulation of end products is the driving force behind microvascular damage in DM and is associated with myocardial stiffness and collagen accumulation in the myocardium. The gradual increase in myocardial stiffness also leads to diastolic dysfunction, decreased myocardial tension, and atrial dilatation, which is associated with an increased prevalence of atrial fibrillation in patients with DM [108].

Mitochondrial dysfunction can also lead to CMiPD development. This happens because of excessive mitophagy causing an imbalance between mitophagy and mitochondrial biogenesis. As a result, myocardial cells are destructed more intensively [109].

It has been established that ketone metabolism can be an alternative to the energy supply of the heart muscle [110]. The concentrations of circulating ketone bodies increase in HF and they enter the cell as an insulin-independent energy substrate. The appearance of ketone enzymes in a hypertrophied and damaged heart leads to energy consumption for the oxidation of ketones with insufficient possibilities for oxidation of fatty acids [111]. The presence of DM contributes to the development of myocardial dysfunction and CHF due to the development and maintenance of endothelial dysfunction, dyslipidemia, hypercoagulation, and the direct effect of hyperglycemia on myocardial function and morphology [112]. At the same time, in HF, as a result of organ hypoperfusion and hyperactivation of neurohumoral systems (decrease in glucose consumption by muscle tissue, increased gluconeogenesis in the liver, contra-insular effects of catecholaminemia), blood glucose levels increase.

Thus, the development of HF in DM is due to the progression of atherosclerosis with subsequent progression of myocardial ischemia and immediate myocardial damage as a result of prolonged hyperglycemia. Myocardial damage against the background of hyperglycemia is mediated by microangiopathy, impaired calcium transport, and fatty acid metabolism. The presence of DM increases the risk of developing HF compared with that in the general population, and there is a significantly higher mortality among DM patients with HF. In addition, an increased risk of developing HF was found in individuals with elevated values of morning glycemia even in the absence of DM. Patients with HF have high insulin resistance and an increased risk of developing DM [113].

6. Screening and diagnosing HF in people with diabetes

6.1 Electrocardiography (ECG)

According to the 2021 ESC guidelines' recommendations, when patients' symptoms signal the presence of acute or chronic HF, ECG is one of the measures used to evaluate their condition [91]. If acute HF is detected, it is recommended to produce an ECG when patients are admitted to the hospital, during their stay, and before they are discharged [91]. Performing electrocardiography is mainly a step toward HF detection, such as changes in the ECG show higher chances of HF in patients and vice versa: HF is not plausible when ECG is normal [91]. Moreover, by looking at the ECG, it is possible to learn about the causes of HF and how to proceed with future treatment [91]. Based on the 2019 ESC-EASD recommendations, ECG is also proposed for "patients with diabetes who have been diagnosed with hypertension" [114].

6.2 Echocardiography

A cardiac injury manifests itself as structural changes and echocardiography is the most effective and non-invasive measure to detect those changes [115], assessing systolic and diastolic dysfunction [116]. Echocardiography is recommended by the 2021 ESC guidelines [91] and the 2019 ESC-EASD recommendations as the first-choice tool for structural and functional evaluation of the heart of diabetic people since it can detect higher LV mass (LVM) and/or diastolic dysfunction when no symptoms of HF are present [114]. It is widely known that LVM is directly proportional with common risk factors for T2D such as age, obesity, and dyslipidemia [117], but it also relies on gender and body size [118]. It is worth mentioning that, LV hypertrophy is a common anomaly seen in asymptomatic T2D patients, such that even after omitting silent coronary disease, it was observed in one-third of individuals without hypertension [119]. Indexed LVM/bovine serum albumin (BSA) enables for the establishment of reference values for comparing subjects of various body sizes [118]. The American Society of Endocrinology defines normal LVM/BSA levels as 43–95 g/m^2 for women and 49–115 g/m^2 for men [118].

6.3 Assessment of biomarkers

The 2021 ESC guidelines [91] and the 2022 AHA/ACC/HFSA updated guidelines [120] recommend natriuretic peptide biomarker screening (either NT-proBNP or BNP) to identify diabetic patients with pre-HF. The 2022 AHA/ACC/HFSA guidelines also recommend routine assessment of circulating biomarkers in general for supporting a diagnosis or exclusion of HF, risk stratification, and prognosis of patients with diabetes [120]. Since HF stages are defined by increased natriuretic peptide levels by the universal definition [90], routine screening of NT-proBNP or BNP is recommended in patients without current or prior HF symptoms or signs. The cut-off levels for BNP and NT-proBNP as settled by the universal definition were as following: 35 pg/mL and 125 pg/mL for ambulatory HF patients and 100 pg/mL and 300 pg/mL for hospitalized/decompensated HF patients, respectively [90]. Nevertheless, natriuretic peptide levels are not sufficient to diagnose HF since CV and non-CV factors diminish explanatory values of those levels under conditions such as AF, increasing age, obesity, and kidney disease [91]. In order to contribute to the informative diagnostic utility of natriuretic peptides, other new biomarkers, such as independent biomarkers for myocardial fibrosis or risk stratification in HF (secreted Frizzled-related proteins) or gut microbiota-derived trimethylamine N-oxide (TMAO), are required [121–124].

6.4 Assessment of glycemic parameters in HF patients

When dysglycemia in patients with HFrEF remains undiagnosed, it is hard to determine a solid prognosis [125]. As a solution, the 2019 ESC-EASD guidelines advise testing HbA1c and FPG levels for detecting diabetes in patients previously diagnosed with CVD [114]. Furthermore, if the aforementioned tests do not yield a concrete result, it is recommended to perform OGTT [114]. The 2021 ESC guidelines recommend to consistently check fasting glucose and HbA1c levels if chronic HF is suspected, to find its treatable causes and related comorbidities [91].

6.5 Strategies in people with diabetes to reduce the risk of HF

The 2019 ESC-EASD guidelines recommend regular microalbuminuria and eGFR screening to identify patients at high risk of renal dysfunction or future CVD. On the other hand, the Standards of Care 2021 from the ADA [126], and the 2019 ESC-EASD guidelines [114] recommend a BP target of <130/80 mmHg (but not <120 mmHg).

Moreover, even though the 2021 ESC guidelines [91] do not recommend a target, the 2022 AHA/ACC/HFSA guidelines [120] do recommend a more stringent target of systolic BP of <120 mmHg in individuals with diabetes at CV risk since hypertension control is associated with a lower HF risk. It is worth noting that masked hypertension (meaning only home, but not office BP levels are hypertensive) [127] is common in T2D patients [128], making out-of-office BP monitoring a viable screening method for this clinical condition [129, 130]. Diabetic and hypertensive patients should have their ECGs checked at rest to identify silent MI, which happens in 4% of diabetic patients and adds an insult to HF [114]. Additionally, for pre-diabetics and hypertensive patients with diabetes, lifestyle adjustments and the use of RAAS blockers as first-line therapy for BP management are advised [114]. RAAS blockers also diminish the incidence of new-onset diabetes and the risk of sudden cardiac death in HFrEF patients [114]. Aside from hypertension, a higher body mass index is thought to be a risk factor for HF, which is why the ESC recommendations for 2021 [91] propose that obesity should be controlled to avoid or delay the onset of HF.

7. Therapeutic considerations of HF in diabetes

Pharmacotherapy is the cornerstone of HFrEF treatment and should be used in conjunction with non-pharmacological therapies before device therapy is considered [130].

Treatment for patients with HFrEF has three key goals: reduction in mortality, avoiding recurrent hospitalizations due to worsening HF, and improving clinical status, functional capacity, and quality of life [130].

Patients with and without diabetes receive similar treatment for HF. On the other hand, anti-diabetic drugs have different effects in patients with HF, and treatments that are both safe and minimize HF-related events should be prioritized [130].

The 2021 ESC guidelines [91] and 2022 ACC/AHA/HFSA guidelines [120] recommend treatment of HFrEF and HFmrEF with a combination therapy of angiotensin-converting-enzyme inhibitors/angiotensin II receptor blockers (ACE-I/ARB), angiotensin-receptor-neprilysin-inhibitors (ARNI), beta-blockers, mineralocorticoid-receptor antagonists (MRA), and SGLT2i. Since there is currently no therapy for HFpEF subjects [91, 131], HFpEF therapy targets only symptom and well-being improvement [91, 94] and treatment of comorbidities [91]. The recently reported EMPEROR-preserved study provides the first proof of improved outcomes in HFpEF individuals [132].

The 2021 ESC guidelines [91] also recommend that patients with improved LVEF should continue to receive HFrEF treatment [91]. On the other hand, the 2021 ESC guidelines recommend to use ICDs in selected patients with HFrEF of an ischemic etiology and to consider using in those with a non-ischemic etiology [91]. Moreover, CRT-P/D is recommended in those patients with HFrEF, in sinus rhythm, with an LBBB ≥150 ms and should be considered in those with an LBBB ≥130–149 ms or non-LBBB ≥150 ms [91]. Advanced HF strategies, such as heart transplantation or MCS may be appropriate in selected patients [91].

ACE-I and ARB: The effect of the ACE-I enalapril was demonstrated in the SOLVD trial. It was shown that compared to placebo, enalapril diminished the incidence of diabetes in subjects with HF [133]. The 2019 ESC-EASD recommendations suggest blood pressure control with ACE-I or an ARB as a measure to lessen the HF risk in diabetes, especially in conditions such as microalbuminuria, albuminuria, proteinuria, or LV hypertrophy [99].

The expediency of using ACE inhibitors in patients with insulin resistance is explained by the activation of the RAAS against the background of hyperinsulinemia and hyperglycemia, as well as by common molecular signal transduction pathways used by the insulin and renin-angiotensin systems. When treating diabetic patients with ACE inhibitors or ARBs, continuous monitoring of potassium levels and renal function is necessary to prevent the development of nephropathy [134].

ARNI: In the PARADIGM-HF trial, it was observed that in comparison with enalapril, sacubitril/valsartan is able to substantially reduce the death and hospitalization risk of HF (HHF) in people with HFrEF, demonstrating its blood pressure lowering effect in the long term [135]. However, in people with HFpEF, this trial showed that sacubitril/valsartan was not effective at reducing the total CV death and HHF rate compared to valsartan alone (regardless of diabetes history in HFpEF patients) [136]. Moreover, the positive impact of sacubitril-valsartan in reducing the risk of HHF was comparable among all PARADIGM-HF trial patients with HFrEF and an HbA1c of 5.4–8.4% [19]. Furthermore, sacubitril-valsartan outperforms enalapril in decreasing HbA1c levels and lowering the rate of insulin treatment initiation in individuals with both diabetes and HFrEF over 3 years [137]. Sacubitril-valsartan is thus expected to enhance glycemic control in these individuals [137].

A significant reduction in NT-proBNP levels was observed in the HFpEF group of the PARADIGM-HF trial [138], demonstrating that sacubitril-valsartan therapy reduces risk. This effect occurred regardless of gender, as sacubitril-valsartan equally reduced NT-proBNP levels in men and women in the PARAGON-HF cohort with HFpEF where 50% of subjects were diabetics [139].

There were a few observed side effects of sacubitril-valsartan therapy in the PARADIGM-HF [135] and the Prospective Comparison of ARNI with ARB Global Outcomes in HF with Preserved Ejection Fraction (PARAGON-HF trial) [136] such as increased prevalence of symptomatic hypertension and angioedema, but this was still lower than with dual inhibition of both ACE and neprilysin, especially in angioedema [135]. In light of these data, the 2019 ESC-EASD Guidelines on diabetes recommend that HF patients with diabetes who remain symptomatic should be treated with sacubitril-valsartan instead of an ACE inhibitor [114].

Beta-blockers: Beta-blockers have been shown to reduce mortality and morbidity in patients with HFrEF, when used together with ACE-I and diuretics [91]. As soon as symptomatic HFrEF is diagnosed, ACE-I and beta-blockers can be started together, according to consensus. However, no evidence proves that starting a beta-blocker before an ACE-I or vice versa is beneficial. Beta-blockers should be given to clinically stable euvolemic patients at low doses and slowly uptitrated to the maximum tolerated dose. Moreover, when patients are admitted with AHF in the hospital, beta-blockers should be given cautiously only after they are hemodynamically stabilized [91].

There is no particular beta-blockade experiment in HFmrEF. The SENIORS trial, in which nebivolol lowered the composite main endpoint of all-cause mortality or CV hospital admissions in the total population, was included in an IPD meta-analysis. There was no interaction between LVEF (35–50% of patients had an LVEF of 35–50%) and the impact of nebivolol on the main outcome. Many patients with HFmrEF may also have another CV reason for a beta-blocker, such as AF or angina. As a result, beta-blocker therapy may be explored in individuals with HFmrEF [91].

MRA: Assessment of MRA therapy efficacy revealed that compared to non-MRA treatment, it improved the clinical outcome of diabetic patients with HF [140]. To be exact, spironolactone or eplerenone was effective at diminishing CV and all-cause mortality and HHF [140]. A non-steroidal MRA finerenone, on the other hand, was able to reduce the incidence of death from any cause, CV-related hospitalization or emergency in subjects with HFrEF, CKD, and/or diabetes when compared to eplerenone MinerAlocorticoid Receptor antagonist Tolerability Study-Heart Failure (ARTS-HF trial) [141].

Adverse events in the ARTS-HF and other MRA trials included in the aforementioned meta-analysis revealed that MRA treatment increases the risk of hyperkalemia [140, 141].

Also, it has been shown that finerenone at doses of 10–20 mg/day may cause hyperkalemia less frequently [142]. The drugs of this group can cause hyperkalemia and deterioration of renal function, especially in the elderly, patients with diabetic and non-diabetic nephropathy, renal failure; therefore, it is recommended to use them only in patients with adequate renal function, while regular monitoring of plasma electrolytes and renal function is mandatory.

Generally, the 2019 ESC-EASD recommendations [114] indicate that diabetic people with HFrEF should be treated with MRAs if their symptoms persist despite therapy with ACE-I or beta-blockers. In these patients, MRAs and sacubitril-valsartan are indicated to minimize the risk of sudden cardiac death [114].

There is no MRA-specific study in HFmrEF. In a retrospective analysis of the TOPCAT trial, spironolactone reduced hospitalizations for HF in patients with an LVEF of ≥45%, but it increased hospitalizations for HF in those with an LVEF of ≥55%. A comparable trend was observed in CV mortality but not in all-cause mortality [91]. Treatment with an MRA may be considered in patients with HFmrEF [91].

SGLT2 inhibitors: Numerous clinical trials have demonstrated the therapeutic impact of SGLT2 inhibitors on CV outcomes in people with T2D and established HF, demonstrating a cardio-protective effect independent of glycemic status [143].

Inhibition of SGLT2 increases the concentration of circulating ketone bodies, and it can become an alternative source of energy for the diabetic heart with insulin resistance. In addition, other potential mechanisms of action of the drug are possible, such as weight loss of the body, BP, sodium levels, oxidative stress, and sympathetic activation [144]. One evidence comes from the DAPA-HF trial demonstrating that dapagliflozin lowered the risk of progressing HF (HHF) and CV-related death in HFrEF people (NYHA class II–IV) independent of the glycemic status [145] and gender [146]. In addition, The Empagliflozin Outcome Trial in Patients with Chronic Heart Failure with Preserved Ejection Fraction (EMPEROR)-preserved trial provided the first evidence of a cardio-protective effect of empagliflozin on the combined risk of HHF and CV death in subjects with HFpEF, an effect that is independent of the presence of diabetes [132]. In other studies, for empagliflozin, a lowered risk of CV death and HHF was also shown in the EMPA-REG OUTCOME trial in people with T2D and a history of CVD [59] and in the EMPEROR-Reduced trial in people with HFrEF regardless of the presence of diabetes [147].

One piece of evidence comes from the Dapagliflozin and Prevention of Adverse Outcomes in Heart Failure (DAPA-HF) study, which found that dapagliflozin reduced the risk of progressive HF (HHF) and CV-related death in patients with HFrEF (NYHA class II–IV) regardless of glycemic status [145] or gender [146]. Furthermore, the EMPEROR-preserved study showed the first indication of empagliflozin's cardioprotective benefit on the combined risk of HHF and CV death in people with HFpEF, a result that is independent of diabetes [132]. In additional trials, empagliflozin was associated with a decreased risk of CV mortality and HHF in the EMPA-REG OUTCOME trial in patients with T2D and a history of CVD [59] and in the EMPEROR-Reduced trial in people with HFrEF regardless of diabetes.

Reducing the risk of CVD in empagliflozin includes combined decrease in blood pressure, body weight (including visceral obesity), albuminuria, glucose levels, stiffness of the arterial wall, activation of the sympathetic part of the autonomic nervous system, oxidative stress, uric acid concentration, and improvement function of the heart [148]. Empagliflozin is able to improve myocardial microvascular perfusion, eNOS activity, and endothelium-dependent relaxation. Empagliflozin may be beneficial by inhibiting induced DM mitochondrial fission dependent on 5'AMP-activated protein kinase (AMPK) way. On the one hand, the action induced by this drug can slow down the aging of endothelial cells by suppressing oxidative stress, which leads to an improvement in their viability and barrier function. On the other hand, empagliflozin-induced migration endothelium as a result of F-actin homeostasis can contribute to angiogenesis [59, 149]. As DM progresses endothelial damage is detected at an early stage. Through these mechanisms, empagliflozin improves myocardial blood supply. Considerable evidence suggests the ability of empagliflozin to reduce systolic blood pressure by facilitating osmotic diuresis, influencing the microvascular diastolic response by stimulation of eNOS phosphorylation, vascular remodeling, reduction of inflammatory proteins, and decrease in collagen synthesis [150]. This drug is promising for the treatment of patients with diabetes and microvascular dysfunction of the heart; this drug can be considered as a drug for protecting the microvascular bed of the heart to maintain its functions and circulatory structures in hyperglycemia [151].

In the Evaluation of Ertugliflozin Efficacy and Safety Cardiovascular Outcomes Trial (VERTIS CV trial), ertugliflozin was non-inferior to placebo in terms of its important secondary outcome of CV mortality or HHF in participants with T2D and atherosclerotic CVD, but the trial findings did not fulfill the superiority requirements (HR = 0.88, 95% CI 0.75–1.03) [61, 149]. However, there was a 30% reduction in the risk of HHF alone, which was similar to the effects of the other SGLT2 inhibitors on this outcome [149, 152]. A pre-specified analysis in VERTIS CV revealed that the subgroups of patients with the largest decrease in HF-related events had an eGFR of <60 mL/min/1.73 m^2 and albuminuria [62]. Furthermore, another evidence from the SOLOIST-WHF trial shows that simultaneous inhibition of both SGLT1 and SGLT2 in people with T2D may reduce CV fatalities, hospitalizations, and urgent visits for either HFpEF or HFrEF [153]. When started before or shortly after discharge, sotagliflozin avoided CV death, HHF, and urgent HF visits in patients with T2D and recent worsening HF compared to placebo.

SGLT2 inhibitors are cardio-protective in patients with T2D and established CVD, also in people who are at high risk of CV events. The CANVAS study demonstrated that canagliflozin lowered the risk of CV-related events in people with T2D and increased CV risk more effectively than placebo [60]. Furthermore, the DECLARE-TIMI 58 study found that use of dapagliflozin reduces HHF and CV-related death in people with T2D who had or are at risk of atherosclerotic CVD [57].

NT-proBNPs have a predictive value for CV events and death in clinical outcome studies. The decreased NT-proBNP concentration in the canagliflozin arm of the CANVAS trial can be ascribed in part to the reduction in CV-related events in patients with T2D and CV risk [154]. In addition, a sub-analysis of the CANDLE study found a tendency toward decreased NT-proBNP levels in the subgroup with lower LV diastolic function in the canagliflozin treated arm compared to the glimepiride treated arm [155]. Dapagliflozin, like canagliflozin, reduced NT-proBNP levels considerably higher than placebo in the DAPA-HF group [145, 149]. Similarly, empagliflozin significantly lowered NT-proBNP levels 7 days after randomization when delivered as add-on treatment to T2D patients hospitalized for acute decompensated HF compared to the group treated conventionally with glucose-lowering drugs [149, 156]. However, another dual SGLT1/2 inhibitor, licogliflozin, has been shown to reduce NT-proBNP in individuals with both T2D and HF when compared to placebo 12 weeks following randomization [149, 157].

Because of the class impact of SGLT2 inhibitors, the 2019 ESC-EASD guidelines on diabetes propose the SGLT2 inhibitors empagliflozin, canagliflozin, and dapagliflozin to reduce the risk of HHF in diabetic individuals [114]. Aside from that, the ESC guidelines for 2021 recommend ertugliflozin and sotagliflozin for patients with T2D who are at high risk of CV events to reduce HHF, major adverse CV events (MACE), end-stage renal disease, and CV death, and sotagliflozin in patients with T2D and HFrEF to reduce HHF and CV death [91]. In order to minimize HHF, MACE, and CV death, the 2019 ADA/EASD consensus suggests SGLT2 inhibitors in addition to metformin in adults with diabetes and HF (particularly HFrEF) [158].

8. Conclusion

HF is still a significant factor in life expectancy, especially among diabetic patients. HF can be viewed as both a cause and a complication of DM at the same time. Evidence strongly suggest that there is negative predictive effect of DM in the course of HF. Therapy for this category of patients should be characterized by a holistic approach, including a thorough glycemic control, as well as an effective blockade of neurohumoral changes. New pharmacological options, such as SGLT2 inhibitors, are allowing for better control of this life-threatening T2D condition. Biomarkers like NT-proBNP can help identify HF early and predict prognosis and therapeutic efficacy of HF or/and diabetes treatment. As a result, NT-proBNP testing should be used early in the monitoring of subjects with diabetes with a high CV risk.

Acronyms and abbreviations

AAEDTE	Azerbaijan Association of Endocrinology, Diabetology and Therapeutic Education
ACC	American College of Cardiology
ACCF	The American College of Cardiology Foundation
ACE-I	angiotensin-converting-enzyme inhibitors
ADA	American Diabetes Association
AF	atrial fibrillation
AHA	American Heart Association
AHF	acute heart failure
AMPK	5′AMP-activated protein kinase
ARB	angiotensin II receptor blockers
ARNI	angiotensin-receptor-neprilysin-inhibitors
ATP	adenosine triphosphate
BNP	brain natriuretic peptide
BP	blood pressure
BSA	bovine serum albumin
CKD	chronic kidney disease
CMiPD	cardiomyopathy in people with diabetes

CRT-P/D	cardiac resynchronization therapy with pacemaker/defibrillator
CVD	cardiovascular disease
DM	diabetes mellitus
DPP4	dipeptidyl peptidase 4 inhibitors
EASD	European Association for the Study of Diabetes
ECG	electrocardiography
eGFR	estimated glomerular filtration rate
eNOS	endothelial nitric oxide synthase
ESC	European Society of Cardiology
FA	fatty acid
FG	fasting glucose
FPG	fasting plasma glucose
GLP-1	glucagon-like peptide 1 receptor agonist
HbA1c	glycohemoglobin
HF	heart failure
HFmrEF	heart failure with mildly reduced ejection fraction
HFpEF	heart failure with preserved ejection fraction
HFrEF	heart failure with reduced ejection fraction
HFSA	Heart Failure Society of America
HHF	hospitalization for HF
HR	hazard ratio
ICD	implantable cardioverter defibrillator
IDF	International Diabetes Federation
IGM	impaired glucose metabolism
IGT	impaired glucose tolerance
IPD	individual patient data
LBBB	left bundle branch block
LVEF	left ventricular ejection fraction
LVM	left ventricle mass
MACE	major adverse cardiovascular events
MCS	mechanical circulatory support
MI	myocardial infarction
MRA	mineralocorticoid-receptor antagonists
NGM	normal glucose metabolism
NT-proBNP	N-terminal pro-b-type natriuretic peptide
NYHA	New York Heart Association
OGTT	oral glucose tolerance test
PD	prediabetes
RAAS	renin-angiotensin-aldosterone system
SGLT1	sodium-glucose cotransporter 1
SGLT2	sodium-glucose cotransporter 2
SGLT2i	sodium glucose co-transporter 2 inhibitors
T2D	type 2 diabetes
TMAO	trimethylamine N-oxide

Author details

Valeh Mirzazada*, Sadagat Sultanova, Natavan Ismayilova, Aygun Huseynova, Gulnara Nurmammadova, Sevil Ismayilova and Aygun Aliyeva
Therapy Department, Azerbaijan State Advanced Training Institute for Doctors named after A. Aliyev, Baku, Azerbaijan

*Address all correspondence to: valehmirzazade@mail.ru

References

[1] International Diabetes Federation. IDF Diabetes Atlas. 10th ed. Brussels, Belgium; 2021. Available from: https://www.diabetesatlas.org

[2] Centers for Disease Control and Prevention. National Diabetes Statistics Report. 2020. Available from: https://www.cdc.gov/diabetes/pdfs/data/statistics/national-diabetes-statistics-report.pdf

[3] WHO Diabetes Mellitus Classification. 2019. Available from: https://www.who.int/publications/i/item/classification-of-diabetes-mellitus

[4] American Diabetes Association Professional Practice Committee. Classification and diagnosis of diabetes: Standards of medical care in diabetes—2022. Diabetes Care. 2022;**45** (Supplement_1):S17-S38. DOI: 10.2337/dc22-S002

[5] Cole JB, Florez JC. Genetics of diabetes mellitus and diabetes complications. Nature Reviews. Nephrology. 2020;**16**(7):377-390. DOI: 10.1038/s41581-020-0278-5

[6] De Rosa S et al. Type 2 diabetes mellitus and cardiovascular disease: Genetic and epigenetic links. Frontiers in Endocrinology. 2018;**9**:2. DOI: 10.3389/fendo.2018.00002

[7] Booth GL, Kapral MK, Fung K, Tu JV. Relation between age and cardiovascular disease in men and women with diabetes compared with non-diabetic people: A population-based retrospective cohort study. Lancet (London, England). 2006; **368**(9529):29-36. DOI: 10.1016?S-0140-6736(06)68967-8

[8] American Diabetes Association. Economic costs of Diabetes in the U.S. in 2017. Diabetes Care. 2018;**41**(5):917-928. DOI: 10.2337/dci18-0007

[9] Dunlay SM et al. Type 2 diabetes mellitus and heart failure: A scientific statement from the American Heart Association and the Heart Failure Society of America: This statement does not represent an update of the 2017 ACC/AHA/HFSA heart failure guideline update. Circulation. 2019;**140**(7):e294-e324. DOI: 10.1161/CIR.0000000000000691

[10] Bertoluci MC, Rocha VZ. Cardiovascular risk assessment in patients with diabetes. Diabetology and Metabolic Syndrome. 2017;**9**:25. DOI: 10.1186/s13098-017-0225-1

[11] Nichols GA et al. The incidence of congestive heart failure in type 2 diabetes: An update. Diabetes Care. 2004;**27**(8):1879-1884. DOI: 10.2337/diacare.27.8.1879]

[12] Bertoni AG et al. Heart failure prevalence, incidence, and mortality in the elderly with diabetes. Diabetes Care. 2004;**27**(3):699-703. DOI: 10.2337/diacare.27.3.699

[13] Control Group et al. Intensive glucose control and macrovascular outcomes in type 2 diabetes. Diabetologia. 2009;**52**(11):2288-2298. DOI: 10.1007/s00125-009-1470-0

[14] Skyler JS, Bergenstal R, Bonow RO, Buse J, Deedwania P, Gale EAM, et al. Intensive glycemic control and the prevention of cardiovascular events: Implications of the ACCORD, ADVANCE, and VA diabetes trials: A position statement of the American Diabetes Association and a scientific statement of the American College of

Cardiology Foundation and the American Heart Association. Circulation. 2009;**119**(2):351-357. DOI: 10.1161/CIRCULATIONAHA.108.191305

[15] Castagno D, Baird-Gunning J, Jhund PS, Biondi-Zoccai G, MacDonald MR, Petrie MC, et al. Intensive glycemic control has no impact on the risk of heart failure in type 2 diabetic patients: Evidence from a 37,229 patient meta-analysis. American Heart Journal. 2011; **162**:938-948.e2. DOI: 10.1016/j.ahj.2011.07.030

[16] Shindler DM et al. Diabetes mellitus, a predictor of morbidity and mortality in the studies of left ventricular dysfunction (SOLVD) trials and registry. The American Journal of Cardiology. 1996;**77**(11):1017-1020. DOI: 10.1016/s0002-9149(97)89163-1

[17] Dries DL et al. Prognostic impact of diabetes mellitus in patients with heart failure according to the etiology of left ventricular systolic dysfunction. Journal of the American College of Cardiology. 2001;**38**(2):421-428. DOI: 10.1016/s0735-1097(01)01408-5

[18] Gustafsson I et al. Influence of diabetes and diabetes-gender interaction on the risk of death in patients hospitalized with congestive heart failure. Journal of the American College of Cardiology. 2004;**43**(5):771-777. DOI: 10.1016/j.jacc.2003.11.024

[19] Kristensen SL et al. Risk related to pre-diabetes mellitus and diabetes mellitus in heart failure with reduced ejection fraction: Insights from prospective comparison of ARNI with ACEI to determine impact on global mortality and morbidity in heart failure trial. Circulation. Heart failure. 2016;**9**(1):e002560. DOI: 10.1161/CIRCHEARTFAILURE.115.002560

[20] Allen LA et al. Risk factors for adverse outcomes by left ventricular ejection fraction in a contemporary heart failure population. Circulation. Heart failure. 2013;**6**(4):635-646. DOI: 10.1161/CIRCHEARTFAILURE.112.000180

[21] MacDonald MR et al. Impact of diabetes on outcomes in patients with low and preserved ejection fraction heart failure: An analysis of the candesartan in heart failure: Assessment of reduction in mortality and morbidity (CHARM) programme. European Heart Journal. 2008;**29**(11):1377-1385. DOI: 10.1093/eurheartj/ehn153

[22] Kristensen SL et al. Clinical and echocardiographic characteristics and cardiovascular outcomes according to Diabetes status in patients with heart failure and preserved ejection fraction: A report from the I-preserve trial (Irbesartan in heart failure with preserved ejection fraction). Circulation. 2017;**135**(8):724-735. DOI: 10.1161/CIRCULATIONAHA.116.024593

[23] Hong J et al. Effects of metformin versus glipizide on cardiovascular outcomes in patients with type 2 diabetes and coronary artery disease. Diabetes Care. 2013;**36**(5):1304-1311. DOI: 10.2337/dc12-0719

[24] Kooy A et al. Long-term effects of metformin on metabolism and microvascular and macrovascular disease in patients with type 2 diabetes mellitus. Archives of Internal Medicine. 2009;**169**(6):616-625. DOI: 10.1001/archinternmed.2009.20

[25] Maruthur NM et al. Diabetes medications as monotherapy or metformin-based combination therapy for type 2 Diabetes: A systematic review and meta-analysis. Annals of Internal

Medicine. 2016;**164**(11):740-751. DOI: 10.7326/M15-2650

[26] Halabi A, Sen J, Huynh Q, et al. Metformin treatment in heart failure with preserved ejection fraction: A systematic review and meta-regression analysis. Cardiovascular Diabetology. 2020;**19**:124. DOI: 10.1186/s12933-020-01100-w

[27] American Diabetes Association Professional Practice Committee et al. 9. Pharmacologic approaches to glycemic treatment: Standards of medical care in diabetes-2022. Diabetes Care. 2022;**45** (Suppl 1):S125-S143. DOI: 10.2337/dc22-S009

[28] Genuth S. Should sulfonylureas remain an acceptable first-line add-on to metformin therapy in patients with type 2 diabetes? No, it's time to move on! Diabetes Care. 2015;**38**(1):170-175. DOI: 10.2337/dc14-0565

[29] Costello RA, Nicolas S, Shivkumar A. Sulfonylureas. [Updated 2021 Aug 23]. In: StatPearls [Internet]. Treasure Island (FL): StatPearls Publishing; 2022. Available from: https://www.ncbi.nlm.nih.gov/books/NBK513225/

[30] Krentz AJ, Bailey CJ. Oral antidiabetic agents: Current role in type 2 diabetes mellitus. Drugs. 2005;**65**(3): 385-411. DOI: 10.2165/00003495-200565030-00005

[31] Abdelmoneim AS et al. Variations in tissue selectivity amongst insulin secretagogues: A systematic review. Diabetes, Obesity & Metabolism. 2012; **14**(2):130-138. DOI: 10.1111/j.1463-1326.2011.01496.x

[32] Bodmer M et al. Metformin, sulfonylureas, or other antidiabetes drugs and the risk of lactic acidosis or hypoglycemia: A nested case-control analysis. Diabetes Care. 2008;**31**(11): 2086-2091. DOI: 10.2337/dc08-1171

[33] Goto A et al. Severe hypoglycaemia and cardiovascular disease: Systematic review and meta-analysis with bias analysis. BMJ (Clinical Research Ed.). 2013;**347**:f4533. DOI: 10.1136/bmj.f4533

[34] Mattishent K, Loke YK. Meta-analysis: Association between hypoglycemia and serious adverse events in older patients treated with glucose-lowering agents. Frontiers in Endocrinology. 2021;**12**:571568. DOI: 10.3389/fendo.2021.571568

[35] Monami M et al. Cardiovascular safety of sulfonylureas: A meta-analysis of randomized clinical trials. Diabetes, Obesity & Metabolism. 2013;**15**(10):938-953. DOI: 10.1111/dom.12116

[36] Rosenstock J et al. Effect of linagliptin vs glimepiride on major adverse cardiovascular outcomes in patients with type 2 diabetes: The CAROLINA randomized clinical trial. JAMA. 2019;**322**(12):1155-1166. DOI: 10.1001/jama.2019.13772

[37] Simpson SH et al. Mortality risk among sulfonylureas: A systematic review and network meta-analysis. The Lancet. Diabetes & Endocrinology. 2015; **3**(1):43-51. DOI: 10.1016/S2213-8587(14)70213-X

[38] Douros A et al. Pharmacologic differences of sulfonylureas and the risk of adverse cardiovascular and hypoglycemic events. Diabetes Care. 2017;**40**(11):1506-1513. DOI: 10.2337/dc17-0595

[39] Bailey CJ. Thiazolidinediones, Reference Module in Biomedical Sciences. United Kingdom: Elsevier; 2015. DOI: 10.1016/B978-0-12-801238-3.10867-0

[40] Singh S et al. Thiazolidinediones and heart failure: A teleo-analysis. Diabetes Care. 2007;**30**(8):2148-2153. DOI: 10.2337/dc07-0141

[41] Lago RM et al. Congestive heart failure and cardiovascular death in patients with prediabetes and type 2 diabetes given thiazolidinediones: A meta-analysis of randomised clinical trials. Lancet (London, England). 2007; **370**(9593):1129-1136. DOI: 10.1016/S0140-6736(07)61514-1

[42] Wallach JD et al. Updating insights into rosiglitazone and cardiovascular risk through shared data: Individual patient and summary level meta-analyses. BMJ (Clinical Research Ed.). 2020;**368**:l7078. DOI: 10.1136/bmj.l7078

[43] Brunton SA, Wysham CH. GLP-1 receptor agonists in the treatment of type 2 diabetes: Role and clinical experience to date. Postgraduate Medicine. 2020;**132**(sup 2):3-14. DOI: 10.1080/00325481.2020.1798099

[44] Aroda VR. A review of GLP-1 receptor agonists: Evolution and advancement, through the lens of randomised controlled trials. Diabetes, Obesity & Metabolism. 2018;**20**(Suppl 1):22-33. DOI: 10.1111/dom.13162

[45] Chatterjee S et al. What have we learnt from "real world" data, observational studies and meta-analyses. Diabetes, Obesity & Metabolism. 2018; **20**(Suppl 1):47-58. DOI: 10.1111/dom.13178

[46] Levin PA et al. Glucagon-like peptide-1 receptor agonists: A systematic review of comparative effectiveness research. Diabetes, Metabolic Syndrome and Obesity: Targets and Therapy. 2017; **10**:123-139. DOI: 10.2147/DMSO.S130834

[47] Trujillo JM et al. GLP-1 receptor agonists: An updated review of head-to-head clinical studies. Therapeutic Advances in Endocrinology and Metabolism. 2021;**12**:2042018821997320. DOI: 10.1177/2042018821997320

[48] Andreadis P et al. Semaglutide for type 2 diabetes mellitus: A systematic review and meta-analysis. Diabetes, Obesity & Metabolism. 2018;**20**(9):2255-2263. DOI: 10.1111/dom.13361

[49] American Diabetes Association Professional Practice Committee. 10. Cardiovascular disease and risk management: Standards of medical care in diabetes—2022. Diabetes Care. 2022; **45**(Supplement_1):S144-S174. DOI: 10.2337/dc22-S010

[50] Marso SP, Holst AG, Vilsbøll T. Semaglutide and cardiovascular outcomes in patients with type 2 diabetes. New England Journal of Medicine. 2017;**376**:891-892. DOI: 10.1056/NEJMc1615712

[51] Demuth H-U et al. Type 2 diabetes—Therapy with dipeptidyl peptidase IV inhibitors. Biochimica et Biophysica Acta. 2005;**1751**(1):33-44. DOI: 10.1016/j.bbapap.2005.05.010

[52] Cahn A et al. An update on DPP-4 inhibitors in the management of type 2 diabetes. Expert Opinion on Emerging Drugs. 2016;**21**(4):409-419. DOI: 10.1080/14728214.2016.1257608

[53] Scirica BM et al. Saxagliptin and cardiovascular outcomes in patients with type 2 diabetes mellitus. The New England Journal of Medicine. 2013;**369**(14):1317-1326. DOI: 10.1056/NEJMoa1307684

[54] McMurray JJV et al. Effects of vildagliptin on ventricular function in patients with type 2 diabetes mellitus

and heart failure: A randomized placebo-controlled trial. JACC. Heart Failure. 2018;**6**(1):8-17. DOI: 10.1016/j.jchf.2017.08.004

[55] McDonagh TA et al. Corrigendum to: 2021 ESC Guidelines for the diagnosis and treatment of acute and chronic heart failure: Developed by the Task Force for the diagnosis and treatment of acute and chronic heart failure of the European Society of Cardiology (ESC) With the special contribution of the Heart Failure Association (HFA) of the ESC. European Heart Journal. 2021;**42**(48):4901. DOI: 10.1093/eurheartj/ehab670

[56] Hsia DS et al. An update on sodium-glucose co-transporter-2 inhibitors for the treatment of diabetes mellitus. Current Opinion in Endocrinology, Diabetes, and Obesity. 2017;**24**(1):73-79. DOI: 10.1097/MED.0000000000000311

[57] Wiviott SD et al. Dapagliflozin and cardiovascular outcomes in type 2 diabetes. The New England Journal of Medicine. 2019;**380**(4):347-357. DOI: 10.1056/NEJMoa1812389

[58] Perkovic V et al. Canagliflozin and renal outcomes in type 2 diabetes and nephropathy. The New England Journal of Medicine. 2019;**380**(24):2295-2306. DOI: 10.1056/NEJMoa1811744

[59] Zinman B et al. Empagliflozin, cardiovascular outcomes, and mortality in type 2 diabetes. The New England Journal of Medicine. 2015;**373**(22):2117-2128. DOI: 10.1056/NEJMoa1504720

[60] Neal B et al. Canagliflozin and cardiovascular and renal events in type 2 diabetes. The New England Journal of Medicine. 2017;**377**(7):644-657. DOI: 10.1056/NEJMoa1611925

[61] Cannon CP et al. Cardiovascular outcomes with Ertugliflozin in type 2 diabetes. The New England Journal of Medicine. 2020;**383**(15):1425-1435. DOI: 10.1056/NEJMoa2004967

[62] Cosentino F et al. Efficacy of Ertugliflozin on heart failure-related events in patients with type 2 diabetes mellitus and established atherosclerotic cardiovascular disease: Results of the VERTIS CV trial. Circulation. 2020;**142**(23):2205-2215. DOI: 10.1161/CIRCULATIONAHA.120.050255

[63] Snell-Bergeon JK, Wadwa RP. Hypoglycemia, diabetes, and cardiovascular disease. Diabetes Technology & Therapeutics. 2012;**14**(Suppl 1):S51-S58. DOI: 10.1089/dia.2012.0031

[64] Shen L et al. Insulin treatment and clinical outcomes in patients with diabetes and heart failure with preserved ejection fraction. European Journal of Heart Failure. 2019;**21**(8):974-984. DOI: 10.1002/ejhf.1535

[65] Echouffo-Tcheugui JB et al. Severe hypoglycemia and incident heart failure among adults with type 2 diabetes. The Journal of Clinical Endocrinology and Metabolism. 2022;**107**(3):e955-e962. DOI: 10.1210/clinem/dgab794

[66] Tuso P. Prediabetes and lifestyle modification: Time to prevent a. preventable disease. The Permanente Journal. 2014;**18**(3):88-93. DOI: 10.7812/TPP/14-002

[67] Centers for Disease Control and Prevention. National Diabetes Statistic Report. Available from: https://www.cdc.gov/diabetes/data/statistics-report/index.html [Accessed: 09 August 2022]

[68] Weatherspoon D, MacGill M. All about borderline diabetes (prediabetes). Medical News Today. 2019. Available

from: https://www.medicalnewstoday.com/articles/311240

[69] Chakraborty M, Singh P, Dsouza J. Fasting and postprandial lipid parameters: A comparative evaluation of cardiovascular risk assessment in prediabetes and diabetes. Journal of Family Medicine and Primary Care. 2020;**9**(1):287-292. DOI: 10.4103/jfmpc.jfmpc_769_19

[70] Sörensen B et al. Prediabetes and type 2 diabetes are associated with generalized microvascular dysfunction. Circulation. 2016;**134**:1339-1352

[71] Papanas N et al. Neuropathy in prediabetes: Does the clock start ticking early? Nature Reviews Endocrinology. 2011;7:682-690

[72] Vistisen D, Kivimäki M, Perreault L, et al. Reversion from prediabetes to normoglycaemia and risk of cardiovascular disease and mortality: The Whitehall II cohort study. Diabetologia. 2019;**62**(8):1385-1390

[73] Classification of Diabetes Mellitus 2019, WHO 2019; 8. Available from: https://www.who.int/publications/i/item/classification-of-diabetes-mellitus

[74] International Diabetes Federation. Recommendations for Managing Type 2 Diabetes in Primary Care. 2017. Available from: https://www.idf.org/managing-type2-diabetes

[75] Diabetes Canada Clinical Practice Guidelines Expert Committee et al. Definition, classification and diagnosis of diabetes, prediabetes and metabolic syndrome. Canadian Journal of Diabetes. 2018;**42**(Suppl 1):s10-s15. DOI: 10.1016/j.jcjd.2017.10.003

[76] Bell K, Shaw J, Brown L, et al. A position statement on screening and management of prediabetes in adults in primary care in Australia. Diabetes Research and Clinical Practice. 2020; **164**:108-188

[77] Prediabetes diagnosis impaired glucose tolerance. 2019. Available from: http://diabetes.co.uk

[78] American Diabetes Association. 2. Classification and diagnosis of diabetes: Standards of Medical Care in Diabetes—2022. Diabetes Care. 2022;**45** (Supplement_1):S17-S38. DOI: 10.2337/dc22-S002

[79] Mirzazade VA, Aliyeva TT, Abbasova NE, Mammadhasanov RM, et al. Standards of Diagnosis Diabetes Mellitus and Prediabetes. Invitation to Discussion. Baku: Azerbaijan Association of Endocrinology, Diabetology and Therapeutic Education "AzerDiab"; 2017

[80] Akter N, Qureshi NK. Comparison of IDRS, ADA and FINDRISC diabetes risk assessment tools: A cross-sectional analysis in a tertiary care hospital. Sri Lanka Journal of Diabetes Endocrinology and Metabolism. 2020;**10**(2):10-20. DOI: 10.4038/sjdem.v10i2.7415

[81] Wong KC et al. Ausdrisk: Application in General Practice. Australian Family Physician. 2011;**40**: 524-526

[82] Schlesinger S, Neuenschwander M, et al. Prediabetes and risk of mortality, diabetes-related complications and comorbidities: Umbrella review of meta-analyses of prospective studies. Diabetologia. 2022;**65**(2):275-285. DOI: 10.1007/s00125-021-05592-3

[83] Sinha A, Ning H, Ahmad FS, et al. Association of fasting glucose with lifetime risk of incident heart failure: The lifetime risk pooling project.

Cardiovascular Diabetology. 2021; **20**(1):66

[84] The association between glucose abnormalities and heart failure in the population-based Reykjavik study. Available from: https://www.hirsla.lsh.is/handle/2336/2706?show=full

[85] Hoffman A, Honigberg M. Glycated hemoglobin as an integrator of cardiovascular risk. İn individuals without diabetes: Lessons from recent epidemiologic studies. Current Atherosclerosis Reports. 2022;**24**:435-442. DOI: 10.1007/s11883-022-01024-8

[86] Pandey A, Vaduganathan M, Patel KV, Ayers C, Ballantyne CM, Kosiborod MN, et al. Biomarker-based risk prediction of incident heart failure in pre-diabetes and diabetes. JACC: Heart Failure. 2021;**9**(3):215-223

[87] Ardissino M et al. Long-term cardiovascular outcomes after orlistat therapy in patients with obesity: A nationwide, propensity-score matched cohort study. European Heart Journal-Cardiovascular Pharmacotherapy. 2021;**8** (2):179-186. DOI: 10.1093/ehjcvp/pvaa133

[88] Margulies KB, Hernandez AF, Redfield MM, Givertz MM, Oliveira GH, Cole R, et al. Effects of liraglutide on clinical stability among patients with advanced heart failure and reduced ejection fraction: A randomized clinical trial. Journal of the American Medical Association. 2016;**316**(5):500-508

[89] Jorsal A, Kistorp C, et al. Effect of liraglutide, a glucagon-like peptide-1 analogue, on left ventricular function in stable chronic heart failure patients with and without diabetes (LIVE)—A multicentre, double-blind, randomised, placebo-controlled trial. European Journal of Heart. Failure. 2016;**19**(1): 69-77. DOI: 10.1002/EJHF.657

[90] Bozkurt B, Coats AJS, Tsutsui H, Abdelhamid M, Adamopoulos S, Albert N, et al. Universal definition and classification of heart failure: A report of the Heart Failure Society of America, heart failure Association of the European Society of cardiology, Japanese heart failure society and writing Committee of the Universal Definition of heart failure. Journal of Cardiac Failure. 2021;**27**(4): 387-413

[91] McDonagh TA, Metra M, Adamo M, Gardner RS, Baumbach A, Böhm M, et al. ESC guidelines for the diagnosis and treatment of acute and chronic heart failure: Developed by the task force for the diagnosis and treatment of acute and chronic heart failure of the European Society of Cardiology (ESC) with the special contribution of the heart failure association (HFA) of the ESC. European Heart Journal. 2021;**2**:hea368

[92] Owan TE, Hodge DO, Herges RM, Jacobsen SJ, Roger VL, Redfield MM. Trends in prevalence and outcome of heart failure with preserved ejection fraction. The New England Journal of Medicine. 2006;**355**(3):251-259

[93] Oktay AA, Rich JD, Shah SJ. The emerging epidemic of heart failure with preserved ejection fraction. Current Heart Failure Reports. 2013;**10**(4):401-410

[94] Ponikowski P, Voors AA, Anker SD, Bueno H, Cleland JGF, Coats AJS, et al. 2016 ESC guidelines for the diagnosis and treatment of acute and chronic heart failure: The task force for the diagnosis and treatment of acute and chronic heart failure of the European Society of Cardiology (ESC) developed with the special contribution of the Heart Failure Association (HFA) of the ESC. European Heart Journal. 2016;**37**(27):2129-2200

[95] Meta-analysis Global Group in Chronic Heart F. The survival of patients

with heart failure with preserved or reduced left ventricular ejection fraction: An individual patient data meta-analysis. European Heart Journal. 2012;**33**(14): 1750-1757

[96] Yancy Clyde W, Jessup M, Bozkurt B, Butler J, Casey Donald E, Drazner Mark H, et al. 2013 ACCF/AHA guideline for the Management of Heart Failure: Executive summary. Circulation. 2013;**128**(16):1810-1852

[97] Simmonds SJ, Cuijpers I, Heymans S, Jones EAV. Cellular and molecular differences between HFpEF and HFrEF: A step ahead in an improved pathological understanding. Cell. 2020;**9**:1

[98] Ho JE, Lyass A, Lee DS, Vasan RS, Kannel WB, Larson MG, et al. Predictors of new-onset heart failure: Differences in preserved versus reduced ejection fraction. Circulation. Heart Failure. 2013;**6**(2):279-286

[99] Type 2 Diabetes Mellitus and Heart Failure. A scientific statement from the American Heart Association and the Heart Failure Society of America. © 2019 by the American Heart Association, Inc., and the Heart Failure Society of America. Circulation. 2019;**140**:e294-e324. DOI: 10.1161/CIR.0000000000000691. Available from: https://www.ahajournals.org/journal/circ

[100] Shimizu I, Minamino T, Toko H, et al. Excessive cardiac insulin signaling exacerbates systolic dysfunction induced by pressure overload in rodents. The Journal of Clinical Investigation. 2010; **120**(5):1506-1514. DOI: 10.1172/JCI40096

[101] Iribarren C, Karter AJ, Go AS, et al. Glycemic control and heart failure among adult patients with diabetes. Circulation. 2001;**103**:2668-2673. DOI: 10.1161/01.CIR.103.22.2668

[102] Nirengi S, Peres Valgas da Silva C, Stanford KI. Disruption of energy utilization in diabetic cardiomyopathy; a mini review. Current Opinion in Pharmacology. 2020;**54**:82-90

[103] Jia G, Hill MA, Sowers JR. Diabetic cardiomyopathy: An update of mechanisms contributing to this clinical entity. Circulation Research. 2018;**122** (4):624-638

[104] Jang SY, Jang J, Yang DH, Cho HJ, Lim S, Jeon ES, et al. Impact of insulin therapy on the mortality of acute heart failure patients with diabetes mellitus. Cardiovascular Diabetology. 2021;**20**(1): 180

[105] Levelt E, Rodgers CT, Clarke WT, et al. Cardiac energetics, oxygenation, and perfusion during increased workload in patients with type 2 diabetes mellitus. European Heart Journal. 2016;**37**:3461-3469. DOI: 10.1093/eurheartj/ehv442

[106] Zaveri MP, Perry JC, Schuetz TM, Memon MD, Faiz S, Cancarevic I. Diabetic cardiomyopathy as a clinical entity: Is it a myth? Cureus. 2020;**12**(10): e11100

[107] Glass CK, Olefsky JM. Inflammation and lipid signaling in the etiology of insulin resistance. Cell Metabolism. 2012;**15**:635-645. DOI: 10.1016/j.cmet. 2012.04.001

[108] Bonapace S, Valbusa F, Bertolini L, et al. Early impairment in left ventricular longitudinal systolic function is associated with an increased risk of incident atrial fibrillation in patients with type 2 diabetes. Journal of Diabetes and its Complications. 2017;**31**:413-418. DOI: 10.1016/j.jdiacomp. 2016.10.032

[109] Zheng H, Zhu H, Liu X, Huang X, Huang A, Huang Y. Mitophagy in diabetic cardiomyopathy: Roles and mechanisms. Frontiers in Cell and Developmental Biology. 2021;**9**:2675

[110] Shah MS, Brownlee M. Molecular and cellular mechanisms of cardiovascular disorders in diabetes. Circulation Research. 2016;**118**:1808-1829. DOI: 10.1161/CIRCRESAHA.116.306923

[111] Bedi KC Jr, Snyder NW, Brandimarto J, et al. Evidence for intramyocardial disruption of lipid metabolism and increased myocardial ketone utilization in advanced human heart failure. Circulation. 2016;**133**:706-716. DOI: 10.1161/CIRCULATIONAHA.115.017545

[112] Campbell P, Krim S, Ventura H. The bi-directional impact of two chronic illnesses: Heart failure and diabetes—A review of the epidemiology and outcomes. Cardiac Failure Review. 2015;**1**(1):8-10. DOI: 10.15420/cfr.2015.01.01.8

[113] Nielson C, Lange T. Blood glucose and heart failure in nondiabetic patients. Diabetes Care. 2005;**28**:3607-3611. DOI: 10.2337/diacare.28.3.607

[114] Cosentino F, Grant PJ, Aboyans V, Bailey CJ, Ceriello A, Delgado V, et al. 2019 ESC guidelines on diabetes, pre-diabetes, and cardiovascular diseases developed in collaboration with the EASD. European Heart Journal. 2020;**41**(2):255-323

[115] Azevedo PS, Polegato BF, Minicucci MF, Paiva SAR, Zornoff LAM. Cardiac remodeling: Concepts, clinical impact, pathophysiological mechanisms and pharmacologic treatment. Arquivos Brasileiros de Cardiologia. 2016;**106**(1):62-69

[116] Cheng JM, Akkerhuis KM, Battes LC, van Vark LC, Hillege HL, Paulus WJ, et al. Biomarkers of heart failure with normal ejection fraction: A systematic review. European Journal of Heart Failure. 2013;**15**(12):1350-1362

[117] Seferovic JP, Tesic M, Seferovic PM, Lalic K, Jotic A, Biering-Sørensen T, et al. Increased left ventricular mass index is present in patients with type 2 diabetes without ischemic heart disease. Scientific Reports. 2018;**8**(1):926

[118] Lang RM, Badano LP, Mor-Avi V, Afilalo J, Armstrong A, Ernande L, et al. Recommendations for cardiac chamber quantification by echocardiography in adults: An update from the American Society of Echocardiography and the European Association of Cardiovascular Imaging. European Heart Journal Cardiovascular Imaging. 2015;**16**(3):233-270

[119] Pham I, Cosson E, Nguyen MT, Banu I, Genevois I, Poignard P, et al. Evidence for a specific diabetic cardiomyopathy: An observational retrospective echocardiographic study in 656 asymptomatic type 2 diabetic patients. International Journal of Endocrinology. 2015;**2015**:743503

[120] Heidenreich PA, Bozkurt B, Aguilar D, Allen LA, Byun JJ, Colvin MM, et al. AHA/ACC/HFSA guideline for the Management of Heart Failure: A report of the American College of Cardiology/American Heart Association Joint Committee on Clinical Practice Guidelines. Circulation. 2022;**145**:e895-e1032. DOI: 10.1161/CIR.0000000000001063

[121] Yang S, Chen H, Tan K, Cai F, Du Y, Lv W, et al. Secreted frizzled-related protein 2 and extracellular volume fraction in patients with heart failure.

Oxidative Medicine and Cellular Longevity. 2020;**2020**:2563508

[122] Wu Y, Liu X, Zheng H, Zhu H, Mai W, Huang X, et al. Multiple roles of sFRP2 in cardiac development and cardiovascular disease. International Journal of Biological Sciences. 2020;**16** (5):730-738

[123] Wu J, Zheng H, Liu X, Chen P, Zhang Y, Luo J, et al. Prognostic value of secreted frizzled-related protein 5 in heart failure patients with and without type 2 diabetes mellitus. Circulation. Heart Failure. 2020;**13**(9):e007054

[124] Huang A, Huang Y. Role of Sfrps in cardiovascular disease. Therapeutic Advances in Chronic Disease. 2020;**11**: 2040622320901990

[125] Kristensen SL, Jhund PS, Lee MMY, Køber L, Solomon SD, Granger CB, et al. Prevalence of prediabetes and undiagnosed diabetes in patients with HFpEF and HFrEF and associated clinical outcomes. Cardiovascular Drugs and Therapy. 2017;**31**(5–6): 545-549

[126] 10. Cardiovascular disease and risk management: Standards of medical care in diabetes—2021. Diabetes Care. 2021; **44**(Supplement 1):S125-SS50

[127] Papadopoulos DP, Makris TK. Masked hypertension definition, impact, outcomes: A critical review. Journal of Clinical Hypertension (Greenwich, Conn.). 2007;**9**(12):956-963

[128] Sabuncu T, Sonmez A, Eren MA, Sahin I, Çorapçioğlu D, Üçler R, et al. Characteristics of patients with hypertension in a population with type 2 diabetes mellitus. Results from the Turkish Nationwide survey of Glycemic and other metabolic parameters of patients with Diabetes Mellitus (TEMD hypertension study). Primary Care Diabetes. 2021;**15**(2):332-339

[129] Zhu H, Zheng H, Liu X, Mai W, Huang Y. Clinical applications for out-of-office blood pressure monitoring. Therapeutic Advances in Chronic Disease. 2020;**11**:2040622320901660

[130] Sharma A, Verma S, Bhatt D, et al. Optimizing foundational therapies in patients with HFrEF. JACC: Basic to Translational Science. 2022;**7**(5):504-517. DOI: 10.1016/j.jacbts.2021.10.018

[131] Yoon S, Eom GH. Heart failure with preserved ejection fraction: Present status and future directions. Experimental & Molecular Medicine. 2019;**51**(12):1-9

[132] Anker SD, Butler J, Filippatos G, Ferreira JP, Bocchi E, Böhm M, et al. Empagliflozin in heart failure with a preserved ejection fraction. The New England Journal of Medicine. 2021;**9**:25

[133] Vermes E, Ducharme A, Bourassa MG, Lessard M, White M, Tardif JC. Enalapril reduces the incidence of diabetes in patients with chronic heart failure: Insight from the studies of left ventricular dysfunction (SOLVD). Circulation. 2003;**107**(9):1291-1296

[134] Waddingham MT, Edgley AJ, Tsuchimochi H, Kelly DJ, Shirai M, Pearson JT. Contractile apparatus dysfunction early in the pathophysiology of diabetic cardiomyopathy. World Journal of Diabetes. 2015;**6**:943-960. DOI: 10.4239/wjd.v6.i7.943

[135] McMurray JJ, Packer M, Desai AS, Gong J, Lefkowitz MP, Rizkala AR, et al. Angiotensin-neprilysin inhibition versus enalapril in heart failure. The New England Journal of Medicine. 2014; **371**(11):993-1004

[136] Solomon SD, McMurray JJV, Anand IS, Ge J, Lam CSP, Maggioni AP, et al. Angiotensin-neprilysin inhibition in heart failure with preserved ejection fraction. The New England Journal of Medicine. 2019;**381**(17):1609-1620

[137] Seferovic JP, Claggett B, Seidelmann SB, Seely EW, Packer M, Zile MR, et al. Effect of sacubitril/valsartan versus enalapril on glycaemic control in patients with heart failure and diabetes: A post-hoc analysis from the PARADIGM-HF trial. The Lancet Diabetes Endocrinology. 2017;**5**(5):333-340

[138] Zile MR, Claggett BL, Prescott MF, McMurray JJ, Packer M, Rouleau JL, et al. Prognostic implications of changes in N-terminal pro-B-type natriuretic peptide in patients with heart failure. Journal of the American College of Cardiology. 2016;**68**(22):2425-2436

[139] Cunningham JW, Vaduganathan M, Claggett BL, Zile MR, Anand IS, Packer M, et al. Effects of sacubitril/valsartan on N-terminal pro-B-type natriuretic peptide in heart failure with preserved ejection fraction. JACC: Heart Failure. 2020;**8**(5):372-381

[140] Chen M-D, Dong S-S, Cai N-Y, Fan M-D, Gu S-P, Zheng J-J, et al. Efficacy and safety of mineralocorticoid receptor antagonists for patients with heart failure and diabetes mellitus: A systematic review and meta-analysis. BMC Cardiovascular Disorders. 2016;**16**:28

[141] Filippatos G, Anker SD, Böhm M, Gheorghiade M, Køber L, Krum H, et al. A randomized controlled study of finerenone vs. eplerenone in patients with worsening chronic heart failure and diabetes mellitus and/or chronic kidney disease. European Heart Journal. 2016;**37**(27):2105-2114

[142] Pitt B, Anker SD, Böhm M. Rationale and design of mineralocorticoid receptor antagonist tolerability study-heart failure (ARTS-HF): A randomized study of finerenone vs eplerenone in patients who have worsening chronic heart failure with diabetes and/or chronic kidney disease. European Journal of Heart Failure. 2015;**17**(2):224-232. DOI: 10.1002/ejhf.218

[143] Zannad F, Ferreira JP, Pocock SJ, Anker SD, Butler J, Filippatos G, et al. SGLT2 inhibitors in patients with heart failure with reduced ejection fraction: A meta-analysis of the EMPEROR-reduced and DAPA-HF trials. The Lancet. 2020;**396**(10254):819-829

[144] Ferrannini E, Mark M, Mayoux E. CV protection in the EMPAREG OUTCOME trial: A "thrifty substrate" hypothesis. Diabetes Care. 2016;**39**:1108-1114. DOI: 10.2337/dci16–0033

[145] McMurray JJV, Solomon SD, Inzucchi SE, Køber L, Kosiborod MN, Martinez FA, et al. Dapagliflozin in patients with heart failure and reduced ejection fraction. The New England Journal of Medicine. 2019;**381**(21):1995-2008

[146] Butt JH, Docherty KF, Petrie MC, Schou M, Kosiborod MN, O'Meara E, et al. Efficacy and safety of dapagliflozin in men and women with heart failure with reduced ejection fraction: A prespecified analysis of the dapagliflozin and prevention of adverse outcomes in heart failure trial. JAMA Cardiology. 2021;**6**(6):678-689

[147] Packer M, Anker SD, Butler J, Filippatos G, Pocock SJ, Carson P, et al. Cardiovascular and renal outcomes with empagliflozin in heart failure. The New England Journal of Medicine. 2020;**383**:1413-1424

[148] Wanner C, Lachin JM, Inzucchi SE, et al. EMPA-REG OUTCOME empagliflozin and clinical outcomes in patients with type 2 diabetes mellitus, established cardiovascular disease, and chronic kidney disease. Circulation. 2018;**137**(2):119-129. DOI: 10.1161/circulationaha. 117.028268

[149] Ceriello A, Catrinoiu D, Chandramouli C, et al. Heart failure in type 2 diabetes: Current perspectives on screening, diagnosis and management. Cardiovascular Diabetology. 2021;**20**:218. DOI: 10.1186/s12933-021-01408-1

[150] Low Wang C, Hess CN, Hiatt WR, Goldfine AB. Atherosclerotic cardiovascular disease and heart failure in type 2 diabetes—Mechanisms, management, and clinical considerations. Circulation. 2016;**133**(24):2459-2502. DOI: 10.1161/circulationaha. 116.022194

[151] Fitchett D, Zinman B, Wanner C, Lachin JM, Hantel S, Salsali A, et al. Heart failure outcomes with empagliflozin in patients with type 2 diabetes at high cardiovascular risk: Results of the EMPA-REG OUTCOME. European Heart Journal. 2016;**37**:1526-1534. DOI: 10.1093/eurheartj/ehv728

[152] McGuire DK, Shih WJ, Cosentino F, Charbonnel B, Cherney DZI, Dagogo-Jack S, et al. Association of SGLT2 inhibitors with cardiovascular and kidney outcomes in patients with type 2 diabetes: A meta-analysis. JAMA Cardiology. 2021;**6**(2):148-158. DOI: 10.1001/jamacardio.2020.4511

[153] Bhatt DL, Szarek M, Steg PG, Cannon CP, Leiter LA, McGuire DK, et al. Sotagliflozin in patients with diabetes and recent worsening heart failure. The New England Journal of Medicine. 2020;**384**:117-128

[154] Januzzi JL Jr, Xu J, Li J, Shaw W, Oh R, Pfeifer M, et al. Effects of canagliflozin on amino-terminal pro-B-type natriuretic peptide: Implications for cardiovascular risk reduction. Journal of the American College of Cardiology. 2020;**76**(18):2076-2085

[155] Kusunose K, Imai T, Tanaka A, Dohi K, Shiina K, Yamada T, et al. Effects of canagliflozin on NT-proBNP stratified by left ventricular diastolic function in patients with type 2 diabetes and chronic heart failure: A sub analysis of the CANDLE trial. Cardiovascular Diabetology. 2021;**20**(1):186

[156] Tamaki S, Yamada T, Watanabe T, Morita T, Furukawa Y, Kawasaki M, et al. Effect of empagliflozin as an add-on therapy on decongestion and renal function in patients with diabetes hospitalized for acute decompensated heart failure. Circulation. 2021;**14**(3):e007048

[157] de Boer RA, Núñez J, Kozlovski P, Wang Y, Proot P, Keefe D. Effects of the dual sodium-glucose linked transporter inhibitor, licogliflozin vs placebo or empagliflozin in patients with type 2 diabetes and heart failure. British Journal of Clinical Pharmacology. 2020;**86**(7):1346-1356

[158] Buse JB, Wexler DJ, Tsapas A, Rossing P, Mingrone G, Mathieu C, et al. 2019 update to: Management of hyperglycemia in type 2 diabetes, 2018. A consensus report by the American Diabetes Association (ADA) and the European Association for the Study of Diabetes (EASD). Diabetes Care. 2020;**43**(2):487-493

Chapter 10

Prevalence and Risk Factors of Cardiovascular Diseases among the Nigerian Population: A New Trend among Adolescents and Youths

Omigbile Olamide, Oni Adebayo, Abe Emmanuel, Lawal Eyitayo, Oyasope Beatrice and Mayaki Tomisin

Abstract

This chapter gives an overview of the prevalence and risk factors of cardiovascular diseases (CVDs) among Nigerian population with emphasis on the younger population. The Nigerian population is largely dominated by youths who contribute significantly toward economic growth of the country. Addressing the issues of cardiovascular diseases among this population offers an opportunity toward increasing life expectancy and building a healthy nation. In order to understand the issues at hand, this chapter detailed the prevalence of cardiovascular diseases among youths, and it also identifies the risk factors that contribute to the development of CVDs among the population. Furthermore, it gave recommendations on how the issue of CVDs among the younger population can be addressed.

Keywords: cardiovascular diseases, Nigeria, adolescents, youths, prevalence, risk factors

1. Introduction

Cardiovascular diseases (CVDs) are a group of illnesses that mostly affect the heart and blood vessels. They are the major causes of death and disability worldwide, particularly in low- and middle-income nations [1, 2]. CVDs claimed the lives of an estimated 17.9 million individuals in 2019, accounting for nearly 32% of all worldwide fatalities that year [1]. Even more concerning was the fact that three-quarters of these deaths occurred in low- and middle-income nations, such as sub-Saharan Africa (SSA), which also supplied 80% of the global illness burden [1, 3]. Not only is the present mortality, prevalence, and disability associated with CVDs great, but there is also an increasing tendency, making future estimates much bleaker than the current scenario. Roth et al. [2] estimated an almost doubling of the global prevalence of CVDs from 1990 to 2019 in their synthesis of data from the Global Burden of Disease 2019 Study. Similarly, the number of fatalities (from 12.1 million in 1990 to

18.6 million in 2019) and years lived with disability (from 17.7 million in 1990 to 34.4 million in 2019) nearly doubled during the same time [2]. Cardiovascular diseases (CVDs) affect 31% of all people globally. The underlying pathology is a lifetime process that begins in childhood and develops throughout adolescence depending on risk factors. Identifying and treating risk factors in teenagers allow for the management of CVDs [4].

The existence of risk factors considerably influences the development of CVD [5]. In emerging nations, the prevalence of CVD has risen among younger individuals aged 25–44 years, who make up the working population, compared to the older population of persons aged 65 years and older in industrialized countries [6]. This shift has been connected to an increase in harmful lifestyle characteristics such as poor food, inactivity, smoking, and alcohol consumption [7]. CVD risk factors are frequently formed during infancy and adolescence and become established in adulthood [8]. As a result, early detection of its risk throughout infancy and adolescence may help avoid or postpone the beginning of CVD [9]. Adolescents aged 10–19 years [10] experience changes in their social surroundings and social lives as they transition to adulthood. This is visible as they fail to develop regular eating and sleeping routines, resulting in a lack of exercise, bad dietary habits, weight gain, and insufficient sleep [11]. CVD and related risk factors are predicted by socioeconomic level (SES). However, the degree of this relationship changes depending on the countries' economic progress [12, 13]. In high-income nations, regardless of the SES measures utilized, evidence suggests to a negative connection between SES and CVD risk factors in the adult population [14]. This tendency contrasts in low-middle-income nations and among people with lower socioeconomic status in developed countries, where lower socioeconomic status is a possible predictor of worse health outcomes [15].

Inadequate general community understanding of CVD and its risk factors is a barrier to successful CVD prevention and treatment [16]. As a result, understanding CVD knowledge gaps and perceptions among teenagers is critical to developing a CVD preventive program for this subpopulation [17]. It has been demonstrated that increased understanding of an illness and propensity to it improves adherence to lifestyle adjustments [18]. Knowledge of CVD and its risk factors is critical for both primary and secondary CVD prevention [19]. At least one in every three teenagers and young adults has insufficient health literacy and, as a result, engages in unhealthy behaviors [19]. Good CVD knowledge and comprehension will lead to better health-seeking behavior, which will affect CVD preventive and control judgments and decisions [20, 21]. Cardiovascular disease imposes a massive economic burden because of its impact on the working population and the high expense of its treatment [22]. CVD prevention is thus the ideal option for a growing country like Nigeria. The goal of this study is to investigate the prevalence and risk factors for CVD among Nigerian adolescents and youths.

2. Types of cardiovascular diseases

There are few surveys on the prevalence of cardiovascular diseases in among Nigerian adolescents. In urban Nigeria, there has been a rising prevalence of hypertension [23]. A 150% increase in the prevalence of cardiovascular disease has also been reported [24]. Hypertension affects up to 46% of Nigerian adults and a rising proportion of Nigerian adolescents [25, 26]. Furthermore, Adedapo et al. [24] reported in a research study that cardiovascular diseases are fully account for more than a 30% of medical admissions, which is in tandem with the sharp rise in the

DOI: http://dx.doi.org/10.5772/intechopen.108180

S/N	Types of CVDs	Description	Symptoms	Risk factors
1	Coronary heart diseases	Ischemic heart disease (IHD)	• Heart attack • Angina at chronic condition	High blood pressure/blood cholesterol (BC), smoking, unhealthy diet, physical inactivity, diabetes, and aging
2	Stroke	• Ischemic stroke • Hemorrhagic stroke • Transient ischemic attack	• Brain damage resulting into sudden injuries • Weakness often on one side of the body	High, tobacco use, unhealthy diet, physical inactivity, diabetes, and aging
3	Rheumatic heart disease	• Inflammation of the heart valves and heart muscle	• Shortness of breath, fatigue, irregular heartbeats, chest pain and fainting.	—
4	Congenital heart disease	• Malformations of heart or central blood vessel at birth or during pregnancy	• Breathlessness or a failure to attain normal growth and development	• Maternal alcohol and medicines use; maternal infection (e.g. rubella) • Poor maternal nutrition
5	Peripheral vascular disease	• Atherosclerosis • Abdominal aortic aneurysm		• Persisting high BP • Tangential heart disorders • Syphilis, and other inflammatory disorders
6	Deep venous thrombosis (DVT) and pulmonary embolism	• The blood clots in the veins, which can dislodge and move to the heart and lungs		• Surgery, obesity, cancer, recent childbirth, use of contraceptives and hormone replacement therapy.
7	Other forms of cardiovascular diseases	• Tumors of the heart • Disorders of heart muscle (cardiomyopathy) • Heart valve diseases		

Behera et al. [35].

Table 1.
Types of cardiovascular diseases (CVDs), symptoms, and risk factors.

burden of cardiovascular diseases, especially in developing countries [27]. This necessitates a realistic approach to the swift deterrence of an impending epidemic. The middle-aged group who account for nearly half of all cardiovascular disease patients form a sizable portion of the workforce driving the Nigerian economy. Given that biological changes occur at a faster rate throughout childhood and adolescence than at any other time in life, it is acceptable to consider this age group to be an important category for examining CVD risk factors [28]. Adedapo [29] observed hypertension to be the leading cardiovascular disease among medical outpatients in a study in southwestern Nigeria. Ischemic heart disease and cardiomyopathies were entirely unusual, accounting for less than 1% of all cardiovascular diseases in the study.

Also, coronary heart disease (CHD), despite being acknowledged to have ramped up in recent time, is still exceptionally rare and has not made a major contribution to cardiovascular mortality rates [30]. Female patients presenting with cardiovascular disease are becoming increasingly prevalent; however, their survival odds are greater than that of males [29]. The most predominant CVDs over the previous half-century were rheumatic heart disease and cardiomyopathies; however, hypertension, rheumatic valvular disease, and cardiomyopathy overtook and became the leading causes of CVDs in the recent decade [30–34]. Hypertension, coronary heart disease (CHD), stroke, hypertensive heart diseases, arrhythmias, heart failure, cardiomyopathies, valvular heart diseases, and congenital heart disorders are among the cardiovascular diseases of high significance (**Table 1**) [36].

3. Demographic overview of youths and adolescents in Nigeria

Nigeria is the most populous country on the African continent and with a population of about 200 million, and it is the seventh largest in the world. Most of

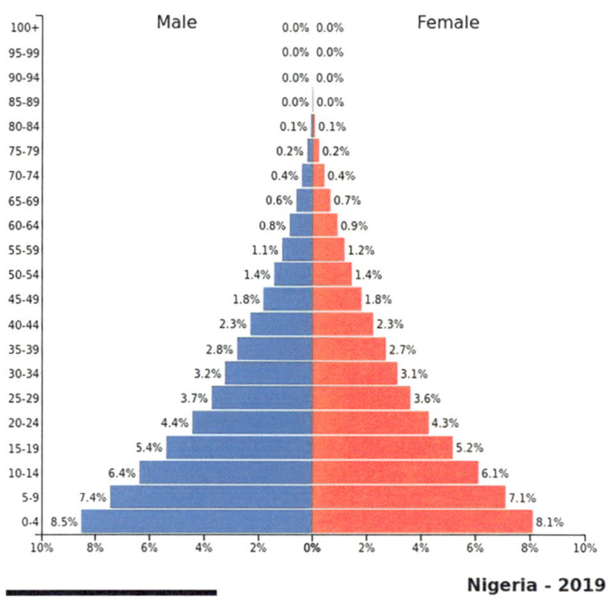

Figure 1.
The population pyramid of Nigeria, the large base representing the large number of young people in the country. Source: US Census Bureau International Data Base.

the population is young, with 42.54% between the ages of 0–14 years and half the population aged below 19 years. As a result, there is a very high dependency ratio in the country at 88.2 dependants per 100 non-dependants (**Figure 1**).

As a result of the large number of young people in the country, there exist specific health and social risks common among people in the early and developmental stage of life. Some of these risks include early pregnancy, sexually transmitted diseases, HIV/AIDS, alcohol and other drug abuse, cybercrime, social exclusion, and youth violence [37, 38]. Responding to all these issues, the Federal government of Nigeria developed a National Youth Policy, designed to address the needs of young people through five priority areas (globalisation, use of communication technology, impact of STDs/HIV/AIDS, and intergenerational issues and youth perpetrators of armed conflict) and thereby enhance youth lives [39].

4. Prevalence of CVD among adolescent

The incidence of risk factors for cardiovascular disease (CVD) is increasing in the world's emerging countries. Worldwide, CVD accounts for the majority of chronic disease mortality [40], with low- and middle-income nations bearing more than 80% of the global CVD burden [41]. According to Oguoma et al. [42], the adult Nigerian population bears a significant burden of modifiable CVD risk factors. Diabetes was thought to be uncommon among Nigerians in the 1960s, with reported prevalence rates of 1% [43]. A few studies in various geopolitical zones of Nigeria found significant prevalence rates of diabetes and prediabetes among study participants. In Nigeria, the first case of prediabetes was reported in 1998 [44]. In a group of urban adults in Nigeria, they discovered a prevalence of 2.2%. In another study conducted in an urban area in Southern Western Nigeria, the overall prevalence of prediabetes was 3.3%, compared to a proven diabetic prevalence of 4.7% [44]. Another research in a remote Nigerian community discovered a diabetes incidence of 4.8% [45]. There is evidence that increased urban migration and urbanisation, which encourage lifestyle changes, contribute to an increase in the prevalence of these modifiable risk factors over time. It is also hoped that increased reporting will reveal the true prevalence of prediabetes and diabetes in Nigeria, particularly among seemingly healthy residents of rural communities.

Females were more obese than their male counterparts, either evaluated by overall obesity or central obesity. This is consistent with the reports of Ogunmola et al. [45] and Adegoke et al. [4] in Nigerian rural communities. In terms of diabetes and prediabetes, urban residents in the study were more obese than rural participants. Early data from Nigeria in the middle and late twentieth century suggested a low prevalence of obesity [46, 47]. In today's world, more areas are becoming urbanised, encouraging sedentary lifestyles and unhealthy eating. Farming and trading are the primary occupations of people living in rural areas, and they require a lot of physical activity. This contributes to their lower obesity prevalence when compared to their urban migrant counterparts. Our study also discovered a significant prevalence of prediabetes, hypercholesterolemia, central obesity, and low HDL in the 18–24 age group. A 10-year study of the incidence of cardiovascular disease risk factors discovered that the elevated risk in people with impaired fasting glucose was majorly driven by the presence of multiple CVD risk factors [48]. This is concerning in a context where procedures for early diagnosis and detection of disease risk factors are underutilized. It is debated that the effect of glucose-lowering drugs can postpone the progression of prediabetes to diabetes [49], but this can only be possible in societies with operational health systems, where people have adequate health care awareness and health-seeking behavior, which will improve the chances of early detection and intervention.

Studies in Nigeria have confirmed that there is variation in the prevalence of hypertension based on gender [50, 51]. Another study in Southeastern Nigeria backs up this finding, noting a high prevalence of hypertension and obesity CVD risks and complications, particularly in low-middle-income countries. Males are more likely than females to have had their blood pressure, blood glucose, and cholesterol levels checked. The reason for this occurrence was unknown. Ahaneku et al. [50] discovered that more females than males in their study had their blood pressure checked. Females are more likely than males to participate in health screening exercises, as observed in both our rural and urban populations. Several studies in Nigeria have found this trend [50, 51]. This could be explained by the characteristics of traditional African societies in which males are the primary breadwinners for their entire family and live in cities, while their wives and children live in villages [52]. Socioeconomic factors across the study population demonstrate that rural populations are more disadvantaged in terms of high-income earnings and post-secondary education. A higher proportion of participants in the rural setting are poor, as defined by the WHO as having an income of less than US$2 per day. The monthly minimum wage in Nigeria is 18,000 Naira, which is approximately US$109.80. In our study population, however, income status was not associated with a high prevalence of hypertension and dyslipidaemia (triglycerides, total cholesterol, and HDL). The high-income group was more diabetic and obese, but the differences between the lower and middle income groups were not statistically significant. Some studies conducted in Western countries found that people with lower incomes were more likely to be obese and diabetic [53, 54].

5. Risk factors for CVD among adolescents and youths

5.1 Unhealthy diets

A host of CVDs has been related to behavioral risk factors such as smoking, excessive alcohol intake, lack of physical exercise, and a high cholesterol diets, age and family history [55, 56]. According to Odunaiya et al. [17], poor dietary habits were widespread among Nigerian teenagers, with low fruit and vegetable intake leading the list, followed by high saturated fatty diets. The trend can be traced to western leisure standards adopted by the majority of the Nigerian populace, as well as major modifications in the quality, content, and quantity of meals consumed, particularly with the expansion of fast-food restaurants [57–59]. Furthermore, the CVD attributable risks at adolescence can either persist into adulthood or turn out to be a considerable predictor of future cardiovascular events, as studies [28, 60] have shown that CVD has its foundations in childhood and adolescence, with variables linked to dietary choices and physical activity, being crucial antecedents of hypertension and obesity. Yilgwan et al. [61] observed high levels of obesity, physical inactivity, hypertension, and dyslipidemia in primary school children, with the pointers dominated by undernutrition. Diet has a significant impact in defining CVD risk factors, and consumption of a diet heavy in saturated fat, particularly palmitic acid, raises total cholesterol and LDL-cholesterol levels [62, 63].

Trans-fatty acids, which are found in relatively high concentrations in processed hydrogenated oils and dairy products common in Nigerian stores and markets, can increase CVD risk by increasing LDL cholesterol and decreasing HDL cholesterol [64]. According to Oguoma et al. [42], high alcohol intake can be connected with a statistically significant risk of hypertension. Similarly, Reynolds et al. [65] found that high alcohol use elevates the incidence of stroke in a meta-analysis. Alcohol intake in Nigeria was previously regulated by customs and traditions [66], but this has changed owing to changes brought about by economic development and westernization. Males are also more likely to consume alcohol than females, according to a WHO report, with 5% of males and 1% of females in Nigeria being regular alcohol consumers [67]. Major cooking oils in Nigeria are palm oil and groundnut oil, which are locally produced and sold at markets. Because these low-cost oils are widely available, people consume them regularly, which contributes to the rise in obesity, metabolic syndrome, and type 2 diabetes [68, 69]. Palm oils are produced locally, but foreign or well-processed groundnut oils, if accessible, are very costly [70].

According to WHO/FAO standards, saturated and monounsaturated fatty acid consumption must not surpass limits of 10% and 15–20%, respectively, to maintain proper total cholesterol levels and lower the risk of CVD [69, 71]. The consumption of fats and oils in Nigeria is an essential subject of research that must be investigated given the constantly growing occurrences of metabolic syndrome and diabetes in the populace.

5.2 Alcohol, tobacco, and other drugs

Harmful use of alcohol and tobacco smoking are established risk factors for the incidence of cardiovascular diseases [1], and studies have also found that all subgroups of recreational drugs are independently associated with a higher likelihood of heart diseases [72]. Over the years, research has found an association between heavy alcohol consumption and tobacco smoking with conditions and events such as hypertension, cardiomyopathy, ischemia, peripheral artery disease, and increased risk of hemorrhage in the blood vessels [73–76]. However, the link between use of some drugs and cardiovascular diseases (CVDs) have not always been clear cut, and some researchers have identified that light to moderate consumption of alcohol might be a protective factor against some cardiovascular conditions like stroke [77]. The reason for this controversy is down to the fact that unlike in other scientific studies in which randomized control trials are the gold standard for concluding causation, it is impractical or even unethical in most cases to use a randomized control trial to investigate whether or not an association exists between drug use and cardiovascular diseases; hence, some uncertainty remains with respect to the causal relationship between some of these drugs, the volume consumed, and the incidence of CVD [78]. Tobacco smoking however has consistently been shown to be linked with heart diseases as seen in longitudinal and cross-generational studies like the British Doctor study and the Framingham Heart study [79, 80].

There has been a rise in CVD in developing countries like Nigeria, with a high mortality rate among young people than in developed countries [81], and this has been linked with both novel and traditional risk factors. One of which is the use of alcohol, tobacco products, and other drugs, which have been shown to be on an upward trajectory among youths in Nigeria, and statistics by the Nigerian Drug Law Enforcement Agency (NDLEA) estimates that about 40% of the country's youths are deeply involved in the use of drugs, with alcohol as the most used substance and cannabis as the most commonly abused illicit drug [82]. The United Nations Office of Drug and Crime [83] has also established that the use of drugs among youths between the ages of 15 and 39 years in Nigeria is high and young people are initiated into use of illicit drugs like cannabis at an average age of 19 years. Using drugs from a young age is associated with poor health outcomes over the long term, and those youths who use four or more psychoactive substances have an increased risk of developing premature atherosclerotic cardiovascular diseases [72]. Although manifestations of CVD mostly occurs in adulthood, risk factors such as drug use develop during adolescence and youth, a critical stage of development, characterized by distinct physical, psychological, cognitive, and social changes [84]. The emergence of CVD among Nigerian adolescents and youths may reflect an increase in the volume and potency of drug use among young people. This increase as described by Dumbili [85] is a result of the normalization of drug use among young people in Nigeria.

S/N	Category	Disease	Gene	Function
1	Congenital Malformations	Atrial septal defect Holt-Oram syndrome (holes between the atria)	NKX2–5 TBX5	• Transcription factor • Transcription factor
2	Cardiomyopathy	Familial hypertrophic Cardiomyopathy Idiopathic dilated cardiomyopathy	β-Myosin Troponin T Troponin I Cardiac myosin-binding protein C α-Tropomyosin Actin Dystrophin	• Muscle contraction(forced generation) • Muscle contraction • (force transduction)
3	Cardiac arrhythmias	Long-QT syndrome Idiopathic ventricular fibrillation (Brugada syndrome) QT-related cardiac arrhythmia with sudden death	KLVQT1 HERG mink SCN5A NOS1AP	• Potassium channel • Sodium channel • The gene is the regulator of neuronal nitric oxide synthase, which modulates cardiac repolarization
4	Myocardial infarction	Early onset Early onset	VAMP8 HNRPUL1	• Platelet degranulation • Encodes a ribonuclear protein
5	Heart failure	Congestive heart failure	KIF6 wild-type gene	• Kinesin family member 6
6	Hypertension	Essential hypertension	AGT	• Contraction of arterial smooth muscle
7	Blood lipid disorders	Familial hypercholesterolemia Familial dyslipoproteinemias	LDL ApoE	• Regulation of low-density lipoprotein • Regulation of plasma lipid concentrations
8	Atherosclerosis	Coronary artery disease Coronary artery inflammatory disease	E-S128R Interleukin-1 receptor antagonist (IL-1ra) gene	• Monitors white blood cell adhesion to the arterial wall IL-1ra is a potent natural mechanism for controlling IL-1 and inflammation

Source: Kewal [87].

Table 2.
Genes that cause cardiovascular diseases.

The 2020 World Drug Report projects the use of drugs among young people to grow in the next decade [86], particularly in low- and middle-income countries, and this will pose more threats to the cardiovascular health of these youngsters. Fortunately, drug use is a modifiable risk factor; thus, it can be prevented and controlled by strengthening early detection [17] and modifying health behavior of young people through adequate health information and health promotion programs designed to improve young people's knowledge and attitudes toward drug use and CVD prevention.

5.3 Genetics

There are multiple causes of cardiovascular diseases, but there is no uncertainty that genetic factors play a crucial role in their development (**Table 2**).

Cardiovascular diseases outcomes in a general population can be complicated by several genetic variables. The study of atypical mendelian types of variations, whereby mutations in single genes create dramatic outcomes, has proved extremely beneficial. These mutations provide a biological framework for understanding CVD development [88]. Mutations in genes that influence certain mechanisms have been found in families with inherited cases of hypertension or hypotension, both are caused by irregularities in the functioning of aldosterone synthase, and this has been observed to be an autosomal dominant trait which is characterized by hypertension, repressed renin activity, and abnormal aldosterone levels. This is induced by an unbalanced overlap between genes encoding enzymes of the adrenal-steroid biosynthesis pathway [89]. Hypertrophic cardiomyopathy is the most prevalent monogenic heart disorder and the leading cause of mortalities from cardiac abnormalities in children and adolescents, with an estimated 1 in 500 people suffering from the condition [90]. The heredity of hypertrophic cardiomyopathy is autosomal dominant in nature, and the condition is associated with mutations of genes that code for proteins in the myocardial contractile apparatus [91].

Arrhythmia predisposing genes have been identified and studied to provide further insight into the molecular pathobiology of arrhythmias [92]. Correspondingly, Gellens et al. [93] reported the SCN5A gene to encode subunits that form Na^+ channels, which is responsible for triggering cardiac action potentials. SCN5A mutations give rise to a number of hereditary arrhythmias, including long-QT syndrome, idiopathic ventricular fibrillation, and cardiac-conduction disorders [94].

6. Strategies to tackle CVD among adolescents and youths in Nigeria (the health-promoting school approach)

Compared to developed nations, developing countries have seen an increase in CVD and associated risk factors, as well as a high death rate among young people. This can be due to the lack of information and practical preventive measures, which is also connected to the high levels of poverty in these nations [81]. Adequate knowledge of CVD risk factors is the first step toward an effective preventive mechanism against the burden of CVD among any population. Studies have identified children, adolescents, and young adults as the target population for the prevention program. Seven essential health conditions and habits, according to the American Heart Association, raise the risk of heart disease and stroke, such as dietary factors, smoking, being overweight or obese, being inactive, uncontrolled blood pressure, high cholesterol, and high blood sugar [95]. Ideal cardiovascular health is in line with the principle of primordial prevention, which refers to the prevention of risk factor development. Additionally, important is primary prevention, which is the management of risk factors in patients who have not yet manifested clinical CVD. The AHA considers persons with risk factors who have received optimal treatment to have intermediate cardiovascular health [96].

Primordial prevention looks to be the higher selection in addressing CVD, and this involves preventing risk factors from occurring by optimizing lifestyles related to smart management of vital signs, low levels of cholesterol, optimum body weight, physical activities and exercise, and elimination of tobacco use. Associate degree intervention of this type involves promoting positive health behaviors, effecting healthy lifestyle policies, and establishing a physical setting that ends up in incorporating and sustaining lifelong heart-healthy lifestyles, from infancy to old age. The American Heart Association guide for improving cardiovascular health at the community level provides a comprehensive list of goals, strategies, and recommendations that may be adopted and domesticated by both developed and developing countries to control cardiovascular diseases. The guide targets not solely health professionals but also government parastatals, nonprofit organizations, community-based organizations, institutions, public health practitioners, and the community [97].

The following strategies could be used to mitigate cardiovascular diseases among adolescents and youths in Nigeria.

6.1 Health promotion and education strategies

Action on the determinants of health is the prime focus of health promotion. It intends to promote efficient and involved public engagement. It integrates a number of different, yet complementary strategies. Included in this are community development, communication, education, legislation, organizational and community improvements, and unscheduled local health hazard prevention actions. Government, both at the provincial and federal levels, and different sectors, all have a part to play, by enhancing CVD prevention efforts through health promotion, environmental change, dietary treatments, and behavioral and lifestyle adjustments [98].

Health education is designed to enhance health literacy through communication to boost knowledge and develop life skills. Health education on the risk factors of CVDs and the ways to improve the health determinants ought to be advocated for. This includes information on the implications of tobacco use, alcohol, unhealthy diet, and lack of physical activities among others. This can be done through mass media campaigns, media adverts, radio chat show programs, bulk SMS, and alternative social networks including social media. This additional could be done by mobilizing communities through advocacy to community leaders and stakeholders and community sensitization meetings. Additionally, public campaigns and social-promoting initiatives to educate and encourage the target audience about healthy dietary habits should be conducted from the states down to the communities using appropriate and acceptable cultural methods. The benefits of physical activity should be taught, and various methods of undertaking them should be demonstrated [99].

6.2 Health-promoting schools

Schools at the primary, secondary, and tertiary levels should be mandated to have research-based, comprehensive, and age-appropriate curricula about cardiovascular health and ways in which to boost health behaviors and scale down CVD risk factors.

The school curriculum should include lessons on the risk factors for CVD and stroke and also the extent of cardiopathy and stroke in the community. Research-based curriculum regarding effective ways of changing health behaviors can be implemented. Students should learn skills needed to achieve the regular practice of healthful behaviors, and parents should learn how to support their children's healthful behaviors. All schools should be mandated to implement an age-appropriate curriculum on changing dietary, physical activity, and smoking behaviors [97].

6.3 Environmental modifications

Strategies to address occupational risks should be primary to the establishment of any workplace. The government should also enact and implement policies that promote smoke-free environments in all work sites, institutions, indoor public places, and other public places. More importantly, policy measures on the creation of health-promoting environments should be implemented before the licencing of any establishment, and means to effectively monitor the adoption of these policies should be put in place [100].

6.4 Nutritional interventions

The effective implementation of WHO recommendations on the marketing of foods and nonalcoholic beverages to children should be a top priority, including adequate mechanisms for monitoring. Effective guidelines should be developed with policy measures that engage different relevant sectors, such as food producers and processors and other relevant commercial operators to produce foods and drinks according to the appropriate terms. The government should effectively collaborate with the agricultural sector to supply policies and reforms for improvement within the provision of fruits and vegetables such that affordability is ensured. Promotion and provision of healthy food and food products should be encouraged by all public institutions including schools and workplaces [101].

6.5 Quality health care delivery

The National Academic Press (US), in 2010, recommends that along with select population-based approaches, a key step in addressing CVD is to strengthen health systems to deliver high-quality, responsive care for the prevention and management of CVD. This can be achieved by implementing provider-level strategies, health financing, and integration of care, workforce development, and access to essential medical products [102].

6.6 Policy change/reform

The primary population approach for the control of CVDs among adolescents and youths is largely dependent on the development and effective implementation of policies and regulations, especially those related to food, physical inactivity, and tobacco. These policy changes may include taxation and regulations on tobacco production and sales; regulations on tobacco and food marketing and labeling; and alterations in subsidies for foods and other food and agricultural policies. Implementation on a sufficient scale and adequate resources for evaluation is highly recommended [103].

7. Challenges to the development and implementation of these strategies

Major obstacles to the development and implementation of effective strategies to reduce the burden of cardiovascular disease among adolescents and youth in Nigeria is as a result of lack of knowledge, ineffective use of available and accessible resources, a dearth of sturdy population-level health and mortality data, insufficient financing for health and health care, suboptimal deployment of available health funding to support health services, and large population inequities [104]. According to Obansa and Orimisan, [105] inadequate laboratory facilities, a lack of basic infrastructure and equipment, poor human resource management, poor pay and motivation, a lack of fair and sustainable health care financing, and unequal and unjust economic and political relations between Nigeria and developed nations are just a few of the major factors that have an impact on the health system's overall contribution to economic growth and development in Nigeria.

8. Conclusion

Since the prevalence of NCDs and their avoidable causes have been documented in Nigeria, the national health system requires targeted individual and population-wide prevention-oriented initiatives. Additionally, the health care system has to be improved in order to effectively handle all types of NCD prevention and control. This should serve as a wake-up call for all sectors, including the government, the general public, nongovernmental organizations, and funding agencies, to adopt an integrated and coordinated preventative strategy [106]. Individualized health education and skill development should be prioritized in order to help people choose and adopt a healthy lifestyle, which includes managing one's nutrition, being active, and abstaining from tobacco and alcohol usage. People and communities should take the appropriate supporting steps to aid in the maintenance of individual choices with the ultimate goal of triggering a good communal impact. This is because individual behavior is influenced by common group practices and beliefs.

Additionally, stakeholder participation in promoting NCD prevention through community participation is also essential to the success of this drive, which may then be gradually integrated into the national health system. In light of the fact that well-designed community programs depend on successful basic and operations research, extensive public health interventions, and government policymaking, it is urgent to increase research funding and ensure that this research has a significant impact on policymaking. This is only achievable if the government is more devoted to providing strong leadership and coordinating the resources required for the prevention and treatment of NCDs [106].

Author details

Omigbile Olamide[1*], Oni Adebayo[2], Abe Emmanuel[2], Lawal Eyitayo[2], Oyasope Beatrice[3] and Mayaki Tomisin[4]

1 Center for Health Ethics Law and Development, Lagos, Nigeria

2 Department of Health Promotion and Education, University of Ibadan, Ibadan, Nigeria

3 Slum and Rural Health Initiative, Ibadan, Nigeria

4 Department of Nutrition and Dietetics, Federal University of Agriculture, Abeokuta, Nigeria

*Address all correspondence to: omigbilelamide@gmail.com

References

[1] World Health Organization. Cardiovascular Diseases (cvds). 2009. Available from: http://www. who. int/mediacentre/factsheets/fs317/en/index.html [Accessed: 12 August 2022]

[2] Roth GA, Mensah GA, Johnson CO, Addolorato G, Ammirati E, Baddour LM, et al. Global burden of cardiovascular diseases and risk factors, 1990-2019: Update from the GBD 2019 study. Journal of the American College of Cardiology. 2020;**76**(25):2982-3021. DOI: 10.1016/j.jacc.2020.11.010

[3] World Health Organization. Global Status Report on Non- communicable Diseases. Geneva, Switzerland: World Health Organization; 2010 Available from: https://www.who.int/health-topics/cardiovascular-diseases

[4] Adegoke OA, Adedoyin RA, Balogun MO, Adebayo RA, Bisiriyu LA, Salawu AA. Prevalence of metabolic syndrome in a rural community in Nigeria. Metabolic Syndrome and Related Disorders. 2010;**8**(1):59-62. DOI: 10.1089/met.2009.0037

[5] Mytton OT, Jackson C, Steinacher A, Goodman A, Langenberg C, Griffin S, et al. The current and potential health benefits of the National Health Service Health Check cardiovascular disease prevention programme in England: a microsimulation study. PLoS Medicine. 6 Mar 2018;**15**(3):e1002517

[6] Leppert MH, Poisson SN, Sillau SH, Campbell JD, Ho PM, Burke JF. Is prevalence of atherosclerotic risk factors increasing among young adults? It depends on how you ask. Journal of the American Heart Association. 2019;**8**(6):e010883. DOI: 10.1161/JAHA.118.010883

[7] Hancock C, Kingo L, Raynaud O. The private sector, international development and NCDs. Globalization and Health. 2011;**7**(1):1-1. DOI: 10.1186/1744-8603-7-23

[8] Bogdanska A, Maniecka-Bryła I, Szpak A. The evaluation of secondary school students' knowledge about risk factors of cardiovascular disease. Roczniki Akademii Medycznej w Białymstoku. 2005;**50**(1):213-215 PMID: 16119669

[9] Hong YM. Atherosclerotic cardiovascular disease beginning in childhood. Korean Circulation Journal. 2010;**40**(1):1-9. DOI: 10.4070/kcj.2010.40.1.1

[10] Obermeyer CM, Bott S, Sassine AJ. Arab adolescents: health, gender, and social context. Journal of Adolescent Health. 1 Sep 2015;**57**(3):252-262

[11] Frech A. Healthy behavior trajectories between adolescence and young adulthood. Advances in Life Course Research. 2012;**17**(2):59-68. DOI: 10.1016/j.alcr.2012.01.003

[12] Secrest AM, Costacou T, Gutelius B, Miller RG, Songer TJ, Orchard TJ. Associations between socioeconomic status and major complications in type 1 diabetes: The Pittsburgh epidemiology of diabetes complication (EDC) study. Annals of Epidemiology. 2011;**21**(5):374-381. DOI: 10.1016/j.annepidem.2011.02.007

[13] Wang Y, Lim H. The global childhood obesity epidemic and the association between socio-economic status and childhood obesity. International Review of Psychiatry. 2012;**24**(3):176-188. DOI: 10.3109/09540261.2012.688195

[14] Cai L, He J, Song Y, Zhao K, Cui W. Association of obesity with socio-economic factors and obesity-related chronic diseases in rural Southwest China. Public Health. 2013;**127**(3):247-251. DOI: 10.1016/j.puhe.2012.12.027

[15] Cunningham J, O'Dea K, Dunbar T, Weeramanthri T, Shaw J, Zimmet P. Socioeconomic status and diabetes among urban indigenous Australians aged 15-64 years in the DRUID study. Ethnicity and Health. 2008;**13**(1):23-37. DOI: 10.1080/13557850701803130

[16] Boateng D, Wekesah F, Browne JL, Agyemang C, Agyei-Baffour P, Aikins AG, et al. Knowledge and awareness of and perception towards cardiovascular disease risk in sub-saharan Africa: A systematic review. PLoS One. 2017;**12**(2):e0189264. DOI: 10.1371/journal.pone.0189264

[17] Odunaiya NA, Louw QA, Grimmer KA. High prevalence and clustering of modifiable CVD risk factors amongst rural adolescents in Southwest Nigeria: Implications for grass root prevention. BMC Public Health. 2015;**15**:6611. DOI: 10.1186/s12889-015-2028-3

[18] Safeer RS, Cooke CE, Keenan J. The impact of health literacy on cardiovascular disease. Vascular Health and Risk Management. 2006;**2**(4):457. DOI: 10.2147/vhrm.2006.2.4.457

[19] Magnani JW, Mujahid MS, Aronow HD, Cené CW, Dickson VV, Havranek E, et al. Health literacy and cardiovascular disease: Fundamental relevance to primary and secondary prevention: A scientific statement from the American Heart Association. Circulation. 2018;**138**(2):e48-e74. DOI: 10.1161/CIR.0000000000000579

[20] Angosta AD, Speck KE. Assessment of heart disease knowledge and risk factors among first-generation Filipino Americans residing in Southern Nevada: A cross-sectional survey. Clinical Nursing Studies. 2014;**2**(2):123-129. DOI: 10.5430/cns.v2n2p123

[21] Kanungo S, Bhowmik K, Mahapatra T, Mahapatra S, Bhadra UK, Sarkar K. Perceived morbidity, healthcare-seeking behavior and their determinants in a poor-resource setting: Observation from India. PLoS One. 2015;**10**(5):e0125865. DOI: 10.1371/journal.pone.0125865

[22] Akintunde AA, Salawu AA, Opadijo OG. Prevalence of traditional cardiovascular risk factors among staff of Ladoke Akintola University of Technology, Ogbomoso, Nigeria. Nigerian Journal of Clinical Practice. 2014;**17**(6):750-755. DOI: 10.4103/1119-3077.144390

[23] Olatunbosun ST, Kaufman JS, Cooper RS, Bella AF. Hypertension in a black population: Prevalence and biosocial determinants of high blood pressure in a group of urban Nigerians. Journal of Human Hypertension. 2000;**14**:249-257. DOI: 10.1038/sj.jhh.1000975

[24] Adedapo AD, Fawole O, Bamgboye AE, Adedapo K, Demmisie K, Osinubi O. Morbidity and mortality patterns of medical admissions in a Nigerian secondary health care hospital. African Journal of Medicine and Medical Sciences. 2012;**41**:13-20

[25] Ogah OS, Okpechi I, Chukwuonye I, Akinyemi J, Onwubere BJC, Falase AO, et al. Blood pressure, prevalence of hypertension and hypertension related complications in Nigerian Africans: A review. World Journal of Cardiology. 2012;**4**(12):327-340. DOI: 10.4330/wjc.v4.i12.327

[26] Senbanjo IO, Osikoya KA. Obesity and blood pressure levels of adolescents in Abeokuta, Nigeria. Cardiovascular Journal of Africa. 2012;**23**(5):260-264. DOI: 10.5830/CVJA-2011-037

[27] He FJ, de Wardener HE, MacGregor GA. Controversies in cardiology. The Lancet. 2006;**367**:1313-1314

[28] Berenson GS, Srnivasan SR, Bogalusa Heart Study Group. Cardiovascular risk factors in youth with implications for aging: The Bogalusa Heart Study. Neurobiology of Aging. 2005;**26**:303-307. DOI: 10.1016/j.neurobiolaging.2004.05.009

[29] Adedapo AD. Rising trend of cardiovascular diseases among South-Western Nigerian female patients. Nigerian Journal of Cardiology. 2017;**14**:71-74. DOI: 10.4103/njc.njc_23_17

[30] Nwaneli CU. Changing trend in coronary heart disease in Nigeria. Afrimedic Journal. 2010;**1**:1-4 ISSN: 2141-162X

[31] Ngwogu KO, Onwuchekwa UN, Ngwogu AC, Ekenjoku AJ. Incidence, pattern and outcome of cardiovascular admissions at the Abia State University Teaching Hospital, Aba: A five year review. International Journal of Basic, Applied and Innovative Research. 2015;**4**:54-61 ISSN: 2315-5388

[32] Oguanobi NI, Ejim EC, Onwubere BJ, Ike SO, Anisiuba BC, Ikeh VO, et al. Pattern of cardiovascular disease amongst medical admissions in a regional teaching hospital in Southeastern Nigeria. Nigerian Journal of Cardiology. 2013;**10**:77-80. DOI: 10.4103/0189-7969.127005

[33] Oke DA, Adebola AP. Myocardial infarction managed in the Lagos university teaching hospital intensive care unit. Nigerian Journal of Postgraduate Medicine. 1999;**6**:83-85

[34] Osuji CU, Onwubuya EI, Ahaneku GI, Omejua EG. Pattern of cardiovascular admissions at Nnamdi Azikiwe University Teaching Hospital Nnewi, South East Nigeria. The Pan African Medical Journal. 2014;**17**:116. DOI: 10.11604/pamj.2014.17.116.1837

[35] Behera SS, Pramanik K, Nayak MK. Recent advancement in the treatment of cardiovascular diseases: Conventional therapy to nanotechnology. Current Pharmaceutical Design. 2015;**21**(30):4479-4497. DOI: 10.2174/1381612821666150817104635

[36] Ike SO, Onyema CT. Cardiovascular diseases in Nigeria: What has happened in the past 20 years? Nigerian Journal of Cardiology. 2020;**17**:21-26. DOI: 10.4103/njc.njc_33_19

[37] Akpor OA, Thupayagale-Tshweneagae G. Teenage pregnancy in Nigeria: professional nurses and educators' perspectives. F1000 Research. 2019;**9**:1-3. DOI: 10.12688/F1000RESEARCH.16893.1

[38] Umar C, Nkosi ZZ, Ndou N. Nigerian university students' practices for preventing sexually transmitted diseases. African Journal for Physical Health Education, Recreation and Dance. 2015;**21**(sup-1):29-40

[39] Ibrahim S, Audu BJ. Youth development policies in Nigeria: Promises, problems, and possibilities. Kenneth Dike Journal of African Studies. 10 Nov 2020;1(1)

[40] Chiolero A, Paradis G, Madeleine G, Hanley JA, Paccaud F, Bovet P. Birth weight, weight change, and blood pressure during childhood and

adolescence: A school-based multiple cohort study. Journal of Hypertension. 2011;**29**(10):1871-1879. DOI: 10.1097/HJH.0b013e32834ae396

[41] Mendis S, Puska P, Norrving B, World Health Organization. Global atlas on cardiovascular disease prevention and control. World Health Organization. 2011. Available from: https://apps.who.int/iris/handle/10665/44701 [Accessed: 13 August 2022]

[42] Oguoma VM, Nwose EU, Skinner TC, Digban KA, Onyia IC, Richards RS. Prevalence of cardiovascular disease risk factors among a Nigerian adult population: Relationship with income level and accessibility to CVD risks screening. BMC Public Health. 2015;**15**:397. DOI: 10.1186/s12889-015-1709-2

[43] Akinkugbe OO, Ojo OA. Arterial pressures in rural and urban populations in Nigeria. British Medical Journal. 1969;**2**(5651):222-224. DOI: 10.1136/bmj.2.5651.222

[44] Olatunbosun ST, Ojo PO, Fineberg NS, Bella AF. Prevalence of diabetes mellitus and impaired glucose tolerance in a group of urban adults in Nigeria. Journal of the National Medical Association. 1998;**90**(5):293-301

[45] Ojewale LY, Adejumo PO. Type 2 diabetes mellitus and impaired fasting blood glucose in urban South Western Nigeria. International Journal of Diabetes and Metabolis. 2012;**21**:1-9

[46] Ogunmola OJ, Olaifa AO, Oladapo OO, Babatunde OA. Prevalence of cardiovascular risk factors among adults without obvious cardiovascular disease in a rural community in Ekiti State, Southwest Nigeria. BMC Cardiovascular Disorders. 2013;**13**:89. DOI: 10.1186/1471-2261-13-89

[47] Lawoyin TO, Asuzu MC, Kaufman J, Rotimi C, Owoaje E, Johnson L, et al. Prevalence of cardiovascular risk factors in an African, urban inner city community. West African Journal of Medicine. 2002;**21**(3):208-211. DOI: 10.4314/wajm.v21i3.28031

[48] Azinge N, Anizor C. Prevalence of obesity among diabetics seen in a tertiary health care Centre in South-South Nigeria. The Nigerian Journal of General Practice. 2013;**11**(1):45-48

[49] Liu J, Grundy SM, Wang W, Smith SC Jr, Vega GL, Wu Z, et al. Ten-year risk of cardiovascular incidence related to diabetes, prediabetes, and the metabolic syndrome. American Heart Journal. 2007;**153**(4):552-558. DOI: 10.1016/j.ahj.2007.01.003

[50] Grundy SM. Pre-diabetes, metabolic syndrome, and cardiovascular risk. Journal of the American College of Cardiology. 2012;**59**(7):635-643. DOI: 10.1016/j.jacc.2011.08.080

[51] Ahaneku GI, Osuji CU, Anisiuba BC, Ikeh VO, Oguejiofor OC, Ahaneku JE. Evaluation of blood pressure and indices of obesity in a typical rural community in Eastern Nigeria. Annals of African Medicine. 2011;**10**(2):120-126. DOI: 10.4103/1596-3519.82076

[52] Onwubere BJ, Ejim EC, Okafor CI, Emehel A, Mbah AU, Onyia U, et al. Pattern of blood pressure indices among the residents of a rural Community in South East Nigeria. International Journal of Hypertension. 2011;**2011**:621074. DOI: 10.4061/2011/621074

[53] Booth GL, Hux JE. Relationship between avoidable hospitalizations for diabetes mellitus and income level. Archives of Internal Medicine. 2003;**163**(1):101-106

[54] Kuntz B, Lampert T. Socioeconomic factors and the distribution of obesity. Deutsches Ärzteblatt. 2010;**107**(30):517-522

[55] Kumar S, Kelly AS. Review of childhood obesity: From epidemiology, etiology, and comorbidities to clinical assessment and treatment. In: Mayo Clinic Proceedings. Vol. 92, No. 2. Elsevier; 1 Feb 2017. pp. 251-265

[56] Redwine KM, Daniels SR. Pre hypertension in adolescents; risk and progression. Journal of Clinical Hypertension. 2012;**14**:360-364. DOI: 10.10.1111/j.1751-7176.2012.00663.x

[57] Kadiri S. Tackling cardiovascular diseases in Africa: Will need much more than just imported measures from more developed countries. BMJ. 2005;**331**:711-712. DOI: 10.1136/bmj.331.7519.711

[58] Yusuf S, Reddy S, Ounpuu S, Anand S. Global burden of cardiovascular diseases: Part I: General considerations, the epidemiologic transition, risk factors, and impact of urbanization. Circulation. 2001;**104**:2746-2753. DOI: 10.1161/hc4601.099487

[59] Lim SS, Vos T, Flaxman AD, Danaei G, Shibuya K, Adair-Rohani H, et al. A comparative risk assessment of burden of disease and injury attributable to 67 risk factors and risk factor clusters in 21 regions, 1990-2010: A systematic analysis for the global burden of disease study 2010. The Lancet. 2012;**380**:2224-2260. DOI: 10.1016/S0140-6736(12)61766-8

[60] Myers L, Strikmiller PK, Webber LS, Berenson GS. Physical and sedentary activity in school children grades 5-8: The Bogalusa Heart Study. Medicine and Science in Sports and Exercise. 1996;**28**:852-859. DOI: 10.1097/00005768-199607000-00012

[61] Yilgwan CS, Hyacinth HI, Ige OO, Abok II, Yilgwan G, John C, et al. Cardiovascular disease risk profile in Nigerian school children. Sahel Medical Journal. 2017;**20**:143-148. DOI: 10.4103/1118-8561.230260

[62] Hu FB, Manson JE, Willett WC. Types of dietary fat and risk of coronary heart disease: A critical review. Journal of the American College of Nutrition. 2001;**20**:5-19. DOI: 10.1080/07315724.2001.10719008

[63] Schaefer EJ. Lipoproteins, nutrition, and heart disease. The American Journal of Clinical Nutrition. 2002;**75**:191-212. DOI: 10.1093/ajcn/75.2.191

[64] de Roos NM, Bots ML, Katan MB. Replacement of dietary saturated fatty acids by trans fatty acids lowers serum HDL-cholesterol and impairs endothelial function in healthy men and women. Arteriosclerosis, Thrombosis, and Vascular Biology. 2001;**21**:1233-1237. DOI: 10.1161/hq0701.092161

[65] Reynolds K, Lewis B, Nolen JD, Kinney GL, Sathya B, He J. Alcohol consumption and risk of stroke: A meta-analysis. JAMA. 2003;**289**:579-588. DOI: 10.1001/jama.289.5.579

[66] Demehin AO. Drug abuse and its social impacts in Nigeria. Public Health. 1984;**98**:109-116. DOI: 10.1016/S0033-3506(84)80105-5

[67] WHOGlobal Status Report on Alcohol 2004. Nigeria, Geneva: World Health Organisation; 2004. Available from: http://whqlibdoc.who.int/publications/2004/9241562722. [Accessed: 14 August 2022]

[68] Tucker KL, Buranapin S. Nutrition and aging in developing countries. The Journal of Nutrition. 2001;**131**:2417S-2423S. DOI: 10.1093/jn/131.9.2417S

[69] Misra A, Singhal N, Khurana L. Obesity, the metabolic syndrome, and type 2 diabetes in developing countries: Role of dietary fats and oils. Journal of the American College of Nutrition. 2010;**29**:289S-301S. DOI: 10.1080/07315724.2010.10719844

[70] Edem DO. Palm oil: Biochemical, physiological, nutritional, hematological and toxicological aspects: A review. Plant Foods for Human Nutrition. 2002;**57**(3):319-341. DOI: 10.1023/a:1021828132707

[71] Elmadfa I, Kornsteiner M. Fats and fatty acid requirements for adults. Annals of Nutrition & Metabolism. 2009;**55**:56-75. DOI: 10.1159/000228996

[72] Mahtta D, Ransey D, Krittanawong C, Al-Rifai M, Khurram N, Samad Z, et al. Recreational substance use among patients with premature atherosclerotic cardiovascular disease. Journal of Health. 2020;**107**:604-606. DOI: 10.1136/heartjnl-2020-3118856

[73] O'Connor AD, Rusyniak DE, Bruno A. Cerebrovascular and cardiovascular complication of alcohol and sympathomimetic drug abuse. The Medical Clinics of North America. 2005;**89**(6):1343-1358. DOI: 10.1016/j.mcna.2005.06.010

[74] Hu N, Zhang Y, Nair S, Culver BW, Ren J. Contribution of ALDH2 polymorphism to alcoholism-associated hypertension. Recent patent on endocrine, metabolic and immune drug discovery. 2014;**8**(3):180-185. DOI: 10.2174/1872214808666141020162000

[75] Kaplan EH, Gottesman RF, Llinas RH, Marsh EB. The association between specific substances of abuse and subcortical intracerebral Heamorrhage versus ischemic lacunar infarction. Frontiers in Neurology. 2014;**2014**(5):174. DOI: 10.3389/fneur.2014.00174

[76] Pineda JR, Kim ES, Osinbowale OO. Impact of pharmacologic interventions on peripheral artery diseases. Progress in Cardiovascular Diseases. 1 Mar 2014;**57**(5):510-520. DOI: 10.1016/j.pcad.2014.12.001

[77] Wakabayashi I, Sotoda Y. Alcohol drinking and peripheral arterial disease of lower extremity. Nihon Arukōru Yakubutsu Igakkai Zasshi. 2014;**49**(1):13-27

[78] Rosoff DB, Smith GD, Mehta N, Clarke T, Lohoff FW. Evaluating the relationship between alcohol consumption, tobacco use, and cardiavascular disease: A multivariate mendelian randomization study. PLoS Medicine. 2020;**17**(12):e1003410. DOI: 10.1371/journal.pmed.1003410

[79] Freund KM, Belanger AJ, D'Agostino RB, Kannel WB. The health risk of smoking the Framingham study: 34 years of follow-up. Annals of Epidemiology. 1993;**3**(4):417-424. DOI: 10.1016/1047-2797(93)90070-k

[80] Doll R, Peto R, Boreham J, Sutherland I. Mortality in relation to smoking: 50 years' observation on male British doctors. BMJ. 2004;**328**(7455):1519. DOI: 10.1136/bmj.38142.554479

[81] Odunaiya NA, Adesanya TB, Okoye EC, Oguntibeju OO. Towards cardiovascular disease prevention in Nigeria: A mixed method study of how adolescents and young adults in a university setting perceive cardiovascular disease and risk factors. The African Journal of Primary Health & Family Medicine. 2021;**13**(1):a2200. DOI: 10.4102/phcfm.v13i1.2200

[82] Onifade PO, Adamson TA, Morankinyo OO, Akinhanmi AO.

Descriptive national survey of substance use in Nigeria. Journal of Addiction Research and Therapy. 2015;**6**:234. DOI: 10.4172/2155-6105.1000234

[83] United Nations World Drug Report. United Nations Office on Drugs and Crime. World Drug Report; 2018

[84] Marcel AV, Jacobson MS, Copperman NM, Klein JD, Santoro K, Pirani H. Prevention of Adult Cardiovascular Diseases among Adolescents: Focusing on Risk Factor Reduction. Washington DC: Publication of the National Institute for Healthcare Management Foundation; 2010

[85] Dumbili EW. Cannabis normalization among young adults in a Nigerian city. Journal of Drug Issues. Jul 2020;**50**(3):286-302. DOI: 10.1177/0022042520912805

[86] Nations U. World drug report. United Nations Publication; 2020

[87] Jain KK. Personalized management of cardiovascular disorders. Textbook of Personalized Medicine. 2015:479-509. DOI: 10.1159/000481403

[88] Lifton RP, Gharavi AG, Geller DS. Molecular mechanisms of human hypertension. Cell. 2001;**104**:545-556. DOI: 10.1016/s0092-8674(01)00241-0

[89] Lifton RP, Dluhy RG, Powers M, et al. Hereditary hypertension caused by chimaeric gene duplications and ectopic expression of aldosterone synthase. Nature Genetics. 1992;**2**:66-74. DOI: 10.1038/ng0992-66

[90] Maron BJ, Gardin JM, Flack JM, Gidding SS, Kurosaki TT, Bild DE. Prevalenceofhypertrophiccardiomyopathy in a general population of young adults: Echocardiographic analysis of 4111 subjects in the CARDIA study: Coronary artery risk development in (young) adults. Circulaton. 1995;**92**:785-789. DOI: 10.1161/01.cir.92.4.785

[91] Kamisago M, Sharma SD, DePalma SR, et al. Mutations in sarcomere protein genes as a cause of dilated cardiomyopathy. The New England Journal of Medicine. 2000;**343**:1688-1696. DOI: 10.1056/NEJM200012073432304

[92] Keating MT, Sanguinetti MC. Molecular and cellular mechanisms of cardiac arrhythmias. Cell. 2001;**104**:569-580. DOI: 10.1016/s0092-8674(01)00243-4

[93] Gellens ME, George AL Jr, Chen LQ, et al. Primary structure and functional expression of the human cardiac tetrodotoxininsensitive voltage-dependent sodium channel. Proceedings of the National Academy of Sciences of the United States of America. 1992;**89**:554-558. DOI: 10.1073/pnas.89.2.554 PMID: 1309946; PMCID: PMC48277

[94] Tan HL, Bink-Boelkens MT, Bezzina CR, et al. A sodium-channel mutation causes isolated cardiac conduction disease. Nature. 2001;**409**:1043-1047. DOI: 10.1038/35059090

[95] World Health Organization. Noncommunicable Diseases Country Profiles; 2018. Key Facts. 2018. Available from: https://www.who.int/news-room/fact-sheets/detail/noncommunicable-diseases [Accessed: 9 August 2022]

[96] Chung RJ, Touloumtzis C, Gooding H. Staying young at heart: Cardiovascular disease prevention in adolescents and young adults. Current Treatment Options in Cardiovascular Medicine. 2015;**17**(12):1-5. DOI: 10.1007/s11936-015-0414-x

[97] Pearson TA, Blair SN, Daniels SR, Eckel RH, Fair JM, Fortmann SP, et al. AHA guidelines for primary prevention of cardiovascular disease and stroke: 2002 update: Consensus panel guide to comprehensive risk reduction for adult patients without coronary or other atherosclerotic vascular diseases. Circulation. Jul 16 2002;**106**(3):388-391. DOI: 10.1161/01.cir.0000020190.45892.75

[98] Kumar S, Preetha G. Health promotion: An effective tool for global health. Indian Journal of Community Medicine. Jan 2012;**37**(1):5-12. DOI: 10.4103/0970-0218.94009

[99] Okafor CN, Young EE, Nwobi AE. Health promotion strategies for the prevention and control of non-communicable diseases in Nigeria. Health Promotion. 2016;**4**(1). DOI: 10.21522/TIJPH.2013.04.01.Art003

[100] Mamudu HM, Owusu D, Asare B, Williams F, Asare M, Oke A, et al. Support for smoke-free public places among adults in four countries in sub-Saharan Africa. Nicotine & Tobacco Research. 2020;**22**(12):2141-2148. DOI: 10.1093/ntr/ntaa008

[101] Patiño SR, Da Silva GF, Constantinou S, Lemaire R, Hedrick VE, Serrano EL, et al. An assessment of government capacity building to restrict the marketing of unhealthy food and non-alcoholic beverage products to children in the region of the Americas. International Journal of Environmental Research and Public Health. 2021;**18**(16):8324. DOI: 10.3390/ijerph18168324

[102] Institute of Medicine (US) Committee on Preventing the Global Epidemic of Cardiovascular Disease: Meeting the Challenges in Developing Countries. In: Fuster V, Kelly BB, editors. Promoting Cardiovascular Health in the Developing World: A Critical Challenge to Achieve Global Health. Epidemiology of Cardiovascular Disease. Vol. 2. Washington (DC): National Academies Press (US); 2010. DOI: 10.17226/12815

[103] Barekatain A, Weiss S, Weintraub WS. Value of primordial and primary prevention for cardiovascular diseases: A global perspective. In: Prevention of Cardiovascular Diseases. Cham: Springer; 2015. pp. 21-28. DOI: 10.1161/CIR.0b013e3182285a81

[104] Abubakar I, Dalglish SL, Angell B, Sanuade O, Abimbola S, Adamu AL, et al. The lancet Nigeria commission: Investing in health and the future of the nation. The Lancet. 2022;**399**(10330):1155-1200. DOI: 10.1016/S0140-6736(21)02488-0

[105] Obansa SA, Orimisan A. Health care financing in Nigeria: prospects and challenges. Mediterranean Journal of Social Sciences. 2013;**4**(1):221

[106] Olukoya O. The war against non-communicable disease: How ready is Nigeria? The Annals of Ibadan Postgraduate Medicine. 2017, 2017;**15**(1):5-6 PMID: 28970764; PMCID: PMC5598443

Chapter 11

Pathophysiology of Preeclampsia: The Role of Adiposity and Serum Adipokines

Ahmed Tijani Bawah, Abdul-Malik Bawah and Ruhaima Issah Zorro

Abstract

The goal of this study was to determine serum adiponectin, leptin, resistin, visfatin, and lipids in pregnant women during the first trimester and to examine the link between these biochemical markers and preeclampsia (PE). Changes in the levels of these adipokines occur in PE, hence this study looked into the possibility of employing these biomarkers to predict the disease. This study compared first-trimester serum biochemical and anthropometric markers in pregnant women with PE to the controls. After 20 weeks of pregnancy, blood pressure and urine protein were measured, and a PE diagnosis was made according to American Heart Association criteria. Generally, there were significant differences ($p < 0.05$) in the biochemical markers between the PEs and the controls. Even after correcting for body mass index (BMI) and family history of hypertension, analyses of area under the receiver operating characteristic curves (AUCs) for the adipokines revealed their capacity to reliably predict PE. After adjusting for BMI, it emerged that adiponectin, leptin, resistin, and visfatin were significant predictors of PE, with resistin being the best predictor. After controlling for BMI, age, parity, and family history of diabetes and preeclampsia, adiponectin was the greatest predictor.

Keywords: preeclampsia, adiponectin, leptin, resistin, visfatin

1. Introduction

Pregnancy is a distinct situation marked by physiological insulin resistance that disappears after delivery. It is also marked by changes in the endocrine, metabolic, and circulatory systems, all of which are intended to supply energy and sustenance to the developing fetus [1]. Gestational diabetes (GDM) and pre-eclampsia (PE) may occur as complications during metabolic dysregulation in pregnancy. GDM is a type of glucose intolerance that develops or is first noticed during pregnancy [2]. A previous diagnosis of gestational or pre-diabetes, impaired fasting glycemia, a family history of type 2 diabetes mellitus (DM) in a first-degree relative, maternal age, ethnic background, being overweight, and a history of previous pregnancy resulting in a child with a high birth weight (>4 kg) are all risk factors for developing GDM [3].

The major goal of this study was to look at the relationship between adipokines, lipids, and preeclampsia, as well as the efficacy and accuracy of these markers in predicting PE [4]. PE is a pregnancy-specific illness in which women who were previously normotensive develop hypertension and proteinuria after 20 weeks of pregnancy [5]. PE affects between 2 and 5% of pregnancies and contributes significantly to fetal, neonatal, and maternal morbidity and mortality. In Ghana, the incidence rate is around 7% [6, 7], however, a prevalence of 8.3% was reported in a study at the Volt Regional Hospital, Ho [8]. PE can develop anywhere from 20 weeks post-conception to 6 weeks post-delivery, and it's commonly considered early inception if it happens before 34 weeks. It shares some of the risk factors of metabolic syndrome, such as insulin resistance, subclinical inflammation, and obesity, and data suggests that women with PE are more likely to develop cardiovascular disease later in life [1].

1.1 Adiponectin

Adiponectin, also known as gelatin-binding protein of 28 kDa (GBP28), adipocyte complement-related protein of 30 kDa (ACRP30), adipoQ, adipose most abundant gene transcript 1 (apM1) is an adipocyte-specific secreted protein with roles in glucose and lipid metabolism [9]. The adiponectin gene is located on chromosome 3q27.3 and it is the most abundant protein released by adipose tissue and circulates in plasma as a low-molecular-weight trimer, a middle-molecular-weight hexamer, and a high-molecular-weight 12–18-mer [10, 11]. The biological activity of various variants varies, with HMW adiponectin being the most physiologically active [12]. The effects of adiponectin on glucose metabolism are mediated by two receptors, AdipoR1 and AdipoR2, respectively [13]. AdipoR2 is particularly abundant in the liver, whereas AdipoR1 is found in almost all bodily tissues [14]. Adiponectin activates adenosine monophosphate protein kinase (AMPK) and peroxisome proliferator-activated receptor alpha (PPAR-) by binding to its receptors AdipoR1 and AdipoR2, which leads to the activation of adenosine monophosphate protein kinase (AMPK) and peroxisome proliferator-activated receptor alpha (PPAR-α). In obesity-related insulin resistance, both adiponectin and its receptors are downregulated [13].

Adiponectin levels in the blood have a positive correlation with HDL cholesterol and a negative correlation with triglycerides [15]. Gender, age, and lifestyle all influence plasma adiponectin levels. Adiponectin gene expression is inhibited by β-adrenergic stimulation, glucocorticoids, and TNF-α [16, 17]. Type 2 diabetes, insulin resistance, obesity, hypertension, and left ventricular hypertrophy are all linked to low adiponectin levels in the blood [18].

Even in the absence of obesity, increased fat buildup in the body during pregnancy leads to a steady drop in adiponectin secretion [19]. Both adiponectin concentration and adiponectin mRNA are negatively correlated with fat mass hence with increased adipose tissue secretion during pregnancy, it's possible that signals are sent to the adipose tissue, resulting in a decrease in adiponectin production even in the absence of obesity [19]. Despite the fact that some researchers have been unable to find adiponectin mRNA expression in the placenta [20, 21], studies show that it could be a source of the hormone [22].

A counterintuitive and considerable increase in adiponectin concentration has been found in several studies during pregnancy complicated with PE [23, 24]. Other researchers, on the other hand, discovered no significant differences in adiponectin mRNA expression in adipose tissue between PE patients and healthy controls [25].

1.2 Leptin

Leptin is a 16 kDa protein product of the ob gene located on chromosome 1p31 and was identified in 1994 [1]. The name "leptin" comes from the Greek word "leptos," which means "thin," because this protein causes increased energy expenditure and reduces calorie intake by acting on satiety signals in the hypothalamus [26]. Its amino acid sequence exhibits no major homologies to other proteins [27] and it's made by differentiated adipocytes, but it's also made in other tissues like the stomach fundus, skeletal muscle, the liver, and the placenta [28]. Leptin suppresses food intake and increases energy expenditure by acting on the hypothalamus [29]. It is also a pro-inflammatory protein and a member of the IL-6 super-family of cytokines [30]. Leptin enhances insulin sensitivity in the periphery and regulates pancreatic β-cell activity [13]. Despite a functioning leptin receptor and high leptin levels, leptin does not cause weight loss in the majority of cases of obesity. This reduced response to the anorexigenic and insulin-sensitizing effects of leptin is called "leptin resistance" [13].

During pregnancy, leptin modulates gonadotrophin-releasing hormone release and facilitates implantation [31]. It also boosts amino acid uptake, regulates placental growth, enhances mitogenesis, and induces human chorionic gonadotrophin synthesis in trophoblast cells [31]. Tumor necrosis factor (TNF) and interleukin (IL)-6 stimulate the synthesis of placental leptin mRNA [32]. Leptin levels begin to rise in the early stages of pregnancy, regardless of maternal weight gain [33], peaking approximately 28 weeks of pregnancy and then dropping to pre-gravid levels shortly after delivery [34]. The placenta, rather than maternal adipose tissue alone, appears to play a significant role in the rise in maternal leptin concentrations throughout pregnancy [35]. The presence of a distinct promoter region in the human placental leptin gene indicates that placental leptin is regulated differently from adipose-derived leptin [36]. The fetus itself contributes to leptin production starting early in the second trimester [37]. In comparison to the placenta, however, the fetus produces a modest amount of it. Furthermore, leptin concentrations in umbilical cord plasma correlate positively with birth weight of newborns [38].

Leptin levels are higher in pregnant women with PE [23] and they may be higher before the disease manifests itself clinically [39, 40], with peaks occurring around 28 weeks of gestation [34]. As a result, leptin may play a role in the disease's pathogenesis. However, other authors have observed lowered [25] or unchanged [41] circulating levels in patients with PE.

1.3 Resistin

Resistin is a 12.5 kDa dimeric protein that circulates in human blood as two 92-amino-acid polypeptides connected by disulfide bridges at Cys-26 [42]. The signaling molecule resistin is found in monocytes, macrophages, and adipocytes [1]. The resistin gene is located on chromosome 19p13.3 and although the exact physiological role in humans is unknown, available evidence suggests that its presence in the blood is linked to a number of inflammatory indicators, including C-reactive protein, soluble TNF-receptor-2, IL-6, and lipoprotein-associated phospholipase A2 [43]. Coronary artery disease has been linked to high levels of resistin in the blood [43], and to severity of disease in sepsis and septic shock [44] and may be involved in the pathogenesis of rheumatoid arthritis [45].

Resistin concentration in PE has been reported by various researchers to remain unchanged [23] decreased [46] or increased [25]. The increased circulating resistin levels in PE could be related to the fact that its concentration in plasma is dependent on glomerular filtration, therefore as renal impairment progresses, resistin levels in plasma may rise [47].

1.4 Visfatin

Visfatin is a 52-kDa protein and is extensively produced in both human and mouse adipose tissue, and its plasma levels rise as obesity progresses [1]. Visfatin gene is located on chromosome 7q22.2 and is widely expressed in adipose tissue but can also be found in the placenta and fetal membranes [48] and myometrium [17]. It is also expressed in bone marrow, liver, muscle, heart, lung, and kidney [49] as well as by the lymphocyte. It is referred to as a pre-B cell colony enhancing factor because it enhances the maturation of B cell precursors [49]. Visfatin is released by amniotic epithelial cells during pregnancy [50] and has nicotinamide phosphoribosyltransferase activity [51].

Some contradictory results have been published on visfatin levels during pregnancy affected by preeclampsia. Some authors published increased visfatin levels in PE [52] while other investigators reported decreased levels [53] or values similar to normal pregnancy [54].

In a normal pregnancy, lipid profile changes are characterized by increases in total plasma cholesterol and triglyceride (TG) levels as a result of increased TG synthesis by the liver and very low-density lipoprotein-cholesterol (VLDL-C) synthesis in response to elevated estrogen levels [55]. The clearance of VLDL-C is reduced when the activity of lipoprotein lipase (LPL) is reduced due to estrogen-induced downregulation of LPL gene expression during pregnancy [56]. Women with PE had higher TG, total cholesterol (TC), low-density lipoprotein cholesterol (LDL-C), and very low-density lipoprotein cholesterol (VLDL-C), according to a study conducted in the Cape Coast metropolis in Ghana [57].

The differences in lipid profiles and abnormalities in certain adipokine metabolism described by different researchers warrant a closer look at their implications in the pathophysiology of PE. The main goal of this study was to see if the metabolism of adiponectin, leptin resistin, and visfatin are affected in the first trimester of pregnancy in pregnancies that go on to develop PE, and if these changes are significant enough in the prediction of PE to prompt interventions early enough to save the mother and baby.

2. Materials and methods

2.1 Study site and design

This case-control study was carried out at the Ho Teaching Hospital (HTH) located in the capital of Volta Region of Ghana between January and December 2016.

2.2 Criteria for selection

Pregnant women over the age of 18 with or without hypertension were included in the study (cases and controls, respectively). Pregnant women without dipstick proteinuria and blood pressures less than 140/90 mmHg were assigned to the control group, whereas those with hypertension and proteinuria were assigned to the case group. Pregnant women with renal disease, diabetes, cancer, multigravida, and pre-gestational hypertension were excluded.

2.3 Study population

We studied first trimester data in 90 pregnant women who later developed PE and 100 women who did not. Participants were chosen from a large prospective observational study of women attending the HTH prenatal clinic for early prediction of pregnancies that are prone to develop problems. Women with pregnancies between 11 and 13 weeks of gestation were invited to take part in the study. Participants' maternal characteristics and medical histories were documented.

2.4 Anthropometric measurement

Participants wore light clothing and after removing their shoes, stood on a Bioimpedance analyzer (BIA; BSD01, Pure Pleasure, a division of the Stingray Group, Cape Town, South Africa) and their weights were recorded to the nearest 0.1 kg. The study participants were made to stand upright, heels together, head in the horizontal plane, and height was measured with a stadiometer to the nearest 0.5 cm without shoes. BMI was estimated as weight/height squared (kg/m^2).

2.5 Blood pressure measurement

Each participant was instructed to sit comfortably, stretch her left arm on a table, and relax for 10 minutes. A mercury sphygmomanometer and stethoscope were used to take measurements from the left upper arm after the subjects had rested for at least 5 minutes. The mean blood pressure was recorded to the closest to 2.0 mmHg in triplicate, with at least 5 minutes of waiting time between tests following the American Heart Association's standards [58].

2.6 Collection and preservation of samples

Five milliliters of blood were drawn between 7:00 and 8:00 a.m. during the first trimester and placed in serum separator tubes before being placed on ice packs. Within an hour, serum samples were separated and stored in aliquots at −80°C for biochemical analysis. Each participant was given a clean, dry, wide mouth, leak-proof container to collect 5 mL of urine sample after the 20th week of pregnancy.

2.7 Biochemical and urine analysis

Sandwich enzyme-linked immunosorbent assay technique (Elabscience Biotechnology Co. Ltd., Wu Han, People's Republic of China) was used to analyze adiponectin, leptin, resistin, and visfatin in the baseline samples of both cases and controls, while the lipid profiles were performed using the Vitros dry chemistry analyzer (Ortho-Clinical Diagnostics, Johnson & Johnson, High Wycombe, UK). None of the samples in this investigation had been thawed and frozen before.

For less than 2 seconds, a urine strip was put into a urine sample up to the test area. To remove surplus urine, the strips' margins were drawn around the brims of the vessels, ensuring that the test areas did not come into contact with them. To eliminate any residual urine, the strips were held vertically and tapped on absorbent papers [59]. Under bright light, the urine strip was horizontally held and compared to the color chart on the vial label.

The intensity of the blue-green color, which was related to the quantity of protein in the urine, was then used to determine the amount of protein. Proteinuria was defined as the presence of urine protein at concentrations of "+" or higher [60].

2.8 Study variables and outcome measurement

After the twentieth week of pregnancy, every pregnant woman in this hospital is screened for PE. PE occurrence (yes/no), as determined by PE diagnosis criteria, was the primary outcome. Urine protein was measured using the dip-stick qualitative/semi-quantitative method (Urit Medical Electronic Co., Ltd., Guangxi, People's Republic of China) after 20 weeks of pregnancy. PE was diagnosed by a qualified Obstetrician/Gynecologist based on systolic and diastolic blood pressures of 140 mmHg or more on two occasions at least 4 hours apart (or both) in addition to proteinuria of + or more.

2.9 Statistical analysis

The SPSS software, version 20, and Graph Pad Prism, version 5.0, San Diego, California, USA, and Systat, Inc. Germany were used to analyze the data. The Shapiro-Wilk test was used to determine the normality of the variables under investigation, followed by a Mann-Whitney *U*-test to compare those with PE to those without. A value of $p < 0.05$ was considered significant in all of the statistical analyses. The AUC (area under the receiver operating characteristic (ROC) curve) is commonly used to assess a test's/accuracy. When the AUC is less than 50%, the result is considered random guessing and thus not meaningful. This is represented by a diagonal line in the ROC plot [61]. The adipokines and lipids were evaluated for their accuracy (AUC 60%) in predicting preeclampsia-like pregnancies.

After correcting for potential confounding variables, multivariate analysis was performed on the individual adipokines as predictors of PE (age, BMI, relatives with hypertension, family history of diabetes mellitus, family history of preeclampsia, and parity). After correcting for confounders, the goal was to determine the independent contribution of each adipokine in predicting PE.

The parameters for the goodness of fit test for the models were −2Log (Likelihood), R2 (Cox and Snell), R2 (Nagelkerke), Akaike Information Criterion (AIC), and Correct Classification Rate (CCR).

The −2Log (Likelihood) statistic indicates how well a model predicts a certain occurrence, the lower the number, the better the model.

The coefficients of determination Cox and Snell R2 and Nagelkerke R2 are used to measure the amount of variation in the dependent variable that is explained by the independent variable. The Cox and Snell R2 has been modified to create the Nagelkerke R2. The AIC is also a relative quality estimator for statistical models. The better the model, the smaller the estimate. The Correct Classification Rate is another valuable metric for evaluating the utility of a logistic regression model (CCR).

3. Results

The baseline demographics, lipids, and adipokine characteristics of those with PE were compared to those without PE (**Table 1**). The mean age of those who acquired PE was significantly greater than that of those who did not (35.1 vs. 28.44 years; $p < 0.0001$), and their BMI was likewise significantly higher (32.63 vs. 24.99 kg/m^2; $P < 0.0001$). Except for HDL, which was considerably lower in the PE group compared to those without PE (1.39 vs. 1.569, $p = 0.043$), the lipid profile parameters did not demonstrate any significant differences between the PE group and those without PE (**Table 1**). Leptin levels were statistically substantially higher in the PE group (39.26 vs. 18.46 ng/mL, $P < 0.0001$) than in the control group. Similarly, resistin and visfatin were considerably higher in PEs compared to normotensives ($p < 0.0001$), although adiponectin was significantly lower in PEs compared to non PEs ($p < 0.0001$).

The ROC curves were used to assess the performance of the screening. **Table 2** shows the areas under the ROC curve, the sensitivities and specificities, as well as the threshold points for detecting PE. The accuracy with which biochemical markers can differentiate on the condition of PE was tested in this study. As shown in **Table 2**, the adipokines leptin (92.0%), resistin (91.4%), and adiponectin (90.5%) have good accuracy levels, whereas visfastin (77.1%) has fair accuracy levels in diagnosing PE, according to **Table 2** ratings. With a cut-off point of 50.55 ng/mL, adiponectin had a sensitivity and specificity of 87.8 and 86%, respectively, while leptin had a sensitivity and specificity of 92% with a threshold of 27 ng/mL. Furthermore, resistin had a sensitivity and specificity of 94 and 91%, respectively, with a cut-off point of around 9 ng/mL, whereas visfatin had a sensitivity and specificity of 69 and 83%, with a threshold of 6.67 ng/mL. This suggests that adiponectin, leptin, resistin, and visfatin are effective PE predictors (**Table 2**).

Furthermore, a detailed examination of the ROC plots (**Figure 1**) reveals that they are all far from the diagonal line, which represents 50%, indicating that they are not random guesses but rather meaningful. This indicates that they are quite good at predicting pregnancies that are likely to result in PE. After adjusting for BMI, none of those in the normal BMI category had PE (**Table 3**); as a result, no AUC values for all of the adipokines studied were obtained. The overweight group, on the other hand, had greater AUCs, sensitivities, and specificities. Obese people, on the other hand, had lower sensitivities and specificities. These findings point to a possible influence of BMI on adiponectin, leptin, resistin, and visfatin, as well as a possible negative feedback mechanism in the metabolism of these adipocytokines during pregnancy. However, BMI does not appear to have an effect on the predictive ability of these PE signaling molecules.

There were minor variations in the AUCs, sensitivities, specificities, and threshold points for predicting PE after controlling for family history of hypertension, which is a known confounding factor, but these variations were minor, and the overall effect of these adipocytokines' predictive abilities remained intact (**Table 4**).

Table 5 shows a multivariate analysis of individual adipokines as PE predictors. Adiponectin, leptin, resistin, and visfatin were included as predictors in Models 1, 2, 3, and 4, respectively, while correcting for confounding factors such as age, parity, BMI, and relative with hypertension, and family history of diabetes and preeclampsia. Based on the criteria analyzed, Model 1 including adiponectin as a predictor was the best model. This means having the greatest Nagelkerke R2 and CCR values of 95 and

Var	BMI		Age		ADP		LP		RTN		VF		TG		TC		HDL		LDL		VLDL	
PE	**No**	**Yes**	**No**	**Yes**	**No**	**Yes**	**No**	**Yes**	**No**	**Yes**	**No**	**Yes**	**No**	**Yes**	**No**	**Yes**	**No**	**Yes**	**No**	**Yes**	**No**	**Yes**
Min	18.9	27.1	16	24	17.7	15.2	2.7	9.9	1.3	4.0	0.3	0.5	0.5	0.5	2.4	2.6	0.1	0.1	0.2	0.2	0.2	0.2
Max	37.3	37.3	41	46	258.2	90.6	40.7	41	12.4	13.9	11.2	19.4	3.3	3.4	9.6	9.3	3.4	3.4	7.8	7.8	1.5	1.4
Mean	25.0	32.6	28.4	35.1	83.6	39.3	18.5	36.3	6.4	10.2	4.4	7.4	1.7	1.6	5.8	5.9	1.6	1.4	3.8	4.0	0.8	0.7
LB	24.2	32.0	27.4	34.0	77.3	35.3	16.8	34.7	6.0	9.8	3.9	6.7	1.5	1.5	5.5	5.5	1.4	1.2	3.5	3.6	0.7	0.6
UB	25.8	33.2	29.5	36.2	90.0	43.2	20.2	37.9	6.8	10.7	5.0	8.0	1.8	1.8	6.1	6.3	1.7	1.7	4.1	4.4	0.9	0.8
P value	**<0.0001****		**<0.0001****		**<0.0001****		**<0.0001****		**<0.0001****		**<0.0001****		0.86		0.826		**0.043***		0.589		0.73	

*significant at $p < 0.05$
**significant at $p < 0.01$
Values in bold are significant at $p < 0.05$
ADP, adiponectin; LP, leptin; RTN, resistin; VF, visfatin; TG, triglyceride; TC, total cholesterol; LDL, low density lipoprotein cholesterol; HDL, high density lipoprotein cholesterol; VLDL, very low density lipoprotein cholesterol.
Reproduced from: Ref. [62].

Table 1.
Mann-Whitney U test for base line biochemical markers and maternal characteristics for study participants.

Variables	AUC (%)	Sensitivity (%)	Specificity (%)	Threshold point
ADP	90.5	87.8	86	≤50.552
LP	92	92.2	92	≥27.273
RTN	91.4	94.4	91.4	≥8.949
VF	77.1	68.9	83	≥6.667

ADP, adiponectin; LP, leptin; RTN, resistin; VF, visfatin.
Reproduced from: Ref. [62].

Table 2.
AUC, sensitivity, specificity, and threshold point for the adipokines in the pregnant women.

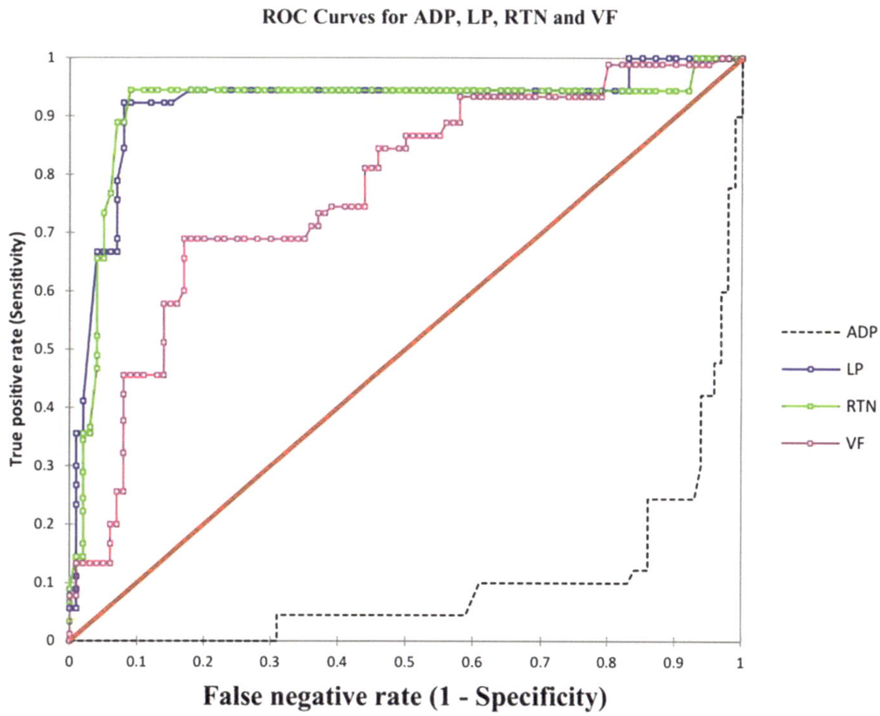

Figure 1.
ROC curves for the adipokines. AUCs (%): ADP (95.0), LP (92.0), RTN (91.4), and VF (77.1). ADP, adiponectin; LP, leptin; RTN, resistin; VF, visfatin.

95.26%, respectively, implying that after correcting for confounders, adiponectin is the strongest predictor of PE. With Nagelkerke R2 and CCR statistics of 89 and 91.58%, respectively, Model 4 with visfatin as a predictor had the least predictive performance.

In their respective models, adiponectin, leptin, resistin, and visfatin were found to be significant predictors of PE ($P < 0.05$). For each unit drop in adiponectin, the probabilities of PE increase by a factor of 1.1, according to the reciprocal of the odds ratio (Model 1). A one-unit increase in leptin increases the risk of PE by 1.15 times (Model 2). Additionally, a unit increase in resistin raises the probabilities of PE by 1.65 (Model 3), whereas visfatin increases the odds of PE by 1.28 (Model 4).

Obesity was revealed to be a significant confounder in all four models, with overweight as the reference category under BMI and parity of four or more with parity one as

Adipokine	BMI category	Prevalence (%)	AUC (%)	Sensitivity (%)	Specificity (%)	Threshold point
ADP	Normal weight	0	—	—	—	—
	Overweight	23	97.7	100	97.7	≤36.163
	Obese	89	83.2	71.4	90	≤44.980
LP	Normal weight	0	—	—	—	—
	Overweight	23	99.3	100	97.7	≥27.245
	Obese	89	70.7	61	80	≥38.482
RTN	Normal weight	0	—	—	—	—
	Overweight	23	95.5	100	90.9	≥8.949
	Obese	89	93.5	93.5	70	≥8.949
VF	Normal weight	0	—	—	—	—
	Overweight	23	89.5	84.6	90.9	≥6.628
	Obese	89	48.2	66.2	60	≥6.243

ADP, adiponectin; LP, leptin; RTN, resistin; VF, visfatin. BMI classification: Normal Weight = (18.5–24.9 kg/m^2), Overweight = (25.0–29.99 kg/m^2), Obese = (Above 30.0 kg/m^2)
Reproduced from: Ref. [62].

Table 3.
AUC, sensitivity, specificity, and threshold point for levels of the adipokines in the pregnant women controlling for BMI.

		Prevalence (%)	AUC (%)	Sensitivity (%)	Specificity (%)	Threshold point
	RWHP					
ADP	YES	73	83.6	84.2	78.6	≤50.552
	NO	38	92.2	84.6	95.3	≤44.980
LP	YES	73	90.6	89.5	92.9	≥25.611
	NO	38	92.2	94.2	91.9	≥27.273
RTN	YES	73	89.8	89.5	85.7	≥9.012
	NO	38	91.6	94.2	93	≥8.949
VF	YES	73	72.5	78.9	78.6	≥6.349
	NO	38	75.1	61.5	83.7	≥6.667

ADP, adiponectin; LP, leptin; RTN, resistin; VF, visfatin; RWHP, relatives with hypertension; YES, those who have relatives with hypertension; NO, those who do not have relatives with hypertension.
Reproduced from: Ref. [62].

Table 4.
AUC, sensitivity, specificity, and threshold point for the adipokines in the pregnant women controlling for those who have relatives with hypertension.

the reference category. In Models 1, 3, and 4, advanced maternal age above 35 years, with the age group 20–35 years as the reference category, was also found to be important.

Although adiponectin showed a mild positive link with HDL and a weak negative correlation with TG and VLDL, it did demonstrate a favorable correlation with HDL. Although leptin and resistin had minor negative relationships with HDL, visfatin had a strong negative link with HDL. Leptin, resistin, and visfatin all had negative correlations with adiponectin. Positive associations were found between leptin, resistin, and visfatin (**Table 6**). These links were weak in those of normal weight, but they were stronger in individuals who were overweight or obese (**Table 7**). This

	Model 1 (ADP)			Model 2 (LP)			Model 3 (RTN)			Model 4 (VF)		
	P-value	OR	OR CI (95%)	*P*-value	OR	OR CI (95%)	*P*-value	OR	OR CI (95%)	*P*-value	OR	OR CI (95%)
Intercept	0.50			**<0.0001**			**<0.0001**			<0.0001		
ADP	**<0.0001**	**0.93**	**(0.9, 0.96)**									
LP				**<0.0001**	1.15	(1.08, 1.22)						
RTN							**<0.0001**	1.65	(1.3, 2.11)			
VF										0.01	1.28	(1.07, 1.55)
Age Cat.												
20–35 years												
Above 35 years	**0.04**	8.86	(1.16, 67.68)	0.07	4.60	(0.88, 24.08)	**0.01**	6.25	(1.46, 26.69)	**0.01**	5.67	(1.41, 22.74)
Less than 20 years	0.89	1.39	(0.01, 135.01)	0.12	32.85	(0.41, 2604.47)	0.39	7.86	(0.07, 901.18)	0.12	27.92	(0.41, 1895.49)
BMI category												
Overweight												
Obese	**<0.0001**	44.24	(7.5, 260.91)	**<0.0001**	20.43	(4.75, 87.87)	**<0.0001**	19.88	(5.06, 78.17)	**<0.0001**	26.52	(7.73, 90.98)
Normal weight	0.16	0.12	(0.01, 2.29)	0.20	0.15	(0.01, 2.62)	0.10	0.08	(0, 1.67)	0.06	0.07	(0, 1.07)
Parity												
1												
2	0.84	1.18	(0.22, 6.41)	0.19	2.76	(0.6, 12.76)	0.08	4.00	(0.84, 19.14)	0.16	2.75	(0.67, 11.2)
3	**0.02**	11.34	(1.53, 84.29)	0.02	7.51	(1.29, 43.58)	0.13	3.73	(0.69, 20.11)	0.05	4.40	(0.99, 19.5)
>4	**0.04**	9.07	(1.03, 80.17)	**<0.0001**	17.35	(2.72, 110.49)	**<0.0001**	14.38	(2.45, 84.57)	**<0.0001**	12.19	(2.41, 61.59)
Family Hist. of Hyp.												
No												
Yes	0.19	2.93	(0.59, 14.48)	**0.04**	4.58	(0.97, 21.64)	0.10	3.84	(0.79, 18.77)	0.07	3.43	(0.89, 13.21)
Family Hist. of DM												
No												

	Model 1 (ADP)			Model 2 (LP)			Model 3 (RTN)			Model 4 (VF)		
	P-value	**OR**	**OR CI (95%)**	**P-value**	**OR**	**OR CI (95%)**	**P-value**	**OR**	**OR CI (95%)**	**P-value**	**OR**	**OR CI (95%)**
Yes	0.40	2.23	(0.35, 14.34)	0.76	1.28	(0.26, 6.21)	0.72	0.75	(0.16, 3.53)	0.88	0.90	(0.21, 3.77)
Family Hist. of PE												
No												
Yes	0.79	0.82	(0.19, 3.52)	0.11	0.34	(0.09, 1.26)	0.22	0.45	(0.12, 1.62)	0.14	0.41	(0.12, 1.36)
Goodness of fit statistics												
	Model 1			Model 2			Model 3			Model 4		
−2Log (Likelihood)	27.186			37.24			40.66			54.11		
R^2 (Cox and Snell)	0.71			0.70			0.69			0.67		
R^2 (Nagelkerke)	0.95			0.93			0.92			0.89		
AIC	51.19			61.24			64.66			78.11		
CCR (%)	95.26			93.16			92.63			91.58		

Reproduced from: Ref. [62].
Values in bold are significant at $p < 0.05$.

Table 5.
Multivariate analysis of clinical factors affecting preeclampsia.

Variables	ADP	LP	RTN	VF	TC	HDL	LDL	VLDL	TG
ADP	**1**	**−0.5403**	**−0.3807**	**−0.2399**	0.0549	0.0531	0.0390	−0.0640	−0.0558
LP	**−0.5403**	**1**	**0.6667**	**0.5460**	0.0629	−0.1333	0.0963	−0.0016	0.0092
RTN	**−0.3807**	**0.6667**	**1**	**0.4510**	0.0911	−0.1248	0.0671	0.0227	0.0395
VF	**−0.2399**	**0.5460**	**0.4510**	**1**	**0.1928**	**−0.1527**	**0.1699**	0.1252	**0.1437**
TC	0.0549	0.0629	0.0911	**0.1928**	**1**	**−0.3359**	**0.8891**	**0.5973**	**0.5912**
HDL	0.0531	−0.1333	−0.1248	**−0.1527**	**−0.3359**	**1**	**−0.3899**	**−0.1508**	−0.1335
LDL	0.0390	0.0963	0.0671	**0.1699**	**0.8891**	**−0.3899**	**1**	**0.3370**	**0.3385**
VLDL	−0.0640	−0.0016	0.0227	0.1252	**0.5973**	**−0.1508**	**0.3370**	**1**	**0.9794**
TG	−0.0558	0.0092	0.0395	**0.1437**	**0.5912**	−0.1335	**0.3385**	**0.9794**	**1**

Values in bold are different from 0 with a significance level alpha = 0.05.
Reproduced from: Ref. [62].

Table 6.
Correlation among adipokines and lipids.

BMI category	Variables	ADP	LP	RTN	VF
	ADP	**1**	0.1259	0.0157	0.1568
Normal weight	LP	0.1259	**1**	−0.1357	**0.305**
	RTN	0.0157	−0.1357	**1**	**−0.426**
	VF	0.1568	**0.305**	**−0.426**	**1**
	ADP	**1**	**−0.6234**	**−0.3162**	−0.2106
Overweight	LP	**−0.6234**	**1**	**0.5556**	**0.4342**
	RTN	**−0.3162**	**0.5556**	**1**	**0.3758**
	VF	−0.2106	**0.4342**	**0.3758**	**1**
	ADP	**1**	**−0.2559**	−0.0167	0.031
Obese	LP	**−0.2559**	**1**	**0.5853**	**0.497**
	RTN	−0.0167	**0.5853**	**1**	**0.4751**
	VF	0.031	**0.497**	**0.4751**	**1**

Values in bold are different from 0 with a significance level alpha = 0.05. ADP, adiponectin; LP, leptin; RTN, resistin; VF, visfatin. BMI classification: Normal Weight = (18.5–24.9 kg/m^2), Overweight = (25.0–29.99 kg/m^2), Obese = (Above 30.0 kg/m^2).
Reproduced from: Ref. [62].

Table 7.
Correlation of adipokines according to BMI category.

		Sum of squares	*df*	Mean square	*F*	Sig.
Age	Between groups	832.197	1	832.197	25.723	<0.0001
	Within groups	10029.175	310	32.352		
	Total	10861.372	311			
BMI	Between groups	1248.068	1	1248.068	76.461	<0.0001
	Within groups	5060.084	310	16.323		
	Total	6308.152	311			
RWHP	Between groups	0.378	1	0.378	1.771	0.184
	Within groups	66.084	310	0.213		
	Total	66.462	311			
NC	Between groups	3.721	1	3.721	6.182	0.013
	Within groups	186.584	310	0.602		
	Total	190.304	311			
MC	Between groups	2.856	1	2.856	6.199	0.013
	Within groups	142.808	310	0.461		
	Total	145.663	311			
SB	Between groups	0.416	1	0.416	3.216	0.074
	Within groups	39.855	308	0.129		
	Total	40.271	309			
CS	Between groups	0.003	1	0.003	0.026	0.871
	Within groups	28.607	300	0.095		
	Total	28.609	301			

		Sum of squares	*df*	Mean square	*F*	Sig.
NP	Between groups	13.344	1	13.344	8.634	0.004
	Within groups	479.105	310	1.545		
	Total	492.449	311			

RWHP, relatives with hypertension; NC, number of children; MC, number of previous miscarriages; SB, number of previous stillbirths; CS, number of previous cesarean operations; NP, number of pregnancies.
Reproduced from: Ref. [63].

Table 8.
Comparison of maternal characteristics and family history of respondents with those who developed PE (N = 312; PE = 26; Without PE = 286).

reemphasizes the link between adiposity and some of these adipokines. We had earlier examined the associations between maternal factors and PE in a report published in the International Journal of Women's Health [63].

"We had earlier examined the associations between maternal factors and PE (**Table 8**) in a report published in the International Journal of Women's Health [63]. That report indicated that those with PE had significantly higher number of miscarriages, number of previous pregnancies and number of children compared to those without PE."

4. Discussion

The goal of this study was to estimate the levels of adiponectin, leptin, resistin, and visfatin, between 11 and 13 weeks of pregnancy and to see how successful it was to predict PE using first trimester levels of these biomarkers together with maternal factors.

Leptin levels were found to be considerably greater in those who developed PE later on compared to those who did not. This is in line with a previous study that found a rise in leptin levels several weeks before a clinical diagnosis of PE [8]. This observation is also consistent with another study that found an imbalance between adiponectin and leptin in the plasma of women with PE, resulting in raised leptin and decreased adiponectin levels; consequently, these two adipose-derived hormones may play a role in the pathogenesis of PE [64]. Similarly, as compared to normal pregnant controls, leptin levels were found to be 78% higher at 13 weeks of gestation in women who ultimately developed PE [65]. When comparing pregnant women whose first-trimester leptin levels were 25 ng/mL to pregnant women whose first-trimester leptin levels were 25 ng/mL, the risk of PE increased 18.8 fold [66]. Other studies have shown that leptin levels rise before the clinical beginning of the disease, and our findings support that theory [39, 40]. The findings of this study, together with prior research, suggest that leptin is involved in the pathophysiology of PE, rather than a rise in leptin as a result of impaired renal clearance. Hyperleptinemia has been shown to promote sodium reabsorption in the renal tubules, leading to water retention and elevated blood pressure [67]. Furthermore, tumor necrosis factor (TNF)-α and interleukin (IL)-6 upregulate placental leptin mRNA synthesis and increase the formation of endothelin, a vasoconstrictive peptide [68]. The constriction of the blood vessels leads to high blood pressure leading to PE.

Adiponectin levels in the first trimester were considerably lower in women with PE compared to the control group in this study. Other research has found that adiponectin levels are inversely proportional to coronary artery disease but not strongly related to blood pressure levels [69]. In another study, individuals with preeclampsia had lower median maternal high molecular weight and low molecular weight adiponectin concentrations than those with normal pregnancies [70]. Previous reports have demonstrated lower first-trimester adiponectin levels in women who subsequently developed PE compared to their peers [71, 72]. However, this study contradicts a publication that stated that circulation levels of adiponectin were higher in preeclamptic patients than in normal pregnant women [73, 74]. In another study, women with preeclampsia had approximately 50% greater third-trimester adiponectin levels than their normotensive counterparts [75]. In a similar study, women with preeclampsia had higher levels of circulating adiponectin [74]. The compensatory feedback mechanisms to the metabolically altered, anti-angiogenic, and pro-atherogenic condition of severe preeclampsia could explain these increases, which normally occur after the first trimester [74]. Hypoadiponectinemia in the first trimester of pregnant women who later developed PE implies that this adipocytokine is involved in PE etiology [16, 17]. Pregnancy is an inflammatory state associated with elevated plasma TNF-α, which could cause adiponectin levels to drop even further. An increase in TNF-α leads to an increase in endothelin levels [68] which constricts the blood vessels leading to high blood pressure [68]. Adiponectin appears to block the synthesis of angiotensin II, according to available evidence [76]. As adiponectin levels fall, angiotensin II levels rise, resulting in an increase in aldosterone levels. Hypertension results from a rise in aldosterone levels, which causes sodium and water retention.

When comparing pregnancies that resulted in PE to those that did not, this study discovered considerably greater resistin levels in PE pregnancies. A recent study found that preeclamptic pregnancies had higher levels of several adipokines, notably resistin, than healthy pregnant women [25]. Other studies, on the other hand, found no significant difference in resistin levels between preeclampsia patients and healthy pregnant women [77, 78]. Women with PE had significantly lower resistin levels than normotensive women of the same gestational age, according to some studies [46]. The involvement of resistin in the pathophysiology of PE is indicated by the rise in resistin levels months before the clinical diagnosis of PE. Resistin levels in the blood have been associated with coronary artery disease [43]. Resistin levels in the blood have been linked to a number of inflammatory indicators, including C-reactive protein, soluble TNF-α receptor-2, IL-6, and lipoprotein-associated phospholipase A2 [43]. Increased levels of endothelin result from increased TNF-α receptor-2 and IL-6 concentrations, resulting in high blood pressure [68].

Plasma visfatin levels were shown to be considerably higher during PE in our research. Visfatin levels rose during PE from the first trimester onwards, suggesting that visfatin may play a role in the disease's development. Visfatin is widely expressed in adipose tissue, placenta, and fetal membranes [48]. Visfatin concentrations in the second and third trimesters of normal pregnancy have been found to be higher than those in the first trimester [79] indicating that this protein is produced by the placenta and fetal membrane. Thus, it's probable that normal visfatin production is regulated to support the growing baby; yet, in some pregnancies, visfatin's supporting role may be interrupted, resulting in PE. Our findings are consistent with one of similar research which showed greater visfatin levels in the PE compared to normal pregnancy [80]. One study found no significant differences between normal and preeclamptic pregnancies [54] while another found lower levels [53]. Different researchers' reports on visfatin levels during pregnancy could be attributed to variances in sample procedures, ethnic or geographical differences, or the specific test methods used. This study's findings imply that visfatin levels rise before preeclampsia develops.

Visfatin's potential as a marker of preeclampsia, particularly in obese women, will need to be explored further with bigger sample size. Such research will add to the body of knowledge on how to predict this disease and how to start intervention programs to reduce maternal and fetal morbidity and mortality from PE.

The fact that the AUCs and respective sensitivities and specificities did not significantly change after controlling for family history of hypertension (**Table 4**) shows that these biomarkers can predict PE independently regardless of family history of hypertension. When maternal weight was taken into account (**Table 3**), these adipokines were found to be ineffective in predicting PE in women of normal weight (BMI 18.5–24.9 kg/m^2). However, the fact that the overweight group (BMI 25–29.9 kg/m^2) fared better in terms of predicting these adipokines than the obese group (BMI 30.0 kg/m^2) implies a possible negative feedback mechanism that lowers plasma concentrations of these peptides as weight rises. To explain this occurrence, more research with bigger sample size is needed.

This study found that overweight pregnant women are more likely than normal-weight pregnant women to get PE during their pregnancy, corroborating an earlier study that found that the likelihood of developing PE increased by two to three times in women with a higher BMI [81] and also similar to another study, which associated higher maternal BMI to a number of pregnancy complications including PE [82]. In addition, this study backs up a recent analysis that showed that advanced maternal age, especially, 35 years or more was a risk factor for preeclampsia [83] as well as a BMI greater than 30 kg/m^2 [84]. Obesity may play a role in the development of PE, according to the findings of this study. Obesity affects nitric oxide production and causes endothelial dysfunction [85] therefore an excessive buildup of fat in a pregnant woman could lead to hypertension during pregnancy which could lead to PE.

With the exception of HDL cholesterol, which was considerably lower in the PE group (**Table 1**) compared to the normotensive group, this investigation found no significant differences in lipids between women who acquired PE and those who remained normotensive during pregnancy. This study contradicts a report by Brazilian researchers who found a substantial difference in TG-rich proteins (VLDL 1) and small dense lipoprotein (LDL III) in women with PE compared to normal pregnant women [86]. Our findings contrast with those published in the Cape Coast region of Ghana, where researchers found substantial dyslipidemia in women with PE compared to women without PE [57]. The variations could be related to the different stages of pregnancy during which the samples were taken. The samples for this study were taken before the commencement of PE, whereas the samples for the other investigations were taken after the disease had begun to manifest. The lack of a significant difference in first trimester lipids between those who got PE and those who did not show that the atherogenic lipid profile commonly seen in pregnant women as reported by other researchers may be insufficient in predicting the chance of getting PE. However, because lower HDL is a substantial risk factor for hypertension, it's probable that the significantly lower HDL seen in individuals who went on to develop PE was linked to the disease's etiology [87]. Adiponectin and resistin were found to be more significant and better predictors of PE than leptin and visfatin after correcting for these potential confounding variables (age, parity, BMI, family history of diabetes, and preeclampsia). Angiotensin II production is reduced by adiponectin [76] while resistin is linked to elevations in TNF-α receptor-2 and IL-6, and so promotes high blood pressure [43], leading to an increased level of endothelin which constricts blood vessels and raises high blood pressure [68]. A family history of PE has been linked to a threefold increase in the chance of developing PE [88, 89] however, we did not detect a significant link between PE and a family history of hypertension which is likely attributable to the fact that the data obtained from the participants in this study was focused on hypertension in general rather than PE.

According to the findings of this study, obesity may play a role in the development of PE. Obesity induces endothelial dysfunction by reducing nitric oxide production [85], hence if a pregnant woman has an excessive amount of fat on her body, she may develop hypertension and, as a result, PE. Obesity and having four or more children were discovered to be significant PE confounders.

4.1 Study limitations

The study's limitations were limited sample size and insufficient information regarding the individuals' nutritional state. Potassium is abundant in leafy greens like spinach and kale, as well as cherries and red beets. Potassium operates on the kidneys, allowing the salt to be excreted more easily through the kidneys, decreasing blood pressure. Because of the small sample size and lack of nutritional data, conclusions about the association between these adipocytokines and preeclampsia may be difficult to draw, since nutritional status could not be controlled in the multivariate analysis.

5. Conclusions

PE was found to be significantly predicted by low adiponectin and high leptin, resistin, and visfatin, with resistin being the greatest predictor when stratified by BMI categories. After controlling for age, parity, BMI, and family history of diabetes and preeclampsia, adiponectin was the greatest predictor.

Adiponectin concentration in patients with PE starts decreasing as early as 11 weeks of pregnancy and continues to decrease until after 24th weeks of pregnancy when proteinuria becomes apparent and blood pressure rises to an abnormal level and consequently, preeclampsia develops. The decrease in adiponectin contributes to the pathogenesis of PE and can be used to predict this disease.

Leptin concentration starts increasing by 11 weeks of pregnancy in patients who subsequently develop PE. The increase in leptin correlates with proteinuria and elevated systolic and diastolic blood pressure irrespective of maternal age and BMI and hence could be involved in the pathogenesis of GDM.

Resistin in pregnant women who go on to develop PE starts increasing between 11 and 13 weeks of gestation culminating in an excessive increase in blood pressure accompanied by proteinuria by 24 weeks of gestation when a diagnosis of PE becomes apparent.

Visfatin in pregnancies complicated by PE starts increasing during the first trimester of pregnancy and continues to increase until the second trimester when blood pressure increases resulting in the diagnosis of PE in women with concomitant proteinuria. This suggests that hypervisfatinemia can be used to predict hypertensive disorders during pregnancy and hence involved in the pathogenesis of PE.

Our findings suggest that BMI may have an effect on adiponectin, leptin, resistin, and visfatin, as well as a possible negative feedback mechanism in the metabolism of these adipocytokines during pregnancy. More importantly, BMI does not appear to have an effect on the predictive ability of these PE signaling molecules. Advanced maternal age was shown to be an important factor in the development of PE.

These biomarkers can be used in combination with maternal characteristics for the early prediction of PE. This will help health care providers to institute measures such as diet control, medication, and exercises tailored for pregnant women with these risk factors so as to reduce the incidence of preeclampsia.

Acknowledgements

i. Prof. Francis Agyemang Yeboah, Department of Molecular Medicine, School Medical Sciences, Kwame Nkrumah University of Science and Technology, Kumasi, Ghana. Telephone: +233 24 5005500. Email: drfay1801@gmail.com.

ii. Prof. Robert Amadu Ngala, Department of Molecular Medicine, School Medical Sciences, Kwame Nkrumah University of Science and Technology, Kumasi, Ghana. Telephone: +233 207722162. Email: rngala2000@yahoo.com.

iii. Mr. Salifu Nanga, School of Basic and Biomedical Sciences, University of Health and Allied Sciences, Ho, Ghana. Telephone: +233 243667951. Email: snanga@uhas.edu.

Conflict of interest

The authors declare no conflict of interest.

Abbreviations

BMI	body mass index
PE	preeclampsia
ADP	adiponectin
LP	leptin
RTN	resistin
VF	visfatin
TG	triglycerides
TC	total cholesterol
HDL	high-density lipoprotein cholesterol
LDL	low-density lipoprotein cholesterol
VLDL	very low-density lipoprotein cholesterol

Author details

Ahmed Tijani Bawah[1]*, Abdul-Malik Bawah[2] and Ruhaima Issah Zorro[3]

1 Faculty of Allied Health and Pharmaceutical Sciences, Department of Medical Laboratory Sciences, Tamale Technical University, Tamale, Ghana

2 Faculty of Allied Health and Pharmaceutical Sciences, Department of Nutrition and Dietetics, Tamale Technical University, Tamale, Ghana

3 Faculty of Allied Health and Pharmaceutical Sciences, Department of Nursing and Midwifery, Tamale Technical University, Tamale, Ghana

*Address all correspondence to: ahmed024gh@yahoo.com

References

[1] Miehle K, Stepan H, Fasshauer M. Leptin, adiponectin and other adipokines in gestational diabetes mellitus and pre-eclampsia. Clinical Endocrinology. 2012;**76**(1):2-11

[2] Zawiejska A, Wender-Ozegowska E, Brazert J, Sodowski K. Components of metabolic syndrome and their impact on fetal growth in women with gestational diabetes mellitus. Journal of Physiology and Pharmacology. 2008;**59**(Suppl 4):5-18

[3] Ross G. Gestational diabetes. Australian Family Physician. 2006;**35**(6):392

[4] Backes CH, Markham K, Moorehead P, Cordero L, Nankervis CA, Giannone PJ. Maternal preeclampsia and neonatal outcomes. Journal of Pregnancy. 2011;**2011**

[5] Wagner LK. Diagnosis and management of preeclampsia. American Family Physician. 2004;**70**(12):2317-2324

[6] Obed SA, Aniteye P. Pregnancy following eclampsia: a longitudinal study at Korle-BU teaching hospital. Ghana medical journal. 2007;**41**(3):139-143

[7] Owiredu W. The prevalence of the metabolic syndrome among Ghanaian pregnancy-induced hypertensive patients using the World Health Organisation and the National Cholesterol Education program III criteria. Journal of Medical Sciences. 2008;**8**(5):443-451

[8] Yeboah FA, Ngala RA, Bawah AT, Asare-Anane H, Alidu H, Hamid A-WM. Wumbee JDK: Adiposity and hyperleptinemia during the first trimester among pregnant women with preeclampsia. International Journal of Women's Health. 2017;**9**:449

[9] Meier U, Gressner AM. Endocrine regulation of energy metabolism: Review of pathobiochemical and clinical chemical aspects of leptin, ghrelin, adiponectin, and resistin. Clinical Chemistry. 2004;**50**(9):1511-1525

[10] Waki H, Yamauchi T, Kamon J, Ito Y, Uchida S, Kita S, et al. Impaired multimerization of human adiponectin mutants associated with diabetes molecular structure and multimer formation of adiponectin. Journal of Biological Chemistry. 2003;**278**(41):40352-40363

[11] Wang Y, Xu LY, Lam KS, Lu G, Cooper GJ, Xu A. Proteomic characterization of human serum proteins associated with the fat-derived hormone adiponectin. Proteomics. 2006;**6**(13):3862-3870

[12] Pajvani UB, Hawkins M, Combs TP, Rajala MW, Doebber T, Berger JP, et al. Complex distribution, not absolute amount of adiponectin, correlates with thiazolidinedione-mediated improvement in insulin sensitivity. Journal of Biological Chemistry. 2004;**279**(13):12152-12162

[13] Rabe K, Lehrke M, Parhofer KG, Broedl UC. Adipokines and insulin resistance. Molecular Medicine. 2008;**14**(11-12):741

[14] Yamauchi T, Kamon J, Ito Y, Tsuchida A, Yokomizo T, Kita S, et al. Cloning of adiponectin receptors that mediate antidiabetic metabolic effects. Nature. 2003;**423**(6941):762-769

[15] Zavalza-Gómez AB, Anaya-Prado R, Rincón-Sánchez AR, Mora-Martínez JM. Adipokines and insulin resistance during pregnancy. Diabetes Research and Clinical Practice. 2008;**80**(1):8-15

[16] Fasshauer M, Klein J, Neumann S, Eszlinger M, Paschke R. Adiponectin

gene expression is inhibited by β-adrenergic stimulation via protein kinase A in 3T3-L1 adipocytes. FEBS Letters. 2001;**507**(2):142-146

[17] Fasshauer M, Klein J, Neumann S, Eszlinger M, Paschke R. Hormonal regulation of adiponectin gene expression in 3T3-L1 adipocytes. Biochemical and Biophysical Research Communications. 2002;**290**(3):1084-1089

[18] Rasouli N, Kern PA. Adipocytokines and the metabolic complications of obesity. The Journal of Clinical Endocrinology & Metabolism. 2008;**93**(11_Supplement_1):s64-s73

[19] Catalano P, Ehrenberg H. Review article: The short-and long-term implications of maternal obesity on the mother and her offspring. BJOG: An International Journal of Obstetrics & Gynaecology. 2006;**113**(10):1126-1133

[20] Lappas M, Permezel M, Rice GE. Leptin and adiponectin stimulate the release of proinflammatory cytokines and prostaglandins from human placenta and maternal adipose tissue via nuclear factor-κB, peroxisomal proliferator-activated receptor-γ and extracellularly regulated kinase 1/2. Endocrinology. 2005;**146**(8):3334-3342

[21] Masuyama H, Segawa T, Sumida Y, Masumoto A, Inoue S, Akahori Y, et al. Different profiles of circulating angiogenic factors and adipocytokines between early-and late-onset pre-eclampsia. BJOG: An International Journal of Obstetrics & Gynaecology. 2010;**117**(3):314-320

[22] Chen J, Tan B, Karteris E, Zervou S, Digby J, Hillhouse EW, et al. Secretion of adiponectin by human placenta: Differential modulation of adiponectin and its receptors by cytokines. Diabetologia. 2006;**49**(6):1292-1302

[23] Hendler I, Blackwell SC, Mehta SH, Whitty JE, Russell E, Sorokin Y, et al. The levels of leptin, adiponectin, and resistin in normal weight, overweight, and obese pregnant women with and without preeclampsia. American Journal of Obstetrics and Gynecology. 2005;**193**(3):979-983

[24] Kajantie E, Kaaja R, Ylikorkala O, Andersson S, Laivouri H. Adiponectin concentrations in maternal serum: Elevated in preeclampsia but unrelated to insulin sensitivity. Journal of the Society for Gynecologic Investigation. 2005;**12**(6):433-439

[25] Haugen F, Ranheim T, Harsem NK, Lips E, Staff AC, Drevon CA. Increased plasma levels of adipokines in preeclampsia: Relationship to placenta and adipose tissue gene expression. American Journal of Physiology. Endocrinology and Metabolism. 2006;**290**(2):E326-E333

[26] Metwally M, Ong KJ, Ledger WL, Li TC. Does high body mass index increase the risk of miscarriage after spontaneous and assisted conception? A meta-analysis of the evidence. Fertility and Sterility. 2008;**90**(3):714-726

[27] Zhang Y, Proenca R, Maffei M, Barone M, Leopold L, Friedman JM. Positional cloning of the mouse obese gene and its human homologue. Nature. 1994;**372**(6505):425-432

[28] Baratta M. Leptin—From a signal of adiposity to a hormonal mediator in peripheral tissues. Medical Science Monitor. 2002;**8**(12):RA282-RA292

[29] Webber J. Energy balance in obesity. Proceedings of the Nutrition Society. 2003;**62**(02):539-543

[30] Yeboah FA. Oxidative stress and adipokines and their health implications. Topical Series in Health Science. 2013;**1**:1-8

[31] Hauguel-de Mouzon S, Guerre-Millo M. The placenta cytokine network and inflammatory signals. Placenta. 2006;**27**(8):794-798

[32] Nuamah MA, Yura S, Sagawa N, Itoh H, Mise H, Korita D, et al. Significant increase in maternal plasma leptin concentration in induced delivery: A possible contribution of pro-inflammatory cytokines to placental leptin secretion. Endocrine Journal. 2004;**51**(2):177-187

[33] Henson MC, Castracane VD. Leptin in pregnancy: An update. Biology of Reproduction. 2006;**74**(2):218-229

[34] Schubring C, Englaro P, Siebler T, Blum W, Demirakca T, Kratzsch J, et al. Longitudinal analysis of maternal serum leptin levels during pregnancy, at birth and up to six weeks after birth: Relation to body mass index, skinfolds, sex steroids and umbilical cord blood leptin levels. Hormone Research in Pædiatrics. 1998;**50**(5):276-283

[35] Masuzaki H, Ogawa Y, Sagawa N, Hosoda K, Matsumoto T, Mise H, et al. Nonadipose tissue production of leptin: Leptin as a novel placenta-derived hormone in humans. Nature Medicine. 1997;**3**(9):1029-1033

[36] Bi S, Gavrilova O, Gong D-W, Mason MM, Reitman M. Identification of a placental enhancer for the human leptin gene. Journal of Biological Chemistry. 1997;**272**(48):30583-30588

[37] Christou H, Serdy S, Mantzoros CS. Leptin in relation to growth and developmental processes in the fetus. Seminars in Reproductive Medicine. 2002;**39**(05/06):123-130

[38] Gross GA, Solenberger T, Philpott T, Holcomb WL, Landt M. Plasma leptin concentrations in newborns of diabetic and nondiabetic mothers. American Journal of Perinatology. 1998;**11**(04):243-247

[39] Anim-Nyame N, Sooranna S, Steer P, Johnson M. Longitudinal analysis of maternal plasma leptin concentrations during normal pregnancy and pre-eclampsia. Human Reproduction. 2000;**15**(9):2033-2036

[40] Chappell LC, Seed PT, Briley A, Kelly FJ, Hunt BJ, Charnock-Jones DS, et al. A longitudinal study of biochemical variables in women at risk of preeclampsia. American Journal of Obstetrics and Gynecology. 2002;**187**(1):127-136

[41] Martinez-Abundis E, Gonzalez-Ortiz M, Pascoe-Gonzalez S. Serum leptin levels and the severity of preeclampsia. Archives of Gynecology and Obstetrics. 2000;**264**(2):71-73

[42] Aruna B, Ghosh S, Singh AK, Mande SC, Srinivas V, Chauhan R, et al. Human recombinant resistin protein displays a tendency to aggregate by forming intermolecular disulfide linkages. Biochemistry. 2003;**42**(36):10554-10559

[43] Reilly MP, Lehrke M, Wolfe ML, Rohatgi A, Lazar MA, Rader DJ. Resistin is an inflammatory marker of atherosclerosis in humans. Circulation. 2005;**111**(7):932-939

[44] Sundén-Cullberg J, Nyström T, Lee ML, Mullins GE, Tokics L, Andersson J, et al. Pronounced elevation of resistin correlates with severity of disease in severe sepsis and septic shock. Critical Care Medicine. 2007;**35**(6):1536-1542

[45] Bokarewa M, Nagaev I, Dahlberg L, Smith U, Tarkowski A. Resistin, an adipokine with potent

proinflammatory properties. The Journal of Immunology. 2005;174(9):5789-95

[46] Cortelazzi D, Corbetta S, Ronzoni S, Pelle F, Marconi A, Cozzi V, et al. Maternal and foetal resistin and adiponectin concentrations in normal and complicated pregnancies. Clinical Endocrinology. 2007;**66**(3):447-453

[47] Kielstein JT, Becker B, Graf S, Brabant G, Haller H, Fliser D. Increased resistin blood levels are not associated with insulin resistance in patients with renal disease. American Journal of Kidney Diseases. 2003;**42**(1):62-66

[48] Kendal-Wright C, Hubbard D, Bryant-Greenwood G. Chronic stretching of amniotic epithelial cells increases pre-B cell colony-enhancing factor (PBEF/visfatin) expression and protects them from apoptosis. Placenta. 2008;**29**(3):255-265

[49] Samal B, Sun Y, Stearns G, Xie C, Suggs S, McNiece I. Cloning and characterization of the cDNA encoding a novel human pre-B-cell colony-enhancing factor. Molecular and Cellular Biology. 1994;**14**(2):1431-1437

[50] Ognjanovic S, Ku TL, Bryant-Greenwood GD. Pre-B-cell colony-enhancing factor is a secreted cytokine-like protein from the human amniotic epithelium. American Journal of Obstetrics and Gynecology. 2005;**193**(1):273-282

[51] Rongvaux A, Shea RJ, Mulks MH, Gigot D, Urbain J, Leo O, et al. Pre-B-cell colony-enhancing factor, whose expression is up-regulated in activated lymphocytes, is a nicotinamide phosphoribosyltransferase, a cytosolic enzyme involved in NAD biosynthesis. European Journal of Immunology. 2002;**32**(11):3225-3234

[52] Fasshauer M, Waldeyer T, Seeger J, Schrey S, Ebert T, Kratzsch J, et al. Serum levels of the adipokine visfatin are increased in pre-eclampsia. Clinical Endocrinology. 2008;**69**(1):69-73

[53] Hu W, Wang Z, Wang H, Huang H, Dong M. Serum visfatin levels in late pregnancy and pre-eclampsia. Acta Obstetricia et Gynecologica Scandinavica. 2008;**87**(4):413-418

[54] Mazaki-Tovi S, Vaisbuch E, Romero R, Kusanovic JP, Chaiworapongsa T, Kim SK, et al. Maternal and neonatal circulating visfatin concentrations in patients with pre-eclampsia and a small-for-gestational age neonate. The Journal of Maternal-Fetal & Neonatal Medicine. 2010;**23**(10):1119-1128

[55] Salameh WA, Mastrogiannis DS. Maternal hyperlipidemia in pregnancy. Clinical Obstetrics and Gynecology. 1994;**37**(1):66-77

[56] Gürsoy A, Kulaksizoglu M, Sahin M, Ertugrul DT, Ozer F, Tutuncu NB, et al. Severe hypertriglyceridemia-induced pancreatitis during pregnancy. Journal of the National Medical Association. 2006;**98**(4):655

[57] Ephraim RK, Doe P, Amoah S, Antoh E. Lipid profile and high maternal body mass index is associated with preeclampsia: A case-control study of the Cape Coast Metropolis. Annals of Medical and Health Sciences Research. 2014;**4**(5):746-750

[58] Kirkendall WM, Burton AC, Epstein FH, Freis ED. Recommendations for human blood pressure determination by sphygmomanometers. Circulation. 1967;**36**(6):980-988

[59] Yeboah F, Ngala R, Bawah A, Mbroh H. Maternal adiposity and serum leptin levels at 11-13 weeks of gestation among pregnant women with gestational diabetes mellitus. International Journal

of Medical and Health Sciences. 2016;**5**(4):197-202

[60] Obstetricians AC. Gynecologists: Hypertension in pregnancy. Report of the American College of Obstetricians and Gynecologists' Task Force on hypertension in pregnancy. Obstetrics and Gynecology. 2013;**122**(5):1122

[61] Jakobsdottir J, Gorin MB, Conley YP, Ferrell RE, Weeks DE. Interpretation of genetic association studies: Markers with replicated highly significant odds ratios may be poor classifiers. PLoS Genetics. 2009;**5**(2):e1000337

[62] Bawah AT, Yeboah FA, Nanga S, Alidu H, Ngala R. Serum adipocytokines and adiposity as predictive indices of preeclampsia. Clinical Hypertension. 2020;**26**(1):1-11

[63] Yeboah FA, Ngala RA, Bawah AT, Asare-Anane H, Alidu H, Hamid AWM, et al. Adiposity and hyperleptinemia during the first trimester among pregnant women with preeclampsia. International Journal of Women's Health. 2017;**9**:449

[64] Ouyang Y, Chen H, Chen H. Reduced plasma adiponectin and elevated leptin in pre-eclampsia. International Journal of Gynecology & Obstetrics. 2007;**98**(2):110-114

[65] Ning Y, Williams M, Muy-Rivera M, Leisenring W, Luthy D. Relationship of maternal plasma leptin and risk of pre-eclampsia: A prospective study. The Journal of Maternal-Fetal & Neonatal Medicine. 2004;**15**(3):186-192

[66] Samolis S, Papastefanou I, Panagopoulos P, Galazios G, Kouskoukis A, Maroulis G. Relation between first trimester maternal serum leptin levels and body mass index in normotensive and pre-eclamptic pregnancies—Role of leptin as a marker of pre-eclampsia: A prospective case–control study. Gynecological Endocrinology. 2010;**26**(5):338-343

[67] Hall JE, Hildebrandt DA, Kuo J. Obesity hypertension: Role of leptin and sympathetic nervous system. American Journal of Hypertension. 2001;**14**(S3):103S-115S

[68] Craici IM, Wagner SJ, Weissgerber TL, Grande JP, Garovic VD. Advances in the pathophysiology of pre-eclampsia and related podocyte injury. Kidney International. 2014;**86**(2):275-285

[69] Cesari M, Pessina A, Zanchetta M, De Toni R, Avogaro A, Pedon L, et al. Low plasma adiponectin is associated with coronary artery disease but not with hypertension in high-risk nondiabetic patients. Journal of Internal Medicine. 2006;**260**(5):474-483

[70] Mazaki-Tovi S, Romero R, Vaisbuch E, Erez O, Mittal P, Chaiworapongsa T, et al. Maternal serum adiponectin multimers in gestational diabetes. Journal of Perinatal Medicine. 2009;**37**(6):637-650

[71] D'Anna R, Baviera G, Corrado F, Giordano D, De Vivo A, Nicocia G, et al. Adiponectin and insulin resistance in early-and late-onset pre-eclampsia. BJOG: An International Journal of Obstetrics & Gynaecology. 2006;**113**(11):1264-1269

[72] D'Anna R, Baviera G, Corrado F, Giordano D, Di Benedetto A, Jasonni VM. Plasma adiponectin concentration in early pregnancy and subsequent risk of hypertensive disorders. Obstetrics & Gynecology. 2005;**106**(2):340-344

[73] Khosrowbeygi A, Ahmadvand H. Maternal serum levels of adiponectin in preeclampsia. Journal of Ayub Medical College Abbottabad. 2009;**21**(3):79-82

[74] Nien JK, Mazaki-Tovi S, Romero R, Erez O, Kusanovic JP, Gotsch F, et al.

Adiponectin in severe preeclampsia. Journal of Perinatal Medicine. 2007;**35**(6):503-512

[75] Ramsay JE, Jamieson N, Greer IA, Sattar N. Paradoxical elevation in adiponectin concentrations in women with preeclampsia. Hypertension. 2003;**42**(5):891-894

[76] Kintscher U, Unger T. Vascular protection in diabetes: A pharmacological view of angiotensin II type 1 receptor blockers. Acta Diabetologica. 2005;**42**:s26-s32

[77] Danqing C, Minyue D, Qin F, Jing H, Zhengping W, Xiaofu Y. Alterations of serum resistin in normal pregnancy and pre-eclampsia. Clinical Science. 2005;**108**(1):81-84

[78] Chen D, Shi Z, Dong M, Fang Q, He J, Wang Z, et al. [Relationship between serum resistin level and preeclampsia]. Zhejiang da xue xue bao Yi xue ban. Journal of Zhejiang University (Medical Science). 2005;**34**(6):503-528

[79] Mastorakos G, Valsamakis G, apatheodorou DC, Barlas I, Margeli A, Boutsiadis A, et al. The role of adipocytokines in insulin resistance in normal pregnancy: Visfatin concentrations in early pregnancy predict insulin sensitivity. Clinical Chemistry. 2007;**53**(8):1477-1483

[80] Fasshauer M, Blüher M, Stumvoll M, Tönessen P, Faber R, Stepan H. Differential regulation of visfatin and adiponectin in pregnancies with normal and abnormal placental function. Clinical Endocrinology. 2007;**66**(3):434-439

[81] Bodnar LM, Ness RB, Markovic N, Roberts JM. The risk of preeclampsia rises with increasing prepregnancy body mass index. Annals of Epidemiology. 2005;**15**(7):475-482

[82] Cedergren MI. Maternal morbid obesity and the risk of adverse pregnancy outcome. Obstetrics & Gynecology. 2004;**103**(2):219-224

[83] Conde-Agudelo A, Belizán JM. Risk factors for pre-eclampsia in a large cohort of Latin American and Caribbean women. BJOG: An International Journal of Obstetrics & Gynaecology. 2000;**107**(1):75-83

[84] Luealon P, Phupong V. Risk factors of preeclampsia in Thai women. Journal of the Medical Association of Thailand = Chotmaihet thangphaet. 2010;**93**(6):661-666

[85] Frühbeck G. Pivotal role of nitric oxide in the control of blood pressure after leptin administration. Diabetes. 1999;**48**(4):903-908

[86] Lima VJD, Andrade CRD, Ruschi GE, Sass N. Serum lipid levels in pregnancies complicated by preeclampsia. São Paulo Medical Journal. 2011;**129**(2):73-76

[87] Onat A, Hergenç G, Sarı I, Türkmen S, Can G, Sansoy V. Dyslipidemic hypertension: Distinctive features and cardiovascular risk in a prospective population-based study. American Journal of Hypertension. 2005;**18**(3):409-416

[88] Arngrimsson R, Björnsson S, Geirsson RT, Björnsson H, Walker JJ, Snaedal G. Gynaecology: Genetic and familial predisposition to eclampsia and pre-eclampsia in a defined population. BJOG: An International Journal of Obstetrics & Gynaecology. 1990;**97**(9):762-769

[89] Cincotta R, Brennecke SP. Obstetrics: Family history of pre-eclampsia as a predictor for pre-eclampsia in primigravidas. Journal of Gynecology & Obstetrics. 1998;**60**(1):23-27

Chapter 12

Cardiovascular Health in Kawasaki Disease

Mitsuru Seki

Abstract

Kawasaki disease (KD) is a self-limiting vasculitis of unknown etiology primarily affecting young children. The most important aspect in the treatment of KD is the prevention of coronary artery lesions (CALs) because myocardial ischemia or infarction due to coronary artery stenosis or occlusion may be lethal. In addition, patients with a history of KD have systemic vasculitis, which indicates vascular endothelial damage. Therefore, patients with CAL are at a high risk of atherosclerosis. While some reports have shown an increase in vascular stiffness, others have not, and the presence of atherosclerotic lesions in patients with KD is controversial. Appropriate acute-phase treatment to prevent CAL and systemic vasculitis and subsequent regular follow-ups are important. This chapter deals with the cardiovascular health of patients with a history of KD.

Keywords: vasculitis, aortic stiffness, atherosclerosis, vascular health, Kawasaki disease

1. Introduction

Kawasaki disease (KD) was first reported as acute febrile mucocutaneous lymph node syndrome by Tomisaku Kawasaki in 1967. KD is a self-limited vasculitis affecting children mainly under 5 years of age, the etiology is still unknown [1, 2]. KD is one of the most common acquired cardiac disorders in children, causing coronary artery dilatation or aneurysms. Coronary artery lesion (CAL) develop in approximately 25% of KD patients who do not receive appropriate treatment [3]. As KD is a systemic vasculitis, vessel walls other than coronary arteries are affected. KD patients with cardiovascular complications should be closely monitored for cardiovascular events throughout their lives. Furthermore, even in the absence of obvious complications, patients with a history of KD are likely to experience underlying vascular endothelial damage. This chapter deals with long-term cardiovascular health in this population.

2. Epidemiology

KD is a systemic vasculitis that mainly affects children younger than 5 years of age. Currently, more than 60 countries in Asia, the Middle East, the Americas, Africa, and Europe have reported KD cases [4]. The incidence of KD is high in Japan, Korea, and Taiwan, but low in North America and European countries. These incidences reported in different regions of the world can be affected by the survey/surveillance methods used, clinical diagnostic and treatment practices, physician awareness of KD, and data sources used to estimate incidence [5].

According to a nationwide epidemiological survey of KD in Japan, more than 15,000 patients were reported annually until 2019, which was before Coronavirus disease 2019 (COVID-19) pandemic [6]. The annual number of patients with KD in Japan was 17,364 in 2019; however, it decreased to 11,173 in 2020. The incidence rate (per 100,000 children aged 0–4 years per year) was 370.8 (410.1 in boys, and 329.4 in girls) in 2019, and 238.8 (267.3 in boys, and 208.9 in girls) in 2020. Although infectious factors or foreign antigens can trigger KD, the cause of this syndrome remains unclear. Several children diagnosed with COVID-19 have developed multisystem inflammatory syndrome in children (MIS-C), which shows KD-like symptoms [7, 8]. On the other hand, the decline in the incidence of KD remains small, despite the extreme reduction in common pediatric infectious diseases during the COVID-19 pandemic period in Japan, KD may be triggered by unidentified respiratory pathogens that can be acquired both within and outside the household [9].

Genetic factors appear to be involved in KD pathogenesis, as suggested by the highest incidence among Asians and Pacific Islanders, and in boys versus girls. In a genome-wide linkage study, several functional polymorphisms such as *inositol 1,4,5-trisphosphate 3-kinase C (ITPKC)* and *caspase-3 (CASP3)* have been identified as common susceptibility genes for KD. Siblings of children with KD have an increased risk of developing the disease [10]. Sibling pairs with KD within a short time interval may be due to environmental triggers, including infectious antigens. Both genetic and environmental factors are thought to interact with each other during the onset of KD; therefore, a detailed study of these contributing factors may help elucidate the pathogenesis of KD.

3. Histopathology of vasculitis

The histopathological characteristics of KD are as follows: (1) major muscular arteries branching from the aorta, including the coronary arteries, are predominantly injured; (2) the damaged arteries are extra-arterial, not arteries within organs; (3) acute vasculitis occurs synchronously throughout the body; and (4) vasculitis is a proliferative inflammation consisting of an abnormal accumulation of monocytes/macrophages.

KD is characterized by inflammation of the coronary artery in the acute phase, which usually lasts for approximately 6 weeks. The earliest histological changes in coronary arteritis are seen on sixth to eighth day of illness, starting with the infiltration of inflammatory cells in the tunica adventitia and tunica intima. Inflammatory cells infiltrate the tunica media, leading to inflammation of all layers of the vessel wall by the tenth day of illness. Subsequently, the artery begins to dilate owing to significant damage to the internal elastic lamina or tunica media. Inflammatory cell infiltration continues for approximately 2 weeks and then gradually fades. If the vessel wall undergoes a certain degree of damage, even after vasculitis subsides, inflammatory scarring of the coronary artery remains for a long time. In particular, in patients with coronary aneurysms, various findings, such as stenotic lesions or extensive calcification of the aneurysm wall, are observed [11].

In addition to the coronary arteries, other systemic blood vessels are injured by vasculitis [12]. Whole-body examination for KD to evaluate systemic vasculitis shows vascular damage at various sites, especially in the subclavian, brachial, axillary, and iliac arteries. Many case reports have revealed that systemic arterial aneurysms are almost always associated with giant coronary arterial aneurysms, and a detailed evaluation should be considered in these patients.

4. Diagnosis and acute therapy for KD

The recent diagnostic guidelines in Japan are shown in **Table 1** [13]. The typical clinical symptoms are shown in **Figure 1**. Acute treatment should be initiated immediately after diagnosis to prevent cardiovascular complications. Although the incidence of CAL was reported in 23–43% of patients treated only with aspirin, treatment with IVIG and aspirin for four consecutive days reduced the incidence of CAL to 8–15% [14, 15]. Moreover, a single infusion of 2 g/kg IVIG, which is the current standard regimen, reduces the incidence of CAL to 4.6% [16]. Therefore, IVIG is currently the standard therapy for acute KD. A systematic review by the Cochrane Collaboration revealed that the development of CAL can be reduced by a single dose of 2 g/kg IVIG administered before the tenth day of illness [17].

The risk of developing CAL is closely related to responsiveness to treatment. KD patients with IVIG resistance are at an increased risk of developing CALs compared

Principal clinical features
1. Fever.
2. Bilateral bulbar conjunctival injection.
3. Changes of lips and oral cavity: reddening of lips, strawberry tongue, diffuse injection of oral and pharyngeal mucosa.
4. Rash (including redness at the site of Bacille Calmette- Guerin (BCG) inoculation).
5. Changes of peripheral extremities: (Initial stage) reddening of palms and soles, edema. (Convalescent stage) periungual desquamation.
6. Non-supparative cervical lymphadenopathy.
Other significant demographic, clinical, echocardiographic, and laboratory features
1. Kawasaki disease may be suspected in the presence of fewer than four principal clinical features when the following findings are observed: • Elevation of hepatic transaminases early in the course of the disease. • Increased leukocytes in the urine sediment of an infant. • Thrombocytosis in the convalescent phase • Elevation of BNP or NT-pro BNP • Mitral valve regurgitation or pericardial effusion by echocardiography • Enlargement of the gallbladder (hydrops of gallbladder) • Hypoalbuminemia or hyponatremia
2. If a KD patient manifests the following findings, the patient should be considered for admission of a critical care unit. • Hemodynamically significant myocarditis • Hypotention (shock) • Paralytic ileus • Decreased level of consciousness

3. Risk scores to predict intravenous immunoglobulin resistance may be applied to guide patient management. The following features are elements of the risk scores for predicting intravenous immunoglobulin resistance.
   - Leukocytosis with left shift
   - thrombocytopenia
   - hypoalbuminemia
   - hyponatremia
   - hyperbilirubinemia (jaundice)
   - elevation of CRP
   - Age <1 year
4. Other non-specific findings which may be observed in Kawasaki Disease and should not exclude the diagnosis.
   - Irritability
   - Cardiovascular: abnormal extra heart sounds, electrocardiogram changes, aneurysm of peripheral arteries other than coronary (axillary etc.),
   - Gastrointestinal: abdominal pain, vomiting, diarrhea
   - Hematologic: increased erythrocyte sedimentation rate, anemia
   - Dermatologic: micropustular rash, transverse grooves across the finger nails.
   - Respiratory: cough, rhinorrhea, retropharyngeal edema, infiltrate on chest radiograph.
   - Rheumatologic: pain, swelling.
   - Neurologic: cerebrospinal fluid pleocytosis, seizures, facial nerve palsy, paralysis of the extremities.

Table 1.
Diagnostic guideline for Kawasaki disease.

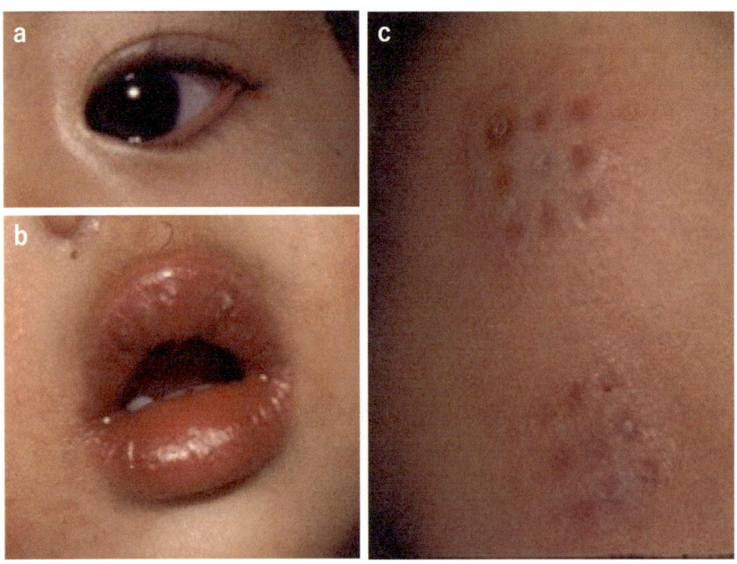

Figure 1.
Typical clinical symptoms of Kawasaki disease. (a) Bulbar conjunctival injection, (b) Reddening of lips, (c) Redness at the site of Bacille Calmette-Guerin inoculation.

to IVIG responders; therefore, various additional treatments such as prednisolone, infliximab, cyclosporine, urinary trypsin inhibitors, and plasma exchange have been established to prevent CAL.

In addition, to improve the prognosis of CALs, several risk-scoring systems to predict IVIG non-responders before initial treatment have been established and are widely used in clinical practice in Japan [18–20]. For patients with a high-risk score, two randomized control trials revealed the efficacy of a first-line combined treatment strategy, IVIG and prednisolone or IVIG and cyclosporin A [21, 22]. As several reports from other countries revealed that these risk-scoring systems are inadaptable to the prediction of IVIG non-responders in regions other than Japan [23, 24], it may be desirable to develop risk-scoring systems that can be used globally or an original scoring system to be adapted to each region for the suppression of KD vasculitis. Although these strategies have improved the prognosis of coronary arteries, the occurrence of giant coronary aneurysms is still observed, and further treatment is desirable.

5. Cardiovascular risk and management

KD is a systemic vasculitis that can lead to atherosclerosis due to vascular dysfunction and damage. Long-term management should consider the cardiovascular risk of atherosclerosis progression in both coronary arteries and systemic vessels.

5.1 Coronary arteries

Coronary artery aneurysms that remain 30 days after the onset of KD are defined as cardiovascular complications of KD. Aneurysms impair vascular endothelial function and thrombus formation. **Figure 2** shows the giant aneurysms identified angiographically in patients with IVIG-resistant KD. This can lead to angina or myocardial infarction owing to coronary artery stenosis or occlusion. In addition, calcification of the vessel wall is frequently observed. However, it is estimated that 75% of coronary aneurysms regress within 3 years of onset [25]. Even when aneurysms remain, they often become smaller in diameter than those in the early stages.

The management strategies in the follow-up stage included (1) prevention of thrombosis in aneurysms and myocardial infarction, (2) early diagnosis of myocardial ischemia and appropriate reperfusion therapy, and (3) management of the risk of atherosclerosis and preventive education.

5.1.1 Prevention of thrombosis in aneurysms and myocardial infarction

In KD patients with CAL, it is important to prevent cardiac events. In general, these patients require aspirin or other antiplatelet agents. Anticoagulants are administered mainly in cases of giant coronary artery aneurysms. Additionally, statin therapy may improve chronic vascular inflammation and endothelial dysfunction, which has been suggested to be useful for vascular health. Statins have multifaceted pharmacological effects, including anti-inflammatory, antioxidant, anticoagulant, and thrombolytic effects, as well as a decrease in serum cholesterol levels. Additionally, statins are expected to be effective in improving vascular endothelial function. According to a statement from the American Heart Association, KD patients with CAL need to be treated prophylactically.

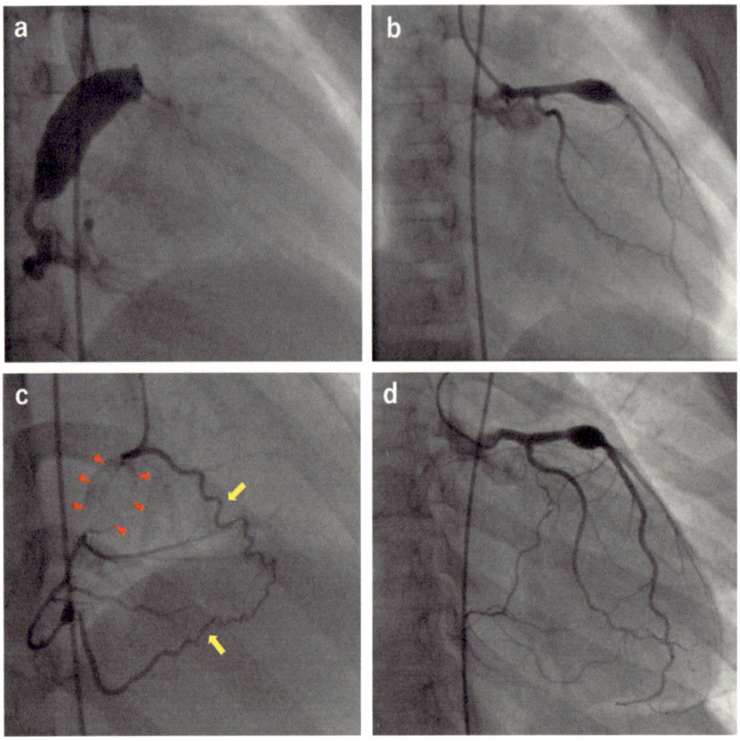

Figure 2.
Giant aneurysms. (a), (b) Coronary angiography in 4-year-old patient with giant aneurysms. This patient was treated with warfarin and aspirin since diagnosis of giant aneurysm. (a) Selective right coronary arteriography. Giant aneurysm was identified. (b) Selective left coronary arteriography. Medium size aneurysm was identified at left anterior descending artery. (c), (d) Follow-up coronary angiography at age 9 (5 years later). (c) Selective right coronary arteriography. Giant aneurysm was occluded (red arrow head) and collateral arteries had developed to the periphery of the right coronary artery (yellow arrow). (b) Selective left coronary arteriography. Medium size aneurysm did not change significantly and no stenotic lesions were detected.

5.1.2 Early diagnosis of myocardial ischemia and appropriate reperfusion therapy

Critical stenotic lesions are sometimes observed at the proximal and distal ends of coronary aneurysms. These findings are believed to be caused by vascular remodeling. Coronary artery stenosis was evaluated using coronary angiography, coronary functional flow reserve, enhanced coronary computed tomography, and stress myocardial scintigraphy. These tests should be performed periodically depending on the severity of the coronary artery aneurysm. Although coronary revascularization is required in less than 1% of patients with a history of KD, percutaneous coronary intervention or coronary artery bypass grafting is required when myocardial ischemia is detected using these modalities.

5.1.3 Management of risk of atherosclerosis and the preventive education

In cases of aneurysms larger than medium size, vascular endothelial dysfunction, chronic inflammation in the vessel wall, and subsequent vascular remodeling continue to occur even late after the onset of KD. Although the details have not yet been elucidated, vascular endothelial damage and chronic inflammation resemble the early lesions of atherosclerosis and may be predisposing factors for future atherosclerosis.

Therefore, it is necessary to actively eliminate cardiovascular risk factors at a younger age. In other words, education on the prevention of hypertension and obesity, smoking cessation, management of blood sugar and lipids, and reduction of psychological stress are important for long-term management.

5.2 Systemic vessels

It is well known that vascular stiffness increases in the atherosclerotic vasculature. Patients with KD have systemic vasculitis because inflammation occurs in medium-sized muscular arteries throughout the body. While some KD patients show vessel lesions throughout the body, the association between KD vasculitis in the acute phase and atherosclerosis in long-term follow-up remains unclear.

The relationship between atherosclerotic lesions and the development of myocardial infarction has long been established in adult patients. It has also been reported that increased aortic stiffness is associated with coronary atherosclerosis, as such, this could be an important predictive marker for cardiovascular events [26]. Given these findings, KD patients with CAL may be at risk of developing atherosclerosis.

It is well known that functional impairment of vascular endothelial cells exists before morphological changes such as vascular intima-media thickening. Recently, the importance of assessment of vascular function has been suggested for vascular health. Although several evaluation methods have been reported, these parameters have mainly been published to understand the pathophysiology of vascular dysfunction in KD. In the future, these indices should be implemented in clinical practice and used for the appropriate follow-up of patients with KD. The following is an overview of each indicator:

5.2.1 Percentage change in flow-mediated dilatation: %FMD

Percentage change in flow-mediated dilatation (%FMD) reflects endothelial nitric oxide-dependent vasodilatation. A significant decrease in %FMD is a common feature of atherosclerosis in adults. Some meta-analyses reported that %FMD was lower in the KD group than in the control group, indicating endothelial damage and a risk of atherosclerosis [27–29]. Several previous studies have reported that the %FMD was significantly lower in patients with a history of KD than in control subjects, showing systemic endothelial dysfunction late after KD onset [30–32]. Interestingly, in pediatric patients with CAL late after KD, there is increased high-sensitivity C-reactive protein in addition to reduced %FMD, indicating the presence of ongoing chronic vascular inflammation and endothelial dysfunction [31].

5.2.2 Pulse wave velocity: PWV

Noninvasive evaluations of vascular elasticity have also been well documented. Pulse-wave velocity (PWV) is a representative parameter for evaluating arterial stiffness. PWV is a simple and noninvasive test for evaluating arterial stiffness. PWV can be measured from various arterial sites, and pressure waveforms are usually obtained percutaneously at the common carotid and femoral arteries. Several methods have been developed to measure PWV, including aortic PWV, brachial-radial PWV, and brachial-ankle PWV. There have been some reports on the measurement of brachial-radial or brachial-ankle PWV, showing a significant increase in arterial stiffness in the KD group compared with the control group, regardless of whether the patients had

CAL [33–35], however, the relationship between vascular stiffness and prognosis is not clear. Although aortic PWV is a known predictor of cardiovascular events [36], no large prognostic studies examining the association between brachial-radial or brachial-ankle PWV and cardiovascular events have been performed. This limitation should be noted when the PWV is used.

5.2.3 Cardio-ankle vascular index: CAVI

The cardio-ankle vascular index (CAVI) is a representative parameter for evaluating arterial stiffness. Because CAVI is obtained by calculating the stiffness parameter β, which indicates the intrinsic stiffness of the blood vessels, CAVI is also theoretically independent of blood pressure. One study reported that there was no significant difference between the KD group without CAL and the control group [37]. CAVI assesses more central vascular stiffness than PVW; therefore, it is speculated that injury to the great vessel may be mild or absent in KD vasculitis. Because CAVI is a relatively new parameter, further studies are needed to elucidate vascular function in patients with a history of KD.

6. Conclusion

In patients with a history of KD, the pathogenesis of vascular complications and long-term prognosis are being elucidated by many studies. This suggests an increased risk of atherosclerosis in these populations. However, there are few reports of an increased incidence of atherosclerotic lesions in adult KD patients. Further studies are needed, and careful management of long-term vascular health is required by evaluating vascular function using these clinical tools.

Author details

Mitsuru Seki
Department of Pediatrics, Jichi Medical University, Tochigi, Japan

*Address all correspondence to: m-seki@jichi.ac.jp

References

[1] Kawasaki T. Acute febrile mucocutaneous syndrome with lymphoid involvement with specific desquamation of the fingers and toes in children. Arerugī. 1967;**16**:178-222

[2] Kawasaki T, Kosaki F, Okawa S, Shigematsu I, Yanagawa H. A new infantile acute febrile mucocutaneous lymph node syndrome (MLNS) prevailing in Japan. Pediatrics. 1974;**54**:271-276

[3] Newburger JW, Takahashi M, Burns JC. Kawasaki disease. Journal of the American College of Cardiology. 2016;**67**:1738-1749

[4] Nakamura Y, Yanagawa H. The worldwide epidemiology of Kawasaki disease. Progress in Pediatric Cardiology. 2004;**19**:99-108

[5] Uehara R, Belay ED. Epidemiology of Kawasaki disease in Asia, Europe, and the United States. Journal of Epidemiology. 2012;**22**(2):79-85

[6] Makino N, Nakamura Y, Yashiro M, et al. Nationwide epidemiologic survey of Kawasaki disease in Japan, 2015-2016. Pediatrics International. 2019;**61**:397-403

[7] Verdoni L, Mazza A, Gervasoni A, et al. An outbreak of severe Kawasaki-like disease at the Italian epicentre of the SARS-CoV-2 epidemic: An observational cohort study. Lancet. 2020;**395**:1771-1778

[8] Belhadjer Z, Meot M, Bajolle F, et al. Acute heart failure in multisystem inflammatory syndrome in children in the context of global SARS-CoV-2 pandemic. Circulation. 2020;**142**:429-436

[9] Ae R, Shibata Y, Kosami K, et al. Kawasaki disease and pediatric infectious diseases during the coronavirus disease 2019 pandemic. The Journal of Pediatrics. 2021;**239**:50-58

[10] Fujita Y, Nakamura Y, Sakata K, et al. Kawasaki disease in families. Pediatrics. 1989;**84**:666-669

[11] Harada M, Yokouchi Y, Oharaseki T, et al. Histopathological characteristics of myocarditis in acute-phase Kawasaki disease. Histopathology. 2012;**61**:1156-1167

[12] Takahashi K, Oharaseki T, Yokouchi Y, Hiruta N, Naoe S. Kawasaki disease as a systemic vasculitis in childhood. Annals of Vascular Diseases. 2010;**3**:173-181

[13] Kobayashi T, Ayusawa M, Suzuki H, et al. Revision of diagnostic guidelines for Kawasaki disease (6th revised edition). Pediatrics International. 2020;**62**:1135-1138

[14] Furusho K, Kamiya T, Nakano H, et al. High-dose intravenous gammaglobulin for Kawasaki disease. Lancet. 1984;**2**:1055-1058

[15] Newburger JW, Takahashi M, Burns JC, et al. The treatment of Kawasaki syndrome with intravenous gamma globulin. The New England Journal of Medicine. 1986;**315**:341-347

[16] Newburger JW, Takahashi M, Beiser AS, et al. A single intravenous infusion of gamma globulin as compared with four infusions in the treatment of acute Kawasaki syndrome. The New England Journal of Medicine. 1991;**324**:1633-1639

[17] Oates-Whitehead RM, Baumer JH, Haines L, et al. Intravenous

immunoglobulin for the treatment of Kawasaki disease in children. Cochrane Database of Systematic Reviews. 2003;**4**:CD004000

[18] Kobayashi T, Inoue Y, Takeuchi K, et al. Prediction of intravenous immunoglobulin unresponsiveness in patients with Kawasaki disease. Circulation. 2006;**113**:2606-2612

[19] Egami K, Muta H, Ishii M, et al. Prediction of resistance to intravenous immunoglobulin treatment in patients with Kawasaki disease. The Journal of Pediatrics. 2006;**149**:237-240

[20] Sano T, Kurotobi S, Matsuzaki K, et al. Prediction of non-responsiveness to standard high-dose gamma-globulin therapy in patients with acute Kawasaki disease before starting initial treatment. European Journal of Pediatrics. 2007;**166**:131-137

[21] Kobayashi T, Saji T, Otani T, et al. Efficacy of immunoglobulin plus prednisolone for prevention of coronary artery abnormalities in severe Kawasaki disease (RAISE study): A randomised, open-label, blinded-endpoints trial. Lancet. 2012;**379**:1613-1620

[22] Hamada H, Suzuki H, Onouchi Y, et al. Efficacy of primary treatment with immunoglobulin plus ciclosporin for prevention of coronary artery abnormalities in patients with Kawasaki disease predicted to be at increased risk of non-response to intravenous immunoglobulin (KAICA): A randomised controlled, open-label, blinded-endpoints, phase 3 trial. Lancet. 2019;**393**:1128-1137

[23] Sleeper LA, Minich LL, McCrindle BM, et al. Evaluation of Kawasaki disease risk-scoring systems for intravenous immunoglobulin resistance. The Journal of Pediatrics. 2011;**158**:831-835e3

[24] Fabi M, Andreozzi L, Corinaldesi E, et al. Inability of Asian risk scoring systems to predict intravenous immunoglobulin resistance and coronary lesions in Kawasaki disease in an Italian cohort. European Journal of Pediatrics. 2019;**178**:315-322

[25] Friedman KG, Gauvreau K, Hamaoka-Okamoto A, et al. Coronary artery aneurysms in Kawasaki disease: Risk factors for progressive disease and adverse cardiac events in the US population. Journal of the American Heart Association. 2016;**15**(5):e003289

[26] Duprez DA, Cohn JN. Arterial stiffness as a risk factor for coronary atherosclerosis. Current Atherosclerosis Reports. 2007;**9**:139-144

[27] Zeng YY, Chen F, Zhang Y, Ji X. Are patients recovering from Kawasaki disease at increased risk for accelerated atherosclerosis? A meta-analysis. World Journal of Pediatrics. 2021;**17**:476-483

[28] Zhang H, Xu MG, Xie LJ, Huang M, Shen J, Xiao TT. Meta-analysis of risk factors associated with atherosclerosis in patients with Kawasaki disease. World Journal of Pediatrics. 2016;**12**:308-313

[29] Dietz SM, Tacke CE, Hutten BA, et al. Peripheral endothelial (dys) function, arterial stiffness and carotid intima-media thickness in patients after Kawasaki disease: A systematic review and meta-analyses. PLoS One. 2015;**10**:e0130913

[30] Dhillon R, Clarkson P, Donald AE, et al. Endothelial dysfunction late after Kawasaki disease. Circulation. 1996;**94**:2103-2106

[31] Huang SM, Weng KP, Chang JS, Lee WY, Huang SH, Hsieh KS. Effects of statin therapy in children complicated with coronary arterial abnormality late

after Kawasaki disease: A pilot study. Circulation Journal. 2008;**72**:1583-1587

[32] Kadono T, Sugiyama H, Hoshiai M, et al. Endothelial function evaluated by flow-mediated dilatation in pediatric vascular disease. Pediatric Cardiology. 2005;**26**:385-390

[33] Ooyanagi R, Fuse S, Tomita H, et al. Pulse wave velocity and ankle brachial index in patients with Kawasaki disease. Pediatrics International. 2004;**46**:398-402

[34] Cheung YF, Yung TC, Tam SC, Ho MH, Chau AK. Novel and traditional cardiovascular risk factors in children after Kawasaki disease: Implications for premature atherosclerosis. Journal of the American College of Cardiology. 2004;**43**:120-124

[35] Cho HJ, Yang SI, Kim KH, Kim JN, Kil HR. Cardiovascular risk factors of early atherosclerosis in school-aged children after Kawasaki disease. Korean Journal of Pediatrics. 2014;**57**:217-221

[36] Vlachopoulos C, Aznaouridis K, Stefanadis C. Prediction of cardiovascular events and all-cause mortality with arterial stiffness: A systematic review and meta-analysis. Journal of the American College of Cardiology. 2010;**55**:1318-1327

[37] Nakagawa R, Kuwata S, Kurishima C, et al. Arterial stiffness in patients after Kawasaki disease without coronary artery involvement: Assessment by performing brachial ankle pulse wave velocity and cardio-ankle vascular index. Journal of Cardiology. 2015;**66**:130-134

Chapter 13

Takayasu Arteritis: Review in Pediatrics

Melisa Rivera, Jose Heriberto López-Beltrán and Blanca Frisia Morales-López

Abstract

Takayasu arteritis (TA) is classified as a large-vessel vasculitis, and it primarily affects the aorta and principal branches. The clinical presentation in pediatric patients is odd and there are few literature about it because of its low incidence and nonspecific clinical presentation. The standardized diagnosis of TA is by imaging support, such as computed tomography (CT) and magnetic resonance imaging (MRI). When using CT, angio-CT is recommended because it will allow us to observe the caliber of the arteries, wall changes, and level of stenosis. The study should include the aortic arch, abdominal aorta, visceral branches, and iliac arteries taking into account that the mainly affected arteries are the left subclavian, abdominal aorta, right renal artery, and descending chest aorta. In the same way in the study, four imaging patterns of TA can be identified: variable decrease in the luminal diameter of the aorta and arteries, total occlusion, fusiform and saccular aneurysm, and irregular contour of the aortic wall. Identifying TA findings is important for early diagnosis, medical management, and proper monitoring specifically in pediatric patients where literature is little available.

Keywords: Takayasu arteritis, large-vessel vasculitis, pediatrics, rheumatology, biological agents

1. Introduction

Takayasu arteritis is a rare vasculitis with no clear etiology presented most of the time in young women. It is even more rare to be presented in children. The clinical characteristics of the disease can be very unspecific and make it harder to diagnose. The diagnosis is done through image criteria along with several clinical data. Treatment is described as multiple options depending on severity and availability. It is important to know the characteristics of this large-vessel vasculitis to be able to identify and treat these patients as soon as possible, the severity and prognosis can vary depending on gender, age, and ethnicity, having a worse prognosis in younger children and African patients. This chapter talks about the characteristics of this disease and how it can be different in adult patients compared to pediatrics.

2. Takayasu arteritis: review in pediatrics

Takayasu arteritis (TA) is classified as a large-vessel vasculitis. It affects the aorta and major branches by causing stenosis, occlusion, and/or aneurysms of the vessel; it is an inflammatory disease with unknown etiology. Predominantly presented in females.

Takayasu arteritis was first described by Doctor Mikito Takayasu, a Japanese ophthalmologist, after a case of changes in the retinal vessels of a 22 year old female in 1908. Since then, there have been many case reports that matched Dr. Takayasu's patient and the disease received many names like pulseless disease, aortic arch syndrome, or obstructive productive arteritis. It was until 1990 when the American College of Rheumatology published and described the disease named "Takayasu arteritis" publishing with it classification criteria for its diagnosis [1].

2.1 Epidemiology

TA is a rare disease and its frequency seems to be influenced by ethnicity. It is generally known to be presented in females under 40 years of age, but it can be seen in older patients as well as children. There is not a statistical value that is acceptable for the general population since the prevalence can vary a lot by ethnicity. TA is known to be a more popular vasculitis in Asia, and their countries have the highest prevalence. In Japan, the prevalence is higher than 4/million. In the United Kingdom, they have an incidence of 0.8/million. North America has an incidence of 2.6/million [2, 3].

Ethnicity does not only affect the incidence and prevalence of the disease, it can also affect the characteristics of presentation, the intensity of symptoms, and the prognosis of the patient. A French retrospective study compared black, white, and North African patients with TA and found that North African patients had lower survival rates in 5 and 10 years than the other two ethnicities, all because North African patients had more ischemic relapses; also white patients seem to have a prolonged diagnosis, according to the mean age of diagnosis, being 10 years later than North African and black patients [4].

The manifestation of TA can also vary, for example, Japanese patients seem to have the aortic arch and branches affected and Indian patients have abdominal aorta and branches more frequently affected [5].

2.1.1 Epidemiology in children

In children, it is very rare to see TA, and because of that there is not a lot of data, there is an estimated incidence of TA in children that is 2.6/ million of all ages. A very limited study of 21 patients in the United States found that it continues to be more common in females, having 71% of their population being females, and having a very large age gap for symptoms on set, from 1.5 months to 17 years, having a median age of 13 years old [6].

2.2 Pathogenesis

The pathogenesis of TA remains unclear, although the involvement of immune mechanisms mediated by cells that secrete proinflammatory cytokines is known to play an important role, so this leads to the use of cytokine-targeting agents, such as TNF or IL-6 inhibitors as treatment [7, 8].

Inflammatory infiltrates of the arterial wall consist of macrophages and lymphoid cells. Th1 and Th17 responses seem to play an important role as demonstrated by an increased expression of Th1 and Th17 immunity in TA, such inflammation that correlates with disease activity [8].

A possible genetic association, a polymorphism of tumor necrosis factor (TNF) has been studied and both human leukocyte antigen (HLA) classes I and II have been associated with TA, and most notably, the HLA-B52 allele has been reported across multiple ethnicities. The genetic contribution to disease pathogenesis is supported by the identification of multiple susceptibility loci in various studies. This disease was also associated with IL-6, RPS9/LILRB3, and an intergenic locus on chromosome 21q22 [7, 8].

Both the innate and adaptive immune systems seem to be involved in the pathogenesis of TA. The inflammatory process usually involves the vasa vasorum, the adventitia, and the outer part of the media and results in vessel wall damage with laminar necrosis and elastic fiber fragmentation, which is eventually replaced by fibrosis and arterial remodeling [8].

The involvement of humoral immune mechanisms is evidenced by the presence of circulating antiendothelial cell antibodies and autoantibody-producing B cells in inflammatory TA lesions that may cause vascular dysfunction. Also, TA patients have also been shown to generate a significantly large number of plasmablasts. These results lend support to the use of anti-B-cell agents in the treatment of TA [8].

2.3 Clinical presentation

TA clinical onset and clinical characteristics can be very hard to describe or identify since it is a compile of nonspecific inflammatory symptoms. We can divide TAK clinical presentation into two phases:

- Active phase or inflammatory phase, where we will have symptoms, such as fever, myalgia, weakness, arthralgias.

- Chronic phase, where it affects the aorta and branches having symptoms of ischemia.

The active phase can be very nonspecific and have different intensity of symptoms, and it seems that the active phase can be more intense in pediatric patients and have different symptoms than in adults (**Table 1**) [9].

2.4 Diagnostic criteria

The diagnosis of TA is made with specific criteria. The initial criteria created by the American College of Rheumatology (ACR) in 1990 has a sensitivity of 91% and a specificity of 98%. The diagnosis is made when the patient has three of the six diagnostic criteria. In 2009, the European Alliance of Associations for Rheumatology (EULAR) published a guide for large-vessel vasculitis, including TA, with an update in 2018. The new guides have greater sensitivity (100%) because they include a diagnostic criteria that is necessary for the diagnosis, which is an angiographic abnormality in any kind of imaging study, with greater accessibility to imaging studies nowadays the EULAR criteria is the go to criteria (**Tables 2** and **3**) [10].

Parameter	Child-onset TA	Adult-onset TA
Median age of onset (years)	14	26
Median symptom duration (months)	12	16
Pulse loss/asymmetry (%)	61.3	70.8
Systolic hypertension (%)	66.4	48.4
Vascular bruit (%)	46.2	51.9
Diastolic hypertension (%)	43.7	38.9
Claudication (%)	38.7	54.6
Malaise/fatigue (%)	33.6	31.5
Headache (%)	31.1	18.2
Fever at presentation (%)	29.4	17.4
Dyspnea (%)	23.5	25.1
Raised creatinine (%)	15.9	4.7
Weight loss (%)	10.1	13.4
Visual disturbance (%)	11.8	7.0
Syncope (%)	7.6	11.8

Table 1.
Comparison of onset symptoms in children with Takayasu arteritis (cTAK) and adults with Takayasu arteritis (aTAK) [9].

ACR diagnostic criteria for Takayasu arteritis. Diagnosis is made with three positive items
<40 years
Claudication of extremities
Decreased brachial pulse
Blood pressure difference >10 mmhg
Arteriographic abnormality
Bruit over subclavian arteries or aorta

Table 2.
ACR diagnosis criteria for Takayasu arteritis.

2.4.1 Imaging diagnosis

There are multiple imaging tools that are useful in these patients. Some are specific to make our diagnosis and others provide a complete evaluation of our patients.

The gold standard in image study is the digital subtraction arteriography since it provides a very specific view of the arteries where the caliber is measurable with more precision, as well as compares the difference in width all along the aorta and branches. Since digital subtraction arteriography is not available in every clinical center, other image studies can help with the diagnosis.

Magnetic resonance imaging (MRI) or computed angiotomography is usually more available and can also be very helpful in assessing the caliber of vessels. A contrast-enhanced MRI will allow to detect vascular abnormalities.

EULAR diagnostic criteria for Takayasu arteritis. Diagnosis is made with arteriographic abnormality plus one of the rest.
Claudication of extremities and/or decreased brachial pulse
Blood pressure difference >10 mmhg
Arteriographic abnormality*
Bruit over subclavian arteries or aorta
Hypertension systolic/diastolic blood pressure >95th percentile for height
Acute phase reactant erythrocyte sedimentation rate >20 mm per hour or C-reactive protein above normal

**obligated criteria.*

Table 3.
EULAR diagnosis criteria for Takayasu arteritis.

In patients with TA, an echocardiogram can be done to completely evaluate the cardiovascular health in our patient evaluating the ventricular function, hypertrophy, aortic valve, and aortic and coronary arteries (**Figures 1** and **2**) [11].

In the image studies, there are multiple patterns of altered anatomy in the vessel, the four principal patterns are: [13]

- Decrease of the luminal diameter.
- Total occlusion.
- Fusiform and saccular aneurysm.
- Irregular contour of the vessel.

Angiographic classification of TA classifies the image findings into five types depending on the part of the aorta that is affected: [11].

I: Branches of the aortic arch.
IIa: Ascending aorta, aortic arch, and its branches.
IIb: Ascending aorta, aortic arch, and its branches, thoracic and descending aorta.
III: Thoracic, descending aorta, abdominal aorta, and/or renal arteries.
IV: Abdominal aorta and/or renal arteries.
V: Combined features of types IIb and IV.

2.4.2 Laboratory findings

Anemia, generally hypochromic normocytic anemia, leukocytosis, and thrombocytosis have been reported in patients in an active phase of the disease or secondary to chronic inflammation [8, 14].

In pediatric cohorts, biologic inflammation is commonly reflected by the elevation of acute phase reactants, such as C-reactive protein (CRP) and erythrocyte sedimentation rate (ESR). However, their sensitivity to reflect active disease remains uncertain, and in addition, they lack specificity as well [8].

C-reactive protein (CRP), more accurately reflects the burden of systemic inflammation and is increasingly measured as a disease activity marker, otherwise, high CRP levels have also been found to be associated with a higher risk of thrombotic complications [2, 3].

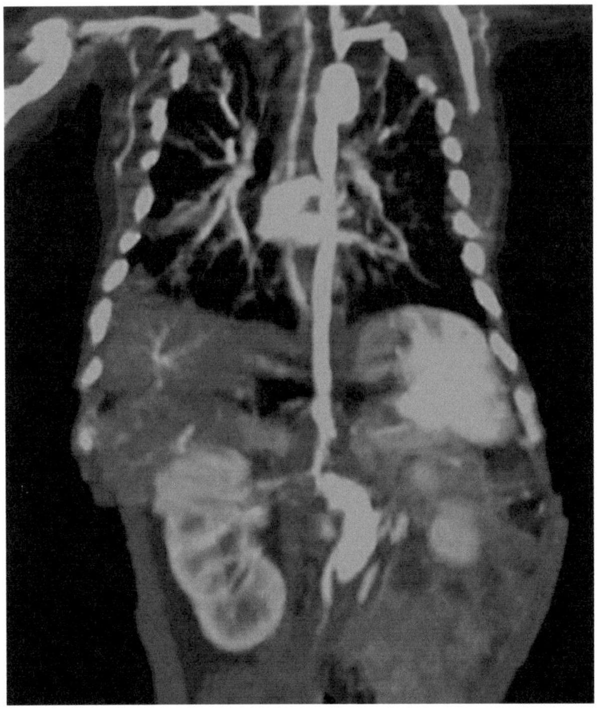

Figure 1.
Vascular abnormalities in computed tomography, such as dilation of the abdominal aorta and stenosis of the renal artery [12].

Erythrocyte sedimentation rate (ESR) increased is common in the acute phases of the disease but without clinical awareness and suspicion. ESR is more sensitive than C-reactive protein in the mentioned phases but both still have poor sensitivity and specificity, the ESR may continue to be elevated in disease remission, but actually, there are cases with active vasculitis without elevation of ESR and/or CRP [3, 7, 11].

Biomarker pentraxin-3 (PTX-3), is a protein rapidly produced in response to an inflammatory reaction, especially by endothelial cells. Levels higher than 1 ng/ml are more accurate than normal thresholds of C-reactive protein or ESR to distinguish active from inactive disease, although we need more reliable biomarkers that reflect vascular wall inflammation. PTX-3 may identify vascular progression only in a subgroup of TA patients not receiving anticytokine treatments. However, in other patients with TA, including those receiving anticytokine treatments, even plasma PTX-3 levels were shown to be normal despite ongoing smoldering vascular inflammation [2, 11].

CD8 cells with reversal of T-cell CD4:CD8 ratio increased is a marker of disease activity [11].

Some authors have suggested new biomarkers correlated with disease activity, such as matrix metalloproteinase (MMP)-2, −3, and – 9, IL-6, IFNg, vascular cell adhesion molecules (VCAM), and pentraxin-3 (PTX-3), but to date, a specific biomarker for TAK does not exist and none of them have yet been validated or implemented as a routine in clinical practice [7, 8].

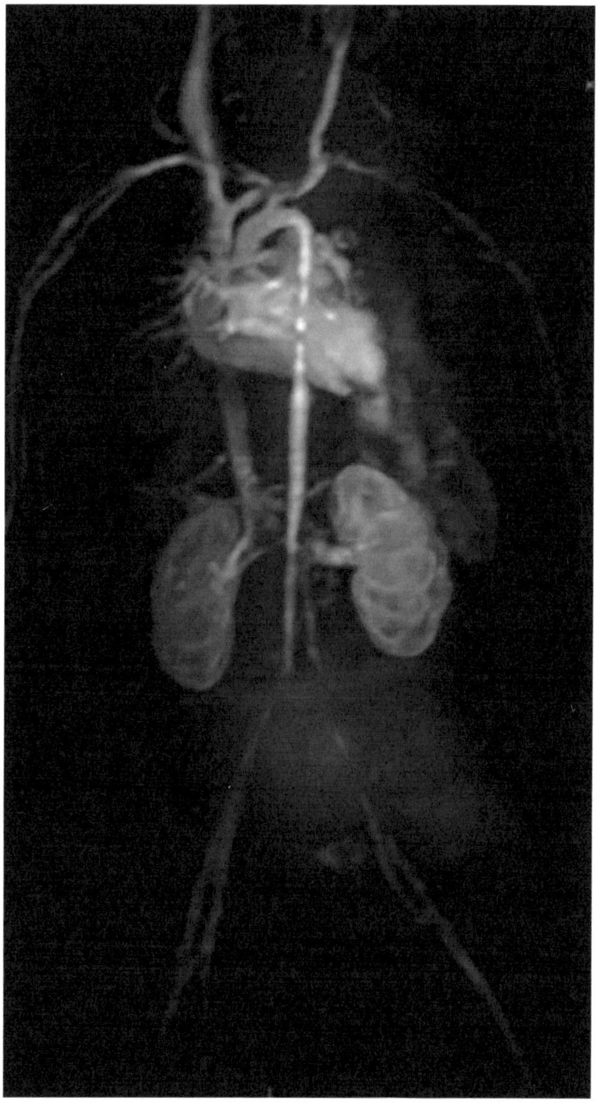

Figure 2.
Vascular abnormalities are shown in magnetic resonance angiography, such as stenosis in the thoracic aorta, iliac artery, and renal artery [12].

2.4.3 Histopathology

A lymphomonocyte infiltrate is observed, and occasionally giant cells with the presence of granulomas, which initially affect the adventitia, but progress toward the arterial lumen, in the form of panarteritis. Over time, there is a reduction in lumen due to thickening, due to fibrosis of the intima and media, thrombotic phenomena appear, and progressively, stenosis, dilation, and aneurysms [7].

A pediatric series from the United Kingdom observed lymphocytic infiltration with incipient neovascularization and the absence of granulomas. This finding contrasts with that observed in adults, in which the presence of granulomas predominates (**Table 4**) [7].

Differential diagnosis	Similar with TA	Dissimilar with TA
Giant cell arteritis (GCA) [2]	• The role of cell-mediated immunity in their pathogenesis. • Pathological findings in the vessel wall, high serum levels, and vascular expressions of cytokines (IL-6, IL-7), this is the major reason why some authors suggested that TA and GCA might exist on a spectrum within the same disease. • IL-12B is the most prominent genetic factor for both diseases.	• TA tends to affect branches of the internal carotid artery, GCA has a tendency to affect branches of the external carotid artery. • On TA, subclavian involvement tended to be asymmetric with a high frequency of left subclavian artery disease. While symmetric subclavian with concomitant axillary involvement was seen more frequently in GCA. • TA is generally seen in young females from far eastern and Asian countries, GCA is generally seen in older patients, especially of Caucasian origin. • On GCA we can find headache, jaw or tongue claudication, and scalp tenderness. • On TA, levels of Th1 cytokines are easily suppressed, and Th17 cytokines are resistant. In patients with GCA Th1 is relatively resistant and Th17 is rapidly suppressed.
Tuberculosis (TB) [2, 3]	• Granulomatous lesions. • Positive tuberculin skin test, on approximately 90% of children with TA has been observed, and about 20% of patients with TA have active tuberculosis.	• TA is associated more often with vascular stenosis, whereas tuberculosis is more often associated with erosion of the vessel wall and aneurysm development. Also, TB particularly affects the descending thoracic and abdominal aorta.

Table 4.
Similarities and differences of some differential diagnosis in comparison with Takayasu arteritis.

2.5 Differential diagnosis

Differential diagnosis are shown in **Table 4**.

2.6 Treatment options

The primary objective of treatment is inducing and maintaining remission of the disease, so early treatment is crucial to resolve or alleviate the inflammation and prevent complications and disease progression. Patient and parent's education, and cooperation between doctor and the patient (including family) are important for compliance and progression [2, 11].

The base of the treatment, at the beginning, is glucocorticoid pulses combined with immunosuppressive drugs (cyclophosphamide) to induce remission, and the use of low doses of corticosteroids and background immunosuppression as maintenance therapy (methotrexate) [7].

2.6.1 Corticosteroids

First-line treatment. Children with corticosteroid resistance should receive high-dose corticosteroids combined with another immunosuppressant agent, usually methotrexate, in order to avoid irreversible vessel damage [11].

2.6.2 Immunosuppressant drugs

Can be used in children as first or second-line agents. Has been shown to be safe and effective as a second agent to achieve sustained remission, decrease steroid dose and improve vascular lesions. This drug include methotrexate, cyclophosphamide, azathioprine, and mycophenolate mofetil [11].

2.6.3 Biological agents

More than one-half (54%) of the patients required treatment with biological agents. Antitumor necrosis factor agents (infliximab, etanercept, and adalimumab), and anti-IL-6 therapy (tocilizumab) have been used with variable effectiveness [11].

Some evidence from the case series suggests that infliximab may be effective in the management of refractory Takayasu arteritis, but has been shown to be effective in inducing and maintaining remission [7, 11].

Due to the fact that in various studies there are theories about the importance of IL-6 in the pathogenesis of this condition, such as the increase in IL-6 expression, blockade with tocilizumab has been shown to be effective in children [7].

Due to the role of Th1 and Th17 cells in the pathogenesis of the disease, there are some published cases with the use of ustekinumab (anti-IL-12/23) [7].

2.7 Prognosis in adults and children

A few studies conclude that the time lapsed from the onset of symptoms to diagnosis of the disease in a period between 2 and 11 years. The development of new drugs and the advances in surgical technology have been an important contribution to the control of disease activity but in spite of these developments, the management of childhood TA remains a challenge as diagnosis and treatment, late diagnosis and progressive disease course resistant to treatment may also cause poor prognosis. Some authors say that the worst prognosis is where patients had systemic and vascular inflammation, vascular lesions, major complications (such as retinopathy, renovascular hypertension, aortic regurgitation, and aortic aneurysm), and progressive course. Also, children under 5 years of age at the onset of the disease have a poor prognosis [2, 7, 11].

TA is associated with significant morbidity and mortality in young patients. Mortality rates vary according to several factors: geographical location, severity and extension of the lesions, treatment strategies, time of follow-up, and whether early or late series are described. Some publications show mortality rates ranging from 16 to 40%, but other ones rate mortality from 3% in the United States of America. Some common causes of death in TA include acute myocardial infarction, congestive heart failure, cerebrovascular accident, renal failure, hemorrhage, lung infection, postoperative complications, and aneurysm rupture [2, 11, 12, 15].

3. Conclusions

Takayasu arteritis continues to be a diagnostic challenge, mostly on the first-line of care, because other pathologies show similar clinical and laboratory findings and there is not a golden standard to diagnose it. In addition, the signs and symptoms are not usually the same in all patients, and it could even be an underdiagnosed disease.

On the other hand, treatment options for TA is an area in which progress has been shown in recent years. However, these options are not yet considered to be accessible to all patients.

This disease still has a field of study in terms of its pathophysiology, diagnosis, and treatment.

Acknowledgements

We would like to acknowledge Dr. Gabriel Vega for introducing us to a new field of study and allowing us to participate in the collaboration of the knowledge of Takayasu arteritis.

Conflict of interests

The authors of this chapter declare to not have a conflict of interest.

Notes/thanks

Thanks to Maria and Roberto Rivera, Daniela and Alonso Rivera, José López.

We would also like to thank our family members who motivate us to keep moving forward.

We would like to prove that women in medicine can do so much for the field and that the difficulties that we face as women every day only make us stronger.

Author details

Melisa Rivera*, Jose Heriberto López-Beltrán and Blanca Frisia Morales-López
Universidad de Guadalajara, Mexico

*Address all correspondence to: riveramelisa4@gmail.com

References

[1] Terao C. History of Takayasu arteritis and Dr. Mikito Takayasu. International Journal of Rheumatic Diseases. 2014;**17**(8):931-935

[2] Keser G, Aksu K, Direskeneli H. Takayasu arteritis: An update. Turkish Journal of Medical Science. 2018;**48**(4):681-697

[3] Brunner J, Feldman BM, Tyrrell PN, Kuemmerle-Deschner JB, Zimmerhackl LB, Gassner I, et al. Takayasu arteritis in children and adolescents. Rheumatology (Oxford, England). 2010;**49**(10):1806-1814

[4] Arnaud L, Haroche J, Limal N, Toledano D, Gambotti L, Chalumeau NC, et al. Takayasu arteritis in France: A single-center retrospective study of 82 cases comparing white, North African, and black patients. Medicine. 2010;**89**:1-17

[5] Moriwaki R, Noda M, Yajima M, et al. Clinical manifestations of Takayasu arteritis in India and Japan – New classification of angiographic findings. Angiology. 1997;**48**:369-379

[6] Szugye HS, Zeft AS, Spalding SJ. Takayasu arteritis in the pediatric population: A contemporary United States-based single center cohort. Pediatric Rheumatology Online Journal. 2014;**12**:21

[7] Lacruz L, Mir M. Arteritis de Takayasu. Protoc diagn ter pediatr. 2020;**2**:259-269

[8] Aeschlimann F, Twilt M, Yeung R. Childhood-onset Takayasu Arteritis. European Journal of Rheumatology. 2020;7(Suppl. 1):S58-S66

[9] Danda D, Goel R, Joseph G, Kumar ST, Nair A, Ravindran R, et al. Clinical course of 602 patients with Takayasu's arteritis: Comparison between childhood-onset versus adult onset disease. Rheumatology (Oxford, England). 2021;**60**(5):2246-2255

[10] Ozen S, Pistorio A, Iusan SM, et al. EULAR/PRINTO/PRES criteria for Henoch–Schönlein purpura, childhood polyarteritis nodosa, childhood Wegener granulomatosis and childhood Takayasu arteritis: Ankara 2008. Part II: Final classification criteria. Annals of the Rheumatic Diseases. 2010;**69**:798-806

[11] Di Santo M, Stelmaszewski EV. Takayasu arteritis in paediatrics. Cardiology in the Young. 2017;**28**(03): 354-361

[12] Vega-Cornejo G, Rivera M, Bañuelos-Zapata J. Case Report: Takayasu Arteritis in a new born, five years follow-up. Revista colombiana de Reumatologia. 2021 [Online]

[13] Hyung PJ. Conventional and CT angiographic diagnosis of Takayasu Arteritis. International Journal of Cardiology. 1996;**54**(Suppl):S135-S141

[14] Dammacco F, Cirulli A, Simeone A, et al. Takayasu arteritis: A cohort of Italian patients and recent pathogenetic and therapeutic advances. Clinical and Experimental Medicine. 2021;**21**:49-62

[15] Seyahi E. Takayasu arteritis: An update. Current Opinion in Rheumatology. 2017;**29**:51-56

Chapter 14

Pulmonary Hypertension

Massimiliano Mulè, Giulia Passaniti and Daniela Giannazzo

Abstract

Pulmonary hypertension (PH) is a complex and multifactorial syndrome, partly unknown, characterized by a profound alteration of pulmonary vasculature and, consequentially, a rise in the pulmonary vascular load, leading to hypertrophy and remodeling of the right heart chambers. The World Health Organization assembles the several forms of PH into five clinical groups: group 1 includes pulmonary arterial hypertension, previously defined as idiopathic forms, group 2 is PH due to left-sided heart diseases, group 3 PH due to lung diseases, hypoxia, or both, group 4 due to pulmonary-artery obstruction, and group 5 PH, which includes forms with multifactorial or unclear mechanisms. In this chapter, we would like to delineate the clinical and hemodynamic definitions of PH and, for each group, we will describe the pathophysiological mechanisms, the diagnostic pathway, and the pharmacological approach and treatment. Finally, we would also like to focus on the latest trials and future therapeutic perspectives for this disease.

Keywords: pulmonary hypertension, pulmonary arterial hypertension, right heart failure, right heart catheterization, pulmonary circulation

1. Introduction

Pulmonary hypertension (PH) is a complex and multifactorial syndrome, partly unknown, characterized by a profound alteration of pulmonary vasculature and, consequentially, a rise in the pulmonary vascular load, leading to hypertrophy and remodeling of the right heart chambers.

1.1 Basic principles of pulmonary circulation

Pulmonary circulation, includes a vast network of arteries, veins, and lymphatic vessels and is unique, both in function and volume: it is a low-pressure, low-resistance, highly distensible system, and it is capable of accommodating large increases in blood flow with none or minimal elevations of its pressure. During embryonic life, the pulmonary circulation is a low-flow and high-resistance circuit. After birth, once the baby takes his first breath, the high resistance in the lungs drops dramatically: from now on, blood can enter lungs for oxygenation. Oxygen relaxes the pulmonary vessels and causes closure of the fetal shunts: at this precise moment, the baby's blood flow is identical to that of an adult [1]. Therefore, this vasculature dilates, in order to take in the entire cardiac output (CO), with high blood flow at low intravascular pulmonary arterial pressure (PAP). Anatomically, pulmonary arteries have thinner walls with less smooth muscle and lack of basal tone: this happens because of the elevated production of endogenous vasodilators and low production of vasoconstrictors from the endothelium of the pulmonary vessel walls. These mechanisms result in the maintenance of a normal pulmonary vascular resistance (PVR) [2]. Pulmonary circulation differs functionally from the systemic one because it carries mixed venous blood. Deoxygenated blood is channeled through the pulmonary artery directly in the alveolar/capillary units where gas exchange occurs and blood releases carbon dioxide and is replenished with oxygen. Then, oxygenated blood is carried back to the left atrium by the pulmonary veins, in order to be distributed to the systemic circulation.

1.2 Physiological bases of hemodynamic classification

In order to better understand the hemodynamic classification of PH, we should recall Poiseuille's law, one of the most important laws of fluid dynamics (1):

$$Q = (P_1 - P_2) \times \pi r^4 / 8\mu l \tag{1}$$

Where Q is flow (l/min) and then Cardiac Output (CO), if we apply the equation to the pulmonary circulation; P_1 is mean pulmonary arterial pressure (mPAP), the pressure at the beginning of the pulmonary circulation, P_2 is the pulmonary artery wedge pressure (PAWP) equivalent to the left atrial pressure, the pressure at the end point of the pulmonary circulation, when measured at right heart catheterization in the absence of pulmonary vein stenosis. $8\mu l/\pi r^4$ is a measure of the pulmonary vasculature resistance (PVR).

According to Poiseuille's law, pulmonary vasculature resistance (PVR) is inversely related to the fourth power of arterial radius: in this equation, l represents the length of the vessel, r its radius, and μ the viscosity of the fluid, in our case, blood. PVR is used to characterize PH because this parameter allows us to quantify abnormalities of the pulmonary vasculature, as it is mainly related to the anatomical geometry of small distal arterioles of the lung. PVR can also be expressed as (2):

$$\text{PVR} = (\text{mPAP–PAWP})/\text{CO} \tag{2}$$

Therefore, PVR reflects the functional status of pulmonary vascular endothelium/smooth muscle cell coupled system, and it is also positively related to blood viscosity. Additionally, PVR may be influenced by changes in perivascular alveolar and pleural pressure. According to Poiseuille's law mPAP depends on cardiac output, left atrial pressure, and PVR (3)

$$\text{mPAP} = (\text{CO} \times \text{PVR}) + \text{PAWP} \tag{3}$$

whereas pressure does not depend on the size of the body, and PAP from different patients can be evaluated without considerable differences in their body size [3, 4]. PAWP is an acceptable estimate of left atrial pressure (LAP) or left ventricular end-diastolic pressure (LVEDP) in the absence of mitral stenosis or pulmonary vein stenosis. Furthermore, PAWP and LVEDP are usually considered to be interchangeable, even if some pathological scenarios, such as atrial fibrillation, rheumatic disease, or large diameter of the left atrium are associated with a PAWP higher than LVEDP. PAWP and LVEDP measurements should be obtained at the end of the expiratory phase and the end of the diastolic phase, QRS gated [4].

2. Haemodynamic classification of PH

According to the European Society of Cardiology 2015 guidelines, PH is defined as an increase in mean pulmonary arterial pressure (mPAP) $\geq$25 mmHg at rest as assessed by right heart catheterization (RHC). Available data have shown that the normal mPAP at rest is 14 $\pm$ 3 mmHg with an upper limit of normal of approximately 20 mmHg [5]. This definition was updated at the sixth world symposium of PH, held in 2018 in Nice: the mPAP threshold was lowered from $\geq$25 to >20 mmHg [6]. Whatever the mPAP cut-off value considered for defining PH, it is important to emphasize that this value used in isolation cannot characterize a clinical condition and does not define the pathological process per se. According to Poiseuille's law mPAP depends on cardiac output, left atrial pressure, and PVR (4).

$$\text{mPAP} = (\text{CO} \times \text{PVR}) + \text{PAWP} \tag{4}$$

Then, mPAP elevation may have several different causes with different prognoses and treatments, including high cardiac output syndromes (anemia, left–to–right shunts, AV fistula, and thyrotoxicosis.) or diseases characterized by high PWAP (left heart diseases) or high PVR because of pulmonary vascular disease [6]. Specifically, precapillary pulmonary hypertension due to pulmonary vascular disease is hemodynamically defined by a pulmonary artery wedge pressure (PAWP) $\leq$15 mmHg and an elevation in PVR of at least three wood units (WU).

Precapillary hypertension contrasts with postcapillary PH in which the PVR is less than 3 WU and the elevation in the mPAP is due to elevated filling pressures on the left side of the heart (PAWP > 15 mmHg) [7].

Postcapillary PH is further subclassified on the basis of the PVR, into isolated postcapillary PH (PAWP > 15 mm Hg and PVR < 3 WU) and combined pre- and post-capillary PH (PAWP > 15 mm Hg and PVR $\geq$ 3 WU). (See **Table 1**).

3. Clinical classification of PH

Besides the haemodynamic classification, the clinical classification of PH is relevant and very helpful to choose the appropriate therapeutic pathway and, consequentially, estimate the prognosis of patients. Since the first world symposium of PH held

Definitions	Characteristics
Pre-capillary PH	mPAP > 20 mmHg
	PAWP ≤ 15 mmHg
	PVR ≥ 3 WU
Isolated post-capillary PH	mPAP > 20 mmHg
	PAWP > 15 mmHg
	PVR < 3 WU
Combined pre- and post-capillary PH	mPAP > 20 mmHg
	PAWP > 15 mmHg
	PVR ≥ 3 WU

Table 1.
Haemodynamic classification of PH.

in 1973, the clinical classification has been reviewed many times: in fact, due to the remarkable spread of PH in the last 40 years, new scientific pieces of evidence have been discovered, leading to a necessary update in the classification. The actual clinical classification was defined by the World Health Organization in 2018, during the Sixth World Symposium in Nice and it includes five major groups, classified according to similar clinical presentation, pathological findings, hemodynamic features, and treatment approaches (see **Table 2**).

Specifically, each group includes:

- Group 1: Pulmonary arterial hypertension (PAH)
- Group 2: PH due to left-sided heart disease
- Group 3: PH due to lung disease, hypoxia, or both
- Group 4: PH due to pulmonary artery obstruction
- Group 5: PH with multifactorial or unclear mechanisms

Making a correct diagnosis of PH is very complex, challenging, and time-demanding, and it can only be made in high expertise centers by a multidisciplinary team of cardiologists, pneumologists, radiologists, and rheumatologists. Diagnostic tools, include EKG, echocardiogram, blood tests analysis, pulmonary function test with diffusing lung capacity test for carbon monoxide, high-resolution CT scan, lung ventilation/perfusion scan, and right heart catheterization (RHC). RHC represents the gold standard for the final diagnosis: while performing it, the expert specialist should also complete the procedure, including a vasoreactivity test with short-acting selective vasodilators agents, in order to predict if patients will respond to treatment. At this point, after ruling out any other causes of increased mPAP, the diagnosis of PAH can be made, as it is a diagnosis of exclusion.

We will now analyze the various groups of PH based on their prevalence.

3.1 PH associated with left heart diseases (group 2)

3.1.1 Epidemiology

Due to the prevalence of left heart diseases in the general population, group 2 PH represents the most prevalent form of PH, responsible for 65% of PH cases [8]. Mostly, it is associated with heart failure (HF), but it can also be a complication in patients with left-side heart valvular and congenital diseases. The exact prevalence of PH is still not known because of variabilities in PH definitions with predominant echo-based literature data and referral bias. It has been estimated that about 60% of patients with heart failure with reduced ejection fraction (HFrEF) have pulmonary hypertension at presentation, while in patients with left ventricular diastolic dysfunction the prevalence of PH is 83% [8, 9].

3.1.2 Pathophysiology

The pathophysiology of this type of PH is multifactorial but mainly based on the effect of the hydrostatic pressure on the pulmonary vasculature, resulting in its

1. Pulmonary arterial hypertension (PAH)	**3. PH due to lung diseases and/or hypoxia**
1.1 Idiopathic PAH	3.1 Obstructive lung disease
1.2 Heritable PAH	3.2 Restrictive lung disease
1.3 Drug- and Toxin-induced PAH	3.3 Other lung disease with mixed restrictive/ obstructive pattern
1.4 PAH associated with	3.4 Hypoxia without lung disease
1.4.1 Connective Tissue Diseases	3.5 Developmental lung disorders
1.4.2 HIV infection	
1.4.3 Portal Hypertension	**4. PH due to pulmonary artery obstruction**
1.4.4 Congenital Heart Disease	4.1 Chronic thromboembolic PH (CTEPH)
1.4.5 Schistosomiasis	4.2 Other pulmonary artery obstructions
1.5 PAH long-term responders to calcium channel blockers	
1.6 PAH with overt features of venous/capillaries (PVOD/ PCH) involvement	**5. PH with unclear and/ or multifactorial mechanisms**
1.7 Persistent PH of the newborn syndrome	5.1 Hematological disorders
2. PH due to left heart diseases	5.2 Systemic and metabolic disorders
2.1 PH due to heart failure with reduced LVEF (HFrEF)	5.3 Others
2.2 PH due to heart failure with preserved LVEF (HFpEF)	5.4 Complex congenital heart diseases
2.3 Mitral and/or Aortic valve diseases	
2.4 Congenital or acquired cardiovascular conditions leading to post-capillary PH	

Table 2.
Updated clinical classification of pulmonary hypertension, according to the 6th PH world symposium of 2018, Nice, France.

change and remodeling. Both types of cardiac heart failure (preserved and reduced ejection fraction), other than valvular disease and congenital heart disease can lead to a passive increase of pressure in the left atrium (LA), and consequently, a decrease in its compliance. The LA has a key role in maintaining normal pulmonary pressure because it constitutes the connection between pulmonary circulation and systemic circulation, through the left ventricle [9]. Any increase in the LA pressure even mild perturbates the pulmonary hemodynamics. According to the Poiseuille's law, the increase of pressure in the LA, the end point of the pulmonary circulation (P_2), will results in a proportional increase of the pressure at the beginning of the pulmonary circulation (P_1), to maintain the forward flow; therefore, the increase of LA pressure will result in a proportional and passive increase of the mPAP. In addition, the increased pressure transmitted back to the pulmonary vasculature promotes significant changes in the structural anatomy. The raised backward pressure causes lung capillary and small artery stress, as the barotrauma breaks the endothelial layer and promotes fluid and protein swelling in the interstitium. Therefore, the intimal layer undergoes fibrosis and the tunica media undergoes hypertrophy [10]. In this setting, the endothelium plays a central role in the local control of tone through the regulated release of nitric oxide (NO) and endothelin (ET): the dysregulation of pulmonary vascular tone involves alterations in these important counterbalancing systems, causing a decrease in the production of endogenous vasodilators NO and an increase in vasoconstrictors ET [10, 11].

The transition from alveolar-capillary stress failure to remodeling is clinically reflected by the rise of PVR in patients with long-standing post-capillary PH who develop combined pre- and post-capillary PH.

3.1.3 Impact on prognosis and clinical picture

PH due to left heart disease results in severe symptoms and worse exercise tolerance and exerts a negative impact on outcome with an evident poor prognosis. These patients are usually elderly, with a high prevalence of cardiovascular co-morbidities, such as obesity, hypertension, atrial fibrillation, diabetes, coronary artery disease, kidney disease, and metabolic syndrome [12]. The patient usually presents with symptoms related to left heart diseases, such as fatigue, exertional dyspnea, orthopnea, paroxysmal nocturnal dyspnea, and peripheral edema. The medical history can reveal a previous diagnosis of heart failure, systolic or diastolic, myocardial infarction, systemic arterial hypertension, or valvular disease (frequently mitral regurgitation). Findings of physical examination, include left-sided gallops, left-sided murmurs (particularly mitral), a displaced or sustained apical impulse, and pulmonary crackles in cases of pulmonary congestion. PH may be a cause of morbidity and mortality in patients with chronic heart failure; death and hospitalization for heart failure are greatly increased in patients with echocardiographic evidence of PH [13]. Apparently, PH has a major impact on right ventricle function, and this is a strong predictor of overall and event-free survival in chronic heart failure patients [14].

3.1.4 Therapy

After the diagnosis is made, the primary need is to start a therapy that has to focus on the global management and improvement of the underlying conditions, before treating the PH; lowering filling pressures in left-heart cavities is the goal of treatment in many forms of group 2 PH.

This can include percutaneous repair or surgery of the valvular heart disease and optimal pharmacological therapy for HF with reduced systolic function [15]. Other cardiovascular risk factors, such as hypertension, dyslipidemia, diabetes, and obesity should be maintained under strict control. In the past years, many trials have been conducted in order to evaluate specific PAH therapies in treating group 2 PH patients: these studies were based on the idea that PH is due to a misbalance between the production of NO and ET. So, it has been supposed that ET receptor antagonists, prostanoids, and phosphodiesterase-5 inhibitors (PDE5-i) can play a role in slowing down the progression of the disease. Several trials were completed using prostanoids and ET receptor antagonists, but none of them have demonstrated the superiority of these treatments in terms of decrease in disease progression or increase in overall survival [16].

3.2 Pulmonary hypertension associated with lung diseases

PH associated with hypoxia and lung diseases is the second most common form of PH worldwide. It is associated with various lung diseases, such as chronic obstructive pulmonary disease (COPD), interstitial lung disease (ILD), obstructive sleep apnea (OSA), and, less frequently, cystic fibrosis [17] and high altitude exposure [18].

PH has a different prevalence in each of the cited lung diseases. Numerous studies in patients with Global Initiative for Chronic Obstructive Lung Disease (GOLD) stage IV revealed that up to 90% of these patients have a mPAP >20 mm Hg [19]. The prevalence of PH in patients with ILD varies greatly according to the underlying disease and the severity of the disease: in idiopathic pulmonary fibrosis (IPF), mPAP values >20 mmHg was reported 8–15% of patients. Higher percentages, ranging from 30% to 50%, are found in advanced and end-stage (>60%) IPF cases [20].

3.2.1 Pathophysiology and differences of PH associated with COPD and ILD

The pathogenesis of the vascular remodeling correlated to COPD has not been fully clarified but appears to be caused by the mutual effects of hypoxia, pulmonary dysfunction with air trapping, and the toxic effects of smoking, leading to inflammation, endothelial dysfunction, and angiogenesis [21]. Hypoxia has both a direct and an indirect effect on pulmonary circulation remodeling: directly, it closes potassium channels of the smooth muscle cells, causing their contraction; indirectly, it acts on the genesis and the production of inducible transcription factors, such as hypoxia-inducible factor-1 (HIF-1), angiotensin II, and more growth factors that have a role in vasoconstriction, vascular remodeling, and neo-angiogenesis [22]. PH in ILD has a different pathogenesis: according to the latest scientific evidence, a recurring stress injury leads to impairment of epithelial cells and basement membranes, and this is consequently followed by exudation of fibrin and focal fibroblast activation and growth, resulting in fibrotic remodeling of lung parenchyma and pulmonary vessels. Specifically, all layers of the muscular pulmonary arteries show concentric and eccentric remodeling. Widespread hyperplasia is present in the intimal layer, media, and adventitia layers are thicker due to hypertrophy and/or hyperplasia of smooth muscle cells and fibroblasts, respectively [23]. Non-muscularized pulmonary arteries demonstrate neo-muscularization of the media and luminal narrowing. In response to these changes, capillary density increases in normal, non-fibrotic areas of the lungs, while in the fibrotic area of the lungs, there is vascular regression [24].

An interesting concept has been presented by Mura et al.: they were one of the first groups to compare gene expression with microarray in the lungs of patients with IPF. In this innovative study, the writers defined particular gene signatures that differentiate IPF patients with and without PH. The authors found that IPF patients without PH predominantly had a pro-inflammatory gene expression, while IPF patients with severe PH (mPAP > 40 mmHg) had a pro-proliferative gene signature expression. This study establishes a strong molecular difference between these two groups of patients, supporting the hypothesis of specific pathway activation during PH development in IPF patients [25]. Finally, with increasing evidence on certain molecular mechanisms driving PH development in IPF patients, the paradigm is slowly changing from a "passive state", where PH development was only due to hypoxic vasoconstriction and loss of vascular bed density, to an "active process" where particular molecular and cellular pathways are involved [24].

PH can also be due to chronic up-regulation of hypoxic pulmonary vasoconstriction, caused by long-term exposure to high altitudes. This particular type of PH affects people residing at an altitude of 2500 meters or higher. The hypoxic stimulus leads to pulmonary vasoconstriction and, consequently, a rise in vascular resistance, in order to decrease perfusion of non-ventilated lung areas and increase blood flow to better-oxygenated areas. Scientific data suggests that genetics plays a role in PH predisposition, but the mechanisms are not clearly understood [18].

3.2.2 Impact on prognosis and clinical picture

PH is a poor prognostic indicator of chronic lung disease. Comparing the 5-year survival rate in patients with COPD, the survival is 36% in patients with PH, compared to the 62% in patients without PH [19]. Patients can present with a variety of symptoms, including shortness of breath, fatigue, cough, reduced exercise capacity, and syncope. Physical examination shows a louder second heart sound with a fixed or paradoxical splitting. Also, a systolic ejection murmur, increased by inspiration, may be heard over the left sternal border. Severe PH eventually leads to right ventricular failure with signs of systemic venous hypertension: this clinical condition was known as core pulmonale. The signs of right ventricular failure, include a high-pitched systolic murmur of tricuspid regurgitation, hepatomegaly, a pulsatile liver, ascites, and peripheral edema.

3.2.3 Therapy

Given the morbidity and mortality associated with PH in pulmonary diseases, there has been great interest in the treatment of these patients with pulmonary vasodilator therapy.

However, nowadays there are still no approved therapies for group 3 PH. In the last few years, many trials have been carried out, in order to examine and analyze if drugs approved for other forms of PH can play a role in the therapeutic pathway of these patients, with conflicting results. In addition to the lack of positive results in terms of prognosis, concerns have been raised about the potentially negative effect of pulmonary vasodilator therapy in worsening hypoxemia due to uncoupling of the ventilation/perfusion (V/Q) ratio in lung diseases. A few studies showed positive effects of pulmonary vasodilators, in the absence of worsening hypoxemia. For example, the SPHERIC-1 (Sildenafil and Pulmonary HypERtension In COPD), explored if Sildenafil can lower PVR and improve the quality of life of group 3 patients. After 16 weeks, the results were that sildenafil safely improved PVR, CO, and symptoms (evaluated with BODE score), in selected patients with COPD-associated severe PH [26]. In patients with ILD, several trials with pulmonary vasodilators have shown detrimental effects of these drugs in terms of symptoms and survival (i.e., Ambrisentan or Riociguat). Positive results have been shown in a randomized controlled trial involving 326 ILD-PH patients, randomized to inhaled treprostinil or placebo: in the inhaled treprostinil group, there was an improvement in exercise capacity, assessed with 6-min walking test [27]. However, more data from larger trials are needed to approve this therapy for COPD- or ILD- PH patients. Currently, therapy for group 3 PH is primarily directed at the treatment of the underlying disease, with general supportive therapy when right ventricular failure develops.

3.3 Pulmonary arterial hypertension

3.3.1 Epidemiology

Group 1 PH (or PAH) is a rare, highly complex, and progressive disorder that is incurable and ultimately can lead to premature death. PAH causes noteworthy physical, social, work, and emotional burdens among affected patients and their caregivers.

PAH affects from 15 to 50 people per million within the United States and Europe, and it usually affects women between 30 and 60 years of age [28]. However, it can occur in males and is often associated with worse clinical outcomes. The National Institutes of Health (NIH) was an important registry that collected PAH data between 1981 and 1985: it included 187 individuals, mostly Caucasian females, having idiopathic PAH. PAH-specific therapies were not available at that time, and registry participants had a median survival of 2.8 years (1 year, 68%; 3 years, 48%; and 5 years, 34%) [29]. Another milestone registry is the Registry to Evaluate Early and Long-Term PAH Disease Management (REVEAL), performed between 2006 and 2009 in the USA: results of this registry showed a 1-year survival rate of 91% among 2716 individuals who were enrolled. A supplementary analysis assessing long-term survival established survival rates of 85% at 3 years, 68% at 5 years, and 49% at 7 years from the time of diagnosis. The increases in survival rates were ascribed to several reasons, including availability of specific drugs, improved patient support, and hypothetically, a change in the PAH population cohort [30].

3.3.2 Pathophysiology

Group 1 PH includes many subgroups, such as idiopathic, heritable, drug, and toxin-induced, and PH associated with other diseases such as connective tissue diseases, HIV infection, portal hypertension, congenital heart disease, and schistosomiasis. However, regardless of the primary conditions, patients show similar pathophysiological pathways, such as augmented pulmonary arterioles contractility, endothelial dysfunction, proliferation of smooth muscle cells, and the presence of in situ thrombi [31]. These lead to an increase in PVR, an increase in mPAP, and, consequently, a raise in right heart afterload. Although the right ventricle initially compensates for this augmented afterload through adaptive hypertrophy and remodeling, this process is not entirely benign and cannot be continued as overload is persistent over time; ultimately, the right ventricle dilates and fails. The ability of the right ventricle to adapt to this afterload is the key element in developing symptoms and determining survival, and eventually, it is the failure of the right ventricle that is the main cause of death in patients with PAH (**Figure 1**). Nowadays, three main pathways are recognized to underline these changes: nitric oxide (NO), endothelin-1 (ET1), and Prostacyclin (PGI_2). As previously explained, NO is a potent pulmonary vasodilator and it also inhibits platelet aggregation. It is produced by the NO synthetase enzyme, by converting L-arginine into L-citrulline. In PAH, there is a notable decrease in the production of NO and this causes vasoconstriction, proliferation of smooth muscle cells, inflammation, and finally thrombosis, due to the lack of platelets' anti-aggregation properties. ET1 is a peptide produced by endothelial cells; it is a potent vasoconstrictor that stimulates smooth muscle cell division and proliferation. Its levels rise in the pulmonary and systemic circulation of PAH patients and its value negatively correlates with patients' survival [32]. PGI_2 is a lipid mediator produced from arachidonic acid in the endothelium: its actions are similar to the NO ones, including reducing smooth muscle cell proliferation, promoting vasodilatation, and inhibiting platelets' aggregation. PGI2 is antagonized by thromboxane A2 (TXA2), which counteracts its effects. In normal conditions, the quantities of these two peptides are in balance; instead, in PAH patients, there is an imbalance between the increased production of TXA2 and the lacking of PGI2. This causes platelet

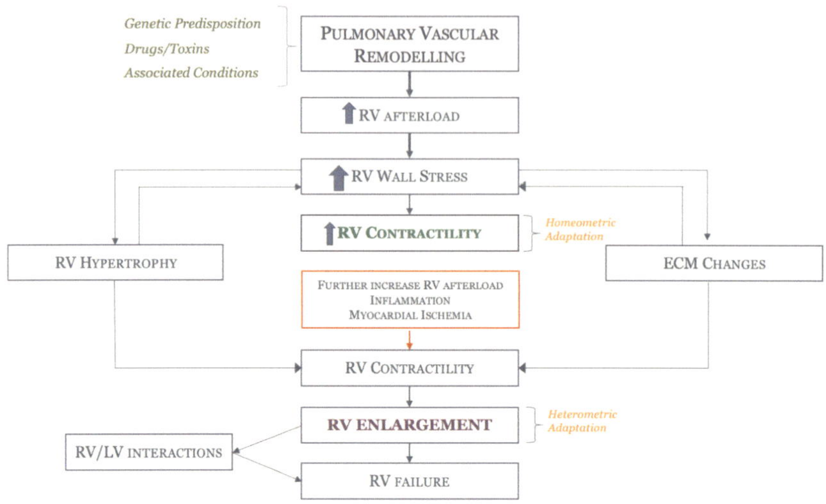

Figure 1.
Pathophysiology of right ventricular failure in PAH. Pulmonary vascular remodeling, the hallmark of PAH, leads to increase RV afterload and RV wall tension. Initially, the right ventricle can cope with the increased RV afterload. Homeometric adaptation consists of adaptive hypertrophy and an increase in contractility of the RV as a response to the rise in RV afterload, with little or no dilatation, hence preserving cardiac output. However, in the long term, prolonged excessive afterload to the RV, maladaptive RV hypertrophy and ECM changes, inflammation and myocardial ischemia together lead to failure of the homeometric adaptation and consequently reduced RV contractility. This increases RV filling pressures and volume (heterometric adaptation) and an attempt to maintain stroke volume through the Starling principle. There is uncoupling of the RV from the pulmonary. RV dilatation and uncoupling, together with a significant negative interaction between the RV and LV, lead to a further increase in RV filling pressure and subsequent drop in cardiac output, precipitating a vicious cycle of events that lead to heart failure, hypotension, and shock. RV: Right ventricle and ECM: Extracellular matrix.

aggregation, proliferation of smooth muscle cells, vasoconstriction, and an increase in PVR. Moreover, patients with PAH have reduced production of prostacyclin as well as reduced expression of prostacyclin receptor and prostacyclin synthase [33].

3.3.3 Clinical picture and prognostic factors of PAH

In the pre-symptomatic stage of PAH, increases in PVR and resting mPAP do not influence resting cardiac function, such as CO. By the time a patient presents with symptoms, even with "early" symptoms, (WHO functional class II) PVR is already significantly above normal, suggesting advanced pulmonary vascular remodeling. Many clinical symptoms or signs, such as peripheral edema and the onset of angina, can mark the moment in which the right ventricle function deteriorates. In particular, patients who begin to experience syncope or who experience an increase in the frequency of syncopal episodes have poor prognoses and require immediate attention: syncope has been proved to be an independent risk of poor survival [34]. Less common symptoms, include cough, hemoptysis, and hoarseness.

Patients must be assessed by:

- WHO functional class (FC) describes patients' symptoms relating to their everyday activities and life. WHO-FC is a strong predictor of survival. Patients in WHO-FC I have no limitation of physical activity; WHO-FC II is characterized by minor limitation in physical activity; WHO-FC III is characterized by a manifest limitation of physical activity with no discomfort at rest; finally,

WHO-FC IV is characterized by an inability to perform any physical activity, with evident signs of right ventricular failure.

- Exercise testing is measured with the 6-min walking test (6MWT) or with the cardiopulmonary exercise testing (CPET), a non-invasive method used to assess the performance of heart and lungs at rest and during exercise. CPET offers several benefits over 6MWT in assessing patients' exercise capacity but requires specific technical equipment and must be performed by highly trained medical personnel.

- Biomarkers: the most used is brain natriuretic peptide (BNP). BNP precursor is secreted by heart cells and it is then splitted in the active BNP and a N-terminal fragment (NT-proBNP). Serum BNP/NT-proBNP levels have been exhibited to reflect right ventricular dysfunction severity in PAH, correlating with mPAP, PVR, and right ventricle mass, and inversely correlating with CO and ejection fraction [35].

- Echocardiography: many echocardiographic parameters can play a role in the assessment of PAH. One of the most important is pericardial effusion, due to decreased venous and lymphatic drainage from the myocardium [36]. Another relevant parameter is TAPSE, a measure of the right ventricular systolic function: a TAPSE < 18 mm is associated with right ventricle systolic and diastolic dysfunction. Both of these factors have a great link with the prognosis of patients.

- Right heart catheterization (RHC), the gold standard method for diagnosing PAH: it should be performed at baseline and 3–4 months after the initiation of therapy, in order to understand if the patient is responding to treatment. Even if it is considered to be the gold standard, RHC has some disadvantages: it has to be performed in high expertise center and it is an invasive procedure.

Many scores can help predict survival and assess patient's risk, such as the REVEAL 2.0 risk score, which takes into consideration 12 variables, such as demographic, comorbidities, NYHA class, vital signs, hospitalization, 6MWT, BNP, echocardiogram, RHC or the ESC/ESR score.

3.3.4 Treatment

PAH treatment is based on the severity of disease at diagnosis and on the evaluation of how the individual will respond to treatment, using a multiparametric risk stratification approach. Clinical, exercise, right ventricular function, and hemodynamic parameters are combined to outline a low-, intermediate- or high-risk status, according to the expected 1-year mortality. PAH remains a severe clinical condition, despite the availability over the past 15 years of multiple drugs interfering with the ET1, NO, and prostacyclin pathways (**Figure 2**). Therefore, the current progress observed in the medical therapy of PAH is not related to the detection of new pathways, but the development of new strategies of combination therapy and escalation of treatments based on clinical response.

The current treatment algorithm provides the most appropriate initial strategy, including monotherapy, or double or triple combination therapy. Additionally, treatment escalation is required in case low-risk status is not achieved in planned follow-up assessments. Usually, treatment starts with general supportive therapies: these

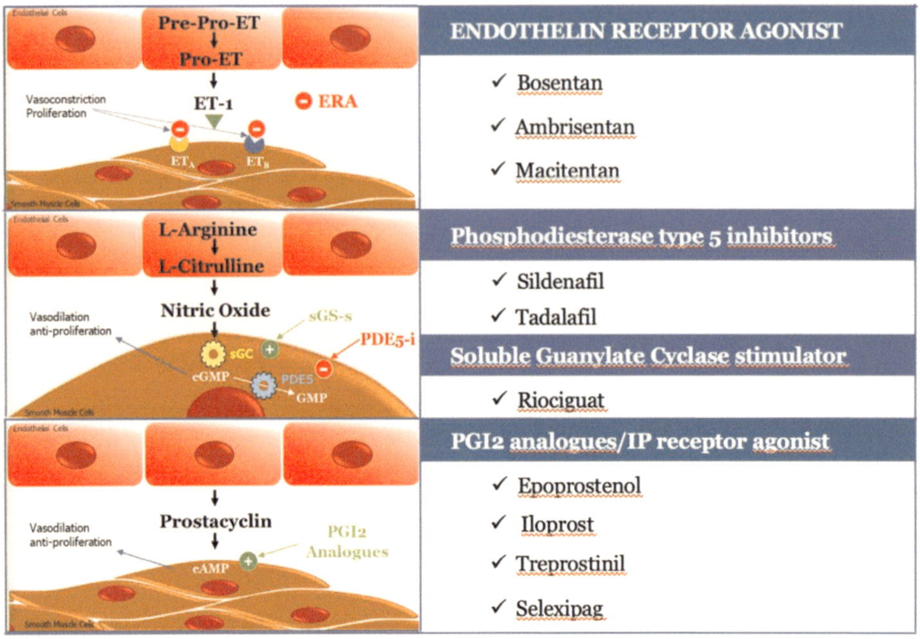

Figure 2.
Biological pathways involved in the pathogenesis of PAH. Pre-pro-ET: Pre-pro-endothelin; pro-ET: Pro-endothelin; ET > −1: Endothelin-1ETA/ETB: ET receptor subtypes A and B; ERA: Endothelin receptor agonist; sGC: Soluble guanylate cyclase; sGCs: sGCs stimulator; PDE5: Phosphodiesterase type 5; PDE-5-i: PDE5 inhibitors; cGMP: Cyclic guanosine monophosphate (GMP); cAMP: Cyclic adenosine monophosphate; PGI2 analogues: Prostaglandin I2 analogues.

measurements, include oxygen supplementation, supervised physical exercise, respiratory rehabilitation, diuretic therapy, and psychosocial support for the patient and his family [37]. Moreover, the fundamental milestone of the treatment is the specific therapy that address the three main specific pathways altered in PAH.

3.3.4.1 Drugs targeting the NO pathway

3.3.4.1.1 Sildenafil

It is a selective inhibitor of type 5 phosphodiesterase (5-PDEi), which specifically degrades cyclic guanosine monophosphate and its level is increased in pulmonary arteries. Normally, NO stimulates intracellular soluble guanylate cyclase resulting in increased levels of cGMP, which then acts to mediate smooth muscle relaxation; in PAH, there is a decrease in NO production from the endothelium. Therefore, sildenafil inhibits 5-PDEi, preventing degradation of cGMP and prolonging its effects. The SUPER-1 trial, a double-blind, and placebo-controlled trial demonstrated a significant increase in the walked distance of the 6MWT, in the WHO functional class and the hemodynamic parameters in the sildenafil group [38]. Thence, the SUPER-2 trial assessed long-term safety and tolerability of sildenafil treatment: it proved that the drug is generally well tolerated, and, after 3 years, the majority of patients (60%) who entered the SUPER-1 trial improved or maintained their functional status, and 46% maintained or improved 6MWT [39]. Common adverse effects of this therapy are diarrhea, dyspepsia, and flushing.

3.3.4.1.2 Tadalafil

It is an alternative molecule and has a better pharmacokinetic profile than sildenafil. In the PHIRST-1 trial, tadalafil demonstrated a significant improvement in 6MWT and hemodynamic parameters, such as mPAP and PVR [40]. Common adverse effects of this therapy are myalgia, flushing, and headache.

3.3.4.1.3 Riociguat

It is a direct activator of guanylate-cyclase, which synthesizes NO. In the 12-week PATENT-1 study, Riociguat was well tolerated and improved several clinically relevant end-points in patients with PAH who had never received a treatment or had been pretreated with endothelin-receptor antagonists or prostanoids. The PATENT-2 trial assessed the long-term safety and efficacy of Riociguat, which resulted to be safe in the long-term treatment of these patients [41].

3.3.4.2 Drugs targeting the ET1 pathway: endothelin receptor antagonist (ERA)

3.3.4.2.1 Bosentan

It is a dual acting ERA, binding to both the ETA and ETB receptors. Two subtypes of ET1 receptor exist: endothelin receptor subtype A (ETA) is mainly found in smooth muscle and also on fibroblasts, while ET 1 receptor subtype B (ETB) is expressed on smooth muscle and endothelial cells. Endothelial ETB activation mediates clearance of ET1 and vasodilatation by NO and prostacyclin release. Bosentan has been studied in several clinical PAH trials, such as BREATHE-1, TRUST, and EARLY [42], with generally positive results. One of the main problems with Bosentan is hepatotoxicity, which initially presents as a raised levels of alanine aminotransferase and aspartate aminotransferase.

3.3.4.2.2 Ambrisentan

It is an ERA that only blocks receptor ETA. It has been shown to increase exercise capacity and hemodynamics with an acceptable side-effect profile. It has also proven to be safely used in combination with other PAH-specific medications, especially with 5-PDEi. In the recent randomized trial ambition, it was proven that upfront dual therapy of ambrisentan and tadalafil considerably decreases the risk of clinical failure compared with monotherapy [43].

3.3.4.2.3 Macitentan

It is a dual ERA developed by adjusting the basic structure of bosentan, in order to increase the efficacity and safety, and it is approved for the treatment of PAH.

In contrast with bosentan, macitentan also has a longer binding with the ET1 receptor and a better tissue penetration [44]. One of the most important trials on Macitentan was the SERAPHIN trial, a multicenter, double-blind, randomized, placebo-controlled, and event-driven phase 3 trial. This trial demonstrated a significant reduction in morbidity and mortality in patients with PAH [45]. Common adverse effect is anemia.

3.3.4.3 Drugs targeting the prostacyclin pathway: prostacyclin analogues and prostacyclin receptor agonist

3.3.4.3.1 Epoprostenol

It is a synthetic prostacyclin, approved by FDA in December 1995 for the treatment of PAH. The pharmacological effects of epoprostenol are due to pulmonary and systemic arterial vasodilation. The effects on platelet aggregation are directly opposite to TXA_2. Epoprostenol has been demonstrated to be one of the safest treatment protocols for PH. It is also one of the best treatments to reduce the mortality rate in patients with idiopathic PAH [46]. Due to its short half-life (3–5 min), epoprostenol must be administered intravenously via continuous infusion pomp and a permanent tunneled catheter and, in order to maintain its safety-efficacy profile dose-dependent adjustments are necessary. Major adverse events are headaches, nausea/vomiting, flushing, myalgias, jaw pain, diarrhea, and upper respiratory tract infections.

3.3.4.3.2 Treprostinil

Treprostinil is an analog of Epoprostenol and can be administered by subcutaneous injection, intravenous infusion, or inhalation.

The several methods of administration, an extended half-life, and its stability at room temperature give treprostinil a pro over Epoprostenol, Iloprost, and Selexipag, the three other FDA-approved drugs targeting the prostacyclin pathway. Moreover, in clinical trials, treprostinil enhanced exercise capacity measured with 6MWT, quality of life, WHO functional class, and the clinical status of patients [47].

Usual adverse effects are dizziness, nausea, pain in the jaw and extremities, diarrhea, flushing, and headache.

3.3.4.3.3 Iloprost

It is a stable prostacyclin analog, available as an inhalant and intravenous preparation for PAH. The principal limitation of this inhaled formulation is the need for daily recurring iloprost inhalations, ranging from 6 to 9, and this can decrease patients' compliance with pharmacological treatment.

3.3.4.3.4 Selexipag

It is an oral, non-prostacyclin, and IP receptor agonist, approved by FDA in December 2015. Its molecule is very stable and has a long half-life: its effects are vasodilation of the pulmonary circulation, inhibition of platelet aggregation, and anti-inflammatory effects. In the GRIPHON study, a phase 3 multicenter, randomized, double-blind, and placebo-controlled trial. 1156 patients with PAH were randomly assigned to receive either placebo or Selexipag. It resulted that among patients with PAH, the risk of the primary composite end point of death or complication related to PAH was significantly lower with Selexipag than with placebo. Instead, there was no significant difference in mortality between the two study groups [48]. Therefore, selexipag is indicated for use in patients with World Health Organization functional class (FC) II or III diseases. Common adverse effects are headache, diarrhea, and nausea.

Treatment is started with an oral combination therapy of two different types of drugs; then, patients are evaluated after 3–6 months. If patients are at high risk, triple therapy can be considered, adding parenteral prostanoids.

3.4 Chronic thromboembolic pulmonary hypertension

Chronic thromboembolic PH (CTEPH) is a specific subtype of PH, included within Group 4. It is characterized by partial obstruction or total occlusion of subsegmental, segmental, or larger pulmonary arteries by post-embolic fibrotic material. CTEPH incidence is uncertain due to difficulties in diagnosing this disease and lack of specific symptoms: incidence is estimated to be 4 cases per million [49]. Incidence after acute pulmonary embolism is estimated to vary between 0.4% and 9.1% [50]. The pathophysiology is peculiar: CTEPH is the result of partial and incomplete resolution of embolic clots after acute pulmonary embolism, because of impaired fibrinolysis.

The residual intraluminal thrombi phenomena of inflammation, fibrosis, and organization lead to development of typical CTEPH lesions characterized by yellow clots highly adherent to the pulmonary vascular wall, containing collagen, elastin, and inflammatory cells (in contrast to fresh and red clots of acute pulmonary embolism, mainly consisting of erythrocytes and platelets in a fibrin mesh). In addition, vascular remodeling characterized by intimal fibrosis and fibromuscular proliferation, similar to idiopathic PAH, has been described in small vessels distal to unoccluded arteries. The pathogenesis of this micro vasculopathy is not clear: it has been proposed that pulmonary blood flow redistribution from occluded vessels to non-obstructed areas leads in the long term to local high-flow pressure and shear stress promoting endothelial dysfunction [51].

Vascular remodeling resulting from incomplete clot resolution and microvasculopathy leads to increased pulmonary vascular resistance and right ventricular failure. Patients affected by CTEPH can display many and non-specific symptoms, such as shortness of breath on exertion in the early stages and at rest in advanced stages, chest pain, and increased fatigue.

Early diagnosis remains a challenge and it affects prognosis and survival rate.

The gold standard for diagnosis is RHC, which displays mPAP >20 mmHg, but it has to be associated with ventilation/perfusion (V/Q) scintigraphy that shows at least one large perfusion defect in one segment or two subsegments. CT scan has also shown an excellent diagnostic efficacy, and it is usually included in the diagnostic pathway of CTEPH. A correct and early diagnosis is of fundamental importance, as CTEPH is the only PH subtype suitable for a surgical treatment and potentially curable.

Treatment of choice is pulmonary endarterectomy (PEA): within the use of circulatory arrest and hypothermia, it implicates the removal of organized tissue from pulmonary vessels. The milestone of the surgical treatment is to define the operability of patient: this is based on age, comorbidities (diabetes mellitus, lung diseases, hypertension, asthma, and coronary heart disease) and anatomical reasons (inaccessible or distal thrombi). Although, the progress in diagnostic pathways and the accumulation of surgical experience have contributed to the latest surgical development, redefining the distal limits of PEA. Therefore, in expert centers, surgery can be performed successfully in patients with thromboembolism of the distal vessels. Balloon pulmonary angioplasty (BPA) is an emerging interventional treatment and has been included in the treatment algorithm of CTEPH: it is reserved for patients that cannot undergo surgical treatment with PEA due to distal thrombi or continuous symptoms after surgery. It involves the insertion of a balloon catheter into pulmonary vessels to dilate pulmonary stenosis in order to improve hemodynamics parameters, clinical symptoms, exercise capacity, and RH compliance, with a low rate of complications [52]. Complications can occur during the procedure (vascular injury, wire perforation, vascular dissection, balloon over dilatation, and others) or after the procedure, and include lung injury, contrast-induced kidney injury, and peripheral access site problems.

Likely between 20% and 40% of patients cannot undergo either of these treatments or show residual PH after interventional therapy and are amenable to medical therapy. This includes diuretics, oxygen therapy, and lifelong anticoagulation. Anticoagulation therapy can be done with either warfarin or direct oral anticoagulants: the choice is up to the doctor, who evaluates bleeding risk, renal impairment, and decides which therapy suits better for the patient.

Riociguat has been approved for the treatment of CTEPH, it determines vasodilatation and has anti-fibrotic, anti-proliferative, and anti-inflammatory activity.

Other specific drugs are currently tested with positive results in these patients, such as Macitentan and Treprostinil [53].

4. A look to the future

PH is a complex and multifactorial disease, triggered and sustained by many pathological alterations. The three main modified pathways in PAH (NO, ET1, and PGI2) have been uncovered and targeted with appropriate pharmacological therapy, leading to an improvement in symptoms, quality of life, and survival of these patients.

In the next few years, scientists will focus their attention on researching new molecular targets that can have a role in the pathogenesis of the disease. For example, there is a trial ongoing on Rho-associated protein kinase (ROCK), which is involved in many cellular functions, such as smooth muscle cell contraction, cell migration, and others. It also has been demonstrated to play a role in the pathogenesis of PH. So, scientists are developing ROCK's inhibitors [54]. Another target is apelin, an endogenous vasodilator, which levels are decreased in PAH. Therefore, apelin infusion is being considered and trials are still ongoing [55].

Other drugs target inflammation and immunity: Ubenimex has been tested in a clinical trial but reported no improvement of symptoms and exercise capacity, tested with 6MWT [56].

Additionally, cytokines like IL-6 are overexpressed in PH, so drugs that function as inhibitors of this cytokine can play a role in future pharmacological treatment and are still going through appropriate development and testing [57].

Also, therapy targeting BMPR2 pathway has been considered: it has been shown that there is a decreased expression of this gene in heritable PAH and 20% of idiopathic PAH [58].

Moreover, there is evidence that PAH patients usually have low levels of iron. Actual guidelines suggest that iron supplementations should be considered. Kramer et al., assessed with a long-term study the use of ferric carboximaltose in PAH patients with iron deficiency: iron supplementation has demonstrated an improvement in clinical status, exercise capacity, and a decrease in hospitalization rate [59]. This resulted in an increase in 6MWT distance and a better WHO-FC and, consequently, a decreased risk calculated by ESC/ESR risk score.

Conflict of interest

The authors declare no conflict of interest.

Author details

Massimiliano Mulè*, Giulia Passaniti and Daniela Giannazzo
AOU Policlinico G. Rodolico—San Marco, Catania, Italy

*Address all correspondence to: studiocardiologicomule@gmail.com

References

[1] Boyette LC, Burns B. Physiology, pulmonary circulation. In: StatPearls [Internet]. Treasure Island, FL: StatPearls Publishing; 2021, 2022 PMID: 30085539

[2] Suresh K, Shimoda LA. Lung Circulation. Comprehensive Physiology. 2016;**6**(2):897-943. DOI: 10.1002/cphy.c140049 PMID: 27065170; PMCID: PMC7432532

[3] Parasuraman S, Walker S, Loudon BL, Gollop ND, Wilson AM, Lowery C, et al. Assessment of pulmonary artery pressure by echocardiography—A comprehensive review. International Journal of Cardiology Heart & vasculature. 2016; **12**:45-51. DOI: 10.1016/j.ijcha.2016.05.011

[4] Simonneau G, Montani D, Celermajer DS, Denton CP, Gatzoulis MA, Krowka M, Williams PG, Souza R. Haemodynamic definitions and updated clinical classification of pulmonary hypertension. European Respiratory Journal. 2019;**53**(1):1801913. DOI: 10.1183/13993003.01913-2018. PMID: 30545968; PMCID: PMC6351336

[5] Galiè N, Humbert M, Vachiery J-L, Gibbs S, Lang I, Torbicki A, et al. ESC/ERS guidelines for the diagnosis and treatment of pulmonary hypertension: The joint task force for the diagnosis and treatment of pulmonary hypertension of the European Society of Cardiology (ESC) and the European Respiratory Society (ERS): Endorsed by: Association for European Paediatric and Congenital Cardiology (AEPC), International Society for Heart and Lung Transplantation (ISHLT). European Heart Journal. 2015, 2016;**37**(1):67-119

[6] Condon DF, Nickel NP, Anderson R, Mirza S, de Jesus Perez VA. The 6th world symposium on pulmonary hypertension: What's old is new. F1000Research. 2019;**8**, F1000 Faculty Rev-:888. DOI: 10.12688/f1000research.18811.1 (European Respiratory Journal Jan 2019, 53 (1) 1801913; DOI: 10.1183/13993003.01913-2018)

[7] Naeije R, Chin K. Differentiating precapillary from postcapillary pulmonary hypertension. Circulation. 2019;**140**(9):712-714. DOI: 10.1161/CIRCULATIONAHA.119.040295 Epub 26 August 2019. PMID: 31449453

[8] Mehra P, Mehta V, Sukhija R, Sinha AK, Gupta M, Girish MP, et al. Pulmonary hypertension in left heart disease. Archives of Medical Science. 2019;**15**(1):262-273. DOI: 10.5114/aoms.2017.68938 Epub 17 July 2017. PMID: 30697278; PMCID: PMC6348356

[9] Widrich J, Shetty M. Physiology, pulmonary vascular resistance. In: StatPearls [Internet]. Treasure Island (FL): StatPearls Publishing; 2022 19 August 2021. PMID: 32119267

[10] Moncada S, Palmer RMJ, Higgs EA. Nitric oxide: Physiology, pathophysiology and pharmacology. Pharmacological Reviews. 1991;**43**: 109-142

[11] Al-Omary MS, Sugito S, Boyle AJ, Sverdlov AL, Collins NJ. Pulmonary hypertension due to left heart disease: Diagnosis, pathophysiology, and therapy. Hypertension. 2020;**75**(6): 1397-1408. DOI: 10.1161/HYPERTENSIONAHA.119.14330 Epub 27 April 2020. PMID: 32336230

[12] Guazzi M, Ghio S, Adir Y. Pulmonary hypertension in HFpEF and

HFrEF: JACC review topic of the week. Journal of the American College of Cardiology. 2020;**76**(9):1102-1111. DOI: 10.1016/j.jacc.2020.06.069 PMID: 32854845

[13] Moraes DL, Colucci WS, Givertz MM. Secondary pulmonary hypertension in chronic heart failure: The role of the endothelium in pathophysiology and management. Circulation. 2000;**102**(14):1718-1723. DOI: 10.1161/01.cir.102.14.1718 PMID: 11015353

[14] Abramson SV, Burke JF, Kelly JJ Jr, et al. Pulmonary hypertension predicts mortality and morbidity in patients with dilated cardiomyopathy. Annals of Internal Medicine. 1992;**116**:888-895

[15] Di Salvo TG, Mathier M, Semigran MJ, et al. Preserved right ventricular ejection fraction predicts exercise capacity and survival in advanced heart failure. Journal of the American College of Cardiology. 1995;**25**: 1143-1153

[16] Desai A, Desouza SA. Treatment of pulmonary hypertension with left heart disease: A concise review. Vascular Health and Risk Management. 2017;**13**: 415-420

[17] Fraser KL, Tullis DE, Sasson Z, Hyland RH, Thornley KS, Hanly PJ. Pulmonary hypertension and cardiac function in adult cystic fibrosis: Role of hypoxemia. Chest. 1999;**115**(5): 1321-1328

[18] Mirrakhimov AE, Strohl KP. High-altitude pulmonary Hypertension: An update on disease pathogenesis and management. Open Cardiovascular Medicine Journal. 2016;**10**:19-27

[19] Chaouat A, Bugnet A-S, Kadaoui N, et al. Severe pulmonary hypertension and chronic obstructive pulmonary disease. American Journal of Respiratory and Critical Care Medicine. 2005;**172**: 189-194

[20] Nathan SD, Shlobin OA, Ahmad S, et al. Serial development of pulmonary hypertension in patients with idiopathic pulmonary fibrosis. Respiration. 2008; **76**:288-294

[21] Santos S, Peinado VI, Ramirez J, et al. Characterization of pulmonary vascular remodeling in smokers and patients with mild COPD. The European Respiratory Journal. 2002;**19**:632-638

[22] Colombat M, Mal H, Groussard O, et al. Pulmonary vascular lesions in end-stage idiopathic pulmonary fibrosis: Histopathologic study on lung explant specimens and correlations with pulmonary hemodynamics. Human Pathology. 2007;**38**:60-65

[23] Kim K-H, Maldonado F, Ryu JH, et al. Iron deposition and increased alveolar septal capillary density in nonfibrotic lung tissue are associated with pulmonary hypertension in idiopathic pulmonary fibrosis. Respiratory Research. 2010;**11**:37

[24] Ruffenach G, Hong J, Vaillancourt M, Medzikovic L, Eghbali M. Pulmonary hypertension secondary to pulmonary fibrosis: Clinical data, histopathology and molecular insights. Respiratory Research. 2020; **21**(1):303. DOI: 10.1186/s12931-020-01570-2

[25] Mura M, Anraku M, Yun Z, et al. Gene expression profiling in the lungs of patients with pulmonary hypertension associated with pulmonary fibrosis. Chest. 2012;**141**:661-673

[26] Patrizio V, Callari A, Martino L, Stanziola A, Oggionni T, Federica M,

et al. SPHERIC-1 (Sildenafil and Pulmonary HypERtension in COPD): Intention-to-Treat (ITT) Analysis of Safety and Efficacy Data. The Journal of Heart and Lung Transplantation. 2014; **33**:S148-S149. DOI: 10.1016/j.healun.2014.01.398

[27] Waxman A, Restrepo-Jaramillo R, Thenappan T, et al. Inhaled Treprostinil in pulmonary hypertension due to interstitial lung disease. New England Journal of Medicine. 2021;**384**(4): 325-334. DOI: 10.1056/NEJMoa2008470

[28] Levine DJ. Pulmonary arterial hypertension: Updates in epidemiology and evaluation of patients. The American Journal of Managed Care. 2021;**27**(3 Suppl):S35-S41. DOI: 10.37765/ajmc.2021.88609 PMID: 33710842

[29] Pauwaa S, Machado RF, Desai AA. Survival in pulmonary arterial hypertension: A brief review of registry data. Pulmonary Circulation. 2011;**1**(3): 430-431. DOI: 10.4103/2045-8932.87314

[30] Farber HW, Miller DP, Poms AD, Badesch DB, Frost AE, Muros-Le Rouzic E, et al. Five-year outcomes of patients enrolled in the REVEAL registry. Chest. 2015;**148**(4):1043-1054. DOI: 10.1378/chest.15-0300 PMID: 26066077

[31] Makino A, Firth AL, Yuan JX. Endothelial and smooth muscle cell ion channels in pulmonary vasoconstriction and vascular remodeling. Comprehensive Physiology. 2011;**1**(3):1555-1602

[32] Galie N, Manes A, Branzi A. The endothelin system in pulmonary arterial hypertension. Cardiovascular Research. 2004;**61**:227-237

[33] Tuder RM, Cool CD, Geraci MW, Wang J, Abman SH, Wright L, et al. Prostacyclin synthase expression is decreased in lungs from patients with severe pulmonary hypertension. American Journal of Respiratory and Critical Care Medicine. 1999;**159**: 1925-1932

[34] Le RJ, Fenstad ER, Maradit-Kremers H, et al. Syncope in adults with pulmonary arterial hypertension. Journal of the American College of Cardiology. 2011;**58**:863-867

[35] Fijalkowska A, Kurzyna M, Torbicki A, et al. Serum N-terminal brain natriuretic peptide as a prognostic parameter in patients with pulmonary hypertension. Chest. 2006;**129**:1312-1321

[36] Raymond RJ, Hinderliter AL, Willis PW, et al. Echocardiographic predictors of adverse outcomes in primary pulmonary hypertension. Journal of the American College of Cardiology. 2002;**39**:1214-1219

[37] Guillevin L, Armstrong I, Aldrighetti R, Howard LS, Ryftenius H, Fischer A, et al. Understanding the impact of pulmonary arterial hypertension on patients' and carers' lives. European Respiratory Review. 2013;**22**:535-542

[38] Galiè N, Ghofrani HA, Torbicki A, Barst RJ, Rubin LJ, Badesch D, et al. Sildenafil use in pulmonary arterial hypertension (SUPER) study group. Sildenafil citrate therapy for pulmonary arterial hypertension. The New England Journal of Medicine. 2005;**353**(20): 2148-2157. DOI: 10.1056/NEJMoa050010 Erratum in: N Engl J Med. 2006;**354**(22): 2400-1. PMID: 16291984

[39] Rubin LJ, Badesch DB, Fleming TR, Galiè N, Simonneau G, Ghofrani HA, et al. Long-term treatment with sildenafil citrate in pulmonary arterial

hypertension: The SUPER-2 study. Chest. 2011;**140**(5):1274-1283. DOI: 10.1378/chest.10-0969 Epub 5 May 2011. PMID: 21546436

[40] Galiè N, Brundage BH, Ghofrani HA, Oudiz RJ, Simonneau G, Safdar Z, et al. Pulmonary Arterial Hypertension and Response to Tadalafil (PHIRST) Study Group. Tadalafil therapy for pulmonary arterial hypertension. Circulation. 2009;**119**(22):2894-903. DOI: 10.1161/CIRCULATIONAHA. 108.839274. Epub 2009 May 26. Erratum in: Circulation. 2011;**124**(10):e279. Dosage error in article text. PMID: 19470885

[41] Rubin LJ, Galiè N, Grimminger F, Grünig E, Humbert M, Jing ZC, et al. Riociguat for the treatment of pulmonary arterial hypertension: A long-term extension study (PATENT-2). The European Respiratory Journal. 2015; **45**(5):1303-1313. DOI: 10.1183/09031936.00090614 Epub 22 January 2015. PMID: 25614164

[42] Valerio CJ, Coghlan JG. Bosentan in the treatment of pulmonary arterial hypertension with the focus on the mildly symptomatic patient. Vascular Health and Risk Management. 2009;**5**:607-619. DOI: 10.2147/vhrm. s4713

[43] Rivera-Lebron BN, Risbano MG. Ambrisentan: A review of its use in pulmonary arterial hypertension. Therapeutic Advances in Respiratory Disease. 2017;**11**(6):233-244. DOI: 10.1177/1753465817696040

[44] Sidharta PN, Treiber A, Dingemanse J. Clinical pharmacokinetics and pharmacodynamics of the endothelin receptor antagonist macitentan. Clinical Pharmacokinetics. 2015;**54**(5):457-471. DOI: 10.1007/s40262-015-0255-5

[45] Jansa P, Pulido T. Macitentan in pulmonary arterial hypertension: A focus on combination therapy in the SERAPHIN trial. American Journal of Cardiovascular Drugs: Drugs, Devices, and Other Interventions. 2018;**18**(1): 1-11. DOI: 10.1007/s40256-017-0260-1

[46] Barst RJ, Rubin LJ, Long WA, McGoon MD, Rich S, Badesch DB, et al. A comparison of continuous intravenous epoprostenol (prostacyclin) with conventional therapy for primary pulmonary hypertension. The New England Journal of Medicine. 1996; **334**(5):296-301. DOI: 10.1056/NEJM199602013340504 PMID: 8532025

[47] Barnes H, Yeoh HL, Fothergill T, Burns A, Humbert M, Williams T. Prostacyclin for pulmonary arterial hypertension. The Cochrane Database of Systematic Reviews. 2019;**5**(5):CD012785

[48] Sitbon O, Channick R, Chin KM, Frey A, Gaine S, Galiè N, et al. Selexipag for the treatment of pulmonary arterial hypertension. The New England Journal of Medicine. 2015;**373**(26):2522-2533. DOI: 10.1056/NEJMoa1503184 PMID: 26699168

[49] Poli D, Grifoni E, Antonucci E, et al. Incidence of recurrent venous thromboembolism and of chronic thromboembolic pulmonary hypertension in patients after a first episode of pulmonary embolism. Journal of Thrombosis and Thrombolysis. 2010; **30**(3):294-299

[50] Marti D, Gomez V, Escobar C, et al. Incidence of symptomatic and asymptomatic chronic thromboembolic pulmonary hypertension. Archivos de Bronconeumología. 2010;**46**(12): 628-633

[51] Lang IM, Pesavento R, Bonderman D, et al. Risk factors and

basic mechanisms of chronic thromboembolic pulmonary hypertension: A current understanding. The European Respiratory Journal. 2013; **41**:462-468

[52] Ogo T. Balloon pulmonary angioplasty for inoperable chronic thromboembolic pulmonary hypertension. Current Opinion in Pulmonary Medicine. 2015;**21**:425-431

[53] Ghofrani HA, Simonneau G, D'Armini AM, Fedullo P, Howard LS, Jaïs X, et al. Macitentan for the treatment of inoperable chronic thromboembolic pulmonary hypertension (MERIT-1): Results from the multicentre, phase 2, randomised, double-blind, placebo-controlled study. The Lancet Respiratory Medicine. 2017;**5**(10):785-794. DOI: 10.1016/S2213-2600(17)30305-3 Epub 11 September 2017. PMID: 28919201

[54] Doggrell SA. Rho-kinase inhibitors show promise in pulmonary hypertension. Expert Opinion on Investigational Drugs. 2005;**14**(9): 1157-1159. DOI: 10.1517/13543784.14.9.1157 PMID: 16144499

[55] Mughal A, O'Rourke ST. Vascular effects of apelin: Mechanisms and therapeutic potential. Pharmacology & Therapeutics. 2018;**190**:139-147. DOI: 10.1016/j.pharmthera.2018.05.013 Epub 25 May 2018. PMID: 29807055; PMCID: PMC6165679

[56] Grinnan D, Trankle C, Andruska A, Bloom B, Spiekerkoetter E. Drug repositioning in pulmonary arterial hypertension: Challenges and opportunities. Pulmonary Circulation. 2019;**9**(1):2045894019832226

[57] Steiner MK, Syrkina OL, Kolliputi N, Mark EJ, Hales CA, Waxman AB. Interleukin-6 overexpression induces pulmonary hypertension. Circulation Research. 2009;**104**(2):236-244

[58] Orriols M, Gomez-Puerto MC, Ten Dijke P. BMP type II receptor as a therapeutic target in pulmonary arterial hypertension. Cellular and Molecular Life Sciences. 2017;**74**(16):2979-2995. DOI: 10.1007/s00018-017-2510-4 Epub 26 April 2017. Erratum in: Cell Mol Life Sci. 23 May 2017; PMID: 28447104; PMCID: PMC5501910

[59] Kramer T, Wissmüller M, Natsina K, Gerhardt F, Ten Freyhaus H, Dumitrescu D, et al. Ferric carboxymaltose in patients with pulmonary arterial hypertension and iron deficiency: A long-term study. Journal of Cachexia, Sarcopenia and Muscle. 2021;**12**(6):1501-1512. DOI: 10.1002/jcsm.12764 Epub 9 September 2021. PMID: 34498427; PMCID: PMC8718050

Chapter 15

Stress-Induced Cardiomyopathy

Jake J. Wen and Ravi S. Radhakrishnan

Abstract

The irreversible termination of individual life activities and metabolism means all fatal problems ultimately terminate the heart function. It's very important to protect the patient's life if we have treatment to maintain heart function and care about patients' heart response. It is known that many diseases induced heart dysfunction including Chagas disease, burn injury, smoking and other bad stresses. Chronic stress causes these physical symptoms and emotional symptoms. Due to the awareness created by the media and internet, patients are generally aware that they should seek help immediately for chest pain. Therefore, attention and studies on stress-induced heart dysfunction would help uncover the pathophysiological mechanisms of cardiac response to non-heart diseases and provide an insight of heart-protection drugs. At the same time, physicians should be aware of this new condition and how to diagnose and treat it, even though the causal mechanisms are not yet fully understood. This special chapter will discuss on the cardiac response to the stresses especially on our associated research in recent decades such as Trypanosoma cruzi (*T. cruzi*)-induced cardiomyopathy and burn injury–induced cardiomyopathy, and on some very popular stresses such as behavior, motion, mental, and smoking.

Keywords: stress, cardiomyopathy, emotional symptom, physical symptom, *Trypanosoma cruzi*, burn injury, Tobacco and E-cigarettes

1. Introduction

Stress-induced cardiomyopathy is caused by intense emotional or physical stress leading to rapid and severe reversible cardiac dysfunction. This condition can occur following a variety of emotional stressors such as grief, fear, extreme anger, and surprise. On the other hand, many physical stressors (i.e., stroke, seizure or acute asthma) can also trigger the condition. Suspicion of stress cardiomyopathy is based on clinical symptoms, abnormal electrocardiogram (ECG), mildly elevated serum cardiac troponin, significantly elevated serum natriuretic peptide levels (BNP or NT-proBNP), and noninvasive cardiovascular imaging. Stress-induced cardiomyopathy symptoms following severe stress are often indistinguishable from a heart attack and may include: (1) chest pain, dyspnea, or both during stress period (often sudden and intense) [1]; (2) shortness of breath, (3) rapid or irregular heartbeat, (4) sweating and (5) dizziness [2]. The exact pathophysiology of stress-induced cardiomyopathy remains elusive, and several mechanisms may be involved (**Figure 1**).

Considering the causes of stress-induced cardiomyopathy, the exact cause of stress-induced cardiomyopathy is unclear. In patients without coronary heart disease, emotional stress can lead to severe, reversible left ventricular dysfunction. Although the mechanism of stress-induced cardiomyopathy is unclear, excessive sympathetic stimulation may be central to its etiology, perhaps involving excess catecholamines (**Figure 1**), but the link between the two is unclear. One possibility is ischemia due to epicardial coronary spasm; additionally increased sympathetic tone can lead to vasoconstriction in patients without coronary artery disease [3]. Other studies have demonstrated that these patients have reduced coronary flow reserve and regional deficits in cardiac imaging [4]. Another possible mechanism for catecholamine-mediated myocardial stunning is direct muscle cell damage, as the density of adrenergic receptors in the apex is higher than in other areas of the myocardium [1]. Elevated levels of catecholamines lead to a concentration-dependent decrease in muscle cell viability, which can be explained

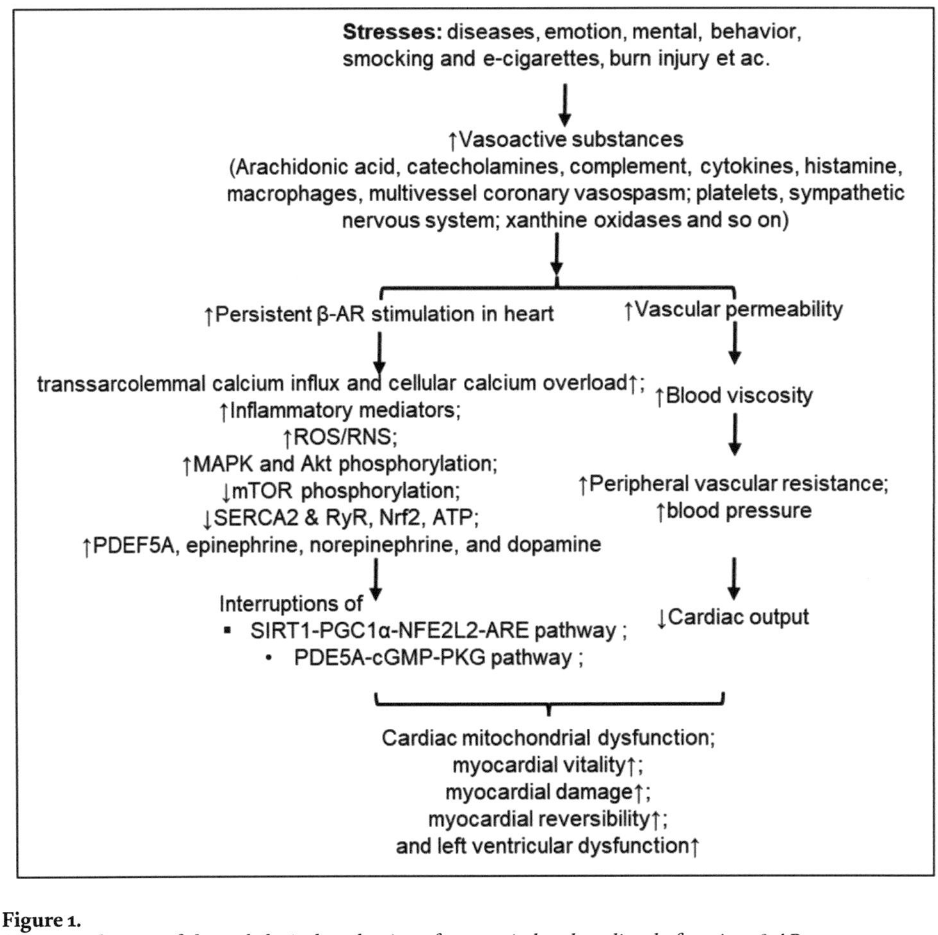

Figure 1.
Schematic diagram of the pathological mechanism of stresses-induced cardiac dysfunction. β-AR, estrogen receptor beta; ROS/RNS, reactive oxygen/nitrogen species; MAPK, mitogen-activated protein kinase; Akt, protein kinase B; mTOR, mammalian target of rapamycin; SERCA2, sarcoplasmic reticulum calcium ATPase 2; RyR, ryanodine receptor; Nrf2, nuclear factor erythroid-derived 2-like 2; ATP, adenosine triphosphate; PDE5A, phosphodiesterase 5A; SIRT1, Sirtuin 1; PGC1-alpha, peroxisome proliferator-activated receptor gamma coactivator 1-alpha; OKG, cGMP-dependent protein kinase or protein kinase G.

by the marked release of creatine kinase in cells and the decreased viability due to calcium overload mediated by circulating AMPs [5]. Animal models suggest that catecholamines are a potential source of free radicals, which in turn may contribute to cardiomyopathy by promoting lipid peroxidation, increasing membrane permeability and muscle cell damage (**Figure 1**) [6]. Myocyte dysfunction may be caused by increased trans-sarcolemmal calcium influx and cellular calcium overload as free radicals interfere with the transport capacity of sodium and calcium transporters (**Figure 1**) [7]. Abnormal coronary blood flow has recently been reported in patients with stress-related myocardial dysfunction in the absence of obstructive disease [8]. Evidence that stress cardiomyopathy may be caused by neurogenic myocardial stunning also revealed a unique pattern of ventricular synergy with meta-iodobenzyl guanidine myocardial scintigraphy, suggesting the presence of cardiac sympathetic hyperactivity and maintaining coronary blood flow [9]. The distribution of primary cardiac injury did not correspond to the perfusion area of a single coronary artery. Plasma levels of catecholamines and stress-related neuropeptides are usually higher than the patient's physiological levels. Unlike polymorphonuclear inflammation in stress cardiomyopathy infarcts, contractile band necrosis is a distinct form of stress-induced cardiomyocyte injury characterized by hypercontraction of sarcomeres, eosinophilic transverse bands, and interstitial mononucleitis, and endomyocardial biopsy shows contractile band necrosis in patients with this syndrome [1]. Research shows that contractile band necrosis is a type of cell death detected as early as 2 min after cell injury, resulting in the release of cardiac enzymes [10]. Excessive circulating catecholamines and focal myocarditis contractile bands were found in the circulatory system of pheochromocytoma, suggesting a circulating catecholamine dependence of focal myocarditis [11], subarachnoid hemorrhage [12, 13], eclampsia [13], and in persons who died from fatal asthma necrosis [14]. All together, these suggest that catecholamines may be the link between emotional stress and heart damage (**Figure 1**).

A surge of stress hormones may temporarily damage the heart, many studies have found. Triggers of stress cardiomyopathy due to stress hormones include: (1) financial stress; (2) surgical stress; (3) bereavement stress; (4) asthma attack stress; (5) chronic disease or diagnostic stress; (6) other. Risk factors for stress cardiomyopathy are also quite different from any physical discomfort, mainly including: (1) age: most cases occur in people over 50; (2) intense physical or emotional events: such as a loved one accidental death, medical diagnosis, sudden economic decline or unemployment, divorce, physical abuse, car accident, major surgery, natural disaster, or intense fear; (3) side effects of certain medications: some are used to treat severe allergic reactions, diabetic neurological problems, depression symptoms or hypothyroidism drugs, etc. may cause a surge in stress hormones, leading to stress cardiomyopathy; (4) gender: this condition affects women much more than men; (5) neurological disorders; (6) previous or current mental illness.

Stress-induced cardiomyopathy is diagnosed by looking for certain markers to distinguish it from other heart conditions. Possible tests should include: (1) blood tests: to check the levels of certain fats, cholesterol, sugars, and proteins in the blood; (2) chest X-ray: common imaging tests of the lungs, heart, and aorta; (3) coronary angiography: this the procedure is usually done in conjunction with cardiac catheterization; (4) echocardiography: this test uses sound waves to take dynamic pictures of the heart's chambers and valves; (5) electrocardiogram (ECG): this test measures the electrical activity of the heart and can help determine whether a part of the heart is enlarged, overworked, or damaged; (6) Magnetic Resonance Imaging (MRI): uses large magnets, radio waves, and a computer to produce images of the heart and blood vessels.

2. Behavior-induced cardiomyopathy

Over the past decade, research on psychosocial risk factors for heart disease has made great strides [15]. According to epidemiological studies [16], behavioral risk factors for heart disease can be divided into five categories [17]: (1) physical health behaviors; (2) negative emotional and mental states; (3) chronic stress; (4) social isolation and lack of social support; and (5) lack of a sense of purpose.

2.1 Physical health behaviors

New research suggests that poor sleep quality and inappropriate rest and relaxation are also behavior-related risk factors for heart disease [18]. As far as sleep is concerned, recent meta-analyses have shown that both insomnia and long or short sleep duration are risk factors for heart disease [19]. Excessive sleep duration can be a potential marker of depression or medical comorbidities, while too short sleep duration can be caused by multiple factors, including sleep deprivation or sleep deprivation due to worrying and other causes of insomnia. As the workload becomes heavier and the pace of life becomes faster, the boundaries between work and leisure are disappearing, and the value of relaxation has become more important. Theoretically, relaxation may benefit physiological and cognitive functions, but so far, epidemiological studies in this area are relatively lacking.

2.2 Affective disorders and negative emotional states

2.2.1 Depression

Studies have consistently shown that depression is an important risk factor for heart disease [20], and a series of meta-analyses have demonstrated a significant effect of depression on prognosis, including a meta-analysis of 54 studies showing that depression nearly doubled the risk of heart disease in a community cohort population [21].

2.2.2 Anxiety symptoms and syndromes

In recent years, studies have identified anxiety as one of the risk factors for heart disease [22]. Many meta-analyses of community cohorts and patient cohorts have shown that anxiety symptoms increase the risk of heart disease [23]. Other studies have shown that patients with generalized anxiety disorder, panic attacks, and post-traumatic stress syndrome have an increased risk of heart disease events [24].

2.2.3 Pessimism

Mental outlook is also one of the determinants of health, with optimists being more positive, having enhanced social functioning and better recovery from myocardial infarction or heart surgery [25]. Recent epidemiological data suggest that pessimism increases the risk of cardiac events, stroke, and/or all-cause mortality [26].

2.2.4 Anger and hostility

Anger and hostility have been extensively studied [27]. However, a meta-analysis of healthy people and patients with heart disease found that anger and/or hostility only increased the rate of cardiac events [28].

2.3 Chronic stress

So far, most studies on chronic stress have focused on situational stress [29], and work stress [30] is the most widely studied one. A recent meta-analysis showed that occupational stress was associated with increase in heart disease events [31]. Separation and divorce are two other common stressors that increase the risk of death [32], and independent epidemiological studies have also shown an association between marital stress and cardiovascular events [33].

It is worth mentioning that personal stress perception may also be one of the important factors affecting health [34]. A study that assessed levels of stress perception and perceptions of whether stress was harmful to health in 28,753 participants showed that stress increased mortality only in those who self-assessed risk harmful to health [35]. A complementary study showed that guiding individuals to understand stress as a positive effect improved cognitive and cardiovascular responses to stress. Combining the above two studies, we should further study the individual's perception of stress and the impact of its regulation on health.

2.4 Social isolation and lack of social support

Epidemiological studies consistently show that small social networks, lack of social support, loneliness, and/or feelings of lack of emotional support increase the risk of cardiac events [36]. Like other psychosocial risk factors, the likelihood of adverse cardiac events increases with the degree of lack of social support, and a positive social overall can nearly triple survival [37].

2.5 Lack of sense of purpose

Observational studies have shown that a strong sense of purpose in life is central to leading an active life, and that a lack of purpose in life can lead to boredom, increase risk of depression, and diminish resilience. Although only a few studies have assessed the pathophysiological outcomes of lack of purpose, a large number of recent studies have shown that lack of purpose increases the risk of death [38].

2.6 Psychosocial functioning

Negative psychosocial factors contribute to the development of disease by forming negative behaviors and direct pathophysiological effects. These effects vary by type of psychosocial stress, but as a whole include autonomic dysfunction, cardiovascular hyperresponsiveness, insulin resistance, central obesity, increased risk of hypertension, endothelial and platelet dysfunction, and brain adverse changes in adaptive and cognitive function, etc. [39].

Conversely, positive psychosocial factors favor healthy behaviors and promote beneficial physiological effects, including enhanced immune and endothelial and autonomic function. In addition, positive psychosocial functioning contributes to increased vitality, which in turn increases presence, purpose, and resistance [40].

3. Bad emotion-induced cardiovascular disease (CVD)

With the transition from the biomedical model to the biopsychosocial medical model, the psychosomatic relationship of cardiovascular disease has attracted more attention. Most cardiovascular diseases have both biomedical and psychosocial factors in the pathogenesis; in terms of clinical symptoms, there are both somatic and psychological symptoms. Growing research is finding a strong link between mood and morbidity and mortality of CVD, as one of the common public health problems worldwide [41], arousing social concern [42]. With the transition from the traditional biomedical model to the modern biopsychosocial medical model, the psychosomatic relationship of CVD has attracted more attention. The effect of emotion on cardiovascular health can be explained by certain association mechanisms, but the specific and clear association mechanism has not yet formed a consensus.

Emotion is a short-lived, strong attitude and experience that an individual is stimulated by the living environment, accompanied by obvious physiological changes and external manifestations of a psychological state [43]. Psychologists divide emotions into two dimensions: negative emotions and positive emotions. Negative emotion is a negative emotion triggered by anticipation of future events and memory of past time, which can manifest in different forms (such as panic, anxiety, depression, hostility, etc.) [44].

3.1 Emotion and cardiomyopathy research

Previous studies have found that patients with acute myocardial infarction are often in varying degrees of negative emotional states after experiencing a sense of near-death [44, 45]. Some studies have also shown that patients with heart failure have poor quality of life, and the incidence of anxiety and depression are 62% and 65%, respectively [46]. On the one hand, negative emotions are one of the independent predictors of poor prognosis in hospitalized patients with CVD [47]. Conversely, positive emotions are associated with a reduced risk of CVD [45, 47]. However, the internal mechanism of the two is still unclear.

3.2 Biological mechanisms of emotional effects on cardiomyopathy

The study found that the biological mechanism of the influence of emotion on cardiomyopathy is mainly reflected in the two aspects of vascular endothelial injury and inflammatory response, as well as the activity of the autonomic nervous system (**Figure 1**) [48].

3.2.1 Emotional changes cause endothelial damage and inflammation

The early manifestation of cardiomyopathy is the damage of the vascular endothelium [49]. Studies have found that there is a correlation between emotional state and the state of the cardiovascular endothelium [50]. Massachusetts area in the United

States found that positive mood (joy) was inversely correlated with inducible nitric oxide synthase promoter methylation [51], which play an important role in maintaining the homeostasis of vascular function.

3.2.2 The autonomic nervous system as a mechanism for the link between mood and cardiomyopathy

The autonomic nervous system has an important regulatory mechanism for the cardiovascular system, including the sympathetic nervous system and the parasympathetic nervous system (**Figure 1**) [52]. Heart rate variability (HRV) is a commonly used index for evaluating autonomic nerve function and the risk of sudden cardiac death. HRV analysis can effectively evaluate the state of cardiac autonomic nerve function. It is a relatively independent index for predicting the short- and long-term prognosis of various CVDs and sudden cardiac death [53]. Liu [54] found that when healthy individuals were exposed to negative emotional stress, the production of cardiac autonomic nerve function was significantly different. Similar changes in the pathological state of coronary heart disease suggest that long-term negative emotions may be one of the reasons for individual parasympathetic nerve damage.

4. Mental stress-induced cardiomyopathy

There is increasing evidence that, in addition to traditional factors, mental stress plays an important role in the occurrence and development of cardiovascular disease [55]. The psychological stress generated in daily life and work can lead to the occurrence of myocardial ischemia, which is clinically referred to as mental stress-induced cardiomyopathy (MSIC) [56]. In addition to affecting the quality of life of patients, mental stress-induced myocardial ischemia (MSIMI) can also lead to a worsening clinical prognosis and an increased risk of death. Its pathogenesis and pathogenesis are different from those of exercise stress or drug-related myocardial ischemia. The incidence of MSIMI is 20–70%, and it will double the adverse cardiac events [57]. Therefore, in-depth understanding of the pathogenesis of MSIMI and timely diagnosis and treatment, is of great clinical significance.

4.1 Features of MSIC

Understanding the clinical features of MSIC will help clinicians identify MSIC patients early and treat them in a timely manner.

4.1.1 Depression or anxiety

Depression and anxiety are risk factors for cardiomyopathy, aggravate the process of heart disease, and affect the prognosis of heart disease. Patients with heart disease complicated by depression or anxiety have a higher incidence of MSIC after mental stress [58].

4.1.2 Brain function

During mental stress, changes in brain function are related to the occurrence of MSIC. Studies have shown that compared with patients with heart disease without depression, patients with heart disease and severe depression have increased activity in the parietal cortex after mental stress stimulation [59]. Another study showed that mental stress-induced vasoconstriction is associated with modulation of brain function, with stress increasing activation in the insula and parietal cortex but decreasing activation in the medial prefrontal cortex [60].

4.1.3 Cardiac markers

Changes in cardiac markers may be associated with MSIC. Highly sensitivity cardiac troponin I (hs-cTnI) is an indicator of myocardial infarction or myocardial injury and is associated with myocardial ischemia caused by mental stress. Studies have shown that compared with heart disease patients without MSIC, patients with heart disease combined with MSIMI have higher serum hs-cTnI levels, and increased N-terminal pro-B-type natriuretic peptide and mean systolic blood pressure after mental stress [55]. Numerous studies have shown that myocardial hypoxia can lead to the elevation of B-type natriuretic peptide (BNP). Elevated BNP levels may be a marker of myocardial ischemia in a meta-analysis of 2784 patients eligible for standard noninvasive stress testing [61].

4.1.4 Other factors

After psychological stress, coronary heart disease patients with severe left ventricular dysfunction have a higher risk of MSIC than patients with normal left ventricular function [62]. The product of heart rate and systolic blood pressure and peripheral arterial tension were measured in resting state and 30 min after mental stress, respectively. It was found that higher hemodynamics and vasoconstriction response were high risk factors for MSIC [63].

4.2 Pathogenesis of MSIC

4.2.1 Hypothalamic-pituitary-adrenal (HPA) axis

When people cope with mental stress, the paraventricular nucleus of the hypothalamus will secrete corticotropin-releasing hormone, which will cause the anterior pituitary to secrete corticotropin, which will stimulate the adrenal cortex to produce cortisol. Decreased baroreceptor reflex sensitivity can lead to myocardial ischemia and even severe arrhythmia and sudden death. Broadley et al. [64] found that the application of metyrapone, a drug that blocks cortisol release, prevented mental stress-related endothelial dysfunction and reduced baroreflex sensitivity. In addition, Seldenrijk et al. [65] showed that, in healthy elderly populations, an enhanced cortisol response to stressful stress was associated with an increased risk of coronary artery calcification.

4.2.2 Sympathetic nervous system

During mental stress, the excitability of the cardiac sympathetic nervous system increases, and the activated sympathetic nervous system promotes the release of catecholamines (including epinephrine, norepinephrine, and dopamine), resulting in increased blood pressure, increased heart rate, increased myocardial contractility, and cardiac output (**Figure 1**) [63]. The study of Wittstein et al. [1] showed that under strong mental stress in patients with stress cardiomyopathy, the level of catecholamines increased rapidly, and the excitability of the sympathetic nervous system was significantly enhanced, which led to the disturbance of neurohumoral regulation, resulting in increased myocardial vitality, myocardial damage, myocardial reversibility and left ventricular dysfunction (**Figure 1**).

4.2.3 Inflammatory factors

Inflammation is closely related to mental stress and cardiovascular disease. When the body responds to mental stress, blood vessels constrict and blood flow increases, prompting white blood cells and platelets to release inflammatory mediators [56]. When the stress is weak, the body can play a defensive role through the inflammatory response. When the stress is strong, excessive inflammatory mediators lead to vascular endothelial damage, which further promotes inflammatory response and inflammatory mediators, as well as promotes inflammatory cells to infiltrate myocardial tissue, leading to myocardial ischemia necrosis and cardiovascular disease [56]. Hammadah et al. [56] showed that the levels of inflammatory factors such as interleukin-6, monocyte chemoattractant protein-1, and matrix metalloproteinase-9, increased in patients with heart disease after mental stress. The level of matrix metalloproteinase-9 was negatively correlated with cortisol after stress. In conclusion, the relationship between inflammation-related factors and MSIC remains to be further explored (**Figure 1**).

4.2.4 Gene polymorphisms

Genetic factors are one of the important reasons for the onset of cardiovascular diseases. Mental and psychological diseases are also closely related to an individual's response to stressful stimuli. For example, the serotonin transporter gene (SLC6A4) polymorphism is associated with emotion regulation in humans, and S allele carriers cause more severe fear and anxiety under mental stress [50]. Studies on the Val66Met single nucleotide polymorphism of brain-derived neurotrophic factor (BDNF) have shown that BDNFMet/Val carriers have a higher incidence of cognitive and mental disorders and coronary heart disease [51, 66].

5. *Trypanosoma cruzi* infection-induced cardiomyopathy

Chagas disease is named after Carlos Ribeiro Justiniano Chagas, a Brazilian doctor and researcher who discovered the disease in 1909. In May 2019, according to the decision of the Seventy-second World Health Assembly, World Day against Chagas Disease was set on April 14 (the day in 1909, when Carlos Chagas diagnosed the first human case of the disease in a two-year-old girl named Berenice). Chagas disease, also known as American trypanosomiasis, is a life-threatening disease caused by the protozoan parasite *Trypanosoma cruzi*. (*T. cruzi*) [67]. An estimated 6–7 million people worldwide are infected with *T. cruzi*, mostly in Latin America, the parasite that causes Chagas disease [68]. Chagas disease is primarily found in endemic areas of 21 countries in the Latin American continent and is mostly transmitted to humans through contact with the feces or urine of triatomine bugs (vector-borne) [69]. Although the majority of these infected individuals reside in Mexico, Central America, and South America, migration patterns have resulted in large numbers of infected individuals in formerly nonaffected areas, including Europe, Japan, Australia, Canada, and the United States [70], with an estimated 300,000 individuals in the United States alone [71]. These bed bugs are also known as “kissing bugs” and have many other names depending on the geographic area.

5.1 Global distribution

Chagas disease was once completely confined to rural areas of the American continent—mostly Latin America (excluding the Caribbean islands). Most of the infected people live in urban environments (urbanization), mainly due to increased population mobility over the past few decades, with an increasing number of infections found in the United States, Canada, many European countries, and some African, Eastern Mediterranean, and Western Pacific countries [72].

5.2 Transmission

In Latin America, *Trigonoscuta cruzi* is mainly transmitted by contact with the feces/urine of infected blood-sucking Triton bugs. These parasite-carrying insects typically live in cracks in the walls or roofs of rural or suburban houses and surrounding structures such as chicken coops, pens and warehouses [71]. Normally, they hide during the day and become active at night, feeding on blood from animals, including humans. They usually bite on exposed areas of the skin, such as the face (hence it is often referred to as a “kissing bug”) and defecate/urine close to the bite. Parasites enter the body when a person involuntarily applies their feces or urine to the bite, eyes, mouth, or any skin breakage. *T. cruzi* can also be spread by: (1) ingestion of food or drink contaminated with *T. cruzi*, such as through contact with the feces or urine of infected Trypanosoma bugs or marsupials (this transmission often results in outbreaks of simultaneous infection of several populations, severe cases or morbidity more frequently and with a higher number of deaths or fatalities); (2) passed from an infected mother to a newborn during pregnancy or childbirth; (3) transfusion of blood or blood products from infected donors; (4) organ transplantation using infected donor organs; and (5) laboratory accident.

5.3 Symptoms and signs

Chagas disease is divided into four phases: incubation phase, acute phase, interminate phase and chronic phase.

5.3.1 Incubation phage

The incubation period for *T. cruzi* ranges from 1 to 2 weeks after vector-borne transmission [69] and up to 3–4 months after transfusion or transplant transmission [73]. The disease in incubation phase is unknown and may be more than a week.

5.3.2 Acute phase

The initial acute phase lasts about 2 months after infection. During the acute phase, a large number of parasites circulate in the blood. However, most cases are asymptomatic or mild and nonspecific. In less than 50% of people bitten by triatomine bugs, the typical first sign seen can be a skin lesion or bruising and swelling on one eyelid. In addition, fever, headache, swollen lymph nodes, pallor, muscle pain, difficulty breathing, swelling, and abdominal or chest pain may also present. In the acute phase, fever (missing or intermittent), rash, hepatosplenomegaly, lymphadenopathy, and non-inflammatory edema may be present and may be limited to the face or systemic. Trypanosoma's enter tissues during or after parasemia, causing myocarditis and endocarditis, sinus tachycardia, mitral systolic murmur, cardiac hypertrophy, and meningoencephalitis. Symptoms disappear after more than 4 to 12 weeks. Severe cases are more common in neonates, young children, the elderly and immunosuppressed. Heart failure or ventricular fibrillation and meningoencephalitis caused by early myocarditis during this period can often lead to death. When more advanced electrocardiographic findings are present, including right bundle-branch block (RBBB), atrial fibrillation, or ventricular arrhythmias, they signal a worse prognosis [74].

5.3.3 Interminate phase

The interminate phase is almost asymptomatic, but progresses to a chronic, symptomatic phase, including the gradual development of irreversible life-threatening and disabling comorbidities, especially to those who are immunosuppressed. Physical examination is normal, and resting electrocardiogram is normal. Only special inspection method can find abnormalities. This is the beginning of the chronic phase. This type can persist for 20 to 30 years, or even life.

5.3.4 Chronic stage

During the chronic phase, the parasite hides mainly in the muscles of the heart and digestive tract. Ten to thirty years later, up to 30% of patients develop cardiac disorders and up to 10% develop gastrointestinal (typically enlarged esophagus or colon), neurological, or mixed lesions. In later years, infections in these patients can lead to myocardial and neurological damage, followed by arrhythmias or progressive heart failure and sudden death. The disease usually begins years or decades after the onset of parasitemia. (1) Cardiomyopathy in endemic areas: trypanosomiasis cardiomyopathy is the main cause of heart disease and sudden death. Patients often develop congestive heart failure with an enlarged heart. Two-thirds of patients have cardiac conduction disorders, often right bundle branch block, polygenic premature contractions, and myocardial necrosis. The disease course can be short and sudden death, or death from long-term heart failure. In addition, emboli from the apex or atrium can cause sudden death due to cerebral or pulmonary embolism. (2) Dilation of multiple organs: in Brazil, Chile, and some parts of Argentina, there are multiple organ expansions, mainly the esophagus and colon. Difficulty swallowing is often caused by esophageal expansion, constipation caused by colon expansion, and volvulus may also occur, such as acute abdomen. As for the giant stomach, giant duodenum, giant bronchus, giant ureter, etc. have been reported but rare.

5.4 Pathogenesis and pathological changes

5.4.1 Research achievements from relevant research institutions

T. cruzi can colonize any nucleated cell. Most of the symptoms in the acute phase of the disease are thought to be caused by damage to host cells by *T. cruzi*. For the chronic phase-related pathogenesis, there are currently two theories. One theory is that *T. cruzi* persists, leading to chronic inflammation [75], and the other theory is that it is caused by autoimmune damage [76]. Possible mechanisms include antigen cross-reactivity [77], direct cell-mediated cytotoxicity [78], antigenic Submitting changes [79], and cardiac mitochondrial dysfunction [80] etc.

Pathological changes in the acute phase showed mononuclear cell infiltration [81], interstitial edema [82], accumulation of amastigotes in muscle cells of subcutaneous tissue [83], and formation of pseudocysts at the invasion site of Trypanosoma [83]. Myocarditis with cardiac enlargement is usually seen in acute-phase deaths. In patients with sudden death in the chronic phase (mostly due to ventricular arrhythmia or conduction block), the heart size is usually normal or only slightly enlarged. In other patients with chronic Chagas heart disease, cardiac hypertrophy, dilation, and thickening can be seen, especially in the apex of the heart, resulting in apical aneurysm. Mural thrombosis and lung and peripheral organ embolism may be seen in some patients. Microscopic examination showed mononuclear cell infiltration, myocardial fiber hypertrophy, degeneration, necrosis and edema. Microscopic changes in megaesophagus or megacolon are similar to those of the heart.

5.4.2 Research achievements from our institution

We firstly have shown that cardiac mitochondria-response plays a very important roles in *T. cruzi*–induced cardiomyopathy [80, 84–92], and established the third theory that oxidative stress was involved in cardiac mitochondrial dysfunction [84, 86, 88] and heart dysfunction [80, 93–97]. In detail, we have contributed to the understanding of the mechanism behind the decline of MnSOD and enhancement of SIRT1/PGC1/PARP-1 in correlation with *T. cruzi*–induced consistently oxidative heart damage [90–92, 97]. From this research, we have observed that (1) MnSODtg mice/MnSOD overexpression in cell lines are beneficial in preserving *T. cruzi*–induced mitochondrial/heart dysfunction [90]; (2) $MnSOD^{-/+}$ mice were worse of *T. cruzi* infection–induced heart dysfunction [91]; and (3) inhibition of PARP-1 would prevent *T. cruzi*–induced heart function [92]. We also have observed *T. cruzi*–induced oxidative stress occurred in adipose tissues by utilizing oxidative markers, which is a novel finding [96, 98]. We have contributed to an understanding of *T. cruzi*–induced oxidative etiopathogenesis [85, 86, 88, 89]. Additionally, we have isolated high quality heart mitochondria to (1) recognize *T. cruzi*–induced oxidative mitochondrial proteins by using combination of BN-PAGE [84] and TOP MALDI MS/MS [88, 95]; (2) ascertain that mitochondrial complex III Qo site was prime source of *T. cruzi*–induced ROS generation [86]; and (3) find that administration of antioxidants improved *T. cruzi*–induced oxidative damage in heart mitochondria and heart tissues [85, 89]. We have conducted a thorough analysis of mitochondrial bioenergetic function as well as the biochemical and molecular factors that are deregulated and contribute to compromised adenosine triphosphate (ATP) production in the myocardium during *T. cruzi* infection. Our team is focused on the discovery and development of novel therapeutics against *T. cruzi*. We found that combination treatment (antioxidants and anti-parasites) is beneficial in arresting the *T. cruzi*–induced inflammatory and oxidative pathology and chronic heart failure in Chagasic rats. We have proven that the *T. cruzi*–induced oxidative alterations in circulation are correlated with heart tissue, suggesting that Chagasic human patients' circulation can replace heart tissue, as issue we are planning to investigate. We also confirmed that this was the case in human patients with Chagasic cardiomyopathy development and assessed different ways to oxidatively modify mitochondrial respiratory complexes (**Figure 1**) [80, 94].

6. Tobacco- and e-cigarettes-induced cardiomyopathy

6.1 Tobacco-induced cardiomyopathy

The tobacco-induced cardiomyopathy accounts for 9.4 million, or 16.6%, of the 56 million deaths worldwide each year [99]. Smoking causes 1.62 million (18%) deaths from heart disease worldwide [100], and cause severe ill health, with an estimated 40.6 million daily lost to heart disease [100].

Tobacco use (smoked and smokeless) and exposure to secondhand tobacco causes heart disease through a variety of mechanisms, including inflammation, blood vessels shrinkage, clot formation, and reduced oxygen supply (**Figure 1**) [101–103]. Smoking-mediated thrombosis appears to be a major factor in the pathogenesis of acute cardiovascular disease [101]. Nicotine stimulates the heart, which increases the demand for oxygen to the heart muscle, triggering angina. Smokers are more likely to develop acute cardiovascular disease at a young age and early in their illness [101]. The associated effects of exposure to secondhand smoke on the heart are almost as severe as the effects of smoking itself, and likely through the same biological mechanisms [104]. Exposure to secondhand smoke in as little as 1 h can increase the risk of heart attack [105].

Risk of damage to the cardiovascular system increases with duration of smoking and the amount and type of smoking tobacco products consumed. However, the close relationship between dose and response is not linear [101]. Even with low exposure levels, the risk increases substantially—people who smoke only one cigarette a day have half the risk of coronary heart disease as those who smoke at least 20 cigarettes a day [106]. In addition to being a major independent risk factor for coronary heart disease, smoking may act synergistically with other major risk factors for coronary heart disease, such as high cholesterol, untreated hypertension, and diabetes [107, 108]. In 2017, an estimated 382 000 deaths from coronary heart disease were attributable to exposure to secondhand smoke [106], accounting for 4.3% of total deaths from coronary heart disease and 31% of total deaths from exposure to secondhand smoke [106]. In the same year, exposure to secondhand smoke was also estimated to be responsible for an estimated 8.8 million disability-adjusted life-years (DALYs) lost to coronary heart disease [106]. Various systematic reviews and meta-analyses have shown that adults exposed to secondhand smoke have a 23–30% increased risk of coronary heart disease in countries with high to low-income levels [101, 109–112]. Cohort studies conducted in multiple countries in the 1970s and 1980s showed that children's exposure to secondhand smoke has adverse effects on cardiovascular disease, including premature atherosclerosis [113, 114]. A major challenge in these studies is accurately assessing lifetime exposure to secondhand smoke. The cumulative total lifetime exposure to secondhand smoke may be much higher than reflected during the study period [104], which may lead to an underestimation of the true risk of exposure to secondhand smoke and the impact on heart disease [104]. A recent study led by the tobacco industry claims that electronic nicotine delivery systems (ENDS) are less harmful than cigarettes [115, 116]. However, ENDS may be more toxic than inhaled ones at low in conventional cigarettes and tobacco products, but they are not harmless, and there are risks associated with use and secondhand exposure [41, 117]. ENDS linked to increased risk of cardiovascular disease Association [118, 119]. The toxic substances contained in these products can lead to causes impaired endothelial function, arterial stenosis, increased heart rate and increased blood pressure [120–122]. Concomitant use with smoking (this is most ENDS common practice of users), effects of a combination of two or more products [123]. Tobacco control measures have been shown to benefit heart health place. For example, raising tobacco taxes is directly related to reducing tobacco consumption. Associated with improved heart health [124].

6.2 E-cigarettes-induced cardiomyopathy

Due to the many pathogenic and negative effects on the heart from smoking on the heart, the market for smoking and nicotine replacement has grown rapidly in recent years. Since 2006, e-cigarettes have become more popular due to their perceived safety profile compared to traditional cigarette smoking. An electronic cigarette (or e-cigarette) is a battery-operated device for heating solutions (or e-liquids) containing nicotine, propanediol alcohol and vegetable glycerin [120, 125, 126]. E-cigarettes not only attract smokers who are trying to quit smoking, but are also becoming more popular among non-smokers, who have even become the main force in the e-cigarette market. Since the advent of electronic cigarettes, its design has constantly changed, but there has been little regulatory control. Common forms of e-cigarettes are the first generation of disposable "Cigalikes", the second generation of rechargeable devices, and the third generation of water tanks, pens and personalized large cigarettes, boxes, and pod-based devices.

The team of Nicholas D Buchanan of The Ohio State University School of Medicine published a paper in the journal Cardiovascular Research, reviewing clinical studies related to the cardiovascular risk of e-cigarettes. This review discusses recent relevant studies from the existing literature, focusing on components and potential cardiovascular risks associated with e-cigarette vapor exposure and on evaluating and broadly discussing data from preclinical and epidemiological studies on the cardiovascular effects of acute (short-term) and chronic (long-term) exposure to e-cigarettes [127]. e-cigarettes increased hyperlipidemia [128], sympathetic dominance [129], endothelial dysfunction [130], DNA damage [131], macrophage activation [132, 133]. Multiple studies suggest e-cigarettes may increase CVD risk.

7. Burn-induced cardiomyopathy

7.1 Research achievements from relevant research institutions

Severe burns can lead to severe hemodynamic and cardiodynamic disturbances, which can lead to sepsis, multiple organ failure, and death. Cardiac stress is a hallmark of acute-phase response to burns, and poorer burn recovery outcomes are associated with severe cardiac insufficiency [134–136]. Severe burn injury has a profound and widespread effect on an individual's cardiovascular system. Early features include myocardial contractile dysfunction and increased vascular permeability.

Plasma levels of catecholamines, vasopressin, angiotensin-II [137] and neuropeptide-Y [138] are significantly elevated after severe burns, which may be responsible for the deleterious effects on cardiovascular function. Nearly 7% of children with 70% burn area develop dilated cardiomyopathy (DCM) [139, 140]. Burn-induced cardiomyopathy usually develops several weeks to several months after injury [139, 141]. The initial cardiac response to severe burns is characterized by reduced cardiac output and metabolic rate (**Figure 1**). Other hemodynamic features of burn shock include stroke volume, venous return, coronary blood flow, peak systolic blood pressure, mean arterial pressure, estimated myocardial work, stroke work, myocardial oxygen consumption, myocardial oxygenation, myocardial contractility, decreased force and myocardial compliance [142]. This initial response will result in left-right heart failure and decreased cardiac contractility and is thought to be mediated by circulating vasoconstrictors (**Figure 1**).

Physiologically, burn-induced myocardial dysfunction is characterized by decreased isovolumic relaxation, impaired contractility, and decreased left ventricular diastolic compliance [143, 144] resulting in decreased cardiac output and metabolic rate [138, 145], leading to myocardial oxygen demand, leading ultimately to right and left heart deficits (**Figure 1**) [143, 146]. Following burn injury, the volume of circulating plasma is markedly reduced due to increased capillary permeability [147] and a concomitant decrease in cardiac output. Depending on the extent of the burn injury, this defect may directly lead to a severe hypermetabolic response [148] and is positively correlated with the size of the original injury [148]. Poor functional recovery from severe burns is associated with high mortality, high infection rates, and cardiac insufficiency [136, 149, 150].

Cardiac stress-induced increases in plasma catecholamines mediate postburn hypermetabolic responses [136, 151, 152]. Upregulation of catecholamines and other catabolic agents such as glucagon and cortisol may induce hyperdynamic cardiovascular responses [134]. Elevated catecholamines and other catabolic agents are further exacerbated by the substantial loss of plasma volume following burns. Hypovolemic shock, typified by severe burns and major tissue trauma, results in marked tachycardia, increased myocardial oxygen demand, and decreased contractility (**Figure 1**) [134]. This eventually leads to increased mortality during acute hospitalization [153]. Severe burns suffer from a profound hypermetabolic response mediated by a surge in plasma catecholamines. Sustained release of large circulating catecholamines may be detrimental to the myocardium, increasing myocardial oxygen delivery and leading to focal degeneration and hypertrophy of the myocardium [134]. Elevated plasma catecholamine levels persist for months to years resulting in cardiac stress and cardiac physiologic disturbance for at least 2 years [154]. This in turn leads to cardiac insufficiency, regional myocardial hypoxia, and cardiac death [155]. Therefore, clinical concern about catecholamine levels is related to burn-induced cardiomyopathy, myocarditis, pathological myocardial injury and necrosis [156, 157].

7.2 Research achievements from our laboratory

We applied mature animal burn models including rat and mouse, established by UTMB Health's Blocker Burn Center, to identify the heart tissue-specific up–/down-regulated genes/proteins/metabolisms via transcriptomics/proteomics/metabolomics, and have many hypothesizes based on the differences. Briefly, the SIRT1-PGC1α-NFE2L2-ARE pathway [158], and PDE5A-cGMP-PKG pathway [159] were involved in the burn-induced cardiomyopathy. To confirm our above observations, we treated burn injury animals with PDE5A inhibitor [159, 160] (Sildenafil), and APMK inhibitor (Domorsorphin)/APMK activator (A769662)/PGC1α activator (ZLN005) [158] to partially/completely recoveries of burn-induced cardiomyopathy. Another important contribution for burn-induced cardiomyopathy was that burn injury disrupts the heart mitochondria (mt) with evidence of cardiomyocyte mtDNA damage [159, 161], mt electron transport chain (ETC) dysfunction, mt membrane potential damage, disrupted mt integrity and significant increase of mt ROS production [159, 161]. Treatment with mitochondrial-target drug (Mito-TEMPO) can be beneficial for burn injury–induced cardiomyopathy (**Figure 1**) [161].

Acknowledgements

We would like to acknowledge David J. Chavarria, who assisted in the correction of the manuscript.

Conflict of interest

The authors declare no conflict of interest.

Acronyms and abbreviations

BNP	B-type natriuretic peptide
CVD	cardiovascular disease
BDNF	brain-derived neurotrophic factor
ECG	electrocardiogram
ENDS	electronic nicotine delivery systems
HRV	heart rate variability
HDL	high-density lipoprotein
hs-cTnI	highly sensitive cardiac troponin I
LDL	low-density lipoprotein
MSIC	mental stress-induced cardiomyopathy
MSIMI	mental stress-induced myocardial ischemia
mt	mitochondria
T. cruzi	*Trypanosoma cruzi*

Author details

Jake J. Wen* and Ravi S. Radhakrishnan
Division of Pediatrics, Department of Surgery, University of Texas Medical Branch at Galveston (UTMB), Galveston, USA

*Address all correspondence to: jiawen@utmb.edu

References

[1] Wittstein IS, Thiemann DR, Lima JA, Baughman KL, Schulman SP, Gerstenblith G, et al. Neurohumoral features of myocardial stunning due to sudden emotional stress. The New England Journal of Medicine. 2005;**352**(6):539-548

[2] Sharkey SW, Lesser JR, Zenovich AG, Maron MS, Lindberg J, Longe TF, et al. Acute and reversible cardiomyopathy provoked by stress in women from the United States. Circulation. 2005;**111**(4):472-479

[3] Lacy CR, Contrada RJ, Robbins ML, Tannenbaum AK, Moreyra AE, Chelton S, et al. Coronary vasoconstriction induced by mental stress (simulated public speaking). The American Journal of Cardiology. 1995;**75**(7):503-505

[4] Sadamatsu K, Tashiro H, Maehira N, Yamamoto K. Coronary microvascular abnormality in the reversible systolic dysfunction observed after noncardiac disease. Japanese Circulation Journal. 2000;**64**(10):789-792

[5] Mann DL, Kent RL, Parsons B, Gt C. Adrenergic effects on the biology of the adult mammalian cardiocyte. Circulation. 1992;**85**(2):790-804

[6] Singal PK, Kapur N, Dhillon KS, Beamish RE, Dhalla NS. Role of free radicals in catecholamine-induced cardiomyopathy. Canadian Journal of Physiology and Pharmacology. 1982;**60**(11):1390-1397

[7] Bolli R, Marban E. Molecular and cellular mechanisms of myocardial stunning. Physiological Reviews. 1999;**79**(2):609-634

[8] Bybee KA, Prasad A, Barsness GW, Lerman A, Jaffe AS, Murphy JG, et al. Clinical characteristics and thrombolysis in myocardial infarction frame counts in women with transient left ventricular apical ballooning syndrome. The American Journal of Cardiology. 2004;**94**(3):343-346

[9] Akashi YJ, Nakazawa K, Sakakibara M, Miyake F, Musha H, Sasaka K. 123I-MIBG myocardial scintigraphy in patients with "takotsubo" cardiomyopathy. Journal of Nuclear Medicine. 2004;**45**(7):1121-1127

[10] Hopster DJ, Milroy CM, Burns J, Roberts NB. Necropsy study of the association between sudden cardiac death, cardiac isoenzymes and contraction band necrosis. Journal of Clinical Pathology. 1996;**49**(5):403-406

[11] Wilkenfeld C, Cohen M, Lansman SL, Courtney M, Dische MR, Pertsemlidis D, et al. Heart transplantation for end-stage cardiomyopathy caused by an occult pheochromocytoma. The Journal of Heart and Lung Transplantation. 1992;**11**(2 Pt 1):363-366

[12] Neil-Dwyer G, Walter P, Cruickshank JM, Doshi B, O'Gorman P. Effect of propranolol and phentolamine on myocardial necrosis after subarachnoid haemorrhage. British Medical Journal. 1978;**2**(6143):990-992

[13] Bauer TW, Moore GW, Hutchins GM. Morphologic evidence for coronary artery spasm in eclampsia. Circulation. 1982;**65**(2):255-259

[14] Drislane FW, Samuels MA, Kozakewich H, Schoen FJ, Strunk RC. Myocardial contraction band lesions in patients with fatal asthma: Possible neurocardiologic mechanisms. The American Review of Respiratory Disease. 1987;**135**(2):498-501

[15] Williams RB, Barefoot JC, Schneiderman N. Psychosocial risk factors for cardiovascular disease: More than one culprit at work. Journal of the American Medical Association. 2003;**290**(16):2190-2192

[16] Neylon A, Canniffe C, Anand S, Kreatsoulas C, Blake GJ, Sugrue D, et al. A global perspective on psychosocial risk factors for cardiovascular disease. Progress in Cardiovascular Diseases. 2013;**55**(6):574-581

[17] Ingles J, Goldstein J, Thaxton C, Caleshu C, Corty EW, Crowley SB, et al. Evaluating the clinical validity of hypertrophic cardiomyopathy genes. Circulation. Genomic and Precision Medicine. 2019;**12**(2):e002460

[18] Hohls JK, Beer K, Arolt V, Haverkamp W, Kuhlmann SL, Martus P, et al. Association between heart-focused anxiety, depressive symptoms, health behaviors and healthcare utilization in patients with coronary heart disease. Journal of Psychosomatic Research. 2020;**131**:109958

[19] Meader N, King K, Wright K, Graham HM, Petticrew M, Power C, et al. Multiple risk behavior interventions: Meta-analyses of RCTs. American Journal of Preventive Medicine. 2017;**53**(1):e19-e30

[20] Jiang W, Krishnan RR, O'Connor CM. Depression and heart disease: Evidence of a link, and its therapeutic implications. CNS Drugs. 2002;**16**(2):111-127

[21] Gathright EC, Goldstein CM, Josephson RA, Hughes JW. Depression increases the risk of mortality in patients with heart failure: A meta-analysis. Journal of Psychosomatic Research. 2017;**94**:82-89

[22] Bradt J, Dileo C, Potvin N. Music for stress and anxiety reduction in coronary heart disease patients. Cochrane Database of Systematic Reviews. 2013;**12**:CD006577

[23] Karlsen HR, Matejschek F, Saksvik-Lehouillier I, Langvik E. Anxiety as a risk factor for cardiovascular disease independent of depression: A narrative review of current status and conflicting findings. Health Psychology Open. 2021;**8**(1):2055

[24] Tully PJ, Cosh SM, Baune BT. A review of the affects of worry and generalized anxiety disorder upon cardiovascular health and coronary heart disease. Psychology, Health & Medicine. 2013;**18**(6):627-644

[25] Pankalainen M, Kerola T, Kampman O, Kauppi M, Hintikka J. Pessimism and risk of death from coronary heart disease among middle-aged and older Finns: An eleven-year follow-up study. BMC Public Health. 2016;**16**(1):1124

[26] Pankalainen MT, Kerola TV, Hintikka JJ. Pessimism and the risk for coronary heart disease among middle-aged and older Finnish men and women: A ten-year follow-up study. BMC Cardiovascular Disorders. 2015;**15**:113

[27] Chida Y, Steptoe A. The association of anger and hostility with future coronary heart disease: A meta-analytic review of prospective evidence. Journal of the American College of Cardiology. 2009;**53**(11):936-946

[28] Chen H, Zhang B, Xue W, Li J, Li Y, Fu K, et al. Anger, hostility and risk of stroke: A meta-analysis of cohort studies. Journal of Neurology. 2019;**266**(4):1016-1026

[29] Biber S, Andonian C, Beckmann J, Ewert P, Freilinger S, Nagdyman N,

et al. Current research status on the psychological situation of parents of children with congenital heart disease. Cardiovascular Diagnosis and Therapy. 2019;**9**(Suppl 2):S369-SS76

[30] Dragano N, Siegrist J, Nyberg ST, Lunau T, Fransson EI, Alfredsson L, et al. Effort-Reward Imbalance at Work and Incident Coronary Heart Disease: A Multicohort Study of 90,164 Individuals. Epidemiology. 2017;**28**(4):619-626

[31] Taouk Y, Spittal MJ, LaMontagne AD, Milner AJ. Psychosocial work stressors and risk of all-cause and coronary heart disease mortality: A systematic review and meta-analysis. Scandinavian Journal of Work, Environment & Health. 2020;**46**(1):19-31

[32] Sbarra DA, Coan JA. Divorce and health: Good data in need of better theory. Current Opinion in Psychology. 2017;**13**:91-95

[33] Dhindsa DS, Khambhati J, Schultz WM, Tahhan AS, Quyyumi AA. Marital status and outcomes in patients with cardiovascular disease. Trends in Cardiovascular Medicine. 2020;**30**(4):215-220

[34] Grauman A, Viberg Johansson J, Falahee M, Veldwijk J. Public perceptions of myocardial infarction: Do illness perceptions predict preferences for health check results. Preventive Medical Reports. 2022;**26**:101683

[35] Kilby CJ, Sherman KA, Wuthrich VM. A scoping review of stress beliefs: Literature integration, measurement issues, and theoretical concerns. Annals of Behavioral Medicine. 2020;**54**(8):595-610

[36] Li H, Xia N. The role of oxidative stress in cardiovascular disease caused by social isolation and loneliness. Redox Biology. 2020;**37**:101585

[37] Golaszewski NM, LaCroix AZ, Godino JG, Allison MA, Manson JE, King JJ, et al. Evaluation of social isolation, loneliness, and cardiovascular disease among older women in the US. JAMA Network Open. 2022;**5**(2):e2146461

[38] Kim ES, Chen Y, Nakamura JS, Ryff CD, VanderWeele TJ. Sense of purpose in life and subsequent physical, behavioral, and psychosocial health: An outcome-wide approach. American Journal of Health Promotion. 2022;**36**(1):137-147

[39] Jaschinski C, Knetsch V, Parzer P, Meyr J, Schroeder B, Fonseca E, et al. Psychosocial impact of congenital heart diseases on patients and their families: A parent's perspective. World Journal of Pediatric Congenit ive and Heart Surgery. 2022;**13**(1):9-15

[40] Kovacs AH, Bellinger DC. Neurocognitive and psychosocial outcomes in adult congenital heart disease: A lifespan approach. Heart. 2021;**107**(2):159-167

[41] Osei AD, Mirbolouk M, Orimoloye OA, Dzaye O, Uddin SMI, Benjamin EJ, et al. Association between E-cigarette use and cardiovascular disease among never and current combustible-cigarette smokers. The American Journal of Medicine. 2019;**132**(8):949-54 e2

[42] Sylvia LG, Faulkner M, Rakhilin M, Amado S, Gold AK, Albury EA, et al. An online intervention for increasing physical activity in individuals with mood disorders at risk for cardiovascular disease: Design considerations. Journal of Affective Disorders. 2021;**291**:102-109

[43] Damasio AR. Emotion in the perspective of an integrated nervous system. Brain Research. Brain Research Reviews. 1998;**26**(2-3):83-86

[44] Sirois BC, Burg MM. Negative emotion and coronary heart disease: A review. Behaviour Modification. 2003;**27**(1):83-102

[45] Tuck NL, Adams KS, Pressman SD, Consedine NS. Greater ability to express positive emotion is associated with lower projected cardiovascular disease risk. Journal of Behavioral Medicine. 2017;**40**(6):855-863

[46] AbuRuz ME. Anxiety and depression predicted quality of life among patients with heart failure. Journal of Multidisciplinary Healthcare. 2018;**11**:367-373

[47] Meyer FA, von Kanel R, Saner H, Schmid JP, Stauber S. Positive affect moderates the effect of negative affect on cardiovascular disease-related hospitalizations and all-cause mortality after cardiac rehabilitation. European Journal of Preventive Cardiology. 2015;**22**(10):1247-1253

[48] Marshall CR, Hardy CJD, Allen M, Russell LL, Clark CN, Bond RL, et al. Cardiac responses to viewing facial emotion differentiate frontotemporal dementias. Annals of Clinical Translational Neurology. 2018;**5**(6):687-696

[49] Knapp M, Tu X, Wu R. Vascular endothelial dysfunction, a major mediator in diabetic cardiomyopathy. Acta Pharmacological Sinica. 2019;**40**(1):1-8

[50] Hassan M, York KM, Li H, Li Q, Gong Y, Langaee TY, et al. Association of beta1-adrenergic receptor genetic polymorphism with mental stress-induced myocardial ischemia in patients with coronary artery disease. Archives of Internal Medicine. 2008;**168**(7):763-770

[51] Chen ZY, Jing D, Bath KG, Ieraci A, Khan T, Siao CJ, et al. Genetic variant BDNF (Val66Met) polymorphism alters anxiety-related behavior. Science. 2006;**314**(5796):140-143

[52] Hajjari P, Mattsson S, McIntyre KM, McKinley PS, Shapiro PA, Gorenstein EE, et al. The effect of hostility reduction on autonomic control of the heart and vasculature: A Randomized Controlled Trial. Psychosomatic Medicine. 2016;**78**(4):481-491

[53] Paine NJ, Watkins LL, Blumenthal JA, Kuhn CM, Sherwood A. Association of depressive and anxiety symptoms with 24-hour urinary catecholamines in individuals with untreated high blood pressure. Psychosomatic Medicine. 2015;**77**(2):136-144

[54] Liu T. Effect of negative emotion evocation on autonomic function activity of hearts in healthy population: An empirical study. Academic Journal of Second Military Medical University. 2011;**12**:1204-1207

[55] Liu MY, Yang Y, Zhang LJ, Pu LH, He DF, Liu JY, et al. Potential predictors for mental stress-induced myocardial ischemia in patients with coronary artery disease. Chinese Medical Journal. 2019;**132**(12):1390-1399

[56] Hammadah M, Sullivan S, Pearce B, Al Mheid I, Wilmot K, Ramadan R, et al. Inflammatory response to mental stress and mental stress induced myocardial ischemia. Brain, Behavior, and Immunity. 2018;**68**:90-97

[57] Jiang W, Velazquez EJ, Samad Z, Kuchibhatla M, Martsberger C, Rogers J,

et al. Responses of mental stress-induced myocardial ischemia to escitalopram treatment: Background, design, and method for the Responses of Mental Stress Induced Myocardial Ischemia to Escitalopram Treatment trial. American Heart Journal. 2012;**163**(1):20-26

[58] Benjamin MM, Bossarte R, Guha A, Shah M, Patel B. Depression and anxiety in patients with heart disease and/or cancer based on the National Health Interview Survey. Proceedings (Baylor University Medical Center). 2020;**34**(1):11-16

[59] Bremner JD, Campanella C, Khan Z, Fani N, Kasher N, Evans S, et al. Brain mechanisms of stress and depression in coronary artery disease. Journal of Psychiatric Research. 2019;**109**:76-88

[60] Shah A, Chen C, Campanella C, Kasher N, Evans S, Reiff C, et al. Brain correlates of stress-induced peripheral vasoconstriction in patients with cardiovascular disease. Psychophysiology. 2019;**56**(2):e13291

[61] Nadir MA, Witham MD, Szwejkowski BR, Struthers AD. Meta-analysis of B-type natriuretic peptide's ability to identify stress induced myocardial ischemia. The American Journal of Cardiology. 2011;**107**(5):662-667

[62] Akinboboye O, Krantz DS, Kop WJ, Schwartz SD, Levine J, Del Negro A, et al. Comparison of mental stress-induced myocardial ischemia in coronary artery disease patients with versus without left ventricular dysfunction. The American Journal of Cardiology. 2005;**95**(3):322-326

[63] Hammadah M, Alkhoder A, Al Mheid I, Wilmot K, Isakadze N, Abdulhadi N, et al. Hemodynamic, catecholamine, vasomotor and vascular responses: Determinants of myocardial ischemia during mental stress. International Journal of Cardiology. 2017;**243**:47-53

[64] Broadley AJ, Korszun A, Abdelaal E, Moskvina V, Jones CJ, Nash GB, et al. Inhibition of cortisol production with metyrapone prevents mental stress-induced endothelial dysfunction and baroreflex impairment. Journal of the American College of Cardiology. 2005;**46**(2):344-350

[65] Seldenrijk A, Hamer M, Lahiri A, Penninx BW, Steptoe A. Psychological distress, cortisol stress response and subclinical coronary calcification. Psychoneuroendocrinology. 2012;**37**(1):48-55

[66] Bozzini S, Gambelli P, Boiocchi C, Schirinzi S, Falcone R, Buzzi P, et al. Coronary artery disease and depression: Possible role of brain-derived neurotrophic factor and serotonin transporter gene polymorphisms. International Journal of Molecular Medicine. 2009;**24**(6):813-818

[67] Busselman RE, Hamer SA. Chagas disease ecology in the united states: Recent advances in understanding trypanosoma cruzi transmission among triatomines, wildlife, and domestic animals and a quantitative synthesis of vector-host interactions. Annual Review of Animal Biosciences. 2022;**10**:325-348

[68] Chagas disease in Latin America: An epidemiological update based on 2010 estimates. Weekly Epidemiological Record. 2015;**90**(6):33-43

[69] Rassi A Jr, Rassi A, Marin-Neto JA. Chagas disease. Lancet. 2010;**375**(9723): 1388-1402

[70] Gascon J, Bern C, Pinazo MJ. Chagas disease in Spain, the United States and

other non-endemic countries. Acta Tropica. 2010;**115**(1-2):22-27

[71] Abras A, Ballart C, Fernandez-Arevalo A, Pinazo MJ, Gascon J, Munoz C, et al. Worldwide control and management of chagas disease in a new era of globalization: A close look at congenital trypanosoma cruzi infection. Clinical Microbiology Reviews. 2022;**35**(2):e0015221

[72] Ramirez JC, Acevedo GR, Torres C, Parrado R, De La Barra A, Villarroel S, et al. Genetic polymorphism of Trypanosoma cruzi bloodstream populations in adult chronic indeterminate Chagas disease patients from the E1224 clinical trial. The Journal of Antimicrobial Chemotherapy. 2022;**77**(3):578-584

[73] Kun H, Moore A, Mascola L, Steurer F, Lawrence G, Kubak B, et al. Chagas disease in transplant recipients investigation T. Transmission of Trypanosoma cruzi by heart transplantation. Clinical Infectious Diseases. 2009;**48**(11):1534-1540

[74] Prata A. Clinical and epidemiological aspects of Chagas disease. The Lancet Infectious Diseases. 2001;**1**(2):92-100

[75] Duthie MS, Kahn M, Zakayan A, White M, Kahn SJ. Parasite-induced chronic inflammation is not exacerbated by immunotherapy before or during Trypanosoma cruzi Infection. Clinical and Vaccine Immunology. 2007;**14**(8):1005-1012

[76] De Bona E, Lidani KCF, Bavia L, Omidian Z, Gremski LH, Sandri TL, et al. Autoimmunity in chronic chagas disease: A road of multiple pathways to cardiomyopathy? Frontiers in Immunology. 2018;**9**:1842

[77] Daltro RT, Leony LM, Freitas NEM, Silva AAO, Santos EF, Del-Rei RP, et al. Cross-reactivity using chimeric Trypanosoma cruzi antigens: Diagnostic performance in settings where chagas disease and American cutaneous or visceral leishmaniasis are coendemic. Journal of Clinical Microbiology. 2019;**57**(8)

[78] Ferreira CP, Cariste LM, Santos Virgilio FD, Moraschi BF, Monteiro CB, Vieira Machado AM, et al. LFA-1 mediates cytotoxicity and tissue migration of specific CD8(+) T cells after heterologous prime-boost vaccination against trypanosoma cruzi infection. Frontiers in Immunology. 2017;**8**:1291

[79] Laucella SA, Mazliah DP, Bertocchi G, Alvarez MG, Cooley G, Viotti R, et al. Changes in Trypanosoma cruzi-specific immune responses after treatment: Surrogate markers of treatment efficacy. Clinical Infectious Diseases. 2009;**49**(11):1675-1684

[80] Wen JJ, Yachelini PC, Sembaj A, Manzur RE, Garg NJ. Increased oxidative stress is correlated with mitochondrial dysfunction in chagasic patients. Free Radical Biology & Medicine. 2006;**41**(2):270-276

[81] Cuervo H, Guerrero NA, Carbajosa S, Beschin A, De Baetselier P, Girones N, et al. Myeloid-derived suppressor cells infiltrate the heart in acute Trypanosoma cruzi infection. Journal of Immunology. 2011;**187**(5):2656-2665

[82] Bonney KM, Luthringer DJ, Kim SA, Garg NJ, Engman DM. Pathology and pathogenesis of chagas heart disease. Annual Review of Pathology. 2019;**14**:421-447

[83] Batista CM, Kessler RL, Eger I, Soares MJ. Trypanosoma cruzi Intracellular amastigotes isolated by nitrogen decompression are capable of endocytosis and Cargo

storage in reservosomes. PLoS One. 2015;**10**(6):e0130165

[84] Wen JJ, Garg N. Oxidative modification of mitochondrial respiratory complexes in response to the stress of Trypanosoma cruzi infection. Free Radical Biology & Medicine. 2004;**37**(12):2072-2081

[85] Wen JJ, Bhatia V, Popov VL, Garg NJ. Phenyl-alpha-tert-butyl nitrone reverses mitochondrial decay in acute Chagas' disease. The American Journal of Pathology. 2006;**169**(6):1953-1964

[86] Wen JJ, Garg NJ. Mitochondrial generation of reactive oxygen species is enhanced at the Q(o) site of the complex III in the myocardium of Trypanosoma cruzi-infected mice: Beneficial effects of an antioxidant. Journal of Bioenergetics and Biomembranes. 2008;**40**(6):587-598

[87] Gupta S, Bhatia V, Wen JJ, Wu Y, Huang MH, Garg NJ. Trypanosoma cruzi infection disturbs mitochondrial membrane potential and ROS production rate in cardiomyocytes. Free Radical Biology & Medicine. 2009;**47**(10):1414-1421

[88] Wen JJ, Garg NJ. Mitochondrial complex III defects contribute to inefficient respiration and ATP synthesis in the myocardium of Trypanosoma cruzi-infected mice. Antioxidants & Redox Signaling. 2010;**12**(1):27-37

[89] Wen JJ, Gupta S, Guan Z, Dhiman M, Condon D, Lui C, et al. Phenyl-alpha-tert-butyl-nitrone and benzonidazole treatment controlled the mitochondrial oxidative stress and evolution of cardiomyopathy in chronic chagasic rats. Journal of the American College of Cardiology. 2010;**55**(22):2499-2508

[90] Wen JJ, Porter C, Garg NJ. Inhibition of NFE2L2-antioxidant response element pathway by mitochondrial reactive oxygen species contributes to development of cardiomyopathy and left ventricular dysfunction in chagas disease. Antioxidants & Redox Signaling. 2017;**27**(9):550-566

[91] Wen JJ, Garg NJ. Manganese superoxide dismutase deficiency exacerbates the mitochondrial ROS production and oxidative damage in Chagas disease. PLoS Neglected Tropical Diseases. 2018;**12**(7):e0006687

[92] Wen JJ, Yin YW, Garg NJ. PARP1 depletion improves mitochondrial and heart function in Chagas disease: Effects on POLG dependent mtDNA maintenance. PLoS Pathogens. 2018;**14**(5):e1007065

[93] Wen JJ, Vyatkina G, Garg N. Oxidative damage during chagasic cardiomyopathy development: Role of mitochondrial oxidant release and inefficient antioxidant defense. Free Radical Biology & Medicine. 2004;**37**(11):1821-1833

[94] Wen JJ, Dhiman M, Whorton EB, Garg NJ. Tissue-specific oxidative imbalance and mitochondrial dysfunction during Trypanosoma cruzi infection in mice. Microbes and Infection. 2008;**10**(10-11):1201-1209

[95] Wen JJ, Garg NJ. Proteome expression and carbonylation changes during Trypanosoma cruzi infection and Chagas disease in rats. Molecular & Cellular Proteomics. 2012;**11**(4):010918

[96] Wen JJ, Nagajyothi F, Machado FS, Weiss LM, Scherer PE, Tanowitz HB, et al. Markers of oxidative stress in adipose tissue during Trypanosoma cruzi infection. Parasitology Research. 2014;**113**(9):3159-3165

[97] Wen JJ, Wan X, Thacker J, Garg NJ. Chemotherapeutic efficacy

of phosphodiesterase inhibitors in chagasic cardiomyopathy. JACC Basic Translational Science. 2016;**1**(4):235-250

[98] Tanowitz HBWJ-J, Machado F-S, Desruisseaux M-S, Robello C, Garg NJ. Trypanosoma cruzi and Chagas disease: Innate immunity, ROS, and cardiovascular system. In: Vascular Responses to Pathogens, Waltham. 2016

[99] Organization WH. Deaths by cause, age, sex, by country and by region, 2000-2016. 2018. Geneva: Global Health Estimates 2016; 2018. [Accessed: 23 October 2019]

[100] Collaborators GBDRF. Global, regional, and national comparative risk assessment of 84 behavioural, environmental and occupational, and metabolic risks or clusters of risks for 195 countries and territories, 1990-2017: A systematic analysis for the Global Burden of Disease Study 2017. Lancet. 2018;**392**(10159):1923-1994

[101] Services. USDoHaH. How tobacco smoke causes disease: The biology and behavioral basis for smoking-attributable disease: A report of the Surgeon General. Atlanta (GA): Centers for Disease Control and Prevention; 2010 [Accessed: 2010]

[102] Csordas A, Bernhard D. The biology behind the atherothrombotic effects of cigarette smoke. Nature Reviews. Cardiology. 2013;**10**(4):219-230

[103] Arteriosclerosis, Thrombosis, and Vascular Biology 2015;35(1):1

[104] Services. USDoHaH. The Health Consequences of Involuntary Exposure to Tobacco Smoke: A Report of the Surgeon General. Atlanta (GA): Centers for Disease Control and Prevention; 2006

[105] Otsuka R, Watanabe H, Hirata K, Tokai K, Muro T, Yoshiyama M, et al. Acute effects of passive smoking on the coronary circulation in healthy young adults. Journal of the American Medical Association. 2001;**286**(4):436-441

[106] Hackshaw A, Morris JK, Boniface S, Tang JL, Milenkovic D. Low cigarette consumption and risk of coronary heart disease and stroke: Meta-analysis of 141 cohort studies in 55 study reports. BMJ. 2018;**360**:j5855

[107] Prevention. Cardiovascular Disease: A Report of the Surgeon General. Atlanta (GA): United States Department of Health and Human Services; 1983

[108] McInnes GT. Hypertension and coronary artery disease: Cause and effect. Journal of Hypertension. Supplement. 1995;**13**(2):S49-S56

[109] Rossi M, Negri E, La Vecchia C, Campos H. Smoking habits and the risk of non-fatal acute myocardial infarction in Costa Rica. European Journal of Cardiovascular Prevention and Rehabilitation. 2011;**18**(3):467-474

[110] Olasky SJ, Levy D, Moran A. Second hand smoke and cardiovascular disease in Low and Middle Income Countries: A case for action. Global Heart. 2012;**7**(2):151-60 e5

[111] Prevention CfDCa. The Health Consequences of Smoking: 50 years of Progress. A Report of the Surgeon General. Atlanta (GA): United States Department of Health and Human Services; 2014

[112] Lv X, Sun J, Bi Y, Xu M, Lu J, Zhao L, et al. Risk of all-cause mortality and cardiovascular disease associated with secondhand smoke exposure: A systematic review and meta-analysis. International Journal of Cardiology. 2015;**199**:106-115

[113] Metsios GS, Flouris AD, Angioi M, Koutedakis Y. Passive smoking and the development of cardiovascular disease in children: A systematic review. Cardiology Research and Practice. 2010;**2011**

[114] West HW, Juonala M, Gall SL, Kahonen M, Laitinen T, Taittonen L, et al. Exposure to parental smoking in childhood is associated with increased risk of carotid atherosclerotic plaque in adulthood: The Cardiovascular Risk in Young Finns Study. Circulation. 2015;**131**(14):1239-1246

[115] Weitkunat R, Lee PN, Baker G, Sponsiello-Wang Z, Gonzalez-Zuloeta Ladd AM, Ludicke F. A novel approach to assess the population health impact of introducing a Modified Risk Tobacco Product. Regulatory Toxicology and Pharmacology. 2015;**72**(1):87-93

[116] Max WB, Sung HY, Lightwood J, Wang Y, Yao T. Modelling the impact of a new tobacco product: Review of Philip Morris International's Population Health Impact Model as applied to the IQOS heated tobacco product. Tobacco Control. 2018;**27**(Suppl. 1):s82-ss6

[117] Organization WH. Electronic nicotine delivery systems and electronic non-nicotine delivery systems (ENDS/ENNDS) (report to the seventh session of the Conference of the Parties to the WHO Framework Convention on Tobacco Control (Delhi, India, 7-12 November 2016)) Geneva: World Health Organization; 2016 (FCTC/COP/7/11; https://wwwwhoint/fctc/cop/cop7/Documentation-Main-documents/en/, accessed 25 October 2019). 2019

[118] Alzahrani T, Pena I, Temesgen N, Glantz SA. Association between electronic cigarette use and myocardial infarction. American Journal of Preventive Medicine. 2018;**55**(4):455-461

[119] Bhatta DN, Glantz SA. Electronic cigarette use and myocardial infarction among adults in the US Population Assessment of Tobacco and Health. Journal of the American Heart Association. 2019;**8**(12):e012317

[120] Qasim H, Karim ZA, Rivera JO, Khasawneh FT, Alshbool FZ. Impact of electronic cigarettes on the cardiovascular system. Journal of the American Heart Association. 2017;**6**(9):1-14

[121] Ikonomidis I, Vlastos D, Kourea K, Kostelli G, Varoudi M, Pavlidis G, et al. Electronic cigarette smoking increases arterial stiffness and oxidative stress to a lesser extent than a single conventional cigarette: An Acute and Chronic Study. Circulation. 2018;**137**(3):303-306

[122] Biondi-Zoccai G, Sciarretta S, Bullen C, Nocella C, Violi F, Loffredo L, et al. Acute effects of heat-not-burn, electronic vaping, and traditional tobacco combustion cigarettes: The Sapienza University of Rome-Vascular Assessment of Proatherosclerotic Effects of Smoking (SUR - VAPES) 2 Randomized Trial. Journal of the American Heart Association. 2019;**8**(6):e010455

[123] Wang JB, Olgin JE, Nah G, Vittinghoff E, Cataldo JK, Pletcher MJ, et al. Cigarette and e-cigarette dual use and risk of cardiopulmonary symptoms in the Health eHeart Study. PLoS One. 2018;**13**(7):e0198681

[124] National Institutes of Health NCIaGWHO. United States National Cancer Institute and World Health Organization. The economics of tobacco and tobacco control (National Cancer Institute Tobacco Control Monograph No. 21; NIH Publication No. 16-CA-8029A). Bethesda, MD: United States Department of Health and Human Services, National Institutes of Health, National Cancer Institute; and Geneva:

World Health Organization; 2016. Available from: https://cancercontrol.cancer.gov/brp/tcrb/monographs/21/ [Accessed: 25 October 2019]

[125] Lippi G, Favaloro EJ, Meschi T, Mattiuzzi C, Borghi L, Cervellin G. E-cigarettes and cardiovascular risk: Beyond science and mysticism. Seminars in Thrombosis and Hemostasis. 2014;**40**(1):60-65

[126] Grana R, Benowitz N, Glantz SA. E-cigarettes: A scientific review. Circulation. 2014;**129**(19):1972-1986

[127] Buchanan ND, Grimmer JA, Tanwar V, Schwieterman N, Mohler PJ, Wold LE. Cardiovascular risk of electronic cigarettes: A review of preclinical and clinical studies. Cardiovascular Research. 2020;**116**(1):40-50

[128] Majid S, Keith RJ, Fetterman JL, Weisbrod RM, Nystoriak J, Wilson T, et al. Lipid profiles in users of combustible and electronic cigarettes. Vascular Medicine. 2021;**26**(5):483-488

[129] Moheimani RS, Bhetraratana M, Yin F, Peters KM, Gornbein J, Araujo JA, et al. Increased cardiac sympathetic activity and oxidative stress in habitual electronic cigarette users: Implications for cardiovascular risk. JAMA Cardiology. 2017;**2**(3):278-284

[130] El-Mahdy MA, Ewees MG, Eid MS, Mahgoup EM, Khaleel SA, Zweier JL. Electronic cigarette exposure causes vascular endothelial dysfunction due to NADPH oxidase activation and eNOS uncoupling. American Journal of Physiology. Heart and Circulatory Physiology. 2022;**322**(4):H549-HH67

[131] Li J, Huynh L, Cornwell WD, Tang MS, Simborio H, Huang J, et al. Electronic cigarettes induce mitochondrial DNA Damage and Trigger TLR9 (Toll-Like Receptor 9)-mediated atherosclerosis. Arteriosclerosis, Thrombosis, and Vascular Biology. 2021;**41**(2):839-853

[132] Espinoza-Derout J, Shao XM, Lao CJ, Hasan KM, Rivera JC, Jordan MC, et al. Electronic cigarette use and the risk of cardiovascular diseases. Frontier in Cardiovascular Medicine. 2022;**9**:879726

[133] Lee WH, Ong SG, Zhou Y, Tian L, Bae HR, Baker N, et al. Modeling cardiovascular risks of E-Cigarettes with human-induced pluripotent stem cell-derived endothelial cells. Journal of the American College of Cardiology. 2019;**73**(21):2722-2737

[134] Williams FN, Herndon DN, Suman OE, Lee JO, Norbury WB, Branski LK, et al. Changes in cardiac physiology after severe burn injury. Journal of Burn Care & Research. 2011;**32**(2):269-274

[135] Hoesel LM, Niederbichler AD, Schaefer J, Ipaktchi KR, Gao H, Rittirsch D, et al. C5a-blockade improves burn-induced cardiac dysfunction. Journal of Immunology. 2007;**178**(12):7902-7910

[136] Jeschke MG, Chinkes DL, Finnerty CC, Kulp G, Suman OE, Norbury WB, et al. Pathophysiologic response to severe burn injury. Annals of Surgery. 2008;**248**(3):387-401

[137] Davies JL. The endocrine response. In: 1982, editor. Physiological Responses to Burning Injury. Orlando: Academic Press

[138] Crum RL, Dominic W, Hansbrough JF, Shackford SR, Brown MR. Cardiovascular and neurohumoral

responses following burn injury. Archives of Surgery. 1990;**125**(8):1065-1069

[139] Mak GZ, Hardy AR, Meyer RA, Kagan RJ. Reversible cardiomyopathy after severe burn injury. Journal of Burn Care & Research. 2006;**27**(4):482-486

[140] Zabala LM, Parray T. Cardiac arrest because of unrecognized delayed dilated cardiomyopathy in a child with severe burn injury. Paediatric Anaesthesia. 2006;**16**(3):358-359

[141] Chen TJ, Shen BH, Yeh FL, Lin JT, Ma H, Huang CH, et al. Delayed dilated cardiomyopathy for major burn injuries. Burns. 2003;**29**(4):343-348

[142] Abu-Sittah GS, Sarhane KA, Dibo SA, Ibrahim A. Cardiovascular dysfunction in burns: Review of the literature. Annals of Burns and Fire Disasters. 2012;**25**(1):26-37

[143] Adams HR, Baxter CR, Izenberg SD. Decreased contractility and compliance of the left ventricle as complications of thermal trauma. American Heart Journal. 1984;**108**(6):1477-1487

[144] Adams HR, Baxter CR, Parker JL. Contractile function of heart muscle from burned guinea pigs. Circulatory Shock. 1982;**9**(1):63-73

[145] Suzuki KOT, Takasu N, et al. Changes in left ventricular preload and contractility following severe bunrs in the dog. Heart and Vessels. 1986;**2**:147-153

[146] Martyn JWR, Burke IF. Right ventricular function and pulmonary hemodynamics during dopamine infusion in burned patients. Chest. 1986;**89**:357-360

[147] Ganrot KJS, Rothman U. Transcapillary passage of plasma proteins in experimental burns. Acta Physiologica Scandinavica. 1974;**91**:497-501

[148] Reiss E, Pearson E, Artz CP. The metabolic response to burns. The Journal of Clinical Investigation. 1956;**35**(1):62-77

[149] Wilmore DW, Aulick LH. Metabolic changes in burned patients. The Surgical Clinics of North America. 1978;**58**(6):1173-1187

[150] Wolf SE, Rose JK, Desai MH, Mileski JP, Barrow RE, Herndon DN. Mortality determinants in massive pediatric burns. An analysis of 103 children with > or = 80% TBSA burns (> or = 70% full-thickness). Annals of Surgery. 1997;**225**(5):554-565

[151] Wilmore DW, Long JM, Mason AD Jr, Skreen RW, Pruitt BA Jr. Catecholamines: Mediator of the hypermetabolic response to thermal injury. Annals of Surgery. 1974;**180**(4):653-669

[152] Goodall M, Stone C, Haynes BW Jr. Urinary output of adrenaline and noradrenaline in severe thermal burns. Annals of Surgery. 1957;**145**(4):479-487

[153] Mohammadi F, Ramachandran J, Woodman R, Muller K, John L, Chen J, et al. Impact of cardiac dysfunction on morbidity and mortality in liver transplant candidates. Clinical Transplantation. 2022:e14682

[154] Jeschke MG, Gauglitz GG, Kulp GA, Finnerty CC, Williams FN, Kraft R, et al. Long-term persistance of the pathophysiologic response to severe burn injury. PLoS One. 2011;**6**(7):e21245

[155] Raab W. Key position of catecholamines in functional and degenerative cardiovascular pathology.

The American Journal of Cardiology. 1960;**5**:571-578

[156] Rona G. Catecholamine cardiotoxicity. Journal of Molecular and Cellular Cardiology. 1985;**17**(4):291-306

[157] Van Vliet PD, Burchell HB, Titus JL. Focal myocarditis associated with pheochromocytoma. The New England Journal of Medicine. 1966;**274**(20):1102-1108

[158] Wen JJ, Cummins CB, Szczesny B, Radhakrishnan RS. Cardiac dysfunction after burn injury: Role of the AMPK-SIRT1-PGC1alpha-NFE2L2-ARE Pathway. Journal of the American College of Surgeons. 2020;**230**(4):562-571

[159] Wen JJ, Cummins CB, Radhakrishnan RS. Burn-induced cardiac mitochondrial dysfunction via interruption of the PDE5A-cGMP-PKG Pathway. International Journal of Molecular Sciences. 2020;**21**(7):2350-2365

[160] Wen JJ, Cummins C, Radhakrishnan RS. Sildenafil recovers burn-induced cardiomyopathy. Cells. 2020;**9**:6

[161] Wen JJ, Mobli K, Rontoyanni VG, Cummins CB, Radhakrishnan GL, Murton A, et al. Nuclear factor erythroid 2-related factor 2 activation and burn-induced cardiac dysfunction. Journal of the American College of Surgeons. 2022;**234**(4):660-671

Section 2

Cardiovascular Diagnostics

Chapter 16

Anthropometrics in Predicting Cardiovascular Disease Risk: Our Research Work Mathematically Demonstrates that Cardiovascular Sciences Were Always Confused for a Long Time

Angel Martin Castellanos

Abstract

Cardiovascular diseases (CVD_S) mainly heart disease and stroke are the leading causes of death globaly. Obesity is a major risk factor for myocardial infarction (MI) and CVD. However, how to measure CVD risk with simple baseline anthropometric characteristics? Besides, association of anthropometrics and CVD may present effects of bias, and in evaluating risk, the lack of balance between simple measurements will be particularly prone to the generation of false-positive results. The purpose of this paper is to provide the key concepts for demonstrating association biases for metrics taken from multiple large-scale studies worldwide. Epidemiologically, waist-to-hip ratio (WHR) is a confounding variable with respect to waist circumference (WC) and waist-to-height ratio (WHtR). This is due to different imbalances between hip circumference (HC)-WC and HC-height, respectively, occurring in a protective overestimation for HC concerning WC and height. Similarly, WC may be a confounding variable with respect to WHtR due to an imbalance in WC-height: This occurs if, and only if, the mean WC > height/2 (WHtR risk cut-off >0.5). This, therefore, overestimates risk in tallest people and lead to underestimations in the shortest people. Anthropometrically, only WHtR is the only measure that is directly associated to a relative risk volume and yields no biases, and it should therefore be the metric used to compare the anthropometrically-measured causal risk.

Keywords: myocardial infarction, cardiovascular disease, risk prediction, obesity, anthropometric indicator, body composition, bias

1. Introduction

Cardiovascular diseases (CVD_S) mainly heart disease and stroke are the leading causes of death globaly [1]. Obesity is a major risk factor for CVD_S such as coronary artery disease. However, overweight/obesity are defined as abnormal or excessive fat accumulation measured by the body mass index (BMI), but it may not correspond to the same degree of fatness and metabolic health in different individuals [2]. Thus, accurate estimation of the body composition (BC) as well as body fat distribution are relevant from a public health perspective [3]. Nevertheless, how can the true unhealthy BC and risk be measured with regard to simple baseline anthropometric measurements? In epidemiology, as in real life, not everything that seems accurate at first glance is true in reality. In medical research, false appearances and biases also occur, which can mean that valuable conclusions may turn out to be worthless. Indeed, bias in research occurs when systematic error is introduced into sampling or testing by selecting or encouraging one outcome or answer over others. Therefore, a thorough understanding about biases, and how it affects study results is essential for medical research because association of anthropometrics does not always equate to causation regarding incidents of myocardial infarction (MI) or CVD. Interestingly, this association may present effects of bias rather than reflecting the true putative risk may be responsible for all or much of the epidemiological causality. In non-randomised study designs, baseline differences in the high BC of risk or in the measured risk when comparing between healthy population and MI/CVD cases may introduce systematic bias in results. Similarly, a different BC between groups with similar baseline confounding variables may provide bias if the risk assignment does not account for the covariates that predict the receiving true risk. Thus, not all anthropometrics are optimal for risk assessment. Critical thinking that covers all potential mechanisms of bias is indispensable to prevent incorrect conclusions being drawn, which may have clinical consequences, especially when predicting MI/CVD causal risk.

Conceptually, each anthropometric provides its own biological meaning depending on the part of the BC that can be distinguished, while the notion of equality in the estimate of risk between body measurements may be respected. If not, the lack of a balanced distribution for the simple measurements between healthy and unhealthy cases will be particularly prone to the generation of false-positive results. Regarding this issue, the mathematical relation of equivalence is a key concept for specifying whether two indicators are the same with respect to a given risk. Thus, any indicator will be comparable to other or not, depending on the measured risk. Therefore, a strong association would lead us to infer or not infer a risk, given that the true nature of risk should come from the selective high risk BC instead the mere findings of the statistical association for each metric. In fact, anthropometrically-measured causal risk depends on specific bodily components; our interpretation may not be confused by the association of arithmetic indicators that suggest a supposed risk that is not verified. Thus, criteria for judgement of causal association must be respected, while also recognising that any association may be bogus, indirect o real.

2. Association of anthropometric measures and MI risk

Various previous studies have recognised the association of a raised BMI with MI, as well as a higher association of abdominal obesity measures with MI [4–10]. Despite this, BMI is an important metric that has been proposed to define ideal cardiovascular health and predict CVD risk [11, 12]. However, it is only a surrogate measure of general body fatness and does not provide accurate information about the true high risk BC, unlike waist circumference (WC). Indeed, evidence is accumulating in support of WC as metric linked to visceral adipose tissue, and the only metric among other simple measurements that predict MI and cardiometabolic risk [4, 7, 9, 13–17]. However, according to the INTERHEART study and others, waist-to-hip ratio (WHR) appeared to have the best predictive value above BMI and WC [4, 18–21]. In addition, results from the UK Biobank have conferred WHR a greater excess risk for MI in women than in men [21].

On the other hand, compound metrics such as waist-to-height ratio (WHtR), whole-body fat percentage (%BF), conicity index, and adiposity measured by technological methods could be better indicators than WC alone to predict cardiovascular events and mortality, even taking consideration of sex differences [5, 14, 20, 22–27]. Furthermore, WHtR and %BF have demonstrated a high level of discrimination in the relationship with a unhealthy BC. WHtR has been more strongly correlated with %BF and adiposity variables in men than it is with WC [24, 27]. WHtR and %BF appear to be strengthened as an anthropometrically valid assessment of biological risk. Thereby, WC and height, and skin folds to a lesser extent, could be taken as basic measurements for evaluating cardiometabolic and MI risk, including cardiovascular mortality, in their relationships with abdominal and relative adiposity [12–16, 20–30]. Complementary, moderate-high endomorphy and high thickness of skinfolds, especially subscapular, have been significantly associated with MI in men [10, 24, 27, 31, 32]. Moreover, patients of both sexes assessed by computed tomography have presented better MI risk prediction as visceral adiposity increases and abdominal subcutaneous area decreases [16, 22].

3. What is new about anthropometrics associated with MI

While overweight/obesity as BMI-measured, enlarged WC, WHR risk cut-off of <1, and WHtR cut-off of $\geq$0.5 have been verified as baseline characteristics for the association of anthropometrics and MI/CVD worldwide, even accounting for differences in strength of association and by sex [4–10, 12–19, 21–24, 27, 32–37]. Similarly, mathematical inequality between the mean simple body measurements as well as non-equivalent relation in the ratios, ratios of ratios and risk cut-offs may also be implicated (**Table 1**). Thus, data from thousands of MI/CVD cases are collated in **Table 1**, where new anthopometrics have been included as mere mathematical expressions derived from original data, demonstrating the inequality and non-equivalence relations between the corresponding mean simple measurements. After associating anthropometrics and MI/CVD risk, since mathematical inequalities between measurements may be demonstrated in any study population, perspective for epidemiological causality should be shifted accordingly. From evidence reflected in **Table 1**, neither WHR risk cutoff <1 (the mean hip circumference (HC) > WC) nor WC risk cut-off (the mean WC > height/2) will adequately describe the risk, because true risk only occurs at the volume measurement WHtR risk cut-off >0.5, where inequality between WC and height (or height/2) matters too. This is because WHtR mathematically represents a volume function with two independent factors: WC and height. These two measurements are also decisive for estimating %BF [23, 24, 27, 36, 37, 45]. In this sense, mathematical and anthropometric observations in our research work have explained the selection bias for WHR with respect to WC and WHtR and, therefore, have revealed that the risk comparison between healthy and unhealthy cases was not the same [23, 24, 27, 36, 37].

Due to anthropometrically-estimated %BF and mesomorphy presenting a high magnitude of association in MI for men [24, 27, 31], there are still uncertainties

Anthropometric	Men	Women	Association findings**
Weight (kg)	Undefined	Undefined	(–) or weak positive
Height (Ht): (cm)	Undefined (Ht >HC >WC)*	Undefined (Ht >HC >WC)*	(–) or weak inverse
HC (cm)	Undefined (HC >WC >Ht/2)*	Undefined (HC >WC >Ht/2)*	(–) or weak positive/inverse
Height/2 (cm)	Undefined (WC >Ht/2)*	Undefined (WC >Ht/2)*	(–) or weak inverse
HtHR: (Ht/HC)	>**1** (Ht >HC)*	>**1** (Ht >HC)*	(–) or weak inverse
HHt/2R: (HC/(Ht/2))	>**1** (HC >Ht/2)*	>**1** (HC >Ht/2)*	(–) or weak positive/inverse
WC (cm)	>94 (102): (WC >Ht/2)*	>80 (88): (WC >Ht/2)*	Strong-moderate positive
BMI (kg/m^2)	>26.5	>25.5	Moderate positive
WHR	≥0.90 <**1** (HC >WC)*	≥0.80 <**1** (HC >WC)*	Strong positive
WHtR	≥**0.5** (Ht >WC >Ht/2)*	≥**0.5** (Ht >WC >Ht/2)*	Strong-moderate positive
WHt/2R: (WC/(Ht/2))	>**1** (WC >Ht/2)*	>**1** (WC >Ht/2)*	Strong-moderate positive
WHR/WHtR	<2 (WHR <WHtR x 2)*	<2 (WHR <WHtR x 2)*	Strong positive

*BMI indicates body mass index; CVD, cardiovascular disease; HC, hip circumference; Ht, body height; HHt/2R, hip-to-height/2 ratio; HtHR, height-to-hip ratio; WC, waist circumference; MI, myocardial infarction; WHR, waist-to-hip ratio; WHtR, waist-to-height ratio; WHt/2R, waist-to-height/2 ratio. *Regardless of risk cutoff values significant inequality between the mean values of the referenced simple measurements and a non-equivalent relation in the ratios is always found. ** Measures of association such as odds ratios, hazard ratios, Receiver Operating Characteristic curves or other statistical models in all studies were used as appropriate. (–): Null or not association. [a] Ethnically-specific risk cutoffs (either in numerical or in undefined values) are taken into account when reflecting inequality between the simple measurements, and therefore non-equivalent risk in the ratios, ratios of ratios and risk cutoffs. [b] Mathematical inequality between the simple measurements and non-equivalence relations are extracted or extrapoled from the differences between the mean (standard deviation) or median values described in thousands of participants in most studies worldwide. Table was elaborated by the author. From the scientific evidence, new metrics were included.*

Table 1.
Defined and undefined risk cut-off points for the association of anthropometrics and MI/CVD. Imbalance between the mean values of the simple body measurements (in parentheses) where appropriate. Risk cut-off values and mathematical inequality between the corresponding simple measurements and ratios where appropriate too [4–10, 14–30, 32–35, 38–44].

regarding the association between BMI and WHR and their relationships with the true high risk BC. Conceptually, the true risk factor regarding BC derives from %BF, fundamentally the part linked to intra-abdominal fat depots functioning as a neuro-endocrine organ that influence CVD risk [46, 47]. On the other hand, mesomorphy represents relative muscularity, but association with MI is artificial and does not equate causation [10, 24, 31, 48]. Thus, seeing as BMI and WHR are anthropometrically linked to musculoskeletal component, and are more weakly correlated with %BF than other metrics, they have presented an information bias and associated a spurious risk for MI in men [23, 24, 27]. Indeed, it is important to understand the discrepancy observed between the strongest association for WHR, and their worst correlations with measures of general and central adiposity in both sexes [4, 17–19, 21, 23, 27]. The discrepancy between the strength of association for WHR and a lower anthropometric coherence as well as the unbalanced distributions for WC and HC between healthy and cases in both sexes, suggest that there where errors regarding the true risk association. Consequently, a systematic error would be introduced regarding the true risk assignment for WHR and BMI, if, when partially capturing a dimension of spurious risk their data were slanted in an artificial direction towards site of cases. In

DOI: http://dx.doi.org/10.5772/intechopen.105098

contrast, a raised WHtR and %BF have demonstrated anthropometric coherence and balanced distribution for the concrete values of volume by unit of height and body fatness for justifying risk excess. This anthropometric profile could help explain the abundance of MI among individuals with raised visceral fat, irrespective of BMI, HC or mesomorphy rating [10, 23, 24, 27, 31, 48].

4. What is the justification for making our arguments?

4.1 Lessons from anthropometry, mathematics, geometry and epidemiology

Arithmetic value and true risk measured from each anthropometric depends on formulae, unit of measure and body measurements derived from different structural components. Mathematical understanding of some concepts turns out to be key to detecting unhealthy BC and anthropometrically-measured risk. From this perspective, weight, height, height/2, WC and HC represent absolute values without expressing equality for risk as a mathematical object. Consequently, in assessing anthropometrics-associated risk, mathematical relation of equivalence between simple measurements and indicators or ratios to be compared should be recognised by the researchers

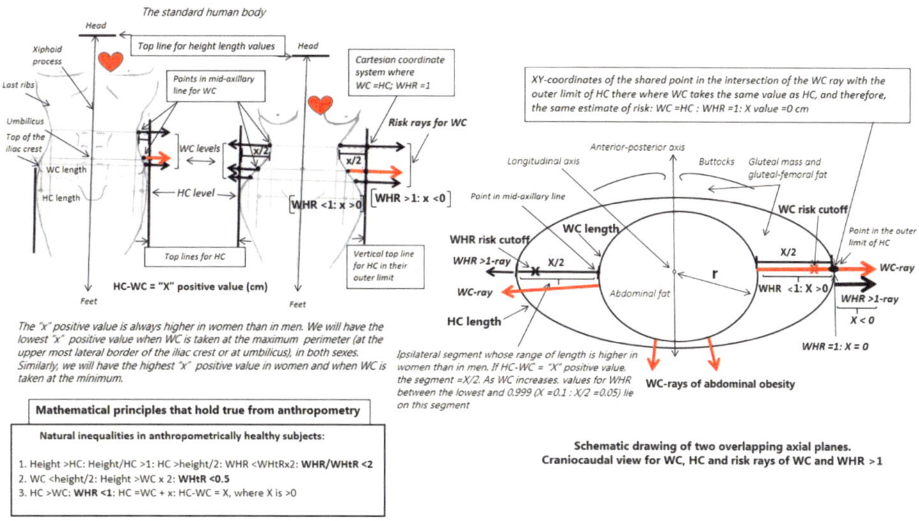

Figure 1.
The standard human body and simple anthropometric measurements. Geometrical lines drawn from anthropometry for understanding metrics and rays of risk for WC and WHR >1. Mathematical principles and anthropometric arguments that hold true in an anthropometrically healthy population. Anthropometrics at baseline would represent mean values per standard deviation for height, height/2, WC, HC, WHR, WHtR and "X" distance being actually valid for any anthropometrically healthy population and ethnicity. On the respective rays of risk for WC (in red colour) and WHR >1 would lie points of increased abdominal obesity representing mean values (SD) for thousands of cases of MI/CVD as well as biological changes pointing towards greater excess risk as WC increases and while height may no condition the whole-risk measured by WC alone. On the ipsilateral segment, which length value is "X" positive (cm)/2 would lie all the points for WHR <1 (including WHR risk cutoff) from the lowest value up to 0.999 (X = 0.1: X/2 = 0.05) just before the outer limit of HC where X = 0. HC indicates hip circumference; WC, waist circumference; WHR, waist-to-hip ratio; WHtR, waist-to-height ratio; X, subtracting HC by WC; X/2, ipsilateral segment as horizontal distance between any point of WC in the mid-axillary line and the vertical top line for HC in their outer limit. Footnote: Original drawings built and designed by the author. Dimensions are not to scale. Anthropometric evidence supports the referred mathematical inequalities between the simple measurements in the standard human body.

(**Figure 1**, **Table 1**). Thus, when comparing with anthropometrically healthy subjects and with the evidence of CVD epidemiology, the rationale is as follows.

Muscle, bone, fat and residual mass as different biological components present no differentiation by body weight (unit of mass), and therefore, a higher BMI does not always involve greater body fat excess, at least in normal or overweight people [2, 24, 27]. Weight and height differences between sexes are not recognised by the BMI formula. Thereby, an equal BMI does not mean the same degree of fatness or unhealthy BC. In this sense, the error of estimation for high risk BC or risk may occur in comparing BMI with others, and either by age or by sex.

Height length depends on the bone structure of the adult. In this sense, height never correlates with adiposity [10, 21, 23, 27, 31, 48], and, therefore, it does not account for the true-risk per se. However, height as a volume factor would exert a modulating effect for conditioning the storage and distribution of the body fat as well as the relative volume that it occupies in the three-dimensional abdominal space [24, 27]. Thereby, a significant difference in height between groups and sexes conditions the risk estimated by each concerned anthropometric, and therefore, height as longitudinal dimension also has important implications.

Mathematically, WC and WHtR would be equivalent for the same estimated risk if, and only if, mean WC = height/2. Therefore, WHtR risk cut-off =0.5 is the entity of risk conditioned on WC, but height/2 taking the same value as WC (e.g., 80/160, 84/168, 85/170, 88/176 etc., all =0.5). If not, the error of estimation for both the true high risk BC and risk may occur in comparing WC alone with WHtR, and either by age or by sex. Thus, if the mean WC is >height/2 (WHtR risk cut-off >0.5) (e.g., 80.5/158, 82.6/162, 82.8/162.4, 95.4/187 etc., all =0.51) protective underestimation occurs for height with respect to WC, whether WC alone assigns the risk from a defined risk cut-off.

In another conceptual consideration, evidence supports that there is a higher excess risk of MI/CVD when abdominal obesity increases [13, 14]. However, when comparing between-groups abdominal obesity may be expressed either in cm^2 (two-dimensional area determined from WC length) or in cm^3 (three-dimensional volume of a solid abdominal disk determined from WC and height of the disk = WHtR cm), (**Figures 2** and **3**) [24, 37]. From this new insight, WC and WHtR do not express the same risk when comparing healthy people and MI/CVD cases. This is because WC < height/2 (WHtR <0.5) is a natural inequality. In this way, WC and WHtR refer to the same risk only if the mean WC = height/2 (WHtR risk cut-off =0.5). However, when the mean WC increases above height/2 (WHtR risk cut-off >0.5), the distribution curves of WC and height/2 appear unbalanced between healthy and cases, and only WHtR as an entity of volume may described the risk that is conditional on both WC and height. Otherwise, if we accept WC alone as an anthropometrically-measured causal risk factor, this will lead to an overestimation of risk for WC concerning height, or a protective underestimation of height with respect to WC. It is clear that, if WHtR risk cut-off is >0.5 (the mean WC > height/2), height appears to be inversely associated with the group of cases, and WHtR is the indicator of risk when comparing by ethnicity and sex, but not WC alone. This is because risk is conditional on both WC and height as independent volume factors.

HC length depends on the breadth between both trochanters, the gluteal mass and the gluteal–femoral fat to determine a two-dimensional geometric area on a transverse plane of defined bodily components, but HC neither discriminates between them nor describes cardiometabolic risk. Therefore, it does not account for the true high risk BC or risk [10, 24, 27, 31, 37, 48]. Thus, either the high risk BC or raised %BF is not affected by

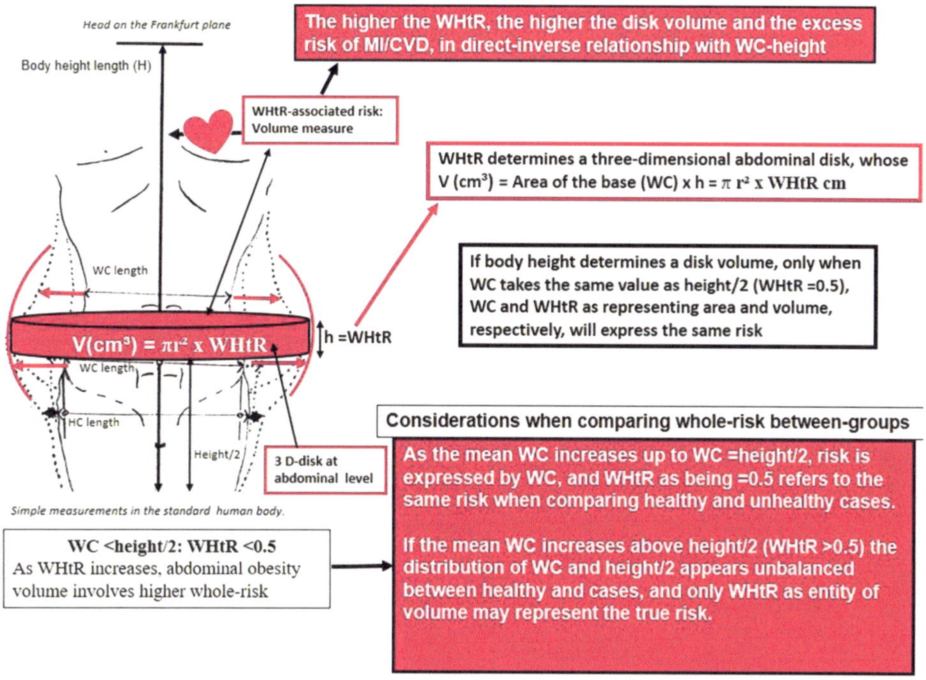

Figure 2.
Anthropometric length measurements in the standard body human and considerations for differencing between volume of a three-dimensional abdominal disk and WC as two-dimensional area. Measurements at baseline would represent mean values per standard deviation for WC, HC, height, height/2 and WHtR being actually valid for any study population and ethnicity. The model of disk for representing volume of an abdominal segment may be applied for both case–control and cohort studies from the respective mean values (SD) and risk cut-offs for WHtR. Anthropometric considerations are explained for understanding volume and excess risk of MI/CVD as WHtR increases. CVD denotes cardiovascular disease; H, body height; height/2, dividing height by 2; h, height of the disk; HC, hip circumference; MI, myocardial infarction, r, radius of the base; V, volume of the disk; WC, waist circumference; WHtR, waist-to-height ratio. Footnote: Original graphical abstract was built and designed by the author.

HC, but vice versa. HC can be modified by physical activity or the ageing process, etc., in both sexes, but this does not justify a direct impact on MI/CVD risk. With modifications in HC, neither WC nor high risk BC and %BF are necessarily affected. In this sense, WC and WHR would be mathematically equivalent for the same estimation of risk if, and only if, the mean HC = WC, and therefore, WHR risk cut-off = 1 being the entity of risk conditional on WC, but HC taking the same value as WC. In this case, subtracting HC by WC we obtain an X value of zero (**Figures 1** and **3**) [36, 37]. If not, the error of estimation for both the true high risk BC and risk may occur in comparing WHR with WC alone, and either by age or by sex. Thus, the mean HC > WC protective overestimation occurs for HC with respect to WC, and WHR <1 may present a risk overestimation by selecting false-positive points as compared to those true-negatives conditional on WC values as the numerator. It is clear that, if WHR risk cut-off is <1 (mean HC > WC: similar to natural inequality), not all subjects in that stratum may present risk because HC as risk factor appears not to be associated with any group when compared. Similarly, if HC > WC (WHR <1: X > 0) is a true premise applicable to a healthy population, the question arises as to how it may be applied to cases of CVD without being a false premise? From an epidemiological viewpoint, effectively only WHR <1 may represent a risk associated to cases when conditioning WC as numerator. This value lies above their

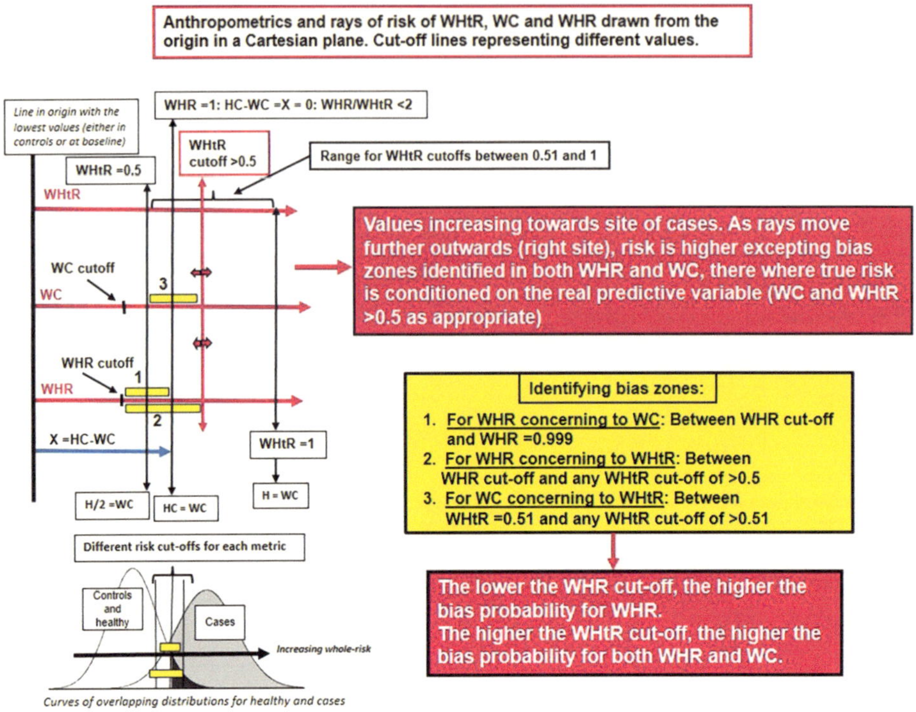

Figure 3.
Number lines in a Cartesian plane for representing values in healthy population and cases of MI/CVD: Metrics-associated risk increases as each anthropometric ray of risk move to the right (site of cases). Subtitled curves of distribution, overlapping area, risk ray and bias zone as appropriate. It is transferable to any study population and ethnicity. All reference values may be represented lying on the respective number lines drawn. We may find the points with the lowest baseline values for WHtR, WC and WHR (healthy/controls or cases) lying on a respective line in the origin. Similarly, risk cut-offs and cutting lines lying where appropriate. The highest baseline values (generally in unhealthy cases) would lie on the arrowhead of the anthropometric rays of risk moving further outwards (right site). Other points would represent mean values per standard deviation for WC, HC, height, height/2, WHR and WHtR in healthy and cases as appropriate. In the respective lines and risk rays drawn in magenta colour would lie points of increased abdominal obesity representing values for thousands of cases of MI/CVD as well as biological changes pointing towards greater excess risk as WC increases and HC and height condition the true risk from WHR and WHtR, respectively. Values for X (between the maximum positive in their origin and zero (WC = HC) would be represented lying on the corresponding partial ray of risk (in blue colour). We have also pointed the theoretical cutting lines for WHtR and WHR there where would occur a balanced distribution of WC-height/2, WC-HC and WC-height mean values (SD) when pooling healthy and unhealthy cases. The model plotted may be applied for both case–control and cohort studies. CVD denotes cardiovascular disease; H, height; HC, hip circumference; MI, myocardial infarction; WC, waist circumference; WHR, waist-to-hip ratio; WHtR, waist-to-height ratio; X, subtracting HC by WC. Footnote: Original graphical abstract was built and designed by the author. Dimensions are not to scale.

defined risk cut-off. Obviously, WHR ≥1 (WC ≥ HC: X ≤ 0) will always represent risk associated to group of cases irrespective of HC value (**Figure 1**). Therefore, the true risk assignment for WHR only depends on WC receiving risk as numerator, and besides, WC as the entity of risk compared according to ethnicity and sex, but never WHR alone as an abstract fraction.

WC length depends on specific biological components that determine a two-dimensional geometric area (cm^2) on a transverse plane. Evidence supports WC as the strongest simple metric linked to visceral adiposity that provides a solid estimation of risk [13, 14, 17, 46, 47, 49]. On the other hand, in the standard human body, WC can be lower than height/2 (WHtR <0.5) without posing any putative risk or protective effect (**Figures 1** and **2**). Only when WC and height/2 are mathematically equivalent (WC = height/2: WHtR = 0.5) is there a notion of equality and balance for the same estimation of risk from WC and WHtR. However, evidence also supports the notion that WHtR >0.5 is strongly associated to cases of MI [15, 18, 21, 23, 27, 37]. When the WHtR risk cut-off is >0.5, equality does not exist between WC and height/2, and only WHtR may be used to draw a valid conclusion for estimating the risk (**Figure 3**, **Table 1**). Thus, if the mean WC > height/2 risk overestimation occurs for WC with respect to height, WC alone will present an overestimation of risk in the tallest people and an underestimation in the shortest. Mathematically, WHtR >0.5 and < 1 is a proper abstract fraction (part/whole) whose decimal value up to 1 (theoretical) tells us the equal parts of WC that we have in height (whole), but never WC (part) referring to the entity of whole-risk as a mathematical object. Quite the opposite is the case; the higher the WHtR (whereas being <1), the higher the risk overestimation for WC as compared to WHtR. Similarly, the higher the WHtR between 0.51 and 0.999, the higher the probability of bias for WC. If WHtR cannot record true risk, WC might capture false risk beyond the true risk of WHtR. Hence, WC might present an error of estimation in women compared to men due to differences in WC and height between both sexes and, therefore, different risks to be compared. Only when the mean WC is lower than height/2 (WHtR risk cut-off <0.5), WC and its risk cut-off would represent the entity of risk without accounting for bias, but only up to WHtR = 0.5 (**Figure 3**). That way, only in unrepresentative, small samples where the mean WC is lower than height/2 or in women where differences between mean WC and height/2 are less important, WC and WHtR would capture similar risk as being close to WHtR = 0.5. However, if WHtR risk cut-off is >0.5 (mean WC > height/2) not all subjects in that stratum will present risk from WC alone because it may not capture true risk, at least without accounting for height. In this regard, if the mean WC > height/2 (WHtR risk cut-off >0.5) is a true premise applicable to MI/CVD cases, how can it be applied to a healthy population without being a false premise? Epidemiologically, those values for WHtR from 0.51 up to any other defined risk cut-off of >0.51, while lying on the overlapping zone of the distribution curves between groups, they may be true-negatives for healthy subjects when conditional on WHtR >0.5 as the true predictive variable, effectively being the mean WC higher than height/2. In this situation, those true-negative points for WHtR always lie before the line of their defined risk cut-off, which is much further on from 0.5 (bias zone for WC, **Figure 3**). Indisputably, if in any study population's WHtR risk cut-off is of >0.5 (mean WC > height/2), the concrete value of this metric while measuring the relative volume and being conditional on both WC and height predicts the received risk, but never WC alone.

The standard human body can have a HC higher than WC without posing any putative risk or protective effect (**Figure 1**). By deduction, HC > WC is an anthropometrically healthy natural inequality, which responds to a linear equation: HC = WC + X, where by subtracting HC from WC we calculate X (>zero) as a unit of length with one decimal digit-tenths; the standard value is higher in women and the middle-aged than in men and elderly subjects, respectively, but higher than zero in all cases. Mathematically, WHR <1 is a proper abstract fraction whose decimal value ranged from hundredths up to 1, which states that equal parts of WC in HC, but it shows no anthropometric consistency or true risk beyond that of WC or X distance. It is clear that WHR <1 is simply a way of representing size (part/whole) that is not a whole number or entity of whole-risk as a mathematical object, unlike WC or X. In this sense, WHR <1 might represent a higher risk than WC and X, when HC has the importance of being overestimated as a protective factor with respect to WC and, therefore, creating bias for WHR. This is because fractions of equal value do not refer to the same risk and the sensitivity of WHR (hundredths) is different from X (tenths). It is clear that between two consecutive values of WHR <1 we have 10 of X (e.g., between 0.95 and 0.96. we have from 5 up to 4.1 for X, but not all referring to the same risk as it is 0.95, which misclassifies risk). Thus, the higher the positive value of X (e.g., in women, middle-aged people, athletes), the higher the probability of bias for WHR when compared to WC, and if values of WC (numerator) and X as true-negatives below their respective risk cut-offs receive no true risk, WHR may effectively capture false-positive points in the stratum of <1. "From a proper abstract fraction, if WHR risk cut-off is of <1, WC turns out to be the entity of risk to be compared, but never WHR performing better than WC, at least while understanding maths and biases" [37].

Anthropometrically, in any study population, from the lowest baseline up to the highest values there is a direct correlation between cardiometabolic risk for WC and WHtR indicating the corresponding risk cut-offs. As WC and WHtR increase, the respective risk cut-offs and points with greater excess risk move further outwards lying on their geometric rays. However, WC may only represent risk when WHtR = 0.5 and the mean WC and height/2 are balanced in their data distribution (**Figure 3**). Similarly, WC alone may represent risk with respect to WHR when the WC cut-off lies before the line where WHR = 1. When the WHR risk cut-off is ≥1 (improper fraction), WC and WHR express the same risk. On the contrary, while WHtR may demonstrate a risk cut-off between 0.51 and 0.999 (<1), neither WC nor WHR will represent risk due to overlapping and bias zones where false-positive points might be selected from both with respect to WHtR, which would receive no risk up to their risk cut-off lying on their ray of risk further outwards (site of cases), (**Figure 3**). Indisputably, the risk points from WHR and WC in bias zones before the WHtR risk cut-off will never capture the true risk while not being true positives lying on their respective rays of risk after the same WHtR risk cut-off. The risk captured by WHR and WC in the identified bias zones will always be false, at least partially.

Epidemiologically, neither height nor HC correlate to cardiometabolic risk. Hence, in predicting MI/CVD risk, HC and height may only be conditional risks for WHR and WHtR as area and volume factors, respectively. HC never appears to take the same cut-off value as height (the mean height is always higher than HC and HC > height/2). WC hardly reaches the same cut-off value as height or HC (mathematically it is always fulfilled as the mean height > HC > WC. The mean HC > WC > height/2, see **Table 1**). In addition, as WC increases, WHR >1 (whole/part) may also draw a similar correlation of risk up to the highest WC values because it directly depends on WC as a total area of risk, irrespective of HC (**Figure 1**). Nevertheless, WHR <1 (part/whole) draws neither ray nor greater excess risk, at least between their risk cut-offs and the 0.999 value where a higher or lesser bias occurs as HC increases or decreases and WC does not move in its respective ray of risk. On the other hand, only WHtR as a relative volume allows a clear indication of risk to be recognised up to value of 1, which theoretically would represent the unity of risk corresponding to the total volume where WC would take the same value as height (in a balanced distribution). In this approach, we will always find the point for WHtR = 0.5 before the line for WHR = 1, and the WHtR risk cut-off lies much more outwards (in the site of cases) than WC and WHR. Thereby, the curves of distribution and overlapping zones explain that, in capturing risk, WHtR presents much more sensitivity (true-positive fraction) than WC or WHR. This is because true-negative values conditioned on the WHtR risk cut-off are not selected as false-positive ones, unlike WC and WHR between their respective risk cut-offs and the end of the bias zones (**Figure 3**).

Anatomically, HC is also higher than height/2 and lower than height (height/HC >1; HC/(height/2) >1) (**Figure 1**). Hence, there would be no equivalent relation between WHR and WHtR risk cut-offs to compare the same risk if the first is lower than the second × 2 (WHR/WHtR <2). According to this premise, WHtR ≥0.5 will always detect risk before WHR ≥1 (see **Figure 3**). Since the balanced distribution between WC and height/2 on the one hand, and between WC and HC on the other hand, may only be found on the risk cut-offs of WHtR =0.5 and WHR =1, respectively, both indices will never capture the same risk because it is anthropometrically impossible and epidemiologically false (**Table 1**). Therefore, bias will occur for WHR with respect to WHtR due to an unbalancing of HC and height/2 values between healthy and unhealthy cases (**Figures 1** and **3**). If WHR risk cut-off is lower than WHtR × 2 and WC does not move, WHR-associated risk above WHtR would be a

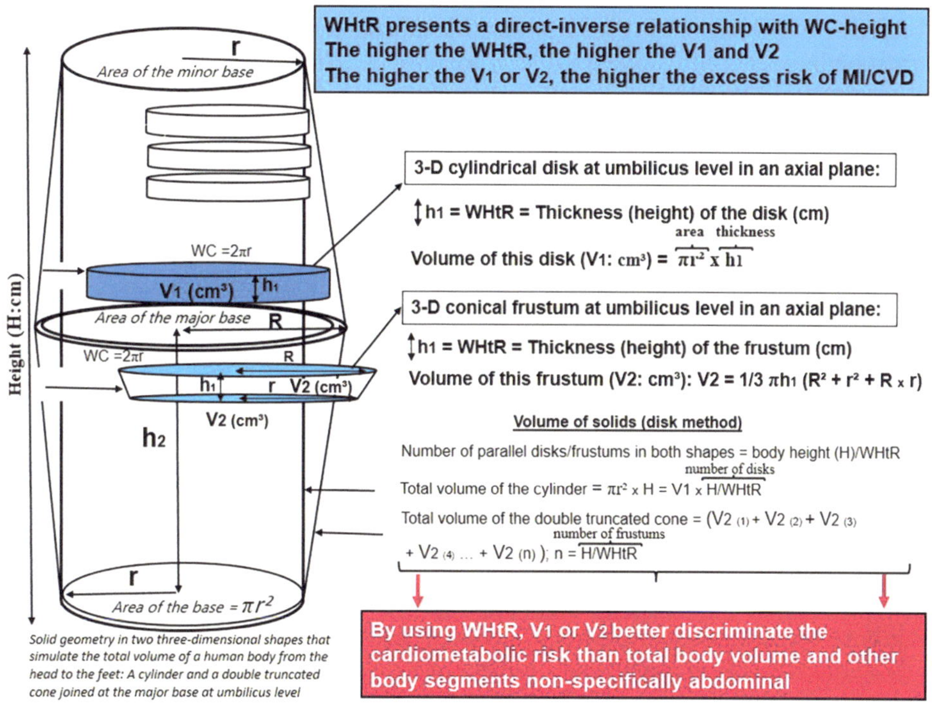

Figure 4.
Lessons from geometry: Volume of solids. Geometric model representing the human body as a solid cylinder or two truncated cones joined together at their major bases. Geometry formulas and explanations for understanding the meaning of WHtR when comparing cardiometabolic risk between healthy population and cases of MI/CVD. Geometric values at baseline would represent the mean values per standard deviation for WC, radius, heights and WHtR being actually valid for any study population and ethnicity. The model may be applied for both case–control and cohort studies from the respective mean values (SD) and risk cut-offs for WHtR. "Volume" refers to the amount of three-dimensional space that bodily components occupy in relation to their mass and density. Volume is determined by geometry formulas. The base of the cylinder and the major base of the truncated cones have a length or perimeter equal to WC as appropriate. Dividing H by WHtR we get the total number of disks that fit into each three-dimensional shape. CVD denotes cardiovascular disease; H, total height corresponding to that of the cylinder or double truncated cone; h_1*, height or thickness of each disk or frustum;* h_2*, height of a single truncated cone (H/2); MI, myocardial infarction, R or r, radius of each base as appropriate;* V_1*, volume of the cylindrical disk;* V_2*, volume of the conical frustum; WC, waist circumference; WHtR, waist-to-height ratio.*

false-positive due a protective overestimation for HC concerning height, either by age or by sex. "From a mathematical conception, ..., if ratio of the risk cut-offs between WHR and WHtR is of <2 (WHR <WHtR x 2), WHtR turns out to be the entity of risk to be compared, but never WHR performing better than WHtR, at least while understanding maths and biases" [37].

From geometry, the concrete volume of a three-dimensional disk or frustum (e.g., at umbilicus level) may be quantified from the WHtR. Simulating a cylinder or truncated cone, the volume of this disk will depend on area of the base$_{(s)}$ (πr^2, where WC $=2\pi r$: $r = WC/2\pi$) and their geometrical height (thickness of the disk = WHtR cm) [36, 37]. Geometrically, the human body as a solid from the head to the feet would have several disks, so that number of disks = body height (H)/WHtR, and the sum of the volume of all the disks would give us the total volume of the body. The total body volume would be the theoretical unity of risk where WC = height: WHtR =1: number of disks =1 (**Figure 4**). Obviously, only from this hypothetical situation WHtR $\geq$1 (improper fraction where the mean WC $\geq$ height) will always represent risk associated to group of cases irrespective of heiht value, and WC and WHtR $\geq$1 refering to the same risk. Thereby, an epidemiologically real WHtR gives us the corresponding relative volume (cm^3) that we have by unit of height or disk in a direct-inverse relationship with WC-height. The higher the WHtR, the higher the volume of the disk. On the other hand, although WC values do not change, the disk volume may be modulated by body height towards a higher or lesser amount of three-dimensional space that risk components occupy and, therefore, modifying their cardiometabolic effect. Epidemiologically, WHtR is important because it captures risk above the WC area, at least when height may have significant differences between groups to be compared and with a WHtR risk cut-off >0.5 and < 1. In this approach, the area and volume from WC and WHtR, respectively, would not be comparable. "From a proper abstract fraction, if WHtR risk cut-off is of >0.5 and <1, the value of this metric is the entity of risk to be compared, but WC never performs better than WHtR, at least while understanding maths and biases" [37].

5. Novel findings in medical research and implications for an anthropometrically correct MI/CVD risk assessment

It is well known BMI depends on weight and it strongly depends on metabolically healthy musculoskeletal components and body fat mass, especially subcutaneous, without discriminating the unhealthy intra-abdominal fat and their volume [2, 14, 23, 24, 37, 48]. Why to choose BMI to assess MI/CVD risk if it captures metabolically contradictory components? The consequence of this chimera is that to describe individuals' risks based on BMI is unfounded and potentially misleading. Accordingly, the concepts of ideal anthropometric health and BMI-classified obesity should not be considered synonymous or interchangeable, unless we accept misclassification and paradoxical information for biological risk assessment. BMI fails to discriminate between harmful body fat and healthy components and is an inappropriate formula to assess the association between excess fat mass and MI/CVD. Besides, while a part of the musculoskeletal component (mesomorphy) may be associated with MI, as %BF increases, a part of the association for BMI would capture a false risk and, therefore, information bias would occur for the true high risk BC in both sexes. The excessive body weight in individuals who have a high BMI and normal %BF (e.g., individuals/athletes with high mesomorphy rating) would indicate a score of spurious risk, but never performing better than WC [24, 27, 37]. With respect to WHR, it is well known that it has demonstrated the highest predictive abilities for MI risk [4, 13, 17–21, 23]. Nevertheless, WHR may present bias with respect to WC when the risk assignment for both does not refer to the same risk, therefore reducing the quality of the comparison [24, 36, 37].

It is noteworthy that WC and HC only may coincide at the same estimation of risk when WC takes the same value as HC (WHR =1; X = 0, see **Figure 1**). Any WHR value of <1 (X > 0) demonstrates no cardiometabolic risk beyond that of WC alone or X. WHR as a proper fraction (<1) will never represent the entity of risk, and any risk-code selected for WHR between their risk cut-off values of <1 and 0.999 will be biased if WC or X receives no risk-code. There would only be a true risk for WHR with respect to WC when WC or X predicts the true risk from their defined risk cut-offs. If not, WHR may select true-negative values as false-positive ones when they merely represent protective overestimation for HC concerning WC and X.

Mathematically, between any WHR risk cut-off <1 (e.g., 0.95) and 0.999, we could always find different individuals and an infinite number of proper fractions whose decimal values receive a risk-code, but that do not refer to the same high risk BC as measured from the WC or X risk cut-off. This discovery arises from rigorous data analysis in the measurements for WC and HC, and where misclassification occurs for WHR-associated risk [23, 24, 36, 37]. As an example, 93.1/98 vs. 93.9/98 vs. 95/100, etc., =0.95: X between 5 and 4.1; 93/95.9 vs. 94.1/96.9 vs. 98/100.9, etc., =0.97: X between 3 and 2.1; 93.8/93.9 vs. 94.2/95 vs. 99/100 etc., =0.99: X between 1 and 0.1. Broadly, there would be five values for WHR between 0.95 and 0.99, and infinite fractions for values of X between 5 and 0.1; HC > WC in all and a WC risk cut-off ≥94.4 in each set. Equal values for WHR (e.g., between 0.82 and 0.999; X between 18 and 0.1) may be transferred to broader populations where the mean values for WC and HC were higher or lower than in the example. In any situation, WC and X values that depend on their own risk cut-offs would reflect different risk-codes in each fraction while WHR would support a unique value for the risk, but any mean value of WHR <1 precludes the same estimation of risk for WC and HC (HC ≠ WC), making the validity of WHR beyond that of WC alone anthropometrically impossible. These observations may help to explain a higher bias for WHR in predicting MI/CVD risk in women because the X positive value is always higher in women than in men. In fact, HC > WC at the baseline involves a positive X value, and the higher the X value, the higher the bias occurs by selecting a higher number of proper fractions and false-positives, so that the protective effect for HC would always be overestimated. Similarly, a higher bias for WHR would occur when the WC is taken at the minimum level vs. the maximum (e.g., at the umbilicus) due to a longer range between the lowest and 0.999 value (see **Figure 1**). "From a proper abstract fraction, if WHR risk cut-off is of <1 all WHR-associated risk above WC as being mathematically incorrect and anthropometrically unjustified provides epidemiological false inferences" [37].

In another mathematical consideration, our research has also revealed that WHR and WHtR contrast by suggesting the same true risk if HC and height present a relationship of height/HC =2. This ratio would occur if and only if WHR/WHtR = 2 (e.g., 0.90/0.45, 0.95/0.475, 1/0.5, 1.2/0.6 etc., HC = height/2 in all). This also appears anthropologically unlikely and selection bias occurred for WHR with respect to WHtR due to the protective overestimation for HC regarding height [23, 37].

As mentioned above, WC and WHtR may only be comparable if the equivalent relationship between WC and height refers to same estimation of risk for both (WC = height/2: WHtR risk cut-off =0.5). If not, between 0.51 and any WHtR risk cut-off up to 1 (e.g., >0.55), we could always find different individuals and an infinite number of fractions receiving the same binary code for WHtR (no risk), but not referring to the same risk-code from the WC risk cut-off (see **Figure 3**). As an example, 82.8/162.4 vs. 88.6/174 vs. 80.6/158 vs. 95.4/187 etc., =0.51; 95.2/178.2 vs. 90/168 vs. 83/156, etc., =0.53; 96.7/178 vs. 92.5/168.2 vs. 98.8/179.6, etc., =0.55. Broadly, there would be no risk-code for WHtR ≤0.55 when the WC represents different risk-codes if their risk cut-offs were > 84 or > 95 on each set, and WC > height/2 in all. Thereby, the higher the WHtR, the higher the risk overestimation for WC occurs by selecting false-positive points as compared to those true-negatives below the WHtR risk cut-off. Equal values for WHtR (e.g., between 0.51 and 0.65) may be transferred to other populations where the mean values for WC and height were higher or lower than in the example. In any situation, WC values depending on their own risk cut-off would reflect different risk-codes into each fraction while WHtR would support a unique, continuous code (no risk) up to their own risk cut-off value. Hence, WC might present bias with respect to WHtR when the risk for both metrics does not refer to the same high risk BC, when compared either in men or in women. Thus, WC might capture risk if there are no differences in height between healthy and unhealthy cases (WHtR risk cut-off close to 0.5). In contrast, the risk captured from WC would be not equivalent when the mean height (WHtR risk cut-off much higher than 0.5) determines a significantly higher relative volume in cases, and therefore a different high risk BC when compared to healthy people (see **Figures 2** and **3**). Regarding this observation, the risk association for WC and WHtR will be equivalent if, and only if, the WHtR risk cut-off is very close to 0.5, but any value >0.5 precludes the same estimation of risk for WC and height (WC ≠ height/2), making the validity of WC alone beyond that of WHtR anthropometrically impossible. Thereby, "when WHtR risk cut-off is of >0.5 and <1 all WC-associated risk above WHtR ... provides epidemiological false inferences" [37].

In another sense, a different cardiometabolic effect among visceral and extra-abdominal fat has been argued when using WC to measure the total abdominal adipose tissue. However, there is evidence that the higher the intra-abdominal fat, the higher the WC value, irrespective of subcutaneous extra-abdominal fat [13–15, 22]. From the Framingham study, visceral fat has been strongly associated with a metabolic risk profile and MI in both sexes and technological studies have also observed that the ratio visceral fat/subcutaneous extra-abdominal fat presented a direct association with MI while subcutaneous area presented the inverse [12, 14, 16, 22, 37, 50]. The anthropometric explanation would be because, as intra-abdominal fat increases, subcutaneous adipose tissue of the extra-abdominal space suffers the mechanical effect of compression, which decreases their relative thickness and volume (tight fat) [37]. Moreover, it is noteworthy that %BF measured by DEXA strongly depends on WC and height rather than BMI in adult individuals [45]. In addition, MI men present high mesomorphy and low ectomorphy ratings, and %BF is more strongly correlated with WHtR than it is with WC (intra-abdominal + subcutaneous area). Therefore, WC does not necessarily refer to risk for an accurate comparison but considering it for a higher relative volume by unit of height, closely linked to a low ectomorphy [10, 24, 27, 31, 48]. Thereby, sophisticated volumetric imaging methods have demonstrated differences in the association of visceral and subcutaneous fat with an adverse metabolic risk profile in both sexes [50].

A novel insight in research, for the first time we have used a propensity score method to address selection biases in balancing the distribution of covariates between anthropometrically healthy subjects and MI cases [36]. It is well known in observational studies, treatment (or exposure) selection is often influenced by subject characteristics [51–53]. As a result, baseline characteristics of treated (or exposed) subjects often differ systematically from those of untreated (or unexposed) subjects. Therefore, one must account for systematic differences in baseline characteristics between treated and untreated (exposed or unexposed) subjects when estimating the effect of treatment (or exposure) on outcomes [53]. Based on our idea of how to reduce the effects of confounding in non-randomised anthropometric studies, we have applied the cited method. Thus, the conditional distribution of risk between groups (healthy and unhealthy cases) should be the same when observed baseline characteristics do not present standardised differences [37, 53]. Thereby, similar baseline characteristics for WHR and WC may provide bias in outcomes of both, if the risk assignment in both does not account for the covariates that predict the receiving true risk, WC as numerator and WHtR as measure volume, respectively. In this sense, as a result, risk assignment for WHR and WC may be systematically biased if values between WC, HC, height/2 and height show no balanced distribution and, therefore, the concerned metrics may not be directly comparable (see **Figure 3** and **Table 1**). Consequently, if the mathematical equivalence between covariates and propensity scores for metrics is not explored, it will be impossible to ensure a balanced distribution of risk between anthropometrics and groups. In agreement with the stratification method, all subjects who have (nearly) similar baseline characteristics and, therefore, similar propensity scores would have the same probability (nonzero) to receive a risk-code, making the risk assignment strongly ignorable [53]. Comparing the similarity of healthy and unhealthy cases in the same strata should begin with a comparison of the means or medians of the simple covariates and the distribution of their categorical counterparts between groups. If, after conditioning on the simple measurements, there remain systematic differences between means or medians, this would be an indication that the propensity score model has not been correctly specified for unbalancing the distribution of the measurements and the risk assignment. Thus, from our research, we have anthropometrically and mathematically demonstrated an association bias of WHR for unbalancing HC with respect to WC and height values in MI men [36, 37]. Besides, results from other larger studies [4–9, 14–22, 28–30, 32–35, 38–44] may be transferred to our analysis as appropriate. In revealing inequality between the simple measurements and risk cut-offs for metrics, our conclusions are not coincidental due to identifying biases and checking the lack of external validity. In brief, we have demonstrated association biases that are extendible to all previous studies and we have proposed the premises to avoid it.

6. Discussion

The anthropometric robustness of BMI and WHR as a link to the true risk of the BC and MI/CVD is unclear and diffuse. Conceptually, each of these provides its own meaning without a verifiable associated risk beyond that of WC. Nevertheless, only a rigorous interpretation removing bias could avoid confusing or paradoxical information, independently focused on the number of lifestyle factors and other established risk factors that influence ideal cardiovascular health [11].

It is well known that BMI has significant association with MI in both sexes, but not the best, and unimportant differences were found when compared by sex [4, 17–19, 21]. From the UK Biobank results, the ratio of women-to-men's hazard ratios for incident MI for the comparison between BMI and WC demonstrated a higher hazard ratio of association for WC in women, and no difference in men. Only WC and WHR, but not BMI and WHtR, were significantly associated with the risk of MI in women compared to men. Moreover, measures of central adiposity, particularly WHR as compared to BMI, showed a higher hazard ratio in women than in men [21]. However, when exploring the association between anthropometrics and obesity, novel findings have explained the reasons why both BMI and WHR are not optimal indicators in predicting MI risk, at least in men [23, 24, 27]. Thereby, it can be reasonably assumed that, since the musculoskeletal component may be artificially or indirectly associated to MI, BMI fails to reveal the true high risk BC by underestimating visceral fat volume and overestimating risk from the mesomorphy component. Thus, in two individuals with mesomorphy dominant and different high risk BC, the same BMI would underestimate the higher body fat volume in one of them. This observation means that BMI has the importance of producing a greater impact and bias in men due to it capturing a dimension of spurious risk beyond that of women. On this basis, from the UK Biobank, the comparison between BMI and WC by sex presented bias. This is because both metrics cannot refer to the same high risk BC when comparing men and women, and WC without accounting for the whole-risk (a 1-SD WHtR was >0.5 and < 1 in both sexes) [21, 37].

To our knowledge, body weight and HC have showed low predictive ability for MI and never justifying true biological plausibility for the risk. On the other hand, height and ectomorphy has been inversely associated to MI with a higher relative risk, although not necessarily referring to a causal relationship [10, 23, 24, 31, 48]. It is clear then that WC would be the only one among the simple measurements for reflecting both the cardiometabolic risk and the highest association discriminative for MI in both sexes [4, 7, 9, 12–21, 23, 24]. Besides, as %BF increases in vivo, the body fat storage is homogeneously distributed and WC, rather than BMI, becomes the best clinical expression of a body fat volume increase. Nevertheless, compound indexes such as WHR, conicity and WHtR have always captured a higher dimension of risk [4, 7, 9, 12, 16–19, 21, 23, 24, 27].

Surprisingly, most studies predicting MI/CVD risk always used a WHR cut-off <1 and/0r WHR/WHtR <2 in both sexes and different ethnicities while selection biases were never discussed [4, 5, 7, 13, 15, 17–19, 21, 28–30, 32, 35, 38–44, 54]. Why, when WHR <1, has the causal relationship between HC and adverse MI/CVD outcomes not clearly been elucidated? From the INTERHEART study [4], the median WHR in the overall population was 0.93 in cases and 0.91 in controls with a significant difference between both values, and therefore for the X distance, so the risk comparison was done without balancing between HC and WC. Besides, WC was obtained at the narrowest point (the longest X distance), and WHtR as entity of risk was not explored. On the other hand, the follow-up in the CONOR study [17] found, for WHR and WC, an association stronger in women and middle-aged than in men and elderly participants, respectively. However, the higher value of X for middle-aged (X = 21) and elderly women (X = 18) with respect to male counterparts (X = 11 and 8, respectively) was not kept in mind, and therefore, biases occurred with respect to WC and X in the risk comparison for unbalancing the mean HC and WC. Additionally, WC would appear to be found with classification bias for the risk in women compared to men if height was not accounted for in the data analysis and WHtR as an entity of risk was not well compared. Similarly, from the UK Biobank study [21], a 1-SD WHR was significantly associated with a higher hazard ratio of MI in women than in men, and with a corresponding women-to-men ratio of hazard ratios of 1.15. Nevertheless, the mean (SD) of WHR was <1 in both sexes (0.82: X = 18 in women, 0.93: X = 7 in men), so the false premise accepted in the risk assignment up to 0.999 value provided a selection bias for WHR when compared to WC or X. Thereby, having a baseline characteristic of WHR <1 either in healthy population or in cases, a different high risk BC as measured by WC and X will provide a higher WHR-associated risk due to the protective overestimation for HC where equal numbers of WHR <1 predict false-positives when accounting for an imbalance of the mean HC and WC or X. Besides, in data distribution and hazard ratios, WHR in the top was always <1 when WHtR in the bottom was >0.45–0.5 and < 1 in both sexes (WHR/WHtR <2), so the risk comparison between both indices was biased and demonstrated a protective overestimation for HC concerning height. Additionally, the strength of association for WC was significantly higher in women than in men while the hazard ratio for WHtR was similar in both sexes (1.34 in women, 1.33 in men). By deduction, height differences were higher in men than in women in occurring similar risk assignments for WC and WHtR in women (hazard ratio of 1.35 and 1.34, respectively), but not in men (hazard ratio of 1.28 and 1.33, respectively). This is because the mean WC and height demonstrated a different relationship, and WC and WHtR was not compared for the same risk [37]. Indeed, the mean (SD) of WHtR at the baseline in women (0.52 ± 0.1) was closer to 0.5 than that of men (0.55 ± 0.1) [21]. This means that, in the stratum between 0.5 and 0.52, WC and WHtR captured a similar dimension of risk in women due to a lower probability of selecting false-positives, while in a higher range up to 0.55, only WHtR captured the highest risk, as it happened in men. Thereby, height differences between women and men involve less chance of bias for WC in women when compared to WHtR, and WHtR more accurately predicts risk in men than WC [21]. By contrast, in the follow up of a Swedish cohort, WC presented less statistical significance for a recurrent MI in the female group [38]. However, the risk the WHtR measured was not explored and, therefore the risk comparison between sexes could not be referred to the same high risk BC and relative volume.

On the other hand, since short-stature has been associated with MI, the WC associated risk that is geometrically-derived from a two-dimensional area will be overestimated in taller individuals with respect to shorter people, including sex differences. In contrast, WHtR has the importance of corresponding to a relative volume where intra-abdominal risk components occupy all the space except for small peripheral-subcutaneous area, which is less deleterious [24, 37, 46, 47]. Unequivocally, WHtR gives us a relative risk volume and the higher the WHtR, the higher the risk. Besides, WHtR yields no bias with respect to others and it may capture a dimension of risk above WC. Obviously, this only happens when WHtR risk cut-off moves too far towards an excess of 0.5, as proven in men [21, 23, 24, 27]. It is also anthropometrically and mathematically demonstrable in most studies (**Table 1**).

In another consideration, some studies have signed a trend towards higher risk of MI as HC decreased (narrow hip) in a relationship with sarcopenia and deficiencies in physical activity [4, 19]. However, despite different values of HC either in the UK, Sweden, Norway, Spain or even in infarcted populations worldwide, studies have always found a WHR risk cut-off <1 and HC never takes the same value as WC [4, 18–21, 23]. On the other hand, HC-adjusted WC has demonstrated the strongest association with coronary disease and cardiovascular mortality [41–44, 53]. Nevertheless, by entering both WC and HC as independent markers of future CVD risk, the causal association for HC-adjusted WC in analytic models also appears to be wrong due to selection bias for the risk. The key lies in the discriminatory risk cut-offs for WC and HC, which reflect different sensitivity and specificity as well as different coherence and biological plausibility from each one. When using HC-adjusted WC, whether considering HC as a protective factor in a WHR risk cut-off of <1 (mean

HC > WC: X > 0) [39–42, 53], this argument becomes a false premise, because we will always find points of spurious risk in any WHR-associated risk above the WC, and therefore draw false conclusions for causation. It would occur even when X values are 0.1: WHR =0.999 (**Figures 1** and **3**). Hence, anthropometric risk evaluation is not subsumable by combining WC and HC data at the same level of equality (WC = HC instead of HC = WC + X), either for WHR <1 or HC-adjusted WC. That way, the paired comparison of two different biological factors would adulterate the associated joint risk and the real effect of HC, which takes a protective role falsely assigned. Then (and only then), when WC takes the same value as HC (risk equivalence) there will be the same (x, y) coordinates in the shared point where WC = HC: WHR = 1: X = 0, and, therefore, the same estimation of risk for WC and HC (**Figure 1**). In the same way, noting that anthropometrically healthy women significantly present lower WHR than men (higher X distance), a higher bias for WHR in predicting MI/CVD risk in women may be explained due to a higher selection of abstract fractions and spurious risk points where HC does not account for the same estimation of risk as WC. Similarly, higher bias would occur when the WC is taken at the minimum perimeter (both sexes), due to a higher X length (**Figure 1**). In this approach, the higher X value, the higher bias may occur. Thus, a higher HC in middle-aged people, physically active subjects or in women with higher gluteal–femoral fat deposits never justify a protective effect that influence MI/CVD, at least anthropometrically and while balancing the mean values of WC, HC, and X in any correct comparison between healthy and unhealthy cases including sex differences.

To our knowledge, using stratification for matching the selection bias of WHR has been demonstrated in men. This was because the same WHR risk-code (yes) on the same matched fractions between 0.95 and 0.999 always found different risk-codes for WC (yes/not) when conditioned on both WC < HC and WC receiving a true risk above their risk cut-off [36, 37].

In agreement with our observations, the strata between the WHR risk cut-off and 0.999 on the one hand, and from 0.51 up to any other WHtR risk cut-off of >0.5 on the other hand, usually coincide on the overlapping areas of the distributions for WHR and WHtR between healthy populations and MI/CVD cases. Thus, for the same binary code of no risk (true-negatives) between 0.51 and any other WHtR risk cut-off of >0.5, we could find the same WHtR value for different fractions from WC and height. However, WC might produce false-positives above their own risk cut-off if conditioned on WC > height/2 and WHtR received no risk (bias zone for WC as explained above). When unbalancing HC vs. WC and height mean values, or the mean WC vs. height/2 false-positive points for WHR and WC, respectively, might be selected for biasing any associated risk above WHtR. Besides, evidence states that, in any study population, HC and height/2 always present different mean values (HC > height/2: WHR/WHtR <2), so a risk assignment for WHR and WHtR always shows an imbalance for overestimating the protective effect of HC with respect to height, and therefore, comparing different risk [4–10, 14–30, 32–35, 38–40], (**Table 1**).

From a syllogistic approach, whether in any study population WHR (risk cut-off <1) shows a higher magnitude of association than WC (the first false major premise for a causal risk), while the mean HC is higher than WC (the second true minor premise), any WHR-associated risk above WC will occur for unbalancing the distribution of WC and HC as covariates. This fact determines false risk assignment for WHR (association bias) with respect to WC, which induces a false inference as the conclusion for causation. In no case WHR <1 would risk be captured above the WC because HC > WC is a natural inequality associated with a healthy population.

Similarly, a WHtR risk cut-off >0.5 occurs, the WC shows higher magnitude of association than WHtR (the first false major premise for a causal risk) and when the mean WC > height/2 (the second true minor premise), any WC-associated risk beyond that of WHtR will occur for unbalancing the distribution of WC and height/2 as covariates. Thus, WC that captures a false risk (association bias) with respect to WHtR would induce a false inference as the conclusion for causation. In no case can WC alone capture the risk above WHtR because WC < height/2 is a natural inequality associated with an anthropometrically healthy population, and only up to a WHtR risk cut-off =0.5 (mean WC = height/2) would WC and WHtR capture the same risk. With the same premise, if any WHR risk cut-off is lower than that of WHtR × 2, and being the mean HC > height/2, any WHR-associated risk beyond that of the WHtR will occur for unbalancing the distribution of HC and height/2 as covariates, but WHR never captures the risk above WHtR. To clarify this, apply the results of the studies referenced in **Table 1** on **Figure 3** and once the simple measurements and their mathematical inequalities in the standard human body are well known, see **Figure 1**).

As a philosophically and anthropometrically correct reflection, not all subjects are at risk as according to their WHR measurement, and with similar baseline characteristics between their risk cut-off of <1 and 0.999 or twice the WHtR value that refer to the same risk as measured from WC or WHtR risk cut-off, respectively (bias zone for WHR). Similarly, not all subjects at risk according to their WC measurement, and with similar baseline characteristics for WC alone above their risk cut-off refer to the same risk as measured from WHtR between 0.51 and any other real risk cut-off >0.5 (bias zone for WC), (**Figure 3**).

Epidemiologically, while a shorter stature may be significantly associated to cases of MI/CVD (WHtR risk cut-off >0.5) and the mean values of HC higher than both WC and height/2 (WHR <1: WHR/WHtR <2: HC > WC > height/2, see **Table 1**), WHtR will always capture the highest dimension of risk above WC and WHR. This is because WHtR as a three-dimensional volume measure would always capture higher a biological risk than WC as a two-dimensional area. Similarly, when balanced distribution between the simple measurements may be checked and the risk may be conditioned on the real predictive variables (WC or WHtR >0.5 as appropriate) [36, 37], WHtR becomes the gold standard for risk assessment. It is geometrically clear. The same values of risk for WC between different individuals refer to a similar risk from WHtR as relative volume if the mean WC is ≤height/2 (WHtR ≤0.5 and unimportant differences for height), but never occur when individuals present a mean WHtR of >0.5 (significant differences for height). Thus, WHtR should be used as the optimal metric when making an anthropometrically and mathematically correct risk prediction, irrespective of the strength of association for other metrics in different studies. In such studies, a spurious risk might be artificially slanted towards the group of cases in the rest of compared metrics when specifically defined or universally categorised risk cut-offs were used [4–10, 14–30, 32–35, 38–44, 49, 54, 55].

Our demonstrations are a touchstone on the risk associated with WHR and WC from many studies, so universal recommendations made on the issues relating to WHR and WC alone for determining abdominal obesity and substantially increased risk of metabolic complications may turn out to be fallacious or at least have information bias [13, 14, 56]. Validity for both WHR and WC depends on the degree for measuring the risk. However, when having a WHR risk cut-off <1 as an abstract fraction or WC alone as a two-dimensional area, it will be impossible to discriminate the risk and relative volume, unlike WHtR, which is a more faithful measure. Thus, a true description of risk for WHR <1 requires of a categorical syllogism, where the risk derives from an affirmative proposition for the WC value as a numerator. On the other hand, any association of risk for WC alone above WHtR will be a false conclusion, if the WHtR risk cut-off is of >0.5 and < 1. Since a part of the assigned risk for WHR and WC may be spurious, the conclusion for the risk will be in error due to a fallacious argument. Similarly, the assumption of risk for categorised risk cut-offs for overweight/obesity when not measuring the true high risk BC nor abdominal obesity volume will be a misleading proposition, which will provide a false conclusion for the associated real risk, or at least provide a conclusion with paradoxical information and bias. Therefore, in any study population, the risk captured by each metric depends on itself, its sensitivity and specificity, consistency, coherence, plausibility and anthropometric validity, rather than on its strength of association with respect to others, at least while predicting risk with simple measurements, where mathematical relationships of inequality provide imbalance and biases for the causal risk association.

In summary, BMI and WC will never refer to the same risk and high risk BC. Regarding that insight, while technological methods are clinically impracticable, to predict MI/CVD risk, WC should be the anthropometric reference for assessing the true high risk BC and risk beyond that of BMI.

It is worthy to note that the universally categorised risk cut-offs for metrics such as overweight/obesity [2], WHR ≥0.90 in men and ≥ 0.85 in women (<1 in both) [14], WC >94 (102) in men and > 80 (88) in women [13, 14, 56], and WHtR >0.5 and < 1 in both sexes, may provide confounding and association biases for causal risk. This occurs when the mathematical relationships are unbalanced between the simple measurements of healthy and unhealthy cases, and a spurious risk assignment being slanted in direction to the group of cases in the confounding metrics. At the same time, in the overlapping areas of the confounding metrics, subjects with similar baseline values must present different risk assignments when conditional on both imbalances between simple measurements and the real predictive variables [37]. Thus, regardless of WC, HC and height should be controlled in data analyses to preclude a different–equal risk assignment between subjects who have equal–different high risk BC and risk. Accordingly, a higher strength of association for WHR or WC with respect to WHtR does not mean higher risk, but association biases where both the high risk BC and relative volume were not well compared. In other words, WHR-associated risk above WC and WC-associated risk beyond that of WHtR were always a bias error, which is evidence that posed issues for the cardiovascular sciences for a long time due to the research process itself. Thus, when ignoring biases in research, false inferences could be drawn to predict MI/CVD risk in both sexes. On the contrary, only WHtR-associated risk above WC and WHR will hold true. Thereby, by identifying and removing biases in research, WHtR will always provide equality and balance between healthy populations and MI/CVD cases to be used as an entity of risk, while also having the importance of being cheap, accessible and easy to measure. Therefore, an appropriate ethnically-based and sex-specific WHtR risk cut-off would be the easiest and most definitive anthropometric tool to meet the best epidemiological criteria for the judgement of causal associations and to identify individuals at risk of MI/CVD. Broadly, it would occur while the degree of adiposity/overweight/obesity still has the importance of accumulating a homogenously distributed body fat volume. A continuous process of accumulating body fat over time provides changes in body shape and a higher degree of adiposity, even with fat flaps that would involve a higher risk and volume excess non-homogeneously distributed and, therefore, non-fully measurable from WC and height. In any case, a high degree of fatness will always keep a high correlation with WHtR, %BF and components of risk of the somatotype [10, 24, 27, 31, 45, 48].

Lastly, after reviewing thousands of cases of MI/CVD, our findings have both internal and external validity, and therefore, they determine the generalisability to any ethnically-based or sex-specific population because they mathematically and epidemiologically satisfy our observations. On this issue, bias and causal associations in observational research must be well known [51–53], and overall, to avoid categorising as risk the value of each metric if their risk cut-off was not well verified and balanced with respect to others and specifically defined and checked in each study population. We also believe that an evolution of findings based on a balanced weighing of potentials for false-positive biases can produce scientific knowledge for the advancement of medical and cardiovascular sciences.

7. Conclusion

Association biases for anthropometrics in predicting MI/CVD risk in both sexes have been demonstrated in anthropometric and mathematical terms. Regardless of BMI, which demonstrates either paradoxical or non-optimal MI/CVD risk prediction in most studies, WHR-associated risk can lead to misleading evidence derived from a generalised mathematical misconception, which overestimates the protective effect of HC concerning WC and height. Until our discoveries by using matching in the overlapping zones between healthy population and cases, no other research has demonstrated biases by assigning spurious risk to true-negative values.

Epidemiologically, in the association of MI/CVD risk, WHR always appears to be a confounding variable with respect to WC and WHtR, due to differences in both the mean X value (HC–WC) and HC – height/2, respectively, either between groups or by sex. This is because there is always a WHR risk cut-off of <1 (mean HC > WC: natural inequality) and WHR/WHtR of <2 (mean HC > height/2: natural inequality). This, therefore, creates a protective overestimation for HC concerning WC and height. Similarly, WC may be a confounding variable with respect to WHtR due to differences for the mean WC and height/2, comparing either by group or by sex. This occurs if, and only if, the WHtR risk cut-off is >0.5 (mean WC > height/2), therefore creating an overestimation of risk for WC with respect to height in the tallest people and an underestimation of risk in the shortest, without accounting for a relative volume by unit of height.

Anthropometrically, the true risk exclusively derives from enlarged WC and abdominal obesity volume. However, accounting for body height as a volume modulator factor rends HC irrelevant or clinically useless, either in women or in men. Any association of MI/CVD causal risk for WHR beyond that of WC and WHtR becomes mathematically biased, anthropometrically inconsistent, biologically less plausible and epidemiologically false. WHtR as a proxy of adiposity and relative volume measure yields no bias and is biologically more plausible and consistent; it may capture a dimension of risk above WC as a two-dimensional transverse area. This only happens when height has an inverse association and the WHtR risk cut-off is >0.5. Thereby, in predicting MI/CVD risk, WHtR is the optimal anthropometric, rather than WC, WHR and BMI. Thus, quoting my own thinking: “Statistics confused medical science and cardiology, but mathematics does not fool the heart”. Hence, researchers have the responsibility to design and conduct studies in a way that makes them capable of balancing the simple body measurements, ratios, ratios of ratios and risk cut-offs, as well as the high risk BC and true risk when predicting anthropometrically-measured causal risk. Once the association biases for anthropometrics have been revealed, the worldwide focus of clinicians and scientists must shift.

8. Recommendation

After decades spent using anthropometrics in medical research and health sciences, our relevant and novel findings with Cartesian demonstrations should be extended to the broader scientific community for the knowledge gained regarding adiposity/overweight/obesity and CVD risk prediction. Many investigations continue to be conducted without consideration of biases, with some studies even spending public resources to obtain unclear or even false conclusions. It is time to avoid such biases in research, as well as in clinical practice.

On the issue relating to anthropometric measures and CVD causal risk, by using non-optimal metrics such as BMI and WHR or even WC alone, public health goals may be impacted by inaccuracies and biased information, especially when tackling prevention and control programmes and gauging CVD risk. It is important to ensure accuracy when measuring each anthropometric characteristic, as well as their relationship as a risk factor for CVD. Thus, monitoring ideal cardiovascular health by measuring body weight (in BMI) or HC (in WHR) will always be less accurate than using abdominal volume measure indirectly obtained from WC and height (in WHtR). Clinical and cardiological protocols should be changed because using misleading metrics will lead to the science remaining anchored in the past and without advancement in the application of the scientific knowledge.

Conflict of interest

The author declares no conflict of interest.

Author details

Angel Martin Castellanos[1,2]

1 Cardiovascular Sciences and Sports Medicine Center, Caceres, Spain

2 Faculty of Nursing and Occupational Therapy, Department of Anatomy, Research Group in Bio-Anthropology and Cardiovascular Sciences, University of Extremadura, Caceres, Spain

*Address all correspondence to: angelmartincastellanos@gmail.com

References

[1] World Health Organization (WHO). Cardiovascular Diseases (CVDS)-WHO/ World Health Organization. Available from: https://www.who.int/news-room/fact-sheets/detail/cardiovascular-diseases-(cvds). [Accessed: February 2022]

[2] World Health Organization (WHO). Obesity and Overweight-WHO/World Health Organization. Available from: https://www.who.int/news-room/fact-sheets/detail/obesity-and-overweight [Accessed: November 2021]

[3] Cornier MA, Després JP, Davis N, et al. Assessing adiposity: A scientific statement from the American Heart Association. Circulation. 2011;**124**(18):1996-2019

[4] Yusuf S, Hawken S, Ounpuu S, et al. Obesity and the risk of myocardial infarction in 27,000 participants from 52 countries: A case-control study. Lancet. 2005;**366**:1640-1649

[5] Gelber RP, Gaziano JM, Orav EJ, et al. Measures of obesity and cardiovascular risk among men and women. Journal of the American College of Cardiology. 2008;**52**(8):605-615. DOI: 10.1016/j.jacc.2008.03.066

[6] Zhu J, Su X, Li G, et al. The incidence of acute myocardial infarction in relation to overweight and obesity: A meta-analysis. Archives of Medical Science. 2014;**10**(5):855-862. DOI: 10.5114/aoms.2014.46206

[7] Gruson E, Montaye M, Kee F, et al. Anthropometric assessment of abdominal obesity and coronary heart disease risk in men: The PRIME study. Heart. 2010;**96**(2):136-140. DOI: 10.1136/hr.2009.171447

[8] Lassale C, Tzoulaki I, Moons KGM, et al. Separate and combined associations of obesity and metabolic health with coronary heart disease: A pan-European case-cohort analysis. European Heart Journal. 2018;**39**(5):397-406. DOI: Doi.10.1093/eurheartj/ehx448

[9] Choi D, Choi S, Son JS, et al. Impact of discrepancies in general and abdominal obesity on major adverse cardiac events. Journal of the American Heart Association. 2019;**8**(18):e013471. DOI 10.1161/JAHA.119.013471

[10] Martín-Castellanos A, Cabañas MD, Martín P, Barca FJ. The body composition in myocardial infarction males. Novel findings in both the association and relationship between anthropometric indicators of risk. JONNPR. 2017;**2**(9): 388-398. DOI: 10.19230/jonnpr.1547

[11] Lloyd-Jones DM, Hong J, Labarthe D, et al. Defining and setting National Goals for Cardiovascular Health Promotion and Disease Reduction: The American Heart Association's strategic impact Goal through 2020 and beyond. Circulation. 2010;**121**:586-613. DOI: 10.1161/CIRCULATIONAHA.109.192703

[12] Fang N, Jiang M, Fan Y. Ideal cardiovascular health metrics and risk of cardiovascular disease or mortality: A meta-analysis. International Journal of Cardiology. 2016;**214**:279-283. DOI: 10.1016/j.ijcard.201603.210

[13] Alberti KG, Eckel RH, Grundy SM, et al. Harmonizing the metabolic syndrome: A joint interim statement of the International Diabetes Federation Task Force on Epidemiology and Prevention; National Heart, Lung, and Blood Institute; American Heart Association; World Heart Federation;

International Atherosclerosis Society; and International Association for the Study of Obesity. Circulation. 2009;**120**(16):1640-1645

[14] World Health Organization. Waist Circumference and Waist-Hip Ratio: Report of a WHO Expert Consultation, Geneva, 8-11 December 2008. World Health Organization 2011. Available from: http://www.who.int/iris/handle/10665/44583 [Accessed: November 2021]

[15] Ladeiras-Lopes R, Sampaio F, Bettencourt N, et al. The ratio between visceral and subcutaneous abdominal fat assessed by computed tomography is an independent predictor of mortality and cardiac events. Review in Espanola Cardiology (Engl Ed). 2017;**70**(5):331-337

[16] Chen Y, Jiang J, Shi J, et al. Association of visceral fat index and percentage body fat and anthropometric measures with myocardial infarction and stroke. Journal of Hypertension. 2016;**5**:235

[17] Brown JC, Harhay MO, Harhay MN. Anthropometrically-predicted visceral adipose tissue and mortality among men and women in the third national health and nutrition examination survey (NHANES III). American Journal of Human Biology. 2017;**29**:e22898. DOI: 10.1002/ajhb.22898

[18] Egeland GM, Igland J, Vollset SE, et al. High population attributable fractions of myocardial infarction associated with waist-hip ratio. Obesity. 2016;**24**(5):1162-1169

[19] Nilson G, Hedberg P, Leppert J, et al. Basic anthropometric measures in acute myocardial infarction patients and individually sex- and age-matched controls from the general population. Journal of Obesity. 2018;**2018**:3839482. DOI: 10.1155/2018/3839482

[20] Cao Q, Yu S, Xiong W, et al. Waist-hip ratio as a predictor of myocardial infarction risk. A systematic review and meta-analysis. Medicine. 2018;**27-30**:e11639. DOI: doi.org/10.1097/MD.0000000000011639

[21] Peters SAE, Bots SH, Woodward M. Sex differences in the association between measures of general and central adiposity and the risk of myocardial infarction: Results from the UK Biobank. Journal of the American Heart Association. 2018;**7**(5):e008507. DOI: 10.1161/JAHA.117.008507

[22] Nicklas BJ, Penninx BH, Cesari M, et al. Association of visceral adipose tissue with incident myocardial infarction in older men and women the health, aging and body composition study. American Journal of Epidemiology. 2004;**160**:741-749. DOI: 10.1093/aje/kwh281

[23] Martín-Castellanos A, Cabañas-Armesilla MD, Barca-Durán FJ, et al. Obesity and risk of myocardial infarction in a sample of european males. Waist to-hip-ratio presents information bias of the real risk of abdominal obesity. Nutrición Hospitalaria. 2017;**34**(1):88-95. DOI: doi.org/10.20960/nh.982

[24] Martin-Castellanos A, Cabañas MD, Martín-Castellanos P, et al. The body composition and risk prediction in myocardial infarction men. Revealing biological and statistical error bias for both general obesity and waist-to-hip ratio. Cardiac Research Medical. 2018;**2**:13-20

[25] Song X, Jousilahti P, Stehouwer CD, et al. Comparison of various surrogate obesity indicators as predictors of cardiovascular mortality in four

European populations. European Journal of Clinical Nutrition. 2013;**67**(12):1298-1302. DOI: 10.1038/ejcn.2013.203

[26] Rost S, Freuer D, Peters A, et al. New indexes of body fat distribution and sex-specific risk of total and cause-specific mortality: A prospective cohort study. BMC Public Health. 2018;**18**(1):427. DOI: 10.1186/s12889-018-5350-8

[27] Martin-Castellanos A, Martin-Castellanos P, Cabañas MD, et al. Adiposity-associated anthropometric indicators and myocardial infarction risk: Keys for waist to-height-ratio as metric in cardiometabolic health. AJFNH. 2018;**3**(5):100-107

[28] Guasch-Ferré M, Bulló M, Martínez-González MA, et al. Waist-to-height ratio and cardiovascular risk factors in elderly individuals at high cardiovascular risk. PLoS One. 2012;**7**(8):e43275. DOI: 10.1371/journal.pone.0043275

[29] Howell CR, Mehta T, Ejima K, et al. Body composition and mortality in Mexican American Adults: Results from the National Health and Nutrition Examination Survey. Obesity (Silver Spring). 2018;**8**:1372-1380. DOI: 10.1002/oby.22251

[30] Liu J, Tse LA, Liu Z, et al. PURE (Prospective Urban Rural Epidemiology) study in China. Predictive Values of Anthropometric Measurements for Cardiometabolic Risk Factors and Cardiovascular Diseases Among 44 048 Chinese. Journal of the American Heart Association. 2019;**8**:e010870

[31] Martín-Castellanos A. Anthropometric profile, body composition and somatotype study in patients with Acute Coronary Syndrome of the Health Area of Caceres [PhD thesis], Complutense University, Madrid, Spain; 2014.

[32] Gavriilidou NN, Pihlsgard M, Elmstahl S. Anthropometric reference data for elderly Swedes and its disease related pattern. European Journal of Clinical Nutrition. 2015;**69**(9):1066-1075

[33] Lee HW, Hong TJ, Hong JY, et al. Waist-hip ratio and 1-year clinical outcome in patients with non-ST-elevation myocardial infarctions. Coronary Artery Disease. 2016;**27**(5):357-364. DOI: 10.1097/MCA.0000000000000369

[34] Medina-Inojosa JR, Batsis JA, Supervia M, et al. Relation of waist-hip ratio to long-term cardiovascular events in patients with coronary artery disease. The American Journal of Cardiology. 2018;**121**(8):903-909. DOI: 10.1016/j.amjcard.2017.12.038

[35] Dhar S, Das PK, Bhattacharjee B, et al. Predictive value of waist height ratio, waist hip ratio and body mass index in assessing angiographic severity of coronary artery disease in myocardial infarction patients. Mymensingh Medical Journal. 2020;**29**(4):906-913

[36] Martin-Castellanos A, Martin-Castellanos P, Martin E, et al. Abdominal obesity and myocardial infarction risk: We demonstrate the anthropometric and mathematical reasons that justify the association bias of waist-to-hip ratio. Nutrición Hospitalaria. 2021

[37] Castellanos AM. Anthropometric measures in predicting myocardial infarction risk. Do we know what we are measuring? Bias in research occurred worldwide when the true unhealthy body composition was not well compared. MRA. 2021;**9**(6):1-19

[38] Campos-Staffico A, Almeida M, Figueiredo V, et al. Anthropometric features and myocardial infarction

in very elderly people. BBA Clinical. 2015;**3**(S):S3

[39] Nalini M, Sharafkhah M, Poustchi H, et al. Comparing anthropometric indicators of visceral and general adiposity as determinants of overall and cardiovascular mortality. Archives of Iranian Medicine. 2019;**22**(6):301-309

[40] Mohammadi H, Ohm J, Discacciati A, et al. Abdominal obesity and the risk of recurrent atherosclerotic cardiovascular disease after myocardial infarction. European Journal of Preventive Cardiology. 2020;**27**(18):1944-1952. DOI: 10.1177/2047487319898019

[41] Canoy D, Boekholdt SM, Wareham N, et al. Body fat distribution and risk of coronary heart disease in men and women in the European Prospective Investigation Into Cancer and Nutrition in Norfolk cohort: A population-based prospective study. Circulation. 2007;**116**(25):2933-2943

[42] Cameron AJ, Magliano DJ, Söderberg S. A systematic review of the impact of including both waist and hip circumference in risk models for cardiovascular diseases, diabetes and mortality. Obesity Reviews. 2013;**14**(1):86-94

[43] Carmienke S, Freitag MH, Pischon T, et al. General and abdominal obesity parameters and their combination in relation to mortality: A systematic review and meta-regression analysis. European Journal of Clinical Nutrition. 2013;**67**(6):573-585. DOI: 10.1038/ejcn.2013.61

[44] Cameron AJ, Magliano DJ, Shaw JE, et al. The influence of hip circumference on the relationship between abdominal obesity and mortality. International Journal of Epidemiology. 2012;**41**(2):484-494. DOI: 10.1093/ije/dyr198

[45] Woolcott OO, Bergman RN. Relative fat mass (RFM) as a new estimator of whole-body fat percentage—A cross sectional study in American adult individuals. ScientificReports. 2018;**8**(1):10980. DOI: 10.1038/s41598-018-29362-1

[46] Tchernof A, Despres JP. Pathophysiology of human visceral obesity: An update. Physiological Reviews. 2013;**93**:359-404

[47] Gruzdeva O, Borodkina D, Uchasova E, et al. Localization of fat depots and cardiovascular risk. Lipids in Health and Disease. 2018;**17**(1):218

[48] Williams SR, Jones E, Bell W, et al. Body habitus and coronary heart disease in men. A review with reference to methods of body habitus assessment. European Heart Journal. 1997;**18**:376-393

[49] Banerjee S, Kumar P, Srivastava S, et al. Association of anthropometric measures of obesity and physical activity with cardio-vascular diseases among older adults: Evidence from a cross-sectional survey, 2017-18. PLoS One. 2021;**16**(12):e0260148. DOI: 10.1371/journal.pone.0260148

[50] Fox CS, Massaro JM, Hoffmann U, et al. Abdominal visceral and subcutaneous adipose tissue compartments: Association with metabolic risk factors in the Framingham Heart Study. Circulation. 2007;**116**(1):39-48

[51] Grimes DA, Schulz KF. Epidemiology series. Bias and causal associations in observational research. The Lancet. 2002;**359**:248-252

[52] Panucci CJ, Wilkins EG. Identifying and avoinding bias in research.

Plastic and Reconstructive Surgery. 2010;**126**(2):619-625

[53] Austin PC. An introduction to propensity score methods for reducing the effects of confounding in observational studies. Multivariate Behavioral Research. 2011;**46**:399-424. DOI: 10.1080/00273171.2011.568786

[54] Streng KW, Voors AA, Hillege HL, et al. Waist-to-hip ratio and mortality in heart failure. European Journal of Heart Failure. 2018;**20**(9):1269-1277. DOI 10.1002/ejhf.1244

[55] Hassan S, Oladele C, Galusha D, et al. Anthropometric measures of obesity and associated cardiovascular disease risk in the Eastern Caribbean Health Outcomes Research Network (ECHORN) Cohort Study. BMC Public Health. 2021;**21**(1):399. DOI: 10.1186/s12889-021-10399-3

[56] National Cholesterol Education Program (NCEP). Executive Summary of the Third Report of the National Cholesterol Education Program. Expert Panel on Detection, Evaluation, and Treatment of High Blood Cholesterol in Adults (Adult Treatment Panel III). Expert Panel on detection, evaluation, and treatment of high blood cholesterol in adults (adult treatment panel III) final report. Circulation. 2002;**106**:3143-3421

Chapter 17

Predicting Risk of Emerging Cardiotoxicity

Megan Goins, Katie Lovell, Greyson Keel, Julia Cook and Robert Lust

Abstract

Smoking, hypercholesterolemia, hyperlipidemia, obesity, diabetes, insulin resistance and family history all are well established general risk factors broadly associated with injury in the cardiovascular system. Similarly, echocardiography, electrocardiography, MRI, PET scans and circulating biomarkers like cardiac Troponin (cTn) provide indications that injury has occurred. Traditionally, cardiovascular injury has been attributed to conditions that exacerbate the potential for ischemia, either by producing excessive metabolic/work demands or by impairing the perfusion necessary to support the metabolic/work demands. This review summarizes additional factors that are underappreciated in contributing to the risk of injury, such as iatrogenic injury secondary to treatment for other conditions, infection, environmental exposures, and autoimmune processes.

Keywords: cardiovascular, cardiac, heart, myocardial, vascular, endothelium, COVID-19, auto-immunity, autoantibody, anthracycline, diabetes, mitochondria, air pollution, nanomaterials, nanoparticles

1. Introduction

The risk factors generally associated with risk for atherosclerotic cardiovascular disease include age, sex, race, systolic and diastolic blood pressure, total, Total cholesterol, high/low density lipoprotein (HDL and LDL) fractions, overweight and obesity, and history of diabetes or smoking [1, 2]. Evidence-based treatment guidelines based on these factors have been established [1]. Apps/tools for use by the general population to predict risk of a cardiovascular event have been published both by the American Heart Association [3], and by the American College of Cardiology [4]. The gold standard for establishing injury is typically direct histologic evidence of injury, which increasingly have become well correlated with surrogate markers such as circulating cardiac troponin (CTnT or cTnI) levels or natriuretic peptide levels (ANP or BNP).

The purpose of this chapter is to highlight potential areas of emerging concern that are not yet established as directly causing increased risk of cardiovascular disease. They may be iatrogenic toxicity effects associated with treatment for non-cardiovascular diseases and therefore no considered a general risk overall [5–7]. They may be effects that alter the progression of an established risk factor, they may be factors that have only recently been considered, or that may not alter the risk of acquiring cardiovascular disease at all but may alter the severity and subsequent mortality of a cardiovascular event, were it to occur secondary to any of the established risk factors. Contributing elements might be disruption of mitochondrial function [8–11], or infectious disease [12–21]. Chronic diseases that have strong systemic inflammatory components such as Systemic Lupus Erythmatosis (SLE) [22–25] or asthma [26–28] may or may not alter the incidence of chronic CVD but may be associated with increased risk of acute events, or may modify the outcome from reperfusion therapies, especially those already known to be complicated by a major inflammatory component [29–32].

In addition, as large-scale health system databases become increasing robust and geo-mapping of environmental influences is increasingly refined, associations between air quality CVD outcomes can now be interrogated with much higher fidelity than before, and what had been experimental and/or local phenomenological observations are becoming increasingly more widely appreciated [33, 34]. Findings previously associated only with air pollution are becoming more generalized to other environmental influences as well [35].

Finally, emerging from across the spectrum of systemic challenges and with wide-ranging targets, the potential role of auto-immune responses as an aggravating risk factor that is becoming increasingly appreciated will be discussed [36–39].

2. Anti-neoplastic agent cardiotoxicity

2.1 Anthracyclines

Cardiovascular risk can be attributed to those things that directly damage the myocyte, those things that increase the likelihood of damage to the myocyte, or those things that impair the recovery following injury to the myocyte. Anthracyclines are effective anti-neoplastic agents, but with efficacy limited by cardiotoxic side effects. Clinically, there are specific guidelines based on serial cTnT levels to monitor of cardiotoxic effects, and experimentally, the cardiotoxicity is well-established enough that doxorubicin, a common anthracycline, is one of the most commonly used approaches to induce experimental heart failure independent of any neoplasm [40]. Anthracyclines cause a type I cardiotoxicity that is dose-limiting, often irreversible, and produces changes demonstrated on biopsy. While previous treatment for cancer is not considered a general cardiovascular risk factor per se, it is clear that at least some cancer therapeutics can produce persistent cardiac effects, and understanding those mechanism provides a great deal of insight regarding underlying mechanisms involved in increasing cardiovascular risk. This is particularly important when anthracyclines were used, but no overt toxicity was noted, which is to say only that ejection fraction, or CTnT NP remained within acceptable limits. It is worth reviewing the many ways that anthracyclines can induce injury so as to better appreciate how a sub-clinical event might have go undetected at the time, but could none-the-less create a vulnerable substrate for injury later.

Doxorubicin is toxic, in itself, and approximately half of the doxorubicin administered into the body is eliminated unchanged. However, the metabolized doxorubicin creates secondary effects/products that are at least as toxic as the parent compound.

Metabolism of doxorubicin occurs in one of three ways: two-electron reduction, one-electron reduction, and deglycosylation [5, 41, 42].

Two-electron reduction is the primary metabolic pathway for doxorubin and results in the formation of active secondary alcohol metabolites. The alcohol metabolites that are produced cause cardiotoxic side effects by disrupting intracellular and especially intramitochondrial calcium and iron homeostasis. Doxorubincinol, a secondary alcohol metabolite of doxorubicin, interacts with aconitase/iron regulatory protein 1 (IRP-1) and converts it to a "null protein". Normally, when iron levels are adequate, aconitase acts within the Krebs cycle to convert citrate to isocitrate. When iron levels are low, this enzyme does not contain a [4Fe-4S] cluster and will act as IRP-1, which has RNA-binding activity. IRP-1 helps to regulate the expression of genes involved in iron metabolism and homeostasis [5, 41, 42].

Doxorubicinol also is an inhibitor of a number of ATPases, including the mitochondria's proton pump and those which regulate intracellular calcium levels, which not only leads to inhibition of cellular oxidative phosphorylation and bioenergetic collapse, but also disrupts calcium homeostasis leading to intracellular calcium overload disruption of excitation-contraction coupling [5, 41, 42]. Anthracyclines, particularly doxorubicin, also increase activity of calpain and may suppress sarcomere protein synthesis via signaling pathways and transcription factors, such as GATA4 [5, 41, 42]. Increased Calpain activity likely is secondary to an increase in intracellular calcium. This increase in activity increases degradation of titin, a major myofilament of sarcomere, which further leads to an impaired diastolic relaxation. Calpain dysregulation is also known to activate caspase-12, which can cause apoptosis. Caspase-12 is localized in the endoplasmic reticulum and is often activated by ER stress [43].

Anthracycline alcohol metabolites also interfere with the activity of iron sequestering proteins which leads to an increase in intracellular free iron. Anthracyclines have a high affinity for ferric iron, forming a free radical that is capable of reducing oxygen [44]. This is one mechanism by which anthracyclines are capable of participating in "redox cycling". Doxorubicin also contributes to the generation of ROS by inactivating the cellular defense enzymes glutathione peroxidase (GPx) and superoxide dismutase (SOD) [5, 41, 42], essential enzymes critical to managing mitochondrial membrane potential.

In one-electron reduction metabolic pathway, doxorubicin's adverse effects are due to redox cycling. The quinone moiety accepts an electron from NADH or NADPH via the use of endothelial nitric oxide synthase (eNOS), leading to the formation of a semiquinone free radical. This free radical reduces oxygen and forms a superoxide radical. This contributes to the increase in ROS observed in cardiomyocytes after doxorubicin exposure [5, 41, 42]. Further, doxorubicin's interaction with eNOS shuttles the enzyme from a NO-producing enzyme to a superoxide-producing enzyme. This could contribute to an impaired cardioprotective mechanism. This "uncoupling of eNOS" has already been shown to be a contributor in heart failure [6].

The deglycosylation pathway is thought to be a less important contributor to anthracycline metabolism, but it creates a lipophilic molecule that has greater accumulation in the mitochondrial membrane than unmetabolized doxorubicin [5, 41, 42], and by interfering with such mitochondrial membrane proteins as cardiolipin, can also disrupt mitochondrial function, which can trigger any number of secondary effects, including energy depletion, ROS generation and DNA damage, as well as apoptosis [7–11].

Topoisomerase IIB is found in all quiescent cells, including cardiomyocytes. Anthracyclines inhibit this enzyme, leading to unrepaired ROS induced double-stranded breaks, DNA damage and transcriptome changes in tissue with little regenerative capability [5, 41, 42]. It was demonstrated that mice with cardiomyocyte specific Top2b deletion were protected from the progressive heart failure effects of doxorubicin [45], clearly suggesting that the inhibition of topoisomerase IIB plays a major role in the cardiotoxicity induced by doxorubicin.

Stress to the heart generally shifts metabolic energy production away from the preferred free fatty acid substrate to one that is glucose based and more prone to lactate production. Typically, those shifts are driven by limitations in perfusion and access to sufficient oxygen to support electron transport chains. The same is true for anthracyclines, except that anthracyclines also directly disrupt multiple aspects of mitochondrial function. Doxorubicin causes p53 activation via its inhibition on topoisomerase IIB, leading to repression of PPARg co-activator alpha and beta, which normally promote mitochondrial biogenesis. Their signaling inhibition leads to aging and heart failure. Thus, doxorubicin's inhibition of topoisomerase IIB leads to a mitochondrial dysfunction that that is known to contribute to development of heart failure in doxorubicin-treated patients [46] and in other models of heart failure as well [7–11].

It has also been suggested that anthracycline-induced cardiotoxicity is partially due to the action of matrix metalloproteinases (MMP's). MMP-2 is highly abundant in cardiac myocytes and increased plasma levels have been observed following heart failure. It is possible that doxorubicin increases the concentration of MMP-2 in cardiac cells. Activation of MMP-2 by doxorubicin has been shown to play a role in the degradation of titin, further suggesting that this mechanism plays a role in sarcomere disruption and cardiac remodeling involved with doxorubicin-induced cardiomyopathy [47]. MMPs play an active role in regulating fibrosis in the heart and dysregulation can lead to disruption of the extracellular matrix, adverse remodeling and impaired relaxation.

Doxorubicin can have genomic effects as well. GATA4 is a zinc finger transcription factor that regulates multiple genes, including anti-apoptotic gene Bcl-x. GATA4 is not only involved in sarcomere integrity, but is also an essential survival factor in cardiomyocytes and has been shown to rapidly deplete after doxorubicin exposure. GATA4 depletion leads to cardiomyocyte apoptosis and is essential for adaptive stress response in the adult heart [48] and decreased GATA4 can occur secondary to p53 accumulation caused by doxorubicin exposure [49]. A GATA motif also was identified in an angiotensin II receptor (ATII-R). When stimulated, this receptor helps regulate the hypertrophic response to pressure overload. Mutations introduced into this binding site eliminated this response, demonstrating a role for GATA4 in the regulation of cardiac hypertrophic response [43].

Doxorubicin has a high affinity for the phospholipid cardiolipin. Cardiolipin is a mitochondrial membrane protein involved in many cellular mechanisms, including mitochondrial cristae morphology, electron transport chain function, steroid synthesis, mitophagy, and apoptosis. Cardiolipin turns over at a slower rate than other phospholipids of the mitochondrial membrane and a change in the cardiolipin pool is observed in multiple cardiovascular diseases and in the aged heart [5, 50]. When complexed to doxorubicin, cardiolipin is unable to perform some of its regular functions such as anchoring cytochrome c [7]. This high affinity for cardiolipin also enables doxorubicin to accumulate in the mitochondria. Additionally, it is possible that anthracyclines possess an affinity to intercalate into mitochondrial DNA and may have a higher affinity for mitochondrial DNA than for nuclear DNA [44], leading to mitochondrial genomic injury as well.

The intimate involvement of mitochondrial dysfunction in progression of cardiovascular injury is becoming increasingly evident [7–11]. It should not be surprising that anthracyclines also interfere with cellular energy metabolism in numerous ways, some of which already have been described. Doxorubicin is known to directly interfere with complex I of the electron transport chain and causes a dose-dependent opening of the mitochondrial permeability transition pore, preventing the mitochondria from creating a proton gradient [7–11]. Furthermore, doxorubicin acutely inhibits AMPK and causes a net metabolic shift from fatty acid oxidation to glucose oxidation and lactic acid production, and the observed alterations in redox and metabolic pathways caused by doxorubicin have been shown to persist beyond the half-life of the drug [7], suggesting a durable effect that would increase both the severity of injury but also recovery from future cardiac events.

In addition to the intracellular mechanisms of apoptosis already discussed, it has been shown that doxorubicin upregulates the expression of several death receptors, including TNFR1, DR4, DR5, and FAS [51]. In one study, Adriamycin was shown to induce apoptosis in a p53-independent mechanism, via a Fas-mediated pathway [52]. The cardiotoxic side effects of doxorubicin are also thought to be partially due to an inflammatory response. Doxorubicin has been shown to increase several specific cytokines, including IL-6 and COX-2, and the inflammatory response induced by doxorubicin can be mediated in part by the activation of the p38 MAPK/NF-κB pathway [53]. The activation of p38 MAPK in cardiac cells has been associated with the accumulation of ROS and the onset of apoptosis in ischemia–reperfusion injured hearts [43] and strategies to limit those effects have been a major feature of cardioprotection in ischemia–reperfusion settings [29–32].

Studies have demonstrated that specific inflammatory biomarkers are predictive of cardiotoxicity in anthracycline-treated patients [44]. For example, one study showed myeloperoxidase levels had predictive value for ANT cardiotoxicity [54]. Another study showed that patients with high baseline levels of IgE were at a lower risk of developing cancer therapy-related cardiotoxicity from doxorubicin and trastuzumab treatment [55]. These results indicate that an inflammatory response likely plays a significant role in the development of anthracycline-induced cardiotoxicity.

2.2 Additional cancer drug treatment related cardiovascular effects

Anti-neoplastic drugs also capable of causing cardiac injury are not limited to the anthracyclines. For example, Trastuzumab causes a type II cardiotoxicity that is often reversible after cessation of therapy; however, some degree of persistent cardiac dysfunction has been documented in a portion of patients [56]. Trastuzumab is a human epidermal growth factor receptor 2 (HER2/ErbB2) inhibitor. In the adult heart, HER2 plays a cardioprotective role and inhibits apoptosis. When the heart is subjected to biomechanical stress, neuregulin-1 (NRG1) secreted from endothelial cells binds to HER2/HER4 heterodimers on cardiomyocytes and activates PI3K and MAPK pathways [57]. ErbB2 inhibition is associated with a significant increase in Bcl-2 family proteins [58]. It has been demonstrated that mice with a cardiac-specific deletion of ErbB2 displayed evidence of dilated cardiomyopathy, suggesting ErbB2 signaling is essential for prevention of dilated cardiomyopathy during remodeling [59]. Further, downregulation of both ErbB2 and ErbB4 has been observed in pathological remodeling of the failing myocardium in humans [60].

Trastuzumab has also been shown to trigger oxidative stress and induce the expression and activation of proapoptotic proteins, ultimately leading to mitochondrial dysfunction, the opening of mitochondrial permeability transition pores, and activation of the cell death pathways [57, 59]. Trastuzumab and anthracycline combination treatment can be powerful in its therapeutic effect, but also is known to significantly aggravate the cardiotoxic effects of anthracyclines. It is thought that anthracycline induced cardiac injury triggers the activation of the HER2 survival pathways. When anthracyclines are treated in combination with trastuzumab, these cardioprotective survival pathways are inhibited and less protection is provided to the heart [57], explaining the aggravated progression of cardiac injury.

Another fairly common therapeutic, cyclophosphamide (CP), is an alkylating agent used to treat diseases such as neuroblastoma, as well as systemic inflammatory conditions such as Systemic Lupus Erythmatosis (SLE), and rheumatoid arthritis [61]. At lower doses, CP has an immunosuppressive effect, while at higher doses, it causes cardiotoxic effects. Cyclophosphamide and its metabolites, 4-hydroxy cyclophosphamide, aldophosphamide, and acrolein are cardiotoxic, with acrolein being the most cardiotoxic [61]. Acrolein forms cytoplasmic and nuclear protein adducts, as well as adducts with lysine and cysteine. When adducted to lysine, Acrolein can react with glutathione to cause oxidative stress. When adducted with cysteine, it leads to activation of caspases and NF-κB. Activation of caspases causes apoptosis and activation of NF-κB causes the production of inflammatory cytokines [61]. Cyclophosphamide also alters the energy pool in cardiomyocytes. Many anticancer drugs, including CP, alter the expression of heart-type fatty acid binding protein (H-FABP) and carnitine palmitoyltransferase 1 (CPT-1), leading to inhibition of fatty acid oxidation and diminished ATP production. When deprived of enough ATP, cardiac tissue alters contraction and relaxation, accumulates calcium in the mitochondria, and undergoes ER stress [61].

Like many other cytotoxic agents, CP causes oxidative stress in cardiomyocytes by decreasing antioxidant levels and generating free radicals. Nrf2 is a leucine zipper protein involved in the regulation of antioxidants. CP decreases antioxidant levels is through its action on Nrf2 [61], and by suppression of intracellular GSH and SOD [62]. In CP-treated rats, additional treatment with cyclosporin-A had a cardioprotective role against CP-induced cytotoxicity [63]. Cyclosporin binds cyclophilin and forms a complex that then binds calcineurin and inactivates it, suggesting that CP induces calcineurin-mediated effects. It is thought that CP causes calcineurin-mediated dephosphorylation of NFAT, which is involved in the transcription of hypertrophic genes and apoptosis via FasL and death receptors. Additionally, calcineurin causes activation of Akt, which participates in phosphorylation of GSK-3B and leads to cardiac hypertrophy [61].

Cyclophosphamide also was shown to increase the expression of pro-apoptotic proteins and decrease the expression of antiapoptotic proteins [64]. p53 inhibition is associated with reduced apoptosis, but CP and anthracyclines both upregulate expression of p53, promoting apoptosis [61], and CP was shown to increase the expression of caspase-3 and decrease the expression of Bcl-2, also pro-apoptotic mechanisms [65, 66]. Ultrastructural changes were observed in rat cardiomyocytes when treated with CP, including lysis of myofibrils, dilation of vesicles in the sarcoplasmic reticulum, and destruction of mitochondria [67] suggesting substantial potential for persistent effects long after therapy has ended.

2.3 Cancer radiation treatment related cardiovascular injury

Additional cancer therapy related adverse cardiovascular effects are not necessarily associated with pharmaceuticals of any kind and can take quite a long time for the association to become evident. In the WECARE prospective clinical trial, women receiving radiation to treat Stage 1 or Stage 2 breast cancer, 10.5% of those receiving left-sided radiation developed coronary artery disease over then next 27 years, nearly double the incidence when compared to those who received right-sided radiation (5.8%). Further, in those patients who were under age 40 at the time of treatment, 5.9% went on to develop heart disease, compared to none in the right-sided radiation treatment group [68]. The association is presumed to relate to the relative position of the underlying cardiac structures predominantly in the left thoracic compared to the right, with coronary artery disease presumed to be the result of direct injury to the coronary arteries. The association has been suggested previously [69] is consistent with findings from a meta-analysis of smaller cohorts [70], and in older patients with a specific subset of breast cancer (estrogen positive) [71]. It remains unclear whether the vascular injury hypothesis is correct, or if the disease progression/complication rate (restenosis, heart failure, arrhythmia) following the incident cardiovascular events also were worse. Perhaps what is becoming increasingly clear is that there is substantial potential for cardiovascular events as a consequence of successful management of other disease processes and heightened routine surveillance of cardiovascular end points may be warranted, even when direct cardiovascular symptoms are not immediately evident.

3. Micronutrient effects and metabolism-targeting drug effects

Micronutrient deficiency is associated with heart failure and is a potential cause of cardiomyopathy. Low vitamin D levels are known to be associated with cardiomyopathy though the mechanism by which vitamin D affects the heart is not fully understood. Vitamin D is known to have an antihypertrophic effect. Vitamin D deficient rats have been shown to have smaller myofibrils than vitamin D sufficient rats. Additionally, vitamin D helps to regulate the expression of MMP's and tissue inhibitors of metalloproteinases (TIMP's). Imbalance in their expression is associated with diastolic and systolic dysfunction [72]. Vitamin D levels are also thought to regulate heart energy metabolism and intracellular calcium handling [73]. Of note, Vitamin D deficits have been strongly identified with morbidity and mortality associated with SARS-2 COVID19 [74]. While COVID19 mortality is not exclusively a cardiovascular event, neither can substantial cardiovascular compromise be excluded as a significant contributing factor, simply suggesting that at least some micronutrient deficiencies likely are emerging as cardiovascular risk factors of note for the future. Consistent with that impression, thiamine deficiency deprives the heart of ATP and can lead to heart failure. Thiamine is an essential cofactor for aerobic metabolism, for example, as a cofactor for the pyruvate dehydrogenase complex.

CoQ10 deficiency may also be capable of causing cardiomyopathy, as it is involved in energy metabolism, stabilization of the cellular membrane, and has antioxidant effects [75]. Blood levels of CoQ10 have been reported to be low in patients taking statin class drugs. Statins are some of the most commonly prescribed drugs to manage risk of ischemic cardiovascular disease, and a recent meta-analysis indicated that

CoQ10 supplementation reduces the risk of Statin-induced peripheral myopathies (muscle weakness, muscle cramp, muscle tiredness) but without changes in creatine kinase levels [76]. Interestingly, while the peripheral myopathies are a known complication of statin therapy, there are few studies specifically questioning whether a cardiomyopathy could also develop in a subset of patients on statins. A recent study examined the potential relationship between heart failure and long-term statin use and reported a statin-associated cardiomyopathy that responded to discontinuation of the statin combined with CoQ10 supplementation. After a mean follow-up of 2.8 years, 34% had normalized diastolic dysfunction, and 25% showed improvement [77]. While encouraging that the adverse outcomes were somewhat reversible, the results also indicate that over 40% of the patients did not improve and had lasting deleterious cardiac effects at least partially attributable to statin therapy originally prescribed to prevent cardiovascular disease [77].

In a similar vein, thiazolidinediones (TZDs) are PPARg agonists used in the treatment of type II diabetes mellitus (DMTII). To the extent that DMTII is one of strongest predictors of cardiovascular risk overall, it makes sense that these would be beneficial drugs for reducing the risk, especially for ischemic heart diseases, and the drugs are effective in that regard. However, in the event an ischemic event occurs anyway, therapeutic doses of TZDs are associated with impaired recovery and increased mortality [78]. Experimental studies indicate that excess stimulation of fatty acid metabolism by upregulating PPAR signaling restricts the heart from transitioning away from fatty acid as a substrate in the setting of ischemia, augmenting injury and subsequent dysfunction [79]. In addition to findings associated with therapeutic doses, there also can be a direct cardiotoxicity associated with TZDs at supratherapeutic levels. At least some of the cardiotoxicity is not PPAR related but remains metabolic/mitochondrial in origin [78]. Thiazolidinediones also bind off-target sites that contribute to the cardiotoxic effects. These off-target sites include mitoNEET, mitochondrial pyruvate carrier 2 (Mpc-2), mitochondrial and cytoplasmic dehydrogenases, ion channels, and enzymes and modulators involved in glucose homeostasis and energy production. MitoNEET is an iron–sulfur cluster transporter on the outer mitochondrial membrane that inhibits mitochondrial iron transport. Altering expression of mitoNEET has been shown to affect ROS levels and damage induced by ROS [78].

Similarly, Rosiglitazone, another DMTII drug, also causes myocardial energy deficiency and oxidative stress in a PPARg-independent mechanism via inhibition of complex I and complex IV of the electron transport chain, resulting in an increase in the NADH/NAD ratio and a reduction in ATP synthesis. Additionally, rosiglitazone potentially decreases mitochondrial ROS-scavenging capacity and increases phosphorylation of p38-MAPK via a PPARg-independent mechanism, as well as inhibiting NF-κB activity, which all can contribute to cardiac hypertrophy [78].

Together, these findings suggest that a host of mechanisms can contribute to adverse cardiovascular outcomes. Many of them impact mitochondrial function, with consequences including excess ROS oxidative stress, decreased capacity to buffer the oxidative stress, energy depletion, and increased apoptosis. In some cases, the cardiovascular risks are unavoidable, but if they could be managed better, the therapeutic efficacy of the drugs might be improved. While managing dosing based on known toxicities and the emergence of symptoms works in some cases, in many cases the emergence of symptoms can be quite delayed, or in some cases, associated with beneficial outcomes in some other aspect of cardiovascular risk. What is increasingly clear is an appreciation that a need for a more sophisticated approach to anticipation and surveillance of cardiovascular risk is emerging.

4. Infectious inflammatory diseases

A more central role for inflammation processes in the progression of chronic cardiovascular disease is becoming increasingly appreciated both as a direct source of the injury, and also as an aggravating condition that accelerates dysfunction in chronic disease [14–16]. There also are concerns that emergence of immunotherapies for a variety of conditions has the potential for adverse cardiovascular impact [80]. Some infections can produce an inflammatory response in the heart that ranges from subclinical to lethal [16]. Persons who become infected with the parasite *Trigonoscuta cruzi* may develop Chagas disease. The acute phase in many is characterized by asymptomatic, mild myocarditis, but a subset can also develop myocarditis that is severe enough to produce irreversible damage and heart failure. If the infection is not identified and treated, it persists in the system and may remain symptomatic for decades. However, 20–30% of chronically infected individuals will develop dilated cardiomyopathy, heart failure with or without arrhythmia, and are at increased risk for sudden cardiac death [12]. The prevalence of Chagas disease is considered endemic in Central America, South America and portions of the United States. A common cardiac feature of the disease is progressive loss of parasympathetic autonomic drive, creating a proarrhythmic substrate, more labile blood pressure control, and increased spasticity in the coronary microvasculature. Persistent sympathetic over-stimulation is known to cause multi-focal micro-infarctions, excess bioenergetic burden and mitochondrial dysfunction, leading to ROS induced DNA damage, apoptosis and progressive loss of function, similar to what has been described with catecholamine cardiotoxicity [12]. Particularly worrisome, however, is that sudden cardiac death is fairly common, and often occurs without previous signs or symptoms of advanced cardiomyopathy.

Similarly, infections caused by the Coxsackie B virus have had a known association with significant cardiovascular complications for over 60 years [81] and account for 25% of all myocarditis in young adults [82]. The early stages of infection can produce directly cytopathic effects, which can progress to a chronic, pathologic immune response if the virus persists, and in a majority of the patients who progress with chronic manifestations, development of a cardiac specific autoimmune response [83]. In fact, Coxsackie N infection has been a well-established mouse model for studying mechanisms associated with the development autoimmune-mediated myocarditis and heart failure (EAM: Experimental Autoimmune Myocarditis) [84].

More recently, the emergence of HIV and then the development of effective anti-retroviral therapies has led to an appreciation that there is an early onset of cardiovascular diseases, complicated by an inability to determine the extent to which the cardiovascular impact is the direct result of the virus, or if the primary factors are more related to the therapies used to treat the infection [13, 85]. HIV has been associated with early onset ischemic heart disease [86], but also with early onset heart failure in patients without evidence of significant coronary artery disease [87].

Most recently, the worldwide experience with SARS2-COVID19 has once again highlighted the capacity for acute infectious effects on exacerbating cardiovascular diseases, highlighted by the increased early mortality rates among those with pre-existing disease [17, 19]. Initially attributed to hypoxia-induced ischemia or hemodynamic failure secondary to the pulmonary impact of the virus, it was established quickly that there was direct cardiac infection [18], and that extrapulmonary effects of the virus were numerous [20, 21]. Given the cellular route of entry vias the Angiotensin 2 Receptor, and the widespread expression of the receptor throughout the body, it should be no surprise really that many tissues would have been impacted by the infection [88]. Driven in part by what was seen largely as microvascular injury, increased thromboembolism, and the prevalence of the receptor in the vasculature, several strong reviews strongly suggested that COVID-19 should be considered as an endothelial disease [89, 90]. The presence of cardiac specific autoantibodies in COVID19 patients [38, 39] together with MRI studies suggesting persistent cardiac dysfunction in recovered COVID patients [91] tend to suggest that there is a larger, more multi-mechanistic cardiovascular profile for the disease [92, 93]. One study is particularly concerning. Ratchford and colleagues studied vascular function in previously healthy, active young adults who had tested positive for the infection but had exhibited only mild symptoms that were resolved quickly. One month after resolution of symptoms, the group (male and female) showed persistent and consistent reductions in vasodilator capacity compared to a matched cohort of control subjects that had never been infected with COVID [94].

By the end of 2022, there will be more than 50 million individuals in the US alone who will have recovered from a COVID19 infection. It was widely observed that when COVID infection occurred in individuals who already had significant cardiovascular disease, they were at higher risk [17, 19]. It is highly likely that COVID infection prior to the subsequent development of cardiovascular disease, even if not directly responsible for the cardiovascular injury, will be associated with increased mortality from whatever disease process does evolve. Determining the best methods for identifying who has the highest future risk, and then considering the possibility of prophylactic risk mitigation could be a significant challenge for the next generation [92, 93], but it strongly highlights the need for an increased appreciation for the potential role of prior infection as an aggravating risk.

5. Non-infectious systemic inflammatory diseases

Systemic Lupus Erythematosus (SLE) also commonly known as lupus, is a chronic autoimmune disease that can affect the joints, skin, brain, lungs, kidneys, and blood vessels. Widespread inflammation and tissue damage occur in these affected organs. Patients with SLE have been reported to have a higher risk of cardiovascular events compared to the general population. Common risk factors known to increase cardiovascular disease are smoking, hypertension, hyperlipidemia, and diabetes, which are also frequent comorbidities in individuals with lupus [24]. Adding to these traditional risk factors, the systemic and vascular inflammation that occurs in individuals with lupus cause the atherosclerotic process to accelerate.

Figure 1 summarizes data indicating that Individuals diagnosed with lupus experience cardiovascular events more frequently. Patients recently diagnosed with lupus had a 3-fold increased risk of myocardial infarction and a 2-fold increased risk of ischemic stroke in the next 5 years [22]. It was also noted that the relative risk for MI and Stroke both were significantly increased within the first year of the diagnosis with lupus. The hazard ratio in the first year for cardiovascular diseases was 5.63 (95% CI 4.02–7.87), for myocardial infarction was 6.47 (95% CI 4.42–9.47), and for stroke was 6.28 (95% CI 4.83–8.17) [22].

When assessing heart failure and its relationship with SLE, patients with lupus are found to have increased short-term and long-term risk of heart failure compared to those without SLE [25]. Due to an increased risk of heart failure within a year of a lupus diagnosis, there is a need for earlier cardiac monitoring in this population.

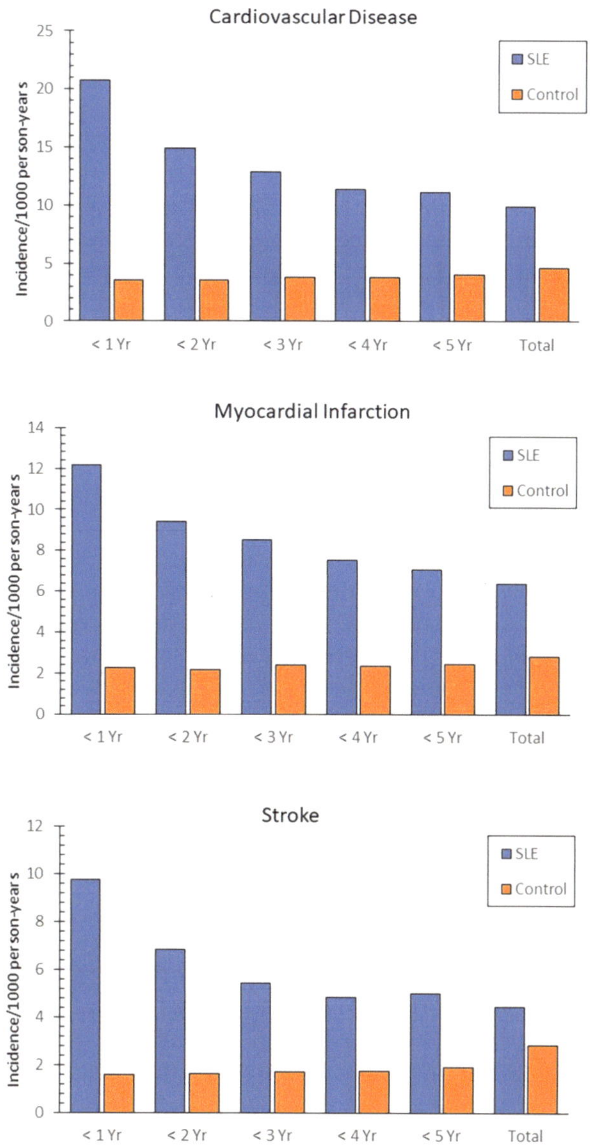

Figure 1.
Summary of cumulative incidence of cardiovascular disease (top panel), myocardial infarction (middle panel), or stroke (bottom panel) in individuals with systemic lupus Erythmatosis (SLE) compared to control (drawn from data in 22).

The median age for patients with SLE diagnosed with heart failure was 65 years old. When comparing this population of patients to those without lupus in any age group, the rate of heart failure still remained higher in those with lupus. Patients younger than the median age of 65 years had a higher rate of heart failure than older patients without lupus. This finding correlates with other research which suggests increased cardiovascular risk in younger patients who have lupus. Although there are no definite conclusions regarding the direct relationship between heart failure and lupus, there are several possible theories that extend beyond the common cardiovascular risk factors. For example, those with lupus who are also taking medications such as glucocorticoids, NSAID's and hydroxychloroquine may enhance their chances of developing heart failure due to specific cardiotoxic drug interactions [25].

Interestingly, SLE affects women more often than men. The association between lupus and cardiovascular disease in women has been shown to be a major cause of premature mortality and morbidity. In a retrospective study looking at women who were diagnosed with lupus within the age range of 35–44 years old, the likelihood of myocardial infarction was increased 52 fold compared to the control group. Comparatively, women diagnosed with lupus who were 45–54 years old, showed a slight decline in the incidence rate for a myocardial infarction. Some plausible explanations include a prothrombic effects of estrogen in combination with hypertension, renal disease, and antiphospholipid antibodies in premenopausal women aged 35–44 years.

In contrast, women of menopausal age (45–54) have declining estrogen levels, which may play a role in providing a cardioprotective effect. While there was a decline in incidence rates for myocardial infarction in the 45–54-year-old women age group, the incidence rates rose again in women 55 and older. Women with SLE display an increase in the estrogen-to-androgen ratio which could explain the increased risk of the SLE during pregnancy and menses. Multivariate analysis of women diagnosed with SLE and having a cardiac event demonstrated that diagnosis of SLE at an older age (39 vs. 34), longer SLE duration (13 vs. 10 years), prolonged use of corticosteroids (11 vs. 7 years), diagnosis of hypercholesterolemia (18 vs. 4%), and postmenopausal status (48 vs. 29%) all contributed significantly to the increased risk of a cardiovascular event in women with SLE [23].

Asthma is a chronic inflammatory airway disease causing around 500,000 hospitalizations per year in America. Because there is a risk of overlapping effects in therapies, individuals with cardiovascular disease often are excluded from asthma studies, and individuals with asthma often are excluded from cardiovascular studies, making a relationship between asthma and cardiovascular disease more difficult to identify.

It is increasingly appreciated that the localized inflammatory airway process is supported by a more generalized systemic inflammatory state and inflammatory processes are major contributors to the evolution and severity of myocardial infarction and their associated reperfusion injuries [29–32]. As such, asthma may be considered as a potential risk factor for enhanced cardiac injury either with an acute myocardial infarction directly, or with reperfusion injury following revascularization therapy. The airway inflammatory response in asthma is driven by T Helper cells type 2 (Th2) and then followed by a systemic inflammatory response characterized by increases in pro-inflammatory biomarkers such as high sensitivity C-reactive protein (hsCRP) and Interleukin 6 (IL-6). Individuals with asthma have higher circulating levels of myeloperoxidase, consistent with higher potential for ROS generation. Asthma-triggered inflammation triggers endothelial release of Platelet-Activating Factor (PAF), which contributes significantly to the airway hyper-responsiveness in asthma, but also may play a role in the increased risk for an acute myocardial infarction in asthmatic patients [26].

Patients with asthma were found to have increased risk of myocardial infarction. Furthermore, the increased MI risk appears to "scale" with the severity of the underlying asthmatic disease. Those with active asthma (individuals on an asthmatic medication) had a risk that was 29% above the increased MI risk seen in patients classified as having non-active asthma (individuals not on asthma medication), but the data are a bit more challenging since those with active asthma also were more likely to be older, diabetic and with increased BMI [26]. In a separate study, it was found that child-onset asthma did not increase the risk of a myocardial infarction, but adult-onset asthma was more likely associated with this elevated risk [27].

The elevated risk that is linked between active asthma and an acute myocardial infarction is primarily increased in the first week after an asthma exacerbation. During this study's reference period, the incident rate of MI was 25/100 person-years, but increased to 120.1/100 person-years in the 1–7 day risk period following an asthma exacerbation. In the 8–14 day risk period after an asthma exacerbation, the incident rate dropped to 50.1/100 person-years and further dropped to 38/100 person-years in the 15–28 days post asthma exacerbation [28].

There are many theories linking asthma exacerbation to increased risk of acute myocardial infarction. Acute respiratory infections are the most common cause of asthma exacerbation. Asthma propagates inflammatory pathways and cytokines leading to systemic vascular inflammation and platelet activation, fibrinolysis inhibition, and elevated CRP. Markers such as hsCRP will cause other inflammatory regulators to be upregulated resulting in leukocyte adhesion to the arterial endothelium. Arterial thrombosis results from platelet activation and endothelial dysfunction. The release of inflammatory cells resulting in the accumulation of neutrophils, platelets, fibrin, and red blood cells are characteristic of a Type 1 myocardial infarction [28]. Experimental studies in our lab, using a rag-weed sensitization to produce a hyper-responsive allergic airway model, demonstrated clearly that myocardial ischemia and reperfusion induced larger infarctions, that were associated with higher inflammatory infiltrates, and increased inducible expression of pro-inflammatory adhesion molecules in the contrary vascular that was present only on reperfusion, but was not expressed under basal sensitized conditions [95–97].

6. Environmental agents in cardiovascular risk

The relationship between air pollution and negative health outcomes has been well established in the literature over the years, first reported with outcomes following the Great London Smog of 1952 when health crises were observed following the event. While the initial correlation was thought to be tied to the pulmonary system, years later the reports were re-examined and showed that cardiac mortality – not pulmonary – was more directly associated with the increase in mortality [98]. In addition, the reexamination has prompted numerous others to delve further into this topic and with technological advancements, research has expanded to include other potential sources of cardiac toxicity such as nanoparticles of various heavy metals. Along with the pulmonary diseases commonly associated with these materials, acute myocardial infarction, atherosclerosis, and increased peripheral resistance have all been implicated with increased exposure [34, 35].

Such findings prompted the WHO to release air pollution guidelines in 2006 in hopes of reducing acute and chronic disease associated with different air pollutants worldwide. Air pollutants can be placed into two broad categories, natural phenomena and human activities [99–101]. Human activities are related to industrial processes and account for pollutants like CO and SO2, which cause most of the harmful adverse health effects. Natural phenomena on the other hand are related to volcanoes, wildfires, and land dust. In addition to this gaseous type of air pollution, particulate matters (PM) are a major player in negative health outcomes. The two major categories of PM are based on size, which are PM2.5 and PM10 – each having a different symptom profile of which the mechanism of action has not completely been resolved. However, with size, the aerodynamic diameter varies. PM10 have an AD range from 2.5 to 10 μm which allows for deposition into nasal and upper airways while PM2.5 have an AD range of less than 2.5 and less than 0.1 μm, which allows them to penetrate lung alveoli and gain access to the bloodstream [33–35].

Likewise, research into the health effects of nanoparticles is more novel and has been less refined; thus, regulations regarding exposure to these materials are not fully resolved. However, there have been numerous studies highlighting the correlation between exposure to these materials and the resultant impacts on cardiovascular function. Six of the most common metal nanoparticles are titanium oxide, zinc oxide, silver, iron oxide, carbon and silicon oxide nanoparticles. Of this list, iron oxide, carbon, and silicon oxide nanoparticles are not only used commercially, but also are used for cancer therapies, drug delivery, as well as other diagnostics. Most of these nanoparticles are associated with increasing the generation of reactive oxygen species or are pro-inflammatory, thus increasing pro-inflammatory cytokines [102].

6.1 Ambient particulate matter

While PM10 has adverse associated health effects, acute exposure to PM2.5 resulted in higher death rate related to cardiovascular disease. Short term exposure to particulate matter can result in induction of the systemic oxidation, inflammation, and increased platelet reactivity as result of elevated serum fibrinogen. However, not all people are impacted to the same magnitude by exposure to these pollutants. Those with pre-existing cardiovascular disease, diabetes, smoking status, age, and pulmonary disease like COPD can have increased responses to exposure.

The relationship between ambient particulates has been most heavily studied in the context of impact on blood pressure. According to a study by Gold et al., with every ~5–6 $\mu g/m^3$ increase in PM2.5, there was a significant increase in cardiovascular disease ranging from 0.5 to 1.5% [103]. In addition, studies have shown that increases in PM2.5 are associated with increases in systolic and diastolic blood pressure. Brook demonstrated that in a period of 5 days in Boston, MA, an increase of 10.5 $\mu g/m^3$ in PM2.5 resulted in a 2.8 mmHg increase in SBP and 2.7 mmHg increase in DBP [98]. The increased blood pressure would be consistent with impaired endothelial reactivity and enhanced constrictor responses that we demonstrated in experimental animals exposed to ambient particulates [104–106]. While is tempting to consider that the effects are attributable to increased sympathetic autonomic balance, we also have demonstrated that in older, heart-failure prone animals, there was increased risk of heart failure exacerbation, but increased risk of brady arrhythmias, and increased cardiac parasympathetic tone [107].

Even when ambient particulates do not alter the incidence of event, we and others have demonstrated that prior exposure can increase the severity of infarction, reduce the effectiveness of reperfusion, and aggravate progression of heart failure [33–35, 99–101, 104–107]. We also have demonstrated that short, episodic exposure to particulates beginning 4–7 days after an ischemia–reperfusion event was associated with increased adverse remodeling in the ventricle, increased fibrosis and decreased cardiac function 30 days post MI, compared to un-exposed animals (**Figure 2**).

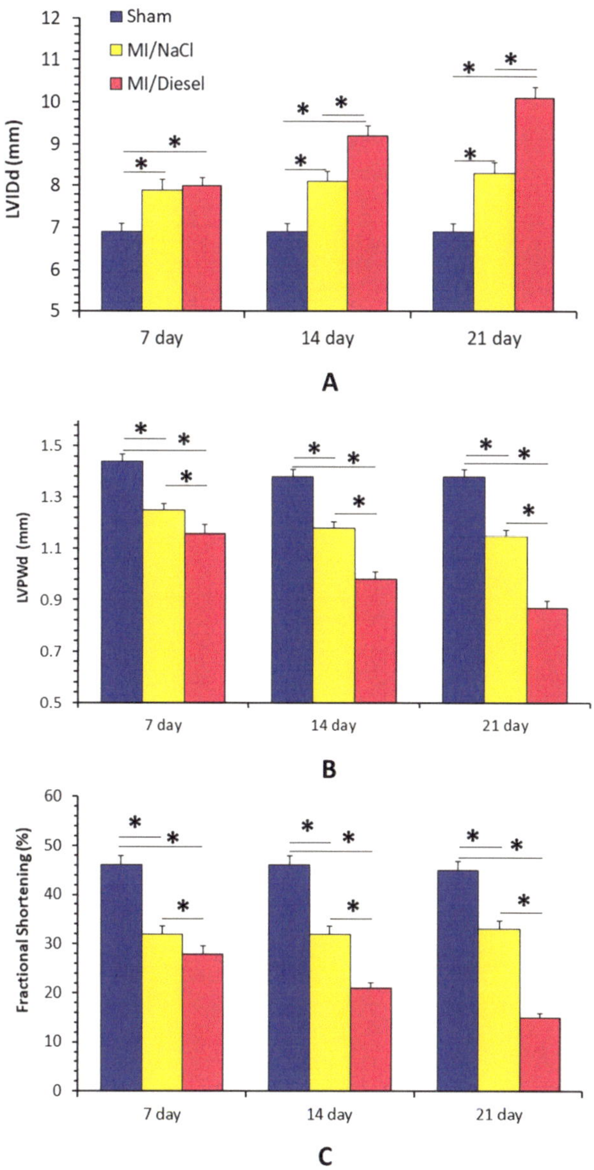

Figure 2.
Summary select echocardiographic findings on days 7, 14 ad 21 after LAD occlusion in a rat model of infarction in sham animals (blue), those with infarction/vehicle exposure (yellow), and those with MI and subsequent exposure to diesel particle on days 4, 11 and 18 (red) following myocardial infraction) on diesel particle exposure on days 4, 11 and 18. MI produced a dilation of the LV that was stable in the sham group, but progressively increased in the diesel exposure group (panel a). MI produced a thinning of the infarcted myocardial wall that was relatively stable in the sham group but progressed substantially in the diesel exposed group (panel B). Consistent with the structural changes, fractional shortening progressively decreased in the diesel group, while the decrease in the sham group was stable. (indicates $p < 0.05$ for the comparison indicated; previously unpublished data).*

6.2 Engineered nanomaterials (nanoparticles)

Nanomaterials have wide and varied commercial applications ranging from athletic equipment to clothing, to sunscreens, to drug delivery systems. Studies

Nanoparticle	Increased	Decreased
Titanium Dioxide	CK-MB	SOD
	Troponin T	GR
	LDH	GST
	Myoglobin	APX
	CK	
	Caspase 3	
	Cyto C release	
	DNA tail length	
Zinc Oxide	CK-MB	Heart rate
	Troponin T	
	CRP	
	IL-6	
	Myoglobin	
	TNF-alpha	
	Caspase-3	
	DNA tail length	
Silver	SOD	FGF-2 expression
	CAT	
	GSH	
	VEGFA expression	
Carbon	ET-1	GSH
	ACE	BFGF expression
	MCP-1	
	IL-6	
	IL-10	
	IO-12	
Silicon Oxide	CK-MB	MEF2C
	Troponin T	NKX2.5
	LDH	
	CRP	
	ET-1	
	D-dimer	
	IL-1 beta	
	TNF-alpha	
	IL-6	
	Inhibition p-VEGFR2	
	inhibition p-ERK1/2	
Iron Oxide	Vascular permeability	Heart rate
		cell proliferation

Table 1.
Summary of active mediators increased in blood or tissue following exposure to various forms of nanomaterials and known to have cardiac effects (assembled from data summarized in 103).

regarding the impact of nanoparticles on the cardiovascular system have shown various mechanisms of action. Three, general, well-accepted mechanisms for pulmonary exposure to nanoparticles have been proposed and demonstrated in several studies: 1) nanoparticles trigger lung-mediated systemic inflammatory response or oxidative stress – altering cardiac functioning 2) translocation of the nanoparticles from the lungs to the circulatory system through the alveoli (as seen with PM2.5) 3) alteration through a neurogenic pathway. These studies demonstrate the deleterious effects on the cardiovascular system from the nanoparticles though the exact mechanisms are not completely clear and likely involve a combination of the general proposed mechanisms [108]. The particular effect for any given nanoparticle varies as a function of its composition and is summarized in **Table 1**.

Iron oxide nanoparticles are commonly used in medicinal applications like drug and gene therapy delivery and cancer therapy [102]. The exposure to iron oxides can result in increased vascular permeability and decreased acute heart rate. However, the mechanism of action is not completely resolved though iron oxides are associated with oxidative damage through the generation of ROS.

Carbon nanoparticles are extremely versatile, resulting in them being found in a large range of substances. In medicine, carbon nanoparticles can be found in cancer therapies, drug delivery, gene therapy, sensors, and plastics. Their small particle size, large surface area, and association with catalytic metals are some of the reasons these nanoparticles (SWCNTs) are considered toxic agents which induce ROS generation and oxidative damage via the Fenton reaction. Exposure to these particles is often through the pulmonary route and due to their size, can be transported to secondary organs. Toxic effects can be oxidative damage and recruitment of inflammatory factors as seen in bronchoalveolar lavage fluids. These effects commonly present as decreases in thiol contents, elevation in lipid-peroxidation produces, and increase in liver and heart inflammatory markers like ET-1, ACE, MCP-1, IL-6, IL-10, and IL-12 [102]. Experimental studies of cardiac ischemia and reperfusion validate the increased risk of cardiac injury and the role of induced inflammatory pathways [109–113].

Silicon oxide nanoparticles are a commonly used commercial nanoparticle as well as their use in drug delivery, gene therapy, and diagnosis. These small particles readily mix in air and the common method of exposure is occupational during production. Ironically, silica NPs have recently been used for adenosine delivery for its cardioprotective effects [102]. However, these nanoparticles can also produce ROS which can lead to the release of cytokines and subsequently apoptosis. Study results in mice show an increase of CRP, TNF-alpha, and IL-6. Cardiac markers like ET-1, D-dimer, LDH, CK-MB, and eTNT increased after the silica exposure [102].

Many of the compounds discussed in this chapter have become ubiquitous today with increasing use of nanoparticles in products and ongoing air pollution of the industrialized world. Though strong correlations exist between common pollutants and cardiotoxicity, further research into the exact mechanisms, safe levels of exposure, and chronic effects need to continue.

7. Autoimmune mechanisms as an emerging source of cardiovascular risk

Idiopathic dilated cardiomyopathy (DCM) is a myocardial disease characterized by a progressive depression of myocardial function and ventricular dilation. DCM is the leading cause of severe heart failure, and the most common cause for heart

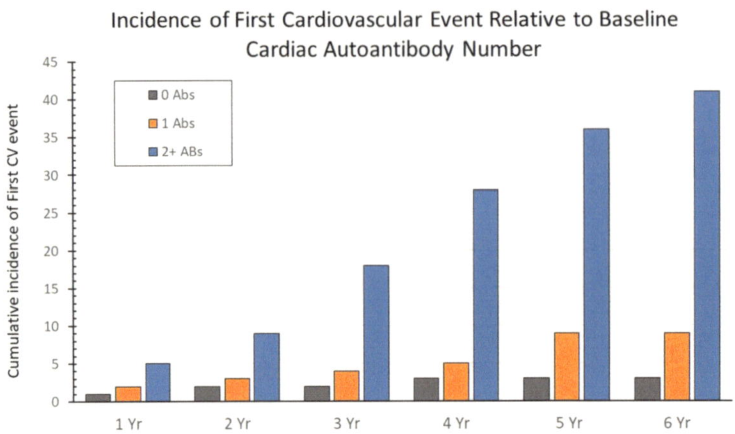

Figure 3.
Cumulative 6 year incidence of a first cardiovascular event in patients with diabetes as a function of pre-existing cardiac autoantibody number at the onset of the study (drawn from data in [117]).

transplantation. Chronic heart failure remains one of the most important sources of "all cause" morbidity and mortality, with a high frequency of hospital readmission, and a total health care expenditure burden more than twice the cost for all forms of cancer combined. The causes of DCM remain unclear, but research has been directed along three major avenues: genetic factors, viral persistence, and immunological abnormalities, including autoimmunity. Myocarditis is an inflammatory disease and some reports suggest that myocarditis and DCM represent acute and chronic stages of organ-specific autoimmune disease of the myocardium.

General characteristics supporting an autoimmune hypothesis are familial aggregation, a weak association with HLA-DR4, abnormal expression of HLA class II antigens on cardiac endothelium on endomyocardial biopsy, and the presence of organ and disease specific cardiac IgG class autoantibodies in the sera of affected patients and symptom free relatives. Supporting the genetic associations are several parallel lines of evidence. The incidence of cardiac complications is significantly higher in patients with Type I diabetes than it is in with other forms of diabetes. Type 1 diabetes is an autoimmune disease and relationship between Type 1 diabetes and autoimmune myocarditis has been suggested [114]. Similarly, Celiac disease, also with autoimmune components, has been associated with autoimmune myocarditis [115]. Type I diabetes and celiac disease, both autoimmune, have been associated with a high prevalence in Saudi children [116].

The incidence of cardiac complications is significantly higher in patients with Type I diabetes than it is in with other forms of diabetes, and the presence of cardiac autoantibodies in diabetic patients is strongly associated with the probability of subsequent cardiac event (**Figure 3**). Autoantibodies are present in between 30 and 90% of all patients with DCM [118–121]. Maguy has shown recently that there is an autoantibody signature associated with sudden cardiac arrest [36], the presence of autoantibodies against HSP65 is strongly associated with post-operative atrial fibrillation [122] and cardiac autoantibodies have been suggested as significant mediators in COVID related cardiac dysfunction and a possible source of increased cardiovascular risk in COVD survivors [38, 39]. Cardiac autoantibodies are present in at least 10% of post-myocardial infarction patients and may explain disproportionate loss of function in a subset of patients relative to that predicated on the ischemic injury per se. Repeated infarctions, stabilized by repeated revascularization may also be repeated episodes for sensitization and expansion of an autoimmune signal leading to increased rates of deteriorating function and heart failure [39].

The possibility that an auto-immune process could complicate post-infraction recovery has been suggested for more than 40 years [123, 124]. High titers of auto-antibodies to the beta-1 adrenergic receptor were identified in patients with Chagas disease. The beta-1 adrenergic autoantibody is the most studied so far. It meets Witebsky's postulates for indirect and direct autoimmune etiology. The autoantibody is stimulatory, ultimately leading to increased apoptosis sufficient to cause loss of function. Those results are consistent with models of catecholamine cardiotoxicity and with premature DCM in transgenic mice with cardiac specific overexpression of beta-1 adrenergic receptors. Signaling may be ERK1/2 dependent, but some evidence suggests that the mechanism is independent/different from standard isoproterenol stimulated beta-adrenergic responses [118–120]. Kaya [37] has demonstrated a strong association between cardiac autoantibodies and heart failure, as have others [125, 126], with an emphasis on the myosin molecules as the primary antigenic drive [118–121, 126–128]. Serum levels of troponin are the single best indicator of myocardial injury, but immunizing mice with Troponin I caused T-cell activation and cardiac inflammation with elevated RANTES, MCP-1, MIP1-alpha, MIP1-beta, MIP2, T-cell activation gene 3, CCR1, CCR2 and CCR5. It's clear that the cardiac autoimmune response can be both antibody and T cell mediated [129]. General anti-inflammatory effects (carvedilol, prednisone) or macrophage dependent inflammation (Olmesartan) all have shown efficacy is reducing the progression in experimental models of DCM.

8. Summary

It appears that many of the risk factors generally associated with cardiovascular risk, like diabetes, endothelial dysfunction, sympathetic over stimulation, all may have an under- appreciated component that is immune/inflammation mediated, and that may include an autoimmune component. Systemic inflammatory diseases without infectious triggers, airborne particles, manufactured nanoparticles, and some therapeutics used in the treatment of other diseases all may exaggerate the consequences of a cardiovascular inflammatory reaction. Some compounds, like doxorubicin, have well established mechanistic profiles that may provide insight as to how each of the mediators is adding to the cardiovascular risk, or injury expansion progression profile. It seems clear that future management of cardiovascular risk will need to become more personalized, and with greater appreciation for a much larger menu of contributing factors, all of which will require development of better biomarker screens than what are currently in use. Immunomodulating agents likely will also have an increasingly important role in limiting progression of heart failure.

Author details

Megan Goins, Katie Lovell, Greyson Keel, Julia Cook and Robert Lust*
Brody School of Medicine, East Carolina University, Greenville, NC, USA

*Address all correspondence to: lustr@ecu.edu

References

[1] Arnett DK, Blumenthal RS, Albert MA, Buroker AB, Goldberger ZD, Hahn EJ, et al. ACC/AHA guideline on the primary prevention of cardiovascular disease: A report of the American College of Cardiology/American Heart Association task Force on clinical practice guidelines. Circulation. 2019, 2019;**140**(11):e596-e646. DOI: 10.1161/CIR.0000000000000678

[2] Available from: https://www.cdc.gov/heartdisease/risk_factors.htm

[3] Available from: https://www.cvriskcalculator.com

[4] Available from: https://tools.acc.org/ascvd-risk-estimator-plus/#!/calculate/estimate/

[5] Mele D, Tocchetti CG, Pagliaro P, Madonna R, Novo G, Pepe A, et al. Pathophysiology of anthracycline cardiotoxicity. Journal of Cardiovascular Medicine (Hagerstown, Md.). 2016;**17**(Suppl. 1):e3-e11. Special issue on Cardiotoxicity from Antiblastic Drugs and Cardioprotection. DOI: 10.2459/JCM.0000000000000378 PMID: 27755237

[6] Octavia Y, Tocchetti CG, Gabrielson KL, Janssens S, Crijns HJ, Moens AL. Doxorubicin-induced cardiomyopathy: From molecular mechanisms to therapeutic strategies. Journal of Molecular and Cellular Cardiology. 2012;**52**(6):1213-1225. DOI: 10.1016/j.yjmcc.2012.03.006

[7] Wallace KB, Sardão VA, Oliveira PJ. Mitochondrial determinants of doxorubicin-induced cardiomyopathy. Circulation Research. 2020;**126**(7):926-941. DOI: 10.1161/circresaha.119.314681

[8] Poznyak AV, Ivanova EA, Sobenin IA, Yet SF, Orekhov AN. The role of mitochondria in cardiovascular diseases. Biology (Basel). 2020;**9**(6):137. Published 2020 Jun 25. DOI: 10.3390/biology9060137

[9] Siasos G, Tsigkou V, Kosmopoulos M, Theodosiadis D, Simantiris S, Tagkou NM, Tsimpiktsioglou A, Stampouloglou PK, Oikonomou E, Mourouzis K, Philippou A, Vavuranakis M, Stefanadis C, Tousoulis D, Papavassiliou AG. Mitochondria and cardiovascular diseases-from pathophysiology to treatment. Annals of Translational Medicine 2018;**6**(12):256. DOI: 10.21037/atm.2018.06.21. PMID: 30069458; PMCID: PMC6046286

[10] Murphy E, Ardehali H, Balaban TS, DiLisa F, Dornel GW, Kitsis RN, et al. Mitochondriql Function. Biology and Role in Diseases. 2016;**188**(2):1960-1991

[11] Brown DA, Perry JB, Allen ME, Sabbah HN, Stuaffer BL, Shaikh SR, et al. Mitochondrial function as a therapeutic target in heart failure. Nature Reviews. Cardiology. 2017;**14**:238-250. DOI: 10.1038/nrcardio.2016.20

[12] Nunes MCP, Beaton A, Acquatella H, Bern C, Bolger AF, Echeverría LE, et al. Chagas cardiomyopathy: An update of current clinical knowledge and management: A scientific statement from the American Heart Association. Circulation. 2018;**138**(12):e169-e209. DOI: 10.1161/CIR.0000000000000599 PMID: 30354432

[13] Triant VA. Cardiovascular disease and HIV infection. Current HIV/AIDS Reports. 2013;**10**(3):199-206. DOI: 10.1007/s11904-013-0168-6 PMID: 23793823; PMCID: PMC3964878

[14] Kawai C, Matsmumori A. Dilated cardiomyopathy update: Infectious-immune theory revisited. Heart Failure

Reviews. Nov 2013;**18**(6):703-714. DOI: 10.1007/s10741-013-9401-z

[15] Trachtenberg B, Hare J. Inflammatory cardiomyopathic syndromes. Circulation Research. 2017;**121**:803-818. DOI: 10.1161/CIRCRESAHA.117.310221

[16] Tschope C, Ammirati E, Bozkurt B, Caforio A, Cooper L. Myocarditis and inflammatory cardiomyopathy: Current evidence and future directions. Nature Reviews. 2021;**18**(3):169-193. DOI: org/10.1038/s41569-020-00435-x

[17] Clerkin K, Fried J, Raikhelkar J, Sayer G, Griffin J, et al. COVID-19 and cardiovascular disease. Circulation. 2020;**141**:1648-1655. DOI: 10.1161/CIRCULATIONAHA.120.046941

[18] Linder D, Fitzek A, Brauninger H, Aleshcheva G, Edler C, et al. Association of cardiac infection with SARS-CoV-2 in confirmed COVID-19 autopsy cases. JAMA Cardiology. 2020;**5**(11):1281-1285. DOI: 10.1001/jamacardio.2020.3551

[19] Shi S, Qin M, Shen B, Cai Y, Liu T, et al. Association of cardiac injury with mortality in hospitalized patients with COVID-19 in Wuhan, China. JAMA Cardiology. 2020;**5**(7): 802-810. DOI: 10.1001/jamacardio.2020.0950

[20] Hendren N, Drazner M, Bozkurt B, Cooper L. Description and proposed management of the acute COVID-10 cardiovascular syndrome. Circulation. 2020;**141**:1903-1914. DOI: 10.1161/CIRCLATIONAHA.120.047349

[21] Gutpa A, Madhaven M, Seghal K, Nair N, Mahajan S, et al. Extrapulmonary manifestations of COVID-19. Nature Medicine. 2020;**26**:1017-1032. DOI: 10.1038/s41591-020-0968-3

[22] Aviña-Zubieta JA et al. Risk of myocardial infarction and stroke in newly diagnosed systemic lupus erythematosus: A general population-based study. Arthritis Care & Research. 2017;**69**(6):849-856. DOI: 10.1002/acr.23018

[23] Manzi S et al. Age-specific incidence rates of myocardial infarction and angina in women with systemic lupus erythematosus: Comparison with the Framingham study. American Journal of Epidemiology. 1997;**145**(5):408-415. DOI: 10.1093/oxfordjournals.aje.a009122

[24] Ke S-R et al. Systemic lupus erythematosus is associated with poor outcome after acute myocardial infarction. Nutrition, Metabolism, and Cardiovascular Diseases. 2019;**29**(12):1400-1407. DOI: 10.1016/j.numecd.2019.08.006

[25] Yafasova A et al. Long-term cardiovascular outcomes in systemic lupus erythematosus. Journal of the American College of Cardiology. 2021;**77**(14):1717-1727. DOI: 10.1016/j.jacc.2021.02.029

[26] Cepelis A et al. Asthma, asthma control and risk of acute myocardial infarction: HUNT study. European Journal of Epidemiology. 2019;**34**(10):967-977. DOI: 10.1007/s10654-019-00562-x

[27] Bang DW et al. Asthma status and risk of incident myocardial infarction: A population-based case-control study. The Journal of Allergy and Clinical Immunology in Practice (Cambridge, MA). 2016;**4**(5):917-923. DOI: 10.1016/j.jaip.2016.02.018

[28] Raita Y et al. Risk of acute myocardial infarction and ischemic stroke in patients with asthma exacerbation: A population-based, self-controlled case series study.

The Journal of Allergy and Clinical Immunology in Practice (Cambridge, MA). 2020;**8**(1):188-194.e8. DOI: 10.1016/j.jaip.2019.06.043

[29] Murphy E, Steenbergen C. Mechanisms underlying acute protection from cardiac ischemia-reperfusion injury. Physiological Reviews. 2008;**88**(2):581-609. DOI: 10.1152/physrev.00024.2007

[30] Heusch G. Myocardial ischemia-reperfusion injury and cardioprotection in perspective. Nature Reviews in Cardiology. 2020;**17**:773-789

[31] Yellon DM, Hausenloy DJ. Myocardial reperfusion injury. The New England Journal of Medicine. 2007;**357**:1121-1135. DOI: 10.1056/NEJMra071667

[32] Hausenloy DJ, Candilio L, Evans R, Cono A, Jenkins DP, Kolvekar S, et al. The New England Journal of Medicine. 2015;**373**:1408-1417. DOI: 10.1056/NEJMoa1413534

[33] Brook RD, Franklin B, Cascio W, Hong Y, Howard G, Lipsett M, et al. Air Polution and cardiovascular disease. Circulation. 2004;**109**(21):2655-2271

[34] Franklin BA, Brook R, Pope CA III. Air pollution and cardiovascular disease. Current Problems in Cardiology. 2015;**40**:207-238

[35] Al-Kindi SG, Brook RD, Bisawal S, Rajagopalan S. Environmental determinants of cardiovascular disease: Lessons learned from air pollution. Nature Reviews Cardiology. 2020;**2020**(17):656-672

[36] Maguy A, Tardif J-C, Busseuil D, Ribi C, Li J. Autoantibody signature in cardiac arrest. Circulation. 2020;**141**:1764-1774. DOI: 10.1661/CIRCULATIONAHA119.044408

[37] Kaya Z, Leib C, Katus H. Autoantibodies in heart failure and cardiac dysfunction. Circulation Research. 2012;**110**(1):145-158. DOI: 10.1161.CIRCRESAHA.111.243360

[38] Khamsi R. Rogue antibodies could be driving severe COVID-19. Nature. 2021;**590**:29-31

[39] Blagova O, Varionchik N, Zaidenov V, Savina P, Sarkisova N. Anti-heart antibodies levels and their correlation with clinical symptoms and outcomes in patients with confirmed or suspected diagnosis COVID-19. European Journal of Immunology. 2021;**51**:893-902. DOI: 10.1002/eji.202048930

[40] Carll AP, Willis MS, Lust RM, Costa DL, Farraj AK. Merits of non-invasive rat models of left ventricular heart failure. Cardiovascular Toxicology. 2011;**11**(2):91-112. DOI: 10.1007/s12012-011-9103-5 PMID: 21279739

[41] Corremans R, Adão R, De Keulenaer GW, Leite-Moreira AF, Brás-Silva C. Update on pathophysiology and preventive strategies of anthracycline-induced cardiotoxicity. Clinical and Experimental Pharmacology & Physiology. 2019;**46**(3):204-215. DOI: 10.1111/1440-1681.13036 PMID: 30244497

[42] Timm KN, Tyler DJ. The role of AMPK activation for Cardioprotection in doxorubicin-induced cardiotoxicity. Cardiovascular Drugs and Therapy 2020;**34**(2):255-269. DOI: 10.1007/s10557-020-06941-x. PMID: 32034646; PMCID: PMC7125062. 8

[43] Kang YJ. Molecular and cellular mechanisms of cardiotoxicity.

Environmental Health Perspectives. 2001;**109**(Suppl. 1):27-34. DOI: 10.1289/ehp.01109s127

[44] Fabiani I, Aimo A, Grigoratos C, et al. Oxidative stress and inflammation: Determinants of anthracycline cardiotoxicity and possible therapeutic targets. Heart Failure Reviews. 2021;**26**:881-890. DOI: 10.1007/s10741-020-10063-9

[45] Zhang S, Liu X, Bawa-Khalfe T, et al. Identification of the molecular basis of doxorubicin-induced cardiotoxicity. Nature Medicine. 2012;**18**:1639-1642. DOI: 10.1038/nm.2919

[46] Zhu H, Sarkar S, Scott L, Danelisen I, Trush MA, Jia Z, et al. Doxorubicin redox biology: Redox cycling, topoisomerase inhibition, and oxidative stress. Reactive Oxygen Species (Apex, N.C.). 2016;**1**(3):189-198. DOI: 10.20455/ros.2016.83513

[47] Rabinovich-Nikitin I, Love M, Kirshenbaum LA. Inhibition of MMP prevents doxorubicin-induced cardiotoxicity by attenuating cardiac intracellular and extracellular matrix remodelling. Cardiovascular Research. 2021;**117**(1):11-12. DOI: 10.1093/cvr/cvaa198

[48] Aries A, Paradis P, Lefebvre C, Schwartz RJ, Nemer M. Essential role of GATA-4 in cell survival and drug-induced cardiotoxicity. Proceedings of the National Academy of Sciences of the United States of America. 2004;**101**(18):6975-6980. DOI: 10.1073/pnas.0401833101

[49] Park AM, Nagase H, Liu L, Vinod Kumar S, Szwergold N, Wong CM, et al. Mechanism of anthracycline-mediated down-regulation of GATA4 in the heart. Cardiovascular Research. 2011;**90**(1):97-104. DOI: 10.1093/cvr/cvq36110

[50] Dudek J, Hartmann M, Rehling P. The role of mitochondrial cardiolipin in heart function and its implication in cardiac disease. Biochimica et Biophysica Acta (BBA) - Molecular Basis of Disease. 2019;**1865**(4):810-821. DOI: 10.1016/j.bbadis.2018.08.025

[51] Zhao L, Zhang B. Doxorubicin induces cardiotoxicity through upregulation of death receptors mediated apoptosis in cardiomyocytes. Scientific Reports. 2017;**7**:44735. DOI: 10.1038/srep44735

[52] Nakamura T, Ueda Y, Juan Y, Katsuda S, Takahashi H, Koh E. Fas-mediated apoptosis in adriamycin-induced cardiomyopathy in rats: In vivo study. Circulation. 2000;**102**(5):572-578. DOI: 10.1161/01.cir.102.5.572

[53] Guo R, Xu W, Lin J, Mo L, Hua X, Chen P, et al. Activation of the p38 MAPK/NF-κB pathway contributes to doxorubicin-induced inflammation and cytotoxicity in H9c2 cardiac cells. Molecular Medicine Reports. 2013;**8**:603-608. DOI: 10.3892/mmr.2013.1554

[54] Putt M, Hahn VS, Januzzi JL, Sawaya H, Sebag IA, Plana JC, et al. Longitudinal changes in multiple biomarkers are associated with cardiotoxicity in breast Cancer patients treated with doxorubicin, Taxanes, and Trastuzumab. Clinical Chemistry. 2015;**61**(9):1164-1172. DOI: 10.1373/clinchem.2015.241232

[55] Beer LA, Kossenkov AV, Liu Q, Luning Prak E, Domchek S, Speicher DW, et al. Baseline immunoglobulin E levels as a marker of doxorubicin- and Trastuzumab-associated cardiac dysfunction. Circulation Research. 2016;**119**(10):1135-1144. DOI: 10.1161/CIRCRESAHA.116.309004

[56] Koutsoukis A, Ntalianis A, Repasos E, Kastritis E, Dimopoulos MA, Paraskevaidis I. Cardio-oncology: A focus on cardiotoxicity. European Cardiology. 2018;**13**(1):64-69. DOI: 10.15420/ecr.2017:17:2

[57] Varga ZV, Ferdinandy P, Liaudet L, Pacher P. Drug-induced mitochondrial dysfunction and cardiotoxicity. American Journal of Physiology. Heart and Circulatory Physiology. 2015;**309**(9):H1453-H1467. DOI: 10.1152/ajpheart.00554.2015

[58] Grazette LP, Boecker W, Matsui T, Semigran M, Force TL, Hajjar RJ, et al. Inhibition of ErbB2 causes mitochondrial dysfunction in cardiomyocytes: Implications for herceptin-induced cardiomyopathy. Journal of the American College of Cardiology. 2004;**44**(11):2231-2238. DOI: 10.1016/j.jacc.2004.08.066

[59] Crone SA, Zhao YY, Fan L, Gu Y, Minamisawa S, Liu Y, et al. ErbB2 is essential in the prevention of dilated cardiomyopathy. Nature Medicine. 2002;**8**(5):459-465. DOI: 10.1038/nm0502-459

[60] Vasti C, Hertig CM. Neuregulin-1/erbB activities with focus on the susceptibility of the heart to anthracyclines. World Journal of Cardiology. 2014;**6**(7):653-662. DOI: 10.4330/wjc.v6.i7.653

[61] Iqubal A, Iqubal MK, Sharma S, Ansari MA, Najmi AK, Ali SM, et al. Molecular mechanism involved in cyclophosphamide-induced cardiotoxicity: Old drug with a new vision. Life Sciences. 2019;**218**:112-131. DOI: 10.1016/j.lfs.2018.12.018

[62] Omole JG, Ayoka OA, Alabi QK, Adefisayo MA, Asafa MA, Olubunmi BO, et al. Protective effect of Kolaviron on cyclophosphamide-induced cardiac toxicity in rats. Journal of Evidence-Based Integrative Medicine. 2018;**23**:2156587218757649. DOI: 10.1177/2156587218757649

[63] Al-Nasser IA. In vivo prevention of cyclophosphamide-induced Ca2+ dependent damage of rat heart and liver mitochondria by cyclosporin a. Comparative Biochemistry and Physiology Part A: Molecular & Integrative Physiology. 1998;**121**(3): 209-214. DOI: 10.1016/s1095-6433(98) 10135-6

[64] Asiri YA. Probucol attenuates cyclophosphamide-induced oxidative apoptosis, p53 and Bax signal expression in rat cardiac tissues. Oxidative Medicine and Cellular Longevity. 2010;**3**(5):308-316. DOI: 10.4161/oxim.3.5.13107

[65] Avci H, Epikmen ET, Ipek E, Tunca R, Birincioglu SS, Akşit H, et al. Protective effects of silymarin and curcumin on cyclophosphamide-induced cardiotoxicity. Experimental and Toxicologic Pathology: Official Journal of the Gesellschaft fur Toxikologische Pathologie. 2017;**69**(5):317-327. DOI: 10.1016/j.etp.2017.02.002

[66] Refaie MMM, Shehata S, El-Hussieny M, et al. Role of ATP-sensitive Potassium Channel (KATP) and eNOS in mediating the protective effect of Nicorandil in cyclophosphamide-induced cardiotoxicity. Cardiovascular Toxicology. 2020;**20**:71-81. DOI: 10.1007/s12012-019-09535-8

[67] Lushnikova EL, Nepomnyashchikh LM, Sviridov EA, et al. Ultrastructural signs of cyclophosphamide-induced damage to cardiomyocytes. Bulletin of Experimental Biology and Medicine. 2008;**146**:366-371. DOI: 10.1007/s10517-008-0287-z

[68] Carlson LE, Watt GP, Tonorezos ES, Chow EJ, Yu AF, Woods M, et al. Coronary artery disease in young women after radiation therapy for breast Cancer: The WECARE study. JACC: CardioOncology. 2021;**3**(3):381-392. DOI: 10.1016/j.jaccao.2021.07.008 PMID: 34604798; PMCID: PMC8463731

[69] Correa CR, Litt HI, Hwang WT, Ferrari VA, Solin LJ, Harris EE. Coronary artery findings after left-sided compared with right-sided radiation treatment for early-stage breast cancer. Journal of Clinical Oncology. 2007;**25**(21):3031-3037. DOI: 10.1200/JCO.2006.08.6595 PMID: 17634481

[70] Sardar P, Kundu A, Chatterjee S, Nohria A, Nairooz R, Bangalore S, et al. Long-term cardiovascular mortality after radiotherapy for breast cancer: A systematic review and meta-analysis. Clinical Cardiology. 2017;**40**(2):73-81. DOI: 10.1002/clc.22631 PMID: 28244595; PMCID: PMC6490535

[71] Jimenez RB, Wong SM, Johnson A, Lalani N, Hughes KS. The association between cardiac mortality and adjuvant radiation therapy among older patients with stage I Estrogen positive breast Cancer: A surveillance, epidemiology, and end results (SEER)-based study on cardiac mortality and radiation therapy. Advances in Radiation Oncology. 2020;**6**(2):100633. DOI: 10.1016/j.adro.2020.100633 PMID: 33912735; PMCID: PMC8071719

[72] Gardner DG, Chen S, Glenn DJ. Vitamin D and the heart. American Journal of Physiology. Regulatory, Integrative and Comparative Physiology. 2013;**305**(9):R969-R977. DOI: 10.1152/ajpregu.00322.2013

[73] Polat V, Bozcali E, Uygun T, Opan S, Karakaya O. Low vitamin D status associated with dilated cardiomyopathy. International Journal of Clinical and Experimental Medicine. 2015;**8**(1):1356-1362

[74] Chiodini I, Gatti D, Soranna D, Merlotti D, Mingiano C, Fassio A, et al. Vitamin D status and SARS-CoV-2 infection and COVID-19 clinical outcomes. Frontiers in Public Health. 2021;**9**:736665. DOI: 10.3389/fpubh.2021.736665 PMID: 35004568; PMCID: PMC8727532

[75] Sciatti E, mbardi C, Ravera A, Vizzardi E, Bonadei I, Carubelli V, et al. Nutritional deficiency in patients with heart failure. Nutrients. 2016;**8**(7):442. DOI: 10.3390/nu8070442

[76] Qu H, Guo M, Chai H, Wang WT, Gao ZY, Shi DZ. Effects of coenzyme Q10 on statin-induced myopathy: An updated Meta-analysis of randomized controlled trials. Journal of the American Heart Association. 2018;**7**(19):e009835. DOI: 10.1161/JAHA.118.009835. PMID: 30371340; PMCID: PMC6404871

[77] Langsjoen PH, Langsjoen JO, Langsjoen AM, Rosenfeldt F. Statin-associated cardiomyopathy responds to statin withdrawal and administration of coenzyme Q10. The Permanente Journal. 2019;**23**:18-257. DOI: 10.7812/TPP/18.257 PMID: 31496499; PMCID: PMC6730959

[78] Jiang J-B, Balschi JA Jr, F. X., & He, H. Thiazolidinediones cause cardiotoxicity via PPARγ- independent mechanism. Cardiotoxicity. 2018. DOI: 10.5772/intechopen.78957

[79] Sambandam N, Morabito D, Wagg C, Finck BN, Kelly DP, Lopaschuk GD. Chronic activation of PPARα is detrimental to cardiac recovery after ischemia. American Journal of Physiology. Heart and Circulatory Physiology. 2006;**290**:H87-H95

[80] Baik A, Oluwole O, Johnson D, Shah N, Salem J-E, et al. Cardiovascular toxicities and immunotherapies. Circulation Research. 2021; **128**(11):1780-1801. DOI: 10.1161/CIRCRESAHA.120.315894

[81] Woodward TE, FR MC Jr, Carey TN, Togo Y. Viral and rickettsial causes of cardiac disease, including the Coxsackie virus etiology of pericarditis and myocarditis. Annals of Internal Medicine. 1960;**53**:1130-1150. DOI: 10.7326/0003-4819-53-6-1130 PMID: 13786607

[82] Kim KS, Hufnagel G, Chapman NM, Tracy S. The group B coxsackieviruses and myocarditis. Reviews in Medical Virology. 2001;**11**(6):355-368. DOI: 10.1002/rmv.326 PMID: 11746998

[83] Tam PE. Coxsackie virus myocarditis: Interplay between virus and host in the pathogenesis of heart disease. Viral Immunology. 2006;**19**(2):133-146. DOI: 10.1089/vim.2006.19.133 PMID: 16817756

[84] Fairweather D, Rose NR. Coxsackievirus-induced myocarditis in mice: A model of autoimmune disease for studying immunotoxicity. Methods. 2007;**41**(1):118-122. DOI: 10.1016/j.ymeth.2006.07.009. PMID: 17161308; PMCID: PMC1764911

[85] Freiberg MS, So-Armah K. HIV and cardiovascular disease: We need a mechanism, and we need a plan. Journal of the American Heart Association. 2016;**4**(3):e003411. DOI: 10.1161/JAHA.116.003411. PMID: 27013540; PMCID: PMC4943288

[86] Freiberg MS, Chang CC, Kuller LH, Skanderson M, Lowy E, Kraemer KL, et al. HIV infection and the risk of acute myocardial infarction. JAMA Internal Medicine. 2013;**173**:614-622

[87] Butt AA, Chang CC, Kuller L, Goetz MB, Leaf D, Rimland D, et al. Risk of heart failure with human immunodeficiency virus in the absence of prior diagnosis of coronary heart disease. Archives of Internal Medicine. 2011;**171**:737-743

[88] Ni W, Yang X, Yang W, Bao J, Xiao Y, et al. Role of angiotensin-converting enzyme 2 (ACE2) in COVID-19. Critical Care. 2020;**24**:422. DOI: doi.org/10.1186/s13054-020-03120-0

[89] Libby P, Lüscher T. COVID-19 is, in the end, an endothelial disease. European Heart Journal. 2020;**41**(32):3038-3044. DOI: 10.1093/eurheartj/ehaa623 PMID: 32882706; PMCID: PMC7470753

[90] Evans PC, Rainger GE, Mason JC, Guzik TJ, Osto E, Stamataki Z, et al. Endothelial dysfunction in COVID-19: A position paper of the ESC working Group for Atherosclerosis and Vascular Biology, and the ESC Council of basic cardiovascular science. Cardiovascular Research. 2020;**116**(14):2177-2184. DOI: 10.1093/cvr/cvaa230 PMID: 32750108; PMCID: PMC7454368

[91] Puntmann V, Carej M, Wieters I, Fahim M, Arendt C, et al. Outcomes of cardiovascular magnetic resonance imaging in patients recently recovered from coronavirus disease 2019 (COVID-19). JAMA Cardiology. **2020**. DOI: 10.1001/jamacardio.2020.3557

[92] Nishiga M, Wang DW, Han Y, Lewis DB, Wu JC. COVID-19 and cardiovascular disease: From basic mechanisms to clinical perspectives. Nature Reviews. Cardiology 2020;**17**(9):543-558. DOI: 10.1038/s41569-020-0413-9. PMID: 32690910; PMCID: PMC7370876.

[93] Guzik TJ, Mohiddin SA, Dimarco A, Patel V, Savvatis K, Marelli-Berg FM,

et al. COVID-19 and the cardiovascular system: Implications for risk assessment, diagnosis, and treatment options. Cardiovascular Research. 2020;**116**(10):1666-1687. DOI: 10.1093/cvr/cvaa106 PMID: 32352535; PMCID: PMC7197627

[94] Ratchford SM, Stickford JL, Province VM, Stute N, Augenreich MA, Koontz LK, et al. Vascular alterations among young adults with SARS-CoV-2. American Journal of Physiology. Heart and Circulatory Physiology. 2021;**320**(1):H404-H410. DOI: 10.1152/ajpheart.00897.2020 PMID: 33306450; PMCID: PMC8083172

[95] Hazarika S, Van Scott MR, Lust RM. Airborne allergen increases severity of myocardial injury following ischemia-reperfusion in allergic mice. American Journal of Physiology. Heart and Circulatory Physiology. 2007;**292**(1):H572-H579. PMID: 16905595

[96] Hazarika S, Van Scott MR, Lust RM, Wingard CJ. Pulmonary allergic reactions impair systemic vascular relaxation in ragweed sensitive mice. Vascular Pharmacology. 2010;**53**(5-6):258-263 PMID: 20888432

[97] Wingard CJ, Cozzi E, van Scott MR, Lust RM. Particulate exposures and cardiovascular inflammation. Chapter 5. In: Meggs W, editor. Toxicant Induction of Irritant Asthma, Rhinitis, and Related Conditions. New York: Springer; 2013. ISBN 978-1-4614-9043-2

[98] Brook RD. Why physicians who treat hypertension should know more about air pollution. The Journal of Clinical Hypertension. 2007;**9**(8):629-635. DOI: 10.1111/j.1524-6175.2007.07187.x

[99] Lee BJ, Kim B, Lee K. Air pollution exposure and cardiovascular disease. Toxicology Research. 2014;**30**(2):71-75. DOI: 10.5487/TR.2014.30.2.071

[100] Simkhovich BZ, Kleinman MT, Kloner RA. Air pollution and cardiovascular injury. Journal of the American College of Cardiology. 2008;**52**(9):719-726. DOI: 10.1016/j.jacc.2008.05.029

[101] Bourdrel T, Bind MA, Béjot Y, Morel O, Argacha JF. Cardiovascular effects of air pollution. Archives of Cardiovascular Diseases. 2017;**110**(11):634-642. DOI: 10.1016/j.acvd.2017.05.003

[102] Bostan HB, Rezaee R, Valokala MG, et al. Cardiotoxicity of nano-particles. Life Sciences. 2016;**165**:91-99. DOI: 10.1016/j.lfs.2016.09.017

[103] Gold DR, Litonjua A, Schwartz J, et al. Ambient pollution and heart rate variability. Circulation. 2000;**101**(11):1267-1273. DOI: 10.1161/01.cir.101.11.1267

[104] Cozzi E, Hazarika S, Stallings HW, Cascio WE, Devlin RB, Lust RM, et al. Ultrafine particulate matter exposure augments ischemia reperfusion injury in mice. American Journal of Physiology. Heart and Circulatory Physiology. 2006;**291**(2):H894-H903. PMID: 16582015

[105] Cascio WE, Cozzi E, Devlin RB, Henriksen RA, Lust RM, Van Scott MR, et al. Cardiac and vascular changes in mice after exposure to ultrafine particulate matter. Inhalation Toxicology. 2007;**19**(Suppl. 1):67-73 PMID: 17886053

[106] Cozzi E, Wingard CJ, Cascio WE, Devlin RB, Miles JJ, Bofferding AR, et al. Effect of ambient particulate matter exposure on hemostasis. Translational Research. 2007;**149**(6):324-332. PMID: 17543851

[107] Carll AP, Lust RM, Hazari MS, Perez CM, Krantz QT, King CJ, et al. Diesel exhaust inhalation increases cardiac output, bradyarrhythmias, and parasympathetic tone in aged heart failure-prone rats. Toxicological Sciences. 2013, 2013;**131**(2):583-595. PMID: 23047911

[108] Kan H, Pan D, Castranova V. Engineered nanoparticle exposure and cardiovascular effects: The role of a neuronal-regulated pathway. Inhalation Toxicology. 2018;**30**(9-10):335-342. DOI: 10.1080/08958378.2018.1535634

[109] Wingard CJ, Walters DM, Cathey BL, Hilderbrand SC, Katwa P, Lin S, et al. Mast cells contribute to altered vascular reactivity and ischemia-reperfusion injury following cerium oxide nanoparticle instillation. Nanotoxicology. 2011;**5**(4):531-545. PMID: 20888432

[110] Thompson LC, Urankar RN, Holland NA, Vidanapathirana AK, Pitzer JE, Han L, et al. C60 exposure augments cardiac ischemia/reperfusion injury and coronary artery contraction in Sprague-Dawley rats. Toxicological Sciences. 2014;**138**(2):365-378. DOI: 10.1093/toxsci/kfu008 PMID: 24431213

[111] Holland NA, Becak DP, Shannahan JH, Brown JM, Carratt SA, Van Winkle LS, et al. Cardiac ischemia reperfusion injury following instillation of 20 nm citrate-capped Nanosilver. Journal of Nanomedicine & Nanotechnology. 2015;**S6**. DOI: 10.4172/2157-7439.S6-006 PMID:26966636

[112] Holland NA, Thompson LC, Vidanapathirana AK, Urankar RN, Lust RM, Fennell TR, et al. Impact of pulmonary exposure to gold core silver nanoparticles of different size and capping agents on cardiovascular injury. Particle and Fibre Toxicology. 2016;**13**(1):48-69. DOI: 10.1186/s12989-016-0159-z PMID:27558113

[113] Urankar RM, Lust RM, Mann E, Katwa P, Wang X, Podila R, et al. Expansion of cardiac ischemia/reperfusion injury after instillation of three forms of multi-walled carbon nanotubes. Particle and Fibre Toxicology. 2012;**16**(9):38 PMID:23072542

[114] Gottumukkala RV, Lv H, Cornivelli L, Wagers AJ, Kwong RY, Bronson R, et al. Myocardial infarction triggers chronic cardiac autoimmunity in type 1 diabetes. Science Translational Medicine. 2012;**4**(138):138ra80. DOI: 10.1126/scitranslmed.3003551 PMID: 22700956; PMCID: PMC4303259

[115] Frustaci A, Cuoco L, Chimenti C, Pieroni M, Fioravanti G, Gentiloni N, et al. Celiac disease associated with autoimmune myocarditis. Circulation. 2002;**105**(22):2611-2618. DOI: 10.1161/01.cir.0000017880.86166.87. PMID: 12045166

[116] Al-Hussaini A, Sulaiman N, Al-Zahrani M, Alenizi A, El Haj I. High prevalence of celiac disease among Saudi children with type 1 diabetes: A prospective cross-sectional study. BMC Gastroenterology. 2012;**12**:180. DOI: 10.1186/1471-230X-12-180. PMID: 23259699; PMCID: PMC3543703

[117] Sousa GR, Niewczas M. Lipes MA; 251-OR: Cardiac autoantibodies (AB) predict cardiovascular disease (CVD) in T1D and are associated with cytokine signatures linked to CVD risk. Diabetes. 2020;**69**(Supplement_1) 251–OR. DOI: 10.2337/db20-251-OR

[118] Caforio A, Mahon N, Tona F, McKenna W. Circulating cardiac autoantibodies in dilated cardiomyopathy and myocarditis: Pathogenetic and

clinical significance. European Journal of Heart Failure. 2002;**411-417**

[119] Caforo A, Tona F, Bottaro S, Vinvi A, Dequal G, et al. Clinical implications of anti-heart autoantibodies in myocarditis and dilated cardiomyopathy. Autoimmunity. 2008;**41**:35-45. DOI: 10.1080.08916930701619235

[120] Moraru M, Roth A, Keren G, George J. Cellular autoimmunity to cardiac myosin in patients with a recent myocardial infarction. International Journal of Cardiology. 2006;**107**:61-66. DOI: 10.1016/j.ijcard.2005.02.036

[121] Calabrese F, Thiene G. Myocarditis and inflammatory cardiomyopathy: Microbiological and molecular biological aspects. Cardiovascular Research. 2003;**60**:11-25. DOI: 10.1016/S008-6363(03)00475-9

[122] Mandal K, Jahangiri J, Mukhin M, Poloniecki J, Camm A, et al. Association of anti-heat shock protein 65 antibodies with development of postoperative atrial fibrillation. Circulation. 2004:2588-2590. DOI: 10.1161/01.CIR.0000136825.96029.A5

[123] Kossowsky W, Epstein J, Levine R. Post myocardial infarction syndrome: An early complication acute myocardial infarction. Chest. 1973;**63**:35-40. DOI: 10.1378/chest.63.1.35

[124] Deubner N, Berliner D, Schlipp A, Gelbrich G, Caforio A, et al. Cardiac B1-adrenoceptor autoantibodies in human heart disease: Rationale and design of the etiology, time-course, and survival (ETiCS) study. European Journal of Heart Failure. 2010;**12**:753-7662. DOI: 10.1093/eurjhf/hfq072

[125] Sahara H, Meltzer A, Weiss M, Iwamoto Y, et al. Autoimmune sensitization to cardiac myosin leads to acute rejection of cardiac allografts in miniature swine. Transplantation. 2011;**91**:1187-1191. DOI: 10.1097/TP.0b013e318218415d

[126] Mascaro-Blanco A, Alvarez K, Yu X, Lindenfeld J, Olansky L, et al. Consequences of unlocking the cardiac myosin molecule in human myocarditis and cardiomyopathies. Autoimmunity. 2008;**41**:442-453. DOI: 10.1080/08916930802031579

[127] Bracamonte-Baran W, Cihakova D. Cardiac autoimmunity; myocarditis. Advances in Experimental Medicine and Biology. 2017;**1003**:187-221. DOI: 10.1007/978-3-319-57613-8_10

[128] Mocumbi A, Latif N, Yacoub M. Presence of circulating anti-myosin antibodies in endomyocardial fibrosis. PLoS Neglected Tropical Diseases. 2010;**4**(4)

[129] Ono M, Shimizu J, Miyachi Y, Sakaguchi S. Control of autoimmune myocarditis and multiorgan inflammation by glucocorticoid-induced TNF receptor family-related protein foxp3-expressing-CD25 and CD25 regulatory T cells. Journal of Immunology. 2006;**176**:4748-4756. DOI: 10.4049/jimmunol.176.4748

Chapter 18

Echocardiographic Prognostic Factors in Pulmonary Hypertension

Gabriela Silvia Gheorghe, Andrei Cristian Dan Gheorghe, Ana Ciobanu and Andreea Simona Hodorogea

Abstract

Pulmonary hypertension (PH) is defined as an increase in mean pulmonary arterial pressure of ≥25 mmHg at rest by right heart catheterization. Echocardiography estimates systolic pulmonary arterial pressure on the tricuspid regurgitation jet velocity, mean and diastolic pressure based on the pulmonary regurgitation jet, and data regarding the function of the right ventricle. ESC guidelines propose an echocardiographic risk assessment in PH according to right atrial area > 26 cm^2 and pericardial effusion. Other risk factors correlated with the severity of the PH include right atrial pressure > 15 mmHg, tricuspid regurgitation more than moderate, TAPSE <18 mm, tricuspid S′ < 11.5 cm/s assessed by TDI, right ventricle ejection fraction <45% using 3D imaging, fractional area change of the right ventricle <35%, dP/dt < 400 mmHg/s on the tricuspid regurgitation flow, reduced strain of the right ventricle, diastolic dysfunction. Left ventricular eccentricity index (EI) >1.7 combined with TAPSE <15 mm was associated with a higher death rate compared to patients with normal values. However, each of these parameters used in the assessment of the right ventricle has technical limitations, and it is necessary to use multiple tests for a correct evaluation of the prognosis of PH.

Keywords: pulmonary hypertension, tricuspid regurgitation, right ventricle, right atrium, global strain

1. Introduction

Pulmonary hypertension (PH) is defined as an increase in mean pulmonary arterial pressure (mPAP) of ≥25 mmHg at rest as assessed by right heart catheterization. Current data have shown that the normal mPAP at rest is 14 ± 3 mmHg with the upper limit of normal of approximately 20 mmHg. The clinical significance of mPAP between 21 and 24 mmHg is unclear [1]. There are also unclear data regarding the normal versus exaggerated elevation of mPAP at physical effort, making it difficult to put the diagnosis of exercise-induced PH. Pulmonary vascular resistance (PVR) with a cut-off of ≥3 Wood units has been included in the hemodynamic diagnosis of PH, and pulmonary artery wedge pressure (PAWP) with a cut-off of ≥15 mmHg is used for the classification of PH in pre-capillary, post-capillary, or combined pre- and post-capillary PH [1]. PH is classified into five groups, depending on the underlying disease [1].

Not all patients with PH perform right heart catheterization, and, in practice, the diagnosis of PH is based on the echocardiographic evaluation of the pulmonary artery pressure. Also, echocardiography can detect the underlying disease and the consequences of the PH on the right and left ventricles (**Table 1**), [2–8]. Nevertheless, the echocardiographic evaluation of the right heart is more difficult than that of the left heart because of the complex shape of the right ventricle (RV) and its load-dependent physiology. Its shape in apical 4-chamber view is more triangular, in contrast to the left ventricle more conical. In the parasternal short axis view, it is like a crescent. The cavity of the RV has three parts: inlet, apical trabeculae, and outlet segments. The outlet segment is not trabeculated and is separated from the inlet segment by the supraventricular crest. The subepicardial myofibrils have a circumferential orientation, and the subendocardial myofibrils have predominantly a longitudinal orientation [9, 10]. The interventricular septum separates the right and left ventricles and bulges into RV during the ventricular systole. From the three leaflets of the tricuspid valve, the septal leaflet is usually visible by echocardiography. The 2D echography has a low sensitivity for defining the RV endocardial border contour of the free wall and of the apex. The complex morphology of the RV makes the correct echocardiographic evaluation difficult and implies great variation in the 2D measurement results of the RV diameters and area. In a study that included 900 patients, Tamborini G. et al. [11] demonstrated high inter- and intraobserver variabilities in the measurements of RV fractional area change (FAC), a parameter of RV systolic function. There are also difficulties in the echocardiographic examination of the right atria (RA). RA has an ellipsoid shape and includes crista terminalis, RA appendage, cavotricuspid isthmus, Eustachian valve, the orifice of the coronary sinus, and Thebesian valve. Echographic data include RA indexed major and minor axis length and systolic RA volume. The values are different in men and women, and the indexed RA volume using the single-plane method of disks has lower values than those obtained by the area-length method [12]. RA becomes dilated, and a process of RA remodeling occurs in longstanding PH. The RA pressure (RAP) increases, and its evaluation according to the diameter and inspiratory changes of the inferior vena cava (IVC) is an important parameter for the evaluation of RV systolic pressure in the absence of significant RV outflow tract obstruction. The RAP estimated non-invasively is the main source of errors in the assessment of both sPAP and mPAP. sPAP is calculated using the maximal velocity of tricuspid regurgitation flow (**Figure 1**) and mPAP by formulas that use pulmonary regurgitation flow velocity at the beginning of the diastole or pulmonary velocity acceleration time. Both can underestimate the PH in case of RV failure. RV failure can impede the left ventricle (LV) function by many mechanisms. So assessing the RV and LV morphology and function is essential for the correct diagnosis and prognostic of PH. The echocardiographic evaluation of the right heart can be improved through other methods, such as agitated saline study, echocardiographic contrast agents, speckle tracking, and 3D echocardiography [13]. 2D RV longitudinal strain of the free wall (RV-FWS) and 2D RV global longitudinal strain (RV-GLS), which includes in the analysis of the interventricular septum, can demonstrate subclinical impairment of the longitudinal contraction in patients with PH. The method is less angle and load-dependent and less influenced by the complex geometry of RV, but it depends on image quality that can be poor because of many artifacts [14, 15]. The analysis of segmental contractility of the RV walls by strain technique offers information about the pattern of RV remodeling in PH. The cut-off value proposed for RV-FWS is −23% and −20% for RV-GLS. For now, there is no consensus on which method to use, but it seems that RV-FWS is more useful. The 3D technique is more accurate than the 2D technique in the evaluation of RV strain.

Parameter	Method	Formula	Normal range	Abnormal values
Pulmonary artery flow evaluation				
Pulmonary velocity acceleration time (PAT)	Time to peak velocity of the pulmonary artery flow in parasternal short axis view (PW)		>130 ms	<105 ms and/or midsystolic notching
Systolic pulmonary arterial pressure	Maximum velocity of tricuspid regurgitation jet (CW)	$4V^2_{maxTRjet} + RAP$	18–25 mmHg; values of 40 mmHg can be normal after 60 years	≤35 mm Hg
Diastolic pulmonary arterial pressure (**Figure 2**)	End diastolic pulmonary regurgitant flow velocity (CW)	$4V^2_{PRenddiastolic} + RAP$	1. mm Hg	> 15 mm Hg
Mean pulmonary arterial pressure	Pulmonary regurgitant flow velocity at the beginning of the diastole (CW)	$4V^2_{PR\ early\ diastolic} + RAP$	10–20 mm Hg	>25 mmHg
	Pulmonary velocity acceleration time (PW)	$79 - 0.45xPAT$		
Pulmonary vascular resistance	Maximum velocity of tricuspid regurgitation (CW)	$0.16 + \frac{Vmax\ of\ TRjet}{VTIRVOT} x10^3$	<3 Wood units	>3 Wood units
Pulmonary velocity acceleration time (PW)	Time to peak the pulmonary flow		>130 ms	<100 ms
Right ventricle and RA evaluation				
RV and RA diameters				
RV diameters	2D	Basal, mid RV, longitudinal diameter, at the end-diastole RV/LV ratio, focused apical 4-chamber view	RV basal diameter 25–41 mm RV mid diameter 19–35 mm RV longitudinal diameter 59–83 mm	RV basal diameter > 41 mm RV mid diameter > 35 mm RV longitudinal diameter > 86 mm
RVOT dimensions	2D	Supra aortic valve diameter in end-systole (RVOT proximal diameter); basal short axis view, Supra pulmonary valve diameter, in end-systole (RVOT distal diameter); basal short axis view	RVOT proximal diameter 21–35 mm RVOT distal diameter 17–27 mm	RVOT proximal diameter > 35 mm RVOT distal diameter > 27 mm

Parameter	Method	Formula	Normal range	Abnormal values
RA dimensions	2D	Minor and major axis, area, volume, apical 4-chamber view, at end-systole	RA minor axis 1.9 ± 0.3 cm/m^2 RA major axis 2.5 ± 0.3 cm/m^2 RA volume 21 ± 6 mL/m^2 in women, 25 ± 7 mL/m^2 in men	RA minor axis > 4.4 cm RA major axis > 5.3 cm RA area > 18 cm^2 RA volume > 34 mL/m^2
RV free wall thickness	2D	Subcostal 4-chamber view, at end-diastole	1–5 mm	>5 mm
Interventricular septum	2D	Flattening, paradoxical movement		In the case of RV pressure overload, "the flattening" of IVS happens in both systole and diastole, in contrast to RV volume overload, with septal flattening predominantly during diastole.
LV maximal and end-systolic of eccentricity index	2D parasternal short-axis view at the mid-papillary level	The ratio of the diameters (from compact myocardium) parallel (D2) and perpendicular (D1) to the ventricular septum, as measured at end-diastole, end-systole, and maximum septal displacement		> 1.1
RV systolic function				
RV fractional area change (RVFAC)	2D, 3D	$\frac{\textit{End distolic area} - \textit{End systolic area}}{\textit{End diastolic area}(cm^2)}$ X100	49% ± 7%	< 35%
RV ejection fraction (**Figure 4**)	2D or 3D; only 3D method has been validated	Must be a good image quality	58% ± 6.5%	< 45%
Tricuspid annular plane systolic excursion (TAPSE)	M mode	Apical 4-chamber view	24 ± 3.5 mm	≤16 mm
Tricuspid annular systolic longitudinal velocity by tissue Doppler (S′)	Pulsed TDI	Apical 4-chamber view	14.1 ± 12.3 cm/s	<9.5 cm/s

Parameter	Method	Formula	Normal range	Abnormal values
RV myocardial performance index (RVMPI)	Measurement of isovolumic contraction time (IVCT $_{RV}$), isovolumic relaxation time (IVRT $_{RV}$), and ejection time (ET) from the same heartbeat using pulsed Doppler or TDI of tricuspid annulus	$(IVCT_{RV} + IVRT_{RV})/ET$		>0.4 for pulsed Doppler RVMPI > 0.55 for TDI RVMPI
Free-wall RV longitudinal strain (RV-FWS) and global RV longitudinal strain (RV – GLS)	Speckle tracking imaging	RV-focused apical 4-chamber view; because the interventricular septum is an integral part of the LV also, RV-GLS might be influenced by LV dysfunction.	RV - FWS 29% ± 4.5% RV-GLS 22.3% ± 2.4%	RV - FWS < 20% RV-GLS <17%
Rate of RV pressure rise during early systole (dP/dt)	TR jet	The value is calculated from the slope of the line between 1 and 2 m/s (4 to 16 mmHg) of the TR spectral envelope		<400 mmHg/s
RV diastolic evaluation				
Tricuspid inflow E/A, TDE	PW Doppler	Apical 4-chamber view	E/A 1.4 ± 0.3 TDE 180 ± 31 ms	E/A < 0.8 or > 2 TDE <119 ms or > 242 ms
RV lateral wall TDI	TDI	Apical 4-chamber view	E/e′ 4 ± 1	E/e' > 6
Inferior vena cava (IVC) diameter and inspiratory collapse are used for the estimation of RA pressure (RAP)		IVC ≤ 2.1 cm, collapses >50% during sniff—RAP 0–5 mm Hg IVC > 2.1 cm, collapses >50% during sniff—RAP 5–10 mm Hg IVC > 2.1 cm, collapses <50% during sniff—RAP 10–20 mm Hg		

RVOT = right ventricle outflow tract; VTIRVOT = velocity time integral in the right ventricle outflow tract; PR = pulmonary regurgitation; TDE = E wave deceleration time; V = velocity; TDI = tissue Doppler imaging; LV = left ventricle; PW = pulse wave; CW = continuous wave; and IVC = inferior vena cava.

Table 1.
Echocardiographic parameters used for the diagnosis of pulmonary hypertension.

Also, right ventricular ejection fraction (RVEF) calculated by the 3D technique (3D-RVEF) is far more accurate than that calculated by the 2D technique (2D-RVEF) because it is independent of geometric assumptions. 3D-RVEF but not 2D-RVEF is validated in relation to cardiac magnetic resonance (CMR) imaging, the "gold standard" for assessing RVEF.

Also, 3D speckle–tracking technique provides a more accurate assessment of ventricular myocardial dynamics than 2D speckle-tracking, which is limited by the out-of-plane motion of different frames. At the same time, measurement of RVEF by 3D echocardiography is not possible in all patients because it requires good image quality [15]. Evaluation of RV shape by 3D technique is not currently used in clinical practice. In patients with a good image of tricuspid regurgitation Doppler signal, one can calculate other parameters with prognostic values, such as right ventricle-pulmonary artery coupling (RV-PA) and myocardial work.

Each technique has its limits, and one must use a multimodal evaluation of the anatomy and function of RV. Furthermore, these new echographic techniques are not standardized between different vendors. Indeed, the gold standard for RVEF evaluation remains for now cardiac magnetic resonance imaging. **Table 1** includes the echocardiographic parameters used in the evaluation of PH and RV.

Table 1 includes the echocardiographic parameters used in the evaluation of PH and RV (**Figures 1–4**).

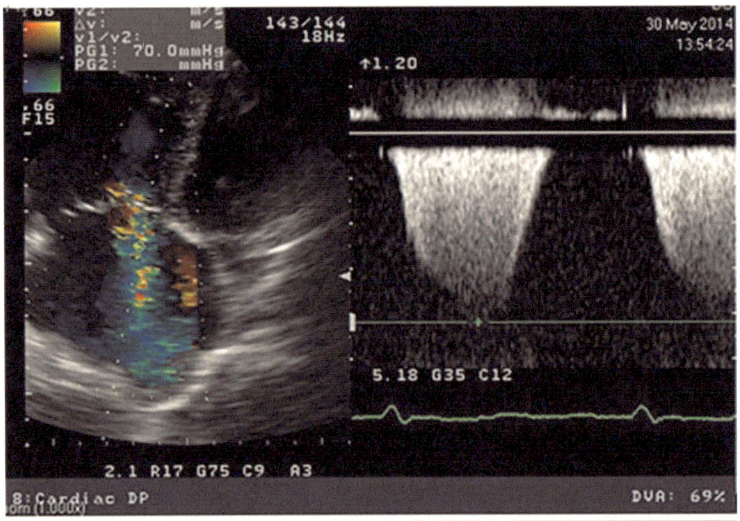

Figure 1.
Parasternal four chamber view. Tricuspid regurgitation (continuous Doppler examination). Right atrial dilation.

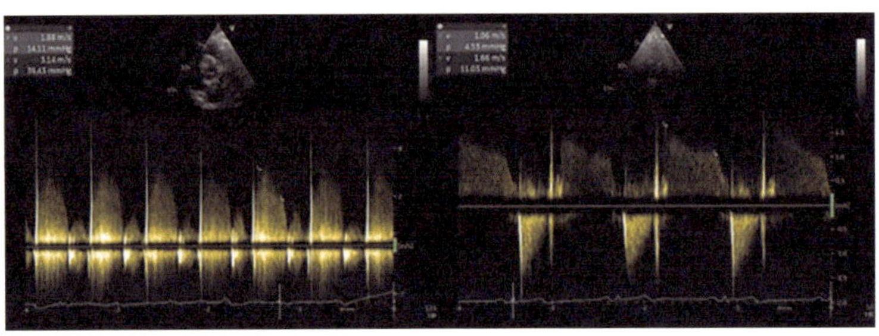

Figure 2.
Example of measurement of mPAP and dPAP in a case with pulmonary hypertension (left) versus a case without pulmonary hypertension (right). Left image: In this case, there was a dilated inferior vena cava with a diameter of 36 mm without respiratory variations. $mPAP = 4\ V^2_{PR\ early\ diastolic} + RAP = 4x3.14^2 + 20 = 54.43$ *mm Hg;* $dPAP = 4\ V^2_{PRenddiastolic} + RAP = 4x1.88^2 + 20 = 34.13$ *mm Hg. Right image: In this case, there was an inferior* vena cava *with a diameter of 16 mm with inspiratory collapse.* $mPAP = 4\ V^2_{PR\ early\ diastolic} + RAP = 4x1.66^2 + 3 = 14$ *mm Hg;* $dPAP = 4\ V^2_{PRenddiastolic} + RAP = 4x1.06^2 + 3 = 7.5$ *mm Hg.*

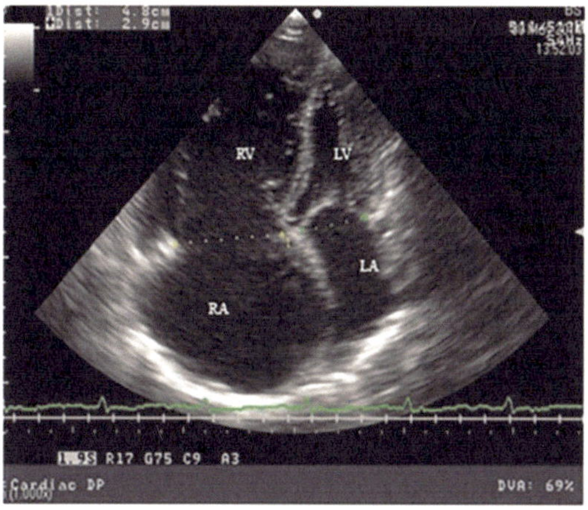

Figure 3.
Apical 4-chamber view. Dilation of the right ventricle (RV) and right atrium (RA). Displacement of the interventricular septum toward the left ventricle (LV) and interatrial septum toward the left atrium (LA).

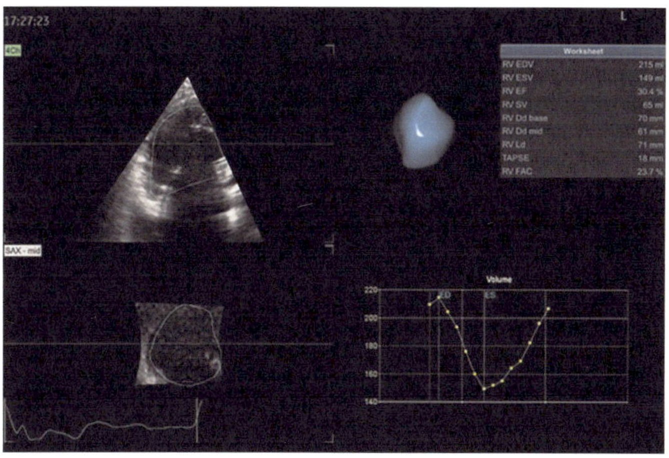

Figure 4.
3D quantification of the right ventricular ejection fraction.

2. Prognostic value of the echocardiographic data in PH

According to the clinical, biochemical, echocardiographic, or other imaging data, patients with PH can be classified as low, intermediate, and high risk of clinical worsening or death [1]. Patients categorized as low risk have estimated 1-year mortality of <5%, those categorized as intermediate risk have estimated 1-year mortality of 5–10%, and those in the high-risk category >10% [1].

The ESC guidelines on pulmonary hypertension propose an echocardiographic risk assessment in PH according to the right atrial area (area over 26 cm^2) (**Figure 1**) and the presence of pericardial effusion (**Figure 2**) [1]. However, many studies demonstrated the usefulness of other echocardiographic parameters as prognostic factors in PH. Patients, with PH and EI above 1.7 (**Figure 2**) combined with TAPSE below 15 mm, have a higher death rate than patients with normal values. The diastolic dysfunction of the RV, expressed by the changes in tricuspid flow E/A ratio and RV relaxation abnormalities by TDI, is associated with a poor prognosis. The systolic dysfunction of the RV is related to a poor prognosis of the PH: TAPSE less than 18 mm, tricuspid S′ < 9.5 cm/s assessed by TDI, 3D - RVEF below 45%, RVFAC less than 35%, dP/dt below 400 mmHg/s on the TR flow, reduced strain of the RV using speckle tracking echocardiography (**Figure 5**).

Many studies support the prognostic role of classical echocardiographic data in PH.

- Raynold RM et al. [16] evaluated the relationships between echocardiographic findings and clinical outcomes in 81 patients with severe primary PH during a mean follow-up period of 36.9–15.4 months. Pericardial effusion and enlarged indexed RA area were independent predictors of a composite end point of death or pulmonary transplantation. They found that septal shift in diastole toward LV is also a predictor of death or pulmonary transplantation. A dilated RA can be a sign of volume and/or pressure overload, and elevated RA pressure is a sign of poor RV ejection fraction [17].

- Austin C et al. [18] performed a retrospective analysis of 121 consecutive patients with pulmonary arterial hypertension during 3 years of follow-up. They demonstrated in a univariate analysis that RA pressure > 15 mmHg, calculated by inferior *vena cava* diameter and collapsibility, RA area > 18 cm^2, the presence of pericardial effusion, RVFAC < 35% and at least moderate TR were predictive of poor survival. However, in the multivariate analysis, RA pressure > 15 mm Hg was the only echocardiographic risk factor predictive of mortality.

- Liu K et al. [19] performed a meta-analysis that included 12 studies totalizing 1085 patients with pulmonary arterial hypertension followed up 9.2 months to 5.0 years. The risk of all-cause mortality and the composite endpoint of death and other PH events was increased in patients with enlarged RA area and RA area index.

- TAPSE less than 1.8 cm was associated with lower RVFAC, lower cardiac index, and reduced survival in 63 patients with PH [20]. The 2 years survival rate was 50% in patients with TAPSE less than 1.8 cm and 88% in those with greater TAPSE. However, TAPSE assessed by M mode cannot discriminate an active contraction from passive entrainment. On the other side, the assessment of TAPSE by RV strain can obtain greater values because TAPSE measures the maximum displacement, and strain measures the peak systolic contraction.

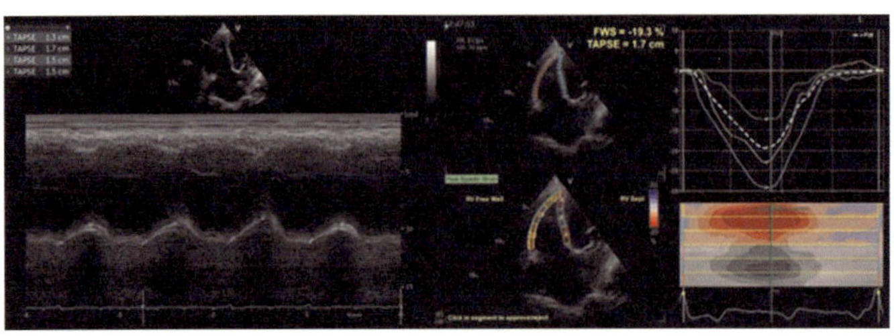

Figure 5.
Example of measurement of free wall right ventricular strain (FWS). Strain-based TAPSE is an approximated M-mode TAPSE, by calculation of the excursion relative to the image apex.

- In a prospective cohort study that included 777 patients with precapillary PH with a follow-up period of 7 years, the multivariable analysis demonstrated that moderate or severe tricuspid regurgitation, RVMPI, presence of pericardial effusion, but not TAPSE were independent predictors of mortality. The authors explained this fact by the presence of severe tricuspid regurgitation in most patients, which can induce a pseudo-normal TAPSE [21].

- Ghio S. et al. [22] examined data from 517 patients, mean age 52 ± 15 years, 64.8% females, included in seven observational studies. They divided patients into three groups according to TAPSE, tricuspid regurgitation, the diameter of inferior *vena cava*, and noted the 5 years cumulative survival. High-risk patients had impaired TAPSE and dilated inferior *vena cava*, and their 5 years cumulative survival rate was 43%, versus 82% in low-risk patients, with normal TAPSE and no tricuspid regurgitation. The intermediate-risk group had normal TAPSE and significant tricuspid regurgitation or impaired TAPSE and non-dilated inferior *vena cava*. Their 5 years cumulative survival rate was 63%. Data from this analysis suggested that the inclusion of the RA area and pericardial effusion did not provide added prognostic value.

- Barket D et al. [23] demonstrated in 78 pediatric patients with PH that an end-systolic EI > 1. 16 identifies the presence of PH, and an end-systolic EI > 1.27 correlates with a higher number of hospitalization and escalation of the therapy.

- RVMPI and the rate of RV pressure rise during early systole (dP/dt) proved to correlate with pulmonary vascular resistance and to predict a reduced RVEF [17].

- Elevated RAP is a sign of poor right ventricular failure [17].

- Blanchard D. et al. [24] demonstrated in 93 patients with chronic thromboembolic pulmonary hypertension that elevated RVMPI measured by TDI correlated with pulmonary vascular resistance but not with mPAP and cardiac output.

- Habbad et al. [25] elaborated a right heart score for the outcome of patients with familial, idiopathic, drug-induced, and toxic PH based on the examination of 95 patients, 43 ± 11 years old, with mean pulmonary arterial pressure of 54 ± 14 mm Hg, and pulmonary vascular resistance index 25 ± 12 Wood units, followed for 5 years. The severity of RV systolic dysfunction, RA enlargement, and systolic blood pressure < 110 mmHg were independently associated with death and lung transplantation.

- Kamimura Y. et al. [26] proposed a prognostic score in chronic thromboembolic pulmonary hypertension calculated as the summation of each point awarded for the presence of four parameters: TAPSE < 16 mm, 1 point, TDI-derived tricuspid lateral annular systolic velocity (S′) < 10 cm/sec, 1 point, RVFAC < 35% 1 point and RVMPI > 0.4, 1 point. An elevated RV dysfunction prognostic score was associated with an advanced functional class of heart failure, elevated mPAP, low cardiac index, high pulmonary vascular resistance, reduced mixed venous oxygen saturation, reduced 6-min walk distance, low maximal O_2 consumption, prolonged slope of minute ventilation/CO_2 production, and elevated plasma brain natriuretic peptide level.

- REVEAL study (US Registry to Evaluate Early and Long-Term PAH Disease Management) [16] enrolled 2716 patients with PAH and assessed predictors of 1-year survival. In the multivariable analysis, variables independently associated with increased mortality included PVR > 32 Wood units, PAH associated with portal hypertension, New York Heart Association functional class IV, men > 60 years of age, and family history of PAH.

- Badagliacca R et al. [27] investigated during 528 ± 304 days 130 patients with idiopathic pulmonary hypertension. They demonstrated that clinical, functional class of heart failure, cardiac index, and RVFAC were the independent predictors of the clinical worsening of the patients.

- The most frequently used parameters for the assessment of prognostic in PH in real-world practice are presented in **Table 2** [28, 29].

Speckle tracking echocardiography applied to the RV has demonstrated its utility in the prognostic stratification of patients with PH:

- Park JH et al. [30] determined RV-GLS in 81 patients with PAH with a follow-up period of 45 ± 15 months. They showed a significant correlation between RV-GLS and RVFAC, TAPSE, RVMPI, pulmonary vascular resistance, and B-natriuretic peptide concentration. In the multivariate analysis, RV-GLS ≥ −15.5% and age were the independent predictor factors for death, lung transplantation, and heart failure hospitalization. Accepted normal values for RV-GLS were − 28%.

- Badagliacca R et al. [31] analyzed RV strain patterns using the speckle tracking technique and identified three post-systolic strain patterns derived from the

Echocardiographic parameters	Abnormal values predicting a poor prognosis of PH
TAPSE	<16 mm
S′	<10 cm/s
RV FAC	<35%
Peak longitudinal RV strain	≥−19%
Isovolumetric contraction velocity (IVCv) by TDI	<9 cm/s
Main PA diameter	>29 mm
LV eccentricity index	>1.4
Pericardial effusion	presence
IVC	>21 mm, inspiratory collapse <50%

TAPSE = tricuspid annular plane systolic excursion; S′ = right ventricle free wall tissue Doppler systolic velocity during ejection period (Lateral tricuspid annulus peak systolic velocity); RVFAC = right ventricle fractional area changes PA = pulmonary artery; LV = left ventricle; and TDI = tissue Doppler imaging.

Table 2.
Echocardiographic parameters recommended in clinical practice for the assessment of PH prognosis.

mid-basal RV free wall segments. Pattern 1 was characterized by a prompt return of strain-time curves to baseline after peak systolic negativity, like in normal control subjects, and corresponded to mild PH. Pattern 2 was characterized by persisting negativity of strain-time curves well into diastole before an end-diastolic returning to baseline and corresponded to more advanced PH with preserved RV function. Pattern 3 was characterized by a slow return of strain-time curves to baseline during diastole corresponded to PH with end-stage RV failure. 60% and respectively 33% of patients with Pattern 3 had a faster-worsening disease assessed at 1 and 2 years

- RV longitudinal strain is superior to TAPSE as a prognostic factor in PH [32]

- RV-arterial coupling reflects both RV after-load and contractility and has prognostic value in PH. It can be assessed using various parameters, such as TAPSE, FAC, 3D-RVEF, which are divided to sPAP [15]. Serkan Unlu et al. [33] determined RA-arterial coupling by the ratio between RV-FWS and sPAP in 65 patients with precapillary PH and found a predictive value for death or heart/lung transplantation with a cut-off of 0.19.

- RV myocardial work enables the evaluation of the contractility of RV independent of the load and a more precise estimate of RV systolic function. It is a promised parameter but not in clinical practice.

3. 3D echocardiography has become increasingly important in the evaluation of RV

- Murata M et al. [34] highlighted the importance of evaluating RV ejection fraction by 3D technique in 85 patients with PH. They showed that patients with 3DRVEF of less than 38% had significantly shorter event-free survival than those with 3DRVEF greater than 38%. A total of 36 patients had mPAP >35 mmHg and a theoretical event-free survival in 2.5 years. Those with greater 3DRVEF had an event-free survival rate of 70% at 2.5 years. This suggests that 3DRVEF is an independent prognosis factor in patients with PH.

- Vitarelli A. et al. [35] studied 73 patients, mean age 53 ± 13 years with chronic PH of different etiologies, and 30 healthy subjects as a control group. They determined RVFAC, TAPSE, mitral and tricuspid TDI annular velocities, 3D RV volumes, 3D RV EF, and RV strains by 2D RV and 3D RV-speckle-tracking echocardiography. RV 3D global-free-wall longitudinal strain (3DGFW-RVLS), 2D global-free-wall longitudinal strain (2DGFW-RVLS), apical-free-wall longitudinal strain, basal-free-wall longitudinal strain, and 3D-RVEF were lower in patients with PH. Also, patients with precapillary PH had lower global and regional peak systolic RV free-wall strain than those with postcapillary PH. 3D-GFW-RVLS and 3D-RVEF were the independent predictors of mortality. 3D RVEF, 2D-STE, and 3D-STE parameters indicate global and regional RV dysfunction associated with RV failure hemodynamics better than conventional echo indices.

- The validity and prognostic importance of 3D-RVEF were recently demonstrated in 446 unselected patients with various cardiac diseases with a follow-up period of 4.1 ± 1.2 years. Patients with 3DRVEF > 45% had the best prognosis, and those with 3DRVEF under 30% had the worst prognosis [36].

4. RV dysfunction as a prognostic factor in patients with cardiac resynchronization therapy (CRT) and cardiac surgery

The evaluation of the RV dysfunction has a prognostic role in the short and long-term outcomes of patients after cardiac resynchronization therapy (CRT). Nagy VC. et al. [37] studied 93 patients with heart failure and low basal value of RV global longitudinal strain and RV free wall strain.

- RV global longitudinal strain below 10.04% before CRT was associated with high 24-month mortality.

- Preoperative RV dysfunction is a prognostic factor for perioperative complications in cardiac surgery [38]. There are studies that demonstrate preoperatory RVFAC <32% and RVMPI >0.5 are prognostic factors for postoperative circulatory failure, higher incidence of postoperative inotropic support, and longer stay in the intensive care unit. Preoperative RVFAC <20% is associated with late postoperative death [39]. The prognostic role of preoperative RV dysfunction is important in both coronary bypass and valvular surgery. Echocardiographic parameters of RV function proposed as preoperative poor prognostic factors included RVFAC<25%, bowing end-systole or end-diastole interventricular septum into left ventricle (flattening or paradoxical movement), TAPSE<1.4 cm, RV longitudinal strain $\leq -15\%$, TAPSE/sPAP [40].

5. Conclusions

The evaluation of the function of RV in PH is essential in establishing the prognosis of PH. In addition to the size of the RA and the presence of pericardial effusion proposed by the guidelines, there are many echocardiographic parameters with prognostic value in PH. They are related to the systolic and diastolic dysfunction of the right ventricle explored by new echocardiographical techniques such as speckle tracking and 3D imaging. These promising techniques investigate in depth the function of the RV and the correlation between RV and pulmonary artery and allow an early diagnosis of the impairment of the RV in PH. Also, the new echographic techniques are useful in the prognostic evaluation of CRT and cardiac surgery. However, each of the echocardiographic parameters used in the assessment of the right ventricle has technical limitations, and it is necessary to use multiple clinical, biological, and echocardiographic tests for a correct evaluation of the prognosis of PH. The complexity of the RV makes useful a multiparametric examination, and modern techniques are increasingly useful. The modern multimodal evaluation of the RV includes not only echocardiography but also cardiac magnetic resonance, nuclear imaging techniques, metabolic imaging techniques, and cardiac scanners. Last but not the least, the influence of RV dysfunction on the LV can be systematically assessed.

Author details

Gabriela Silvia Gheorghe[1], Andrei Cristian Dan Gheorghe[2*], Ana Ciobanu[1,2] and Andreea Simona Hodorogea[1,2]

1 Cardiology and Internal Medicine Department, Theodor Burghele Clinical Hospital, Bucharest, Romania

2 Carol Davila University of Medicine and Pharmacy, Bucharest, Romania

*Address all correspondence to: acd2403@yahoo.com

References

[1] Galie N, Humbert M, Vachiery J-L, Gibbs S, Lang I, Torbicki A, et al. 2015 ESC/ERS guidelines for the diagnosis and treatment of pulmonary hypertension the joint task force for the diagnosis and treatment of pulmonary hypertension of the european society of cardiology (ESC) and the european respiratory society (ERS). European Heart Journal. 2016;**37**(1):67-119. DOI: 10.1093/eurheartj/ehv317

[2] Armstrong WF. Thomas Ryan Feigenbaum's Echocardiography. eight ed. Wolters-Kluwer; 2019. ISBN-13 978-1-4511-9427-2

[3] Lang RM, Goldstein SA, Kronzon I, Khanderhia BA, Saric M, Mor-Avi V. ASE's Comprehensive Echocardiography. third ed. Philadelphia, PA: Elsevier; 2022. pp. 19103-2899. ISBN 9780323698306 Library of Congress Control Number 2020945518, printed in Canada

[4] Ginghină C, Popescu B. Ruxandra Jurcuț Esențialul în ECOCARDIOGRAFIE. Editura Medicala Antaeus. 2nd ed. 2013. pp. 259-274. www.antaeus.ro. ISBN 24 978-606-8470-02-3

[5] Grünig E, Henn P, D'Andrea A, Claussen M, Ehlken N, Maier F, et al. Reference values for and determinants of right atrial area in healthy adults by 2-dimensional echocardiography. Circulation: Cardiovascular Imaging. 2013;**6**:117-124. DOI: 10.1161/CIRCIMAGING.112.978031

[6] Parasuraman S, Walker S, Loudon BL, Gollop ND, Wilson AM, Lowery C, et al. Assessment of pulmonary artery pressure by echocardiography—A comprehensive review. IJC Heart & Vasculature. 2016; **6**(12):45-51

[7] DiLorenzo MP, Bhatt SM. Laura Mercer-Rosa How best to assess right ventricular function by echocardiography. Cardiology in the Young. 2015;**25**(8):1473-1481. DOI: 10.1017/S1047951115002255

[8] Benza RL, Miller DP, Gomberg-Maitland M, Frantz RP, Foreman AJ, Coffey CS, et al. Predicting survival in pulmonary arterial hypertension insights from the registry to evaluate early and long-term pulmonary arterial hypertension disease management (REVEAL). Circulation. 2010;**122**:164-172

[9] Ho SY, Nihoyannopoulos P. Anatomy, echocardiography, and normal right ventricular dimensions. Heart. 2006;**92**(Suppl. 1):i2-i13. DOI: 10.1136/hrt.2005.077875

[10] Zaidi A, Knight DS, Augustine DX, Harkness A, Oxborough D, Pearce K, et al., editors. Vishal Sharma echocardiographic assessment of the right heart in adults: A practical guideline from the British Society of Echocardiography, 2020 British Society of Echocardiography. Echo Research & Practice. 2020;**7**:G19-G41. DOI: 10.1530/ERP-19-0051

[11] Tamborini G, Pepi M, Galli CA, Maltagliati A, Celeste F, Muratori M, et al. Feasibility and accuracy of a routine echocardiographic assessment of right ventricular function. International Journal of Cardiology. 2007;**115**(1):86-89. DOI: 10.1016/j.ijcard.2006.01.017

[12] Lang RM, Cameli M, Sade LE, Faletra F, Fortuni F, Rossi A, et al. Imaging assessment of the right atrium: anatomy and function. European Heart Journal-Cardiovascular Imaging. 2022;**23**:867-884. DOI: 10.1093/ehjci/jeac011

[13] Jones N, Burns AT, Prior DL. Echocardiographic assessment of the right ventricle–state of the art. Heart, Lung and Circulation. 2019;**28**: 1339-1350. DOI: 10.1016/j.hlc.2019.04.016

[14] Gripari P, Muratori M, Fusini L, Tamborini G, Ali SG, Brusoni D, et al. Right ventricular dimensions and function: Why do we need a more accurate and quantitative imaging? Journal of Cardiovascular Echography. 2015;**25**(1):19-25. DOI: 10.4103/2211-4122.158420

[15] Surkova E, Cosyns B, Gerber B, Gimelli A, La Gerche A, Marsan NA. The dysfunctional right ventricle: The importance of multi-modality Imaging. European Heart Journal - Cardiovascular Imaging. 2022;**23**:885-897. DOI: 10.1093/ehjci/jeac037)

[16] Raymond RJ, Hinderliter AL, Willis PW, IV DR, Caldwell EJ, Williams W, et al. Echocardiographic Predictors of Adverse Outcomes in Primary Pulmonary Hypertension. Journal of the American College of Cardiology. 2002;**39**(7):1214-1219

[17] Schneider OM, Binder T. Echocardiographic evaluation of the right heart. Wiener Klinische Wochenschrift. 2018;**130**:413-420. DOI: 10.1007/s00508-018-1330-3

[18] Austin C, Alassas K, Burger C, Safford R, Pagan R, Duello K, et al. Echocardiographic assessment of estimated right atrial pressure and size predicts mortality in pulmonary arterial hypertension. Chest. 2015;**147**(1): 198-208. DOI: 10.1378/chest.13-3035

[19] Liu K, Zhang C, Chen B, Li M, Zhang P. Association between right atrial area measured by echocardiography and prognosis among pulmonary arterial hypertension: A systematic review and meta-analysis. BMJ Open. 2020;**10**: e031316. DOI: 10.1136/bmjopen-2019-031316

[20] Forfia PR, Fisher MR, Thai SC, Housten-Harris T, Hemnes AR, Borlaug BA, et al. Tricuspid annular displacement predicts survival in pulmonary hypertension. American Journal of Respiratory and Critical Care Medicine. 2006;**174**:1034-1041

[21] Grapsa J, Nunes MCP, Tan TC, Cabrita IZ, Coulter T, Smith BCF, et al. Echocardiographic and hemodynamic predictors of survival in precapillary pulmonary hypertension seven-year follow-up. Circulation: Cardiovascular Imaging. 2015;**8**:45-54. DOI: 10.1161/CIRCIMAGING.114.002107

[22] Ghio S, Mercurio V, Fortuni F, Forfia PR, Gall H, Ghofrani A, et al. A comprehensive echocardiographic method for risk stratification in pulmonary arterial hypertension. European Respiratory Journal. 2020;**56**(3):2000513. DOI: 10.1183/13993003.00513-2020

[23] Burkett DA, Patel SS, Mertens L, Friedberg MK, Ivy D. Relationship between left ventricular geometry and invasive hemodynamics in pediatric pulmonary hypertension. Circulation: Cardiovascular Imaging. 2020;**13**: e009825. DOI: 10.1161/CIRCIMAGING.119.009825

[24] Blanchard DG, Malouf PJ, Gurudevan SV, Auger WR, Madani MM, Thistlethwaite P, et al. Utility of right ventricular tei index in the noninvasive evaluation of chronic thromboembolic pulmonary hypertension before and after pulmonary thromboendarterectomy A C. Cardiovascular Imaging. 2009;**2**(2): 143-149

[25] Haddad F, Spruijt OA, Denault AY, Mercier O, Brunner N, Furman D, et al. Right heart score for predicting outcome in idiopathic, familial, or drug- and toxin-associated pulmonary arterial hypertension JACC. Cardiovascular Imaging. 2015;**8**(6):627-638

[26] Kamimura Y, Okumura N, Adachi S, Shimokata S, Tajima F, Nakano Y, et al. Usefulness of scoring right ventricular function for assessment of prognostic factors in patients with chronic thromboembolic pulmonary hypertension. Heart and Vessels. 2018; **33**:1220-1228. DOI: 10.1007/s00380-018-1168-7

[27] Badagliacca R, Papa S, Valli G, Pezzuto B, Poscia R, Manzi G, et al. Echocardiography combined with cardiopulmonary exercise testing for the prediction of outcome in idiopathic pulmonary arterial hypertension. Chest. 2016;**150**(6):1313-1322. DOI: 10.1016/j.chest.2016.07.036

[28] Moceri P, Baudouy D, Chiche O, Cerboni P, Bouvier P, Chaussade C, et al. Imaging in pulmonary hypertension: Focus on the role of echocardiography. Archives of Cardiovascular Disease. 2014;**107**:261-271

[29] Frost A, Badesch D, Simon J, Gibbs R, Gopalan D, Khanna D, et al. Diagnosis of pulmonary hypertension. European Respiratory Journal. 2019;**53**: 1801904. DOI: 101183/13993003.01904-20180

[30] Park J-H, Park MM, Farha S, Sharp J, Lundgrin E, Comhair S, et al. Impaired global right ventricular longitudinal strain predicts long-term adverse outcomes in patients with pulmonary arterial hypertension. Journal of Cardiovascular Ultrasound. 2015;**23**(2): 91-99

[31] Badagliacca R, Pezzuto B, Papa S, Poscia R, Manzi G, Pascaretta A, et al. Right ventricular strain curve morphology and outcome in idiopathic pulmonary arterial hypertension. Cardiovascular Imaging. 2021;**14**(1): 162-172

[32] Muraru D, Haugaa K, Donal E, Stankovic I, Voigt JU, Petersen SE, et al. Right ventricular longitudinal strain in the clinical routine: A state-of-the-art review. European Heart Journal - Cardiovascular Imaging. 2022;**23**(7): 898-912. DOI: 10.1093/ehjci/jeac022

[33] Ünlü S, Bézy S, Cvijic M, Duchenne J, Delcroix M, Voigt JU. Right ventricular strain related to pulmonary artery pressure predicts clinical outcome in patients with pulmonary arterial hypertension. European Heart Journal – Cardiovascular Imaging. 2022;jeac136. DOI: 10.1093/ehjci/jeac136

[34] Murata M, Tsugu T, Kawakami T, Kataoka M, Minakata Y, Endo J, et al. Prognostic value of three-dimensional echocardiographic right ventricular ejection fraction in patients with pulmonary arterial hypertension. Oncotarget. 2016;**7**(52):86781-86790

[35] Vitarelli A, Mangieri E, Terzano C, Gaudio C, Salsano F, Rosato E, et al. Three-dimensional echocardiography and 2D-3D speckle-tracking imaging in chronic pulmonary hypertension: Diagnostic accuracy in detecting hemodynamic signs of right ventricular (RV) failure. Journal of the American Heart Association. 2015;**4**: e001584

[36] Muraru D, Badano LP, Nagata Y, Surkova E, Nabeshima Y, Genovese D, et al. Development and prognostic validation of partition values to grade right ventricular dysfunction severity using 3D echocardiography. European

Heart Journal - Cardiovascular Imaging. 2020;**21**:10-21

[37] Nagy VK, Széplaki G, Apor A, Kutyifa V, Kovács A, Kosztin A, et al. Role of right ventricular global longitudinal strain in predicting early and long-term mortality in cardiac resynchronization therapy patients. PlosOne. 2015. DOI: 10.1371/journal.pone.0143907

[38] Haddad F, Couture P, Tousignant C, Denault AY. The right ventricle in cardiac surgery, a perioperative perspective: II. Pathophysiology, clinical importance, and management. Anesthesia and Analgesia. 2009;**108**(2): 422-433

[39] Wencker D, Borer JS, Hochreiter C, Devereux RB, Roman MJ, Kligfield P, et al. Preoperative predictors of late postoperative outcome among patients with nonischemic mitral regurgitation with 'high risk' descriptors and comparison with unoperated patients. Cardiology. 2000;**93**:37-42

[40] Navaratnam M, DiNardo JA. Perioperative right ventricular dysfunction - The anesthesiologist's view. Cardiovascular Diagnosis and Therapy. 2020;**10**(5):1725-1734. DOI: 10.21037/cdt-20-426)

Chapter 19

The Association of Hair Cortisol and Cardiometabolic Risk Factors in Cardiovascular Disease

Jennifer C. Van Wyk

Abstract

Hair cortisol is increasingly becoming a reliable measure of long-term cortisol concentration and is thought to be a suitable biomarker for chronic stress. Further, a growing amount of scientific literature links elevated hair cortisol concentration with well-known cardiometabolic risk factors such as hypertension, obesity, dyslipidemia, and diabetes. This has important implications for the prognosis, treatment, and prevention of cardiovascular disease. This review focuses on the association between increased hair cortisol and stress-related cardiometabolic risk factors for cardiovascular disease. While the evidence for the relationship between cardiometabolic risk and elevated hair cortisol is clear and compelling, the data is inconsistent. Further studies are needed to support the use of hair cortisol as a biomarker of cardiometabolic risk in cardiovascular disease.

Keywords: cardiovascular disease, hair cortisol, cardiometabolic risk, obesity, hypertension, dyslipidemia, diabetes

1. Introduction

Cardiovascular disease (CVD) continues to be the primary cause of morbidity and mortality worldwide [1]. In 2019, approximately 17.9 million people died from CVDs, representing 32% of all global deaths [2]. Eighty-five percent of CVD deaths resulted from heart attack and stroke. These high numbers are especially concerning since most CVDs are preventable or modifiable by addressing behavioral risk factors, such as a sedentary lifestyle, unhealthy diet, tobacco use, and harmful use of alcohol [1–3]. Early detection is essential in eradicating or in beginning management of cardiovascular disease with counseling and medications.

Cardiometabolic risk (CMR) refers to the risk factors that increase the likelihood of experiencing cardiovascular events or developing metabolic disease [4]. Besides the traditional cardiovascular risk factors (age, gender, family history, hypertension, diabetes, and smoking), CMR factors include abdominal obesity, insulin resistance, inflammation, unhealthy eating habits, and a sedentary lifestyle (**Figure 1**). Several cross-sectional clinical studies have shown a positive association between cortisol and cardiometabolic risk factors. With stress being an integral part of modern life that has become a significant health problem [5, 6], the importance of biomarkers that can assist in the treatment of stress-related diseases should only increase.

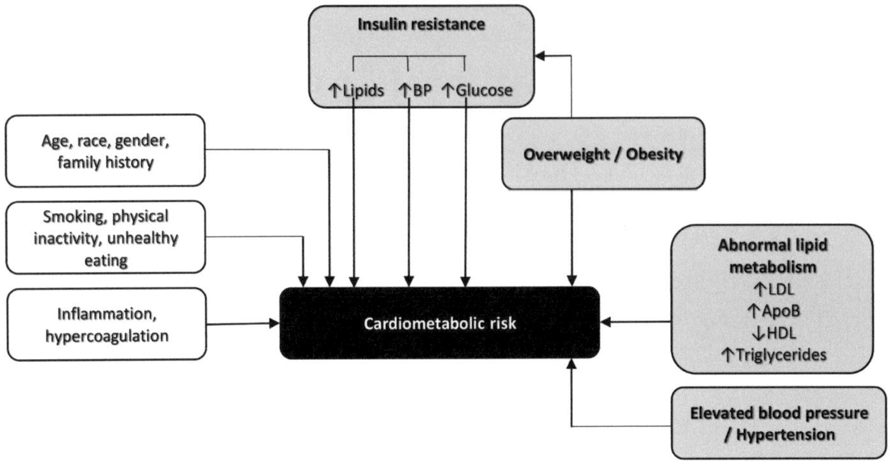

Figure 1.
Factors contributing to cardiometabolic risk.

In particular, hair cortisol concentration (HCC) is gaining interest as a promising biomarker for cardiometabolic risk [7]. However, research investigating the direct association between HCC and cardiometabolic risk factors is still in its infancy, and more extensive prospective cohort studies are needed to gain further insight into the relationship between HCC, CMR, and the development of CVD. Unhealthy lifestyles such as physical inactivity, smoking, and excessive alcohol use also result in elevated cortisol levels and are associated with cardiometabolic risk and cardiovascular disease [4]. However, this review focuses on biological factors linked to high cortisol levels and stress that are activated through the hypothalamic-pituitary-adrenal (HPA) axis pathway, including hypertension, obesity, dyslipidemia, and diabetes.

2. Laboratory determination of hair cortisol concentration (HCC)

Different laboratories use similar methods to measure HCC with minor variations in experimental procedures. Usually, the proximal 3 cm of hair which represents the last 3 months of cortisol production, is collected [8, 9]. Using the most proximal segments reduces the potential for a 'wash-out effect' which relates to a decline in cortisol levels in distal segments due to ultraviolet radiation and hair care practices [8]. The hair sample is carefully sectioned into segment lengths that approximate the period of interest, for example, cut into 1 cm fragments, or whole hair samples are used. Hair grows approximately 1 cm per month, so this is a convenient approximation of changes in HCC each month [9].

The hair is then either finely minced with scissors or pulverized with a ball mill. The mass of hair used for analysis varies between studies, with a range of 2.5–50 mg for ELISA and 1.25–20 mg for LCMS [10]. Next, the samples are incubated in a solvent such as methanol for a set period to extract the cortisol. The extraction medium is evaporated to dryness and the extracted cortisol is reconstituted in a solution such as phosphate-buffered saline or distilled water. HCC is typically measured using two types of analyses: immunoassays or mass spectrometry [9, 10]. Immunoassays used for the analysis include enzyme-linked immunosorbent assay (ELISA), immunoassay with chemiluminescence detection (CLIA), and radioimmunoassay (RIA).

Alternatively, liquid chromatography-mass spectrometry (LCMS) is used to determine HCC. Typically, the inter- and intra-assay coefficients of variability (cvs) are reported to indicate variability between measurements using different plates or tests and between duplicate samples on the same plate, respectively [10].

As the clinical utilization of HCC increases, it is important to establish an international benchmark [8, 9, 11]. Russell *et al.* conducted a study comparing the cortisol testing protocols of four leading laboratories, which include four ELISA methods and two LCMS methods, by analyzing the same hair samples representing the low, intermediate, and high ranges of hair cortisol concentrations (HCC) [9]. This study showed significant positive correlations between the four different immunoassay methods, while the results for the LCMS methods were almost identical. Further, the study concluded that laboratories using immunoassays could use a correction factor to convert results into standard LCMS equivalents.

3. The role of long-term hair cortisol levels in CVD risk

Stress can be defined as any stimuli that can alter homeostasis and causes physical, emotional, or psychological strain. It impairs both physical and physiological health [6], resulting in a higher risk for obesity, type 2 diabetes mellitus, and cardiovascular diseases [5, 6]. Stress can be the result of psychosocial factors like anxiety, social isolation, and traumatic life events. Although some stress is beneficial and helps the body cope (e.g., with inflammation), excessive/prolonged stress can be harmful [12–15]. The response to stress is mediated by the "stress hormone" cortisol, which is released in higher doses under an excessive amount of stress [12]. Cortisol is a lipid-soluble glucocorticoid hormone that regulates a wide range of basal processes throughout the body, including metabolism, and immune response, and, most importantly, it helps the body to respond to stress and to maintain homeostasis. Cortisol does this by increasing blood sugar through gluconeogenesis, suppressing the immune system, and increasing the metabolism of fat, glucose, protein, and carbohydrates [13]. The production of cortisol is housed in the cortex of the adrenal glands and then released into the bloodstream, which transports it throughout the body [12]. Cortisol is an end product of the Hypothalamic-Pituitary-Adrenal (HPA) axis; its secretion in response to biochemical stress may influence health and cognitive events [12, 13].

The hypothalamic-pituitary-adrenal (HPA) axis is a crucial stress response system in the human body [12]. The primary function of the HPA axis is to maintain homeostasis and facilitate successful adaption to the surrounding environment through an intricate cascade of hormonal reactions. The stress response initiates when a stressor triggers the hypothalamus, releasing corticotropin-releasing factor (CRF) and vasopressin (AVP). These hormones stimulate the production of adrenocorticotropic hormone (ACTH) from the pituitary gland, eliciting the release of glucocorticoids, most notably cortisol, from the adrenal glands (**Figure 2**). Chronic stress has been well-documented as increasing the risk of cardiovascular disease through sustained exposure to increased levels of endogenous cortisol [6, 13]. The elevation of plasma cortisol levels is one of the best-studied components of the stress response, and this hormone is one of the best indicators of acute stress in humans.

Elevated cortisol leads to downregulation of the glucocorticoid receptor and potently affects lipid and carbohydrate metabolism [6]. Repeated or chronic stress can result in HPA axis dysfunction and cortisol remaining at high levels [12]. Clinical and population studies have shown that excessive cortisol levels are associated with

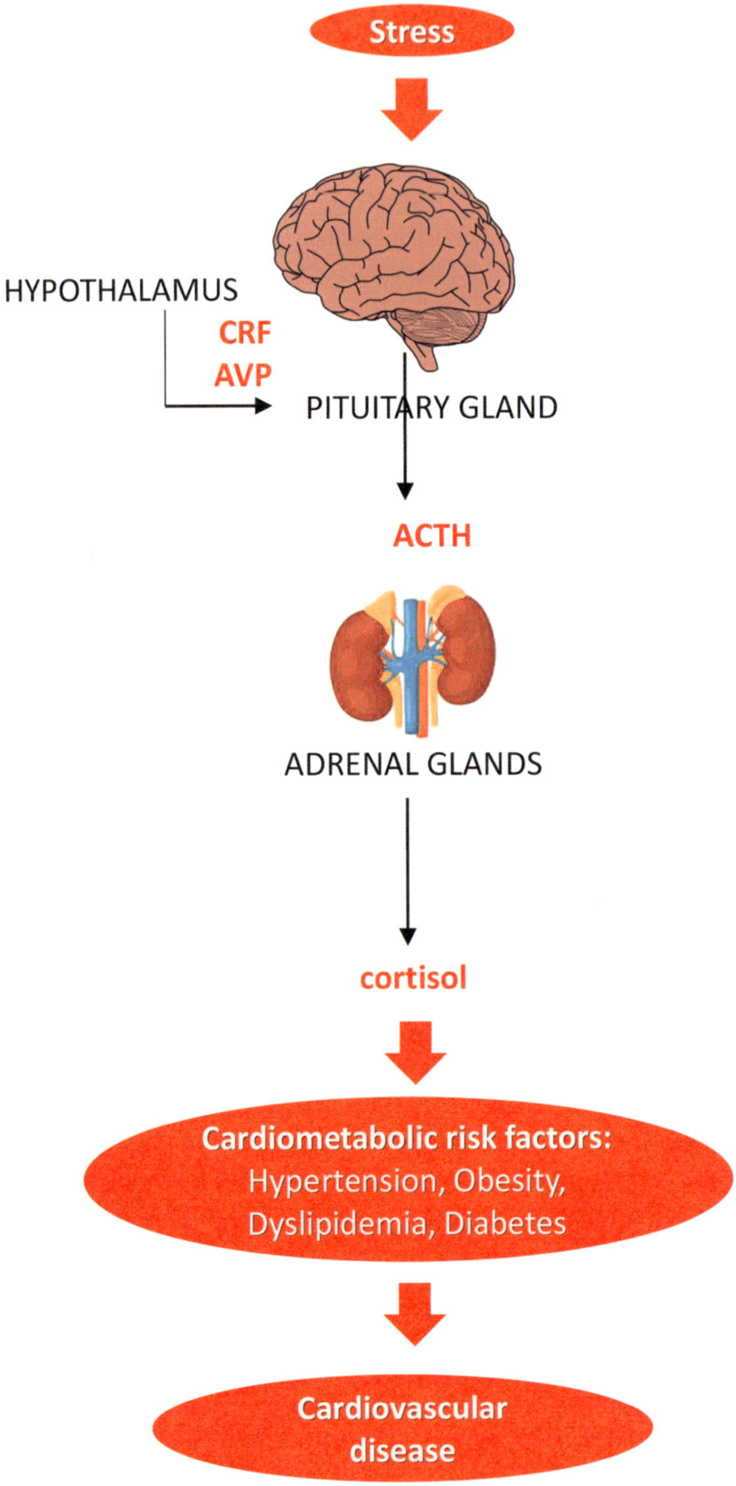

Figure 2.
The HPA axis response to stress resulting in elevated cortisol, increased cardiometabolic risk (CMR), and cardiovascular disease (CVD).

developing central adiposity, insulin resistance and hyperglycemia, hypertension, and dyslipidemia [14, 15]. Traditionally these studies measured cortisol levels in body fluids, including saliva, blood, and urine [16]. While blood and saliva samples provide a cortisol measurement of a single timepoint, urine reflects the total exposure to bioactive cortisol over 12 or 24 hours. In contrast, hair allows for retrospective assessment of long-term cortisol concentrations over weeks, months, and even years [11, 17], potentially providing a better measure of an individual's long-term exposure to stress. HCC is increasingly important in establishing and providing significant insight into cardiovascular disease prognosis, diagnosis, and management [13]. Elevated cortisol has been shown to be associated with an increased risk of cardiovascular diseases (9). Also, several cross-sectional studies found positive associations of hair cortisol with adverse cardiometabolic outcomes, including higher systolic blood pressure [18], diabetes, metabolic syndrome [18], and adiposity [18, 19].

4. Association of hair cortisol with cardiometabolic risk factors

4.1 Hypertension

Hypertension is also known as high or raised blood pressure, in which the blood vessels have persistently raised pressure. A patient is diagnosed with hypertension when the systolic blood pressure (SBP) is above or equal to 140 mm Hg and/or diastolic blood pressure (DBP) is above or equal to 90 mm Hg [20]. If left unmanaged, hypertension can lead to a heart attack, an enlarged heart, and heart failure [21]. Hypertension can also result in kidney failure, blindness, rupture of blood vessels, and cognitive impairment. Hypertension is a critical public health and clinical condition affecting billions worldwide, including approximately the 2 million Americans diagnosed annually [22]. Hypertension is one of the most prevalent risk factors for almost all cardiovascular diseases [23].

Chronic psychosocial stress is believed to increase the risk of hypertension through sustained exposure to elevated cortisol levels [21]. Cortisol is essential for maintaining normal blood pressure but, in excess, produces hypertension [24]. In 2002, the Prospective Studies Collaboration published a meta-analysis based on 61 cohort studies showing that the risk of CVD increased steadily with progressively higher levels of baseline SBP and DBP; a 20 mm Hg higher level of SBP and a 10 mm Hg higher level of DBP resulted in a 2-fold higher BP-related absolute risk of CVD [25]. While research exploring an independent association between HCC and hypertension is still a new research area, several cross-sectional studies found a positive correlation between hair cortisol and hypertension [18, 21]. Still, the data on the relationship between blood pressure and hair cortisol level is inconsistent. While some studies reported a positive association between mean arterial or systolic blood pressure and HCC, other studies failed to demonstrate a relationship. In addition, Feller et al. found no association between prevalent hypertension and HCC and a negative relationship between objectively measured diastolic blood pressure and HCC. Hypertension prevalence was 2.23 times higher in participants with CVD [21].

4.2 Obesity

Cardiovascular disease (CVD) is one of the primary causes of increased morbidity and mortality in people with obesity [26, 27]. Obesity is defined as an excessive accumulation of body fat, with the amount of this excess fat being directly responsible for most obesity-associated health risks [27]. Although body mass index (BMI) is the established clinical measurement to estimate CVD risk associated with excess body weight, increasing evidence suggests that abdominal obesity, as assessed by the waist-hip ratio (WHR), could represent a better marker of CVD risk than BMI [28].

The incidence of obesity is increasing at a rapid and concerning rate in most regions worldwide, with direct consequences on the risk of developing several chronic diseases such as systemic hypertension [29] and type 2 diabetes [30]. More seriously, obesity usually occurs with a cluster of metabolic disturbances such as impaired glucose metabolism, atherogenic dyslipidemia, and hypertension, and obese individuals have an increased risk of CVD [26]. Interestingly, perceived societal stigma due to weight discrimination was shown to contribute to HCC [31], complicating the association of elevated cortisol with obesity. Still, HCC was associated with higher BMI in obese individuals (BMI > 30 kg/m2) compared to average weight (BMI: 18.5–24.9) and nonobese overweight (BMI: 25.0–29.9) people [19]. A meta-analysis confirmed the positive associations between HCC and stress-related anthropometric measures (BMI and WHR) and reported a 9.8% increase in HCC per 2.5 points BMI [18].

4.3 Dyslipidemia

Dyslipidemia is a common metabolic disorder and an established risk factor for cardiovascular disease [32]. The condition is characterized by high-risk lipid levels with an increased level of serum total cholesterol (TC), triglycerides (TG), low-density lipoprotein cholesterol (LDL-C), or a decreased concentration of serum high-density lipoprotein cholesterol (HDL-C) [33]. Dyslipidemia is closely linked with obesity, a disease characterized by an adverse effect on lipoproteins a known cardiometabolic risk factor [34].

The relationship between hair cortisol with lipids varied considerably across studies. The MASHAD study, a prospective cohort population study, found that increased serum total cholesterol levels were positively associated with absolute CVD risk among men and women [33]. However, after adjusting for confounding factors, high serum TC only significantly increased the risk of myocardial infarction in men. Kuehl *et al.* reported a positive association between triglycerides and HCC [35]. Another study found a positive association between low-density lipoprotein cholesterol (LDL-C) and HCC [3]. Since dyslipidemia is one of the main cardiovascular risk factors, further research is needed to examine chronic cortisol exposure and its effect on lipid metabolism.

4.4 Diabetes

Cardiovascular diseases are the most common cause of morbidity and mortality among patients with diabetes mellitus [36]. More than 90% of people with diabetes mellitus suffer from type 2 diabetes (T2D), a disease characterized by hyperglycemia, insulin resistance, and impaired glucose tolerance [37]. T2D and CVD have several shared characteristics; both conditions increase with age, are associated with an adverse lipid profile, obesity, and a sedentary lifestyle, and lifestyle modifications of common risk factors can reduce the risk of both [38]. Generally, patients with T2D also display other comorbidities such as obesity, hypertension, and dyslipidemia, increasing the risk for CVD [36].

Recently the CAPTURE study, a study assessing the prevalence of established CVD and its management in adults with T2D across 13 countries and five continents, reported that CVD was prevalent in 34.8% of patients with T2D [39]. Elevated cortisol levels are consistently associated with glycated hemoglobin, the diagnostic measure of T2D [18, 40] or diabetes [41–43]. Manenschijn *et al*. reported that HCC is associated with CVD and diabetes [13]. Since CVD and T2D share so many characteristics, further study of HCC measurements could be interesting in trying to discriminate between the two diseases or show that they are inextricably linked.

5. Conclusion

The prevention and sensible management of cardiometabolic risk factors such as hypertension, obesity, dyslipidemia, and diabetes can markedly alter cardiovascular morbidity and mortality. Interestingly, cardiovascular risk is often associated with more than one cardiometabolic risk factor related to elevated cortisol levels. The metabolic syndrome describes this group of interrelated disorders such as insulin resistance, abdominal obesity, glucose intolerance, dyslipidemia, and hypertension [18]. HCC levels provide a measure of long-term exposure to chronic stress and have the potential as a suitable biomarker of CMR and contribute to the prevention, early diagnosis, treatment, and management of CVD. Hair cortisol measurements potentially reduce the variability associated with self-reported measures and provide a more robust view than the acute cortisol determinations in urine, saliva, and blood samples. While the evidence for the relationship between cardiometabolic risk and cortisol is clear and compelling, inconsistencies in the data must be addressed and understood.

A recent meta-analysis showed that adherence to several healthy lifestyle behaviors simultaneously reduced cardiovascular disease risk by 66% compared with adopting none or only one behavior [44]. However, no evidence exists that interventions that reduce cardiometabolic risk factors decrease hair cortisol levels in preventing or treating CVD [7]. More extensive studies are needed to ascertain the use of hair cortisol as an effective measure of stress reduction interventions. Also, further research is required to delineate whether HCC is a biomarker of CVD or CVD risk to utilize HCC in clinical settings effectively. Further insight into the mechanisms underlying increased cortisol exposure is necessary for the more effective implementation of cortisol-lowering therapies and potential new treatment targets.

Acknowledgements

I express my sincere gratitude to Francina (Riah) Van Wyk and Momar Milliones for their continued support.

Conflict of interest

The author declares no conflict of interest.

Author details

Jennifer C. Van Wyk
Keratech LLC, Hair and Skin Testing and Research Lab, Pittsburgh, USA

*Address all correspondence to: jvanwyk@keratechllc.com

References

[1] Centers for Disease Control and Prevention. Underlying Cause of Death, 1999-2018. 2018. Available from: https://www.cdc.gov/heartdisease/facts.htm. [Accessed: May 6, 2022]

[2] World Health Organization. Cardiovascular Diseases (CVDs). 2022; Available from: https://www.who.int/health-topics/cardiovascular-diseases#tab=tab_1

[3] Mazgelytė E et al. Association of hair cortisol concentration with prevalence of major cardiovascular risk factors and allostatic load. Medical Science Monitor: International Medical Journal of Experimental and Clinical Research. 2019;**25**:3573

[4] Cannon CP. Cardiovascular disease and modifiable cardiometabolic risk factors. Clinical Cornerstone. 2007;**8**(3):11-28

[5] Varvogli L, Darviri C. Stress management techniques: Evidence-based procedures that reduce stress and promote health. Health Science Journal. 2011;**5**(2):74

[6] Steptoe A, Kivimäki M. Stress and cardiovascular disease. Nature Reviews Cardiology. 2012;**9**(6):360-370

[7] Iob E, Steptoe A. Cardiovascular disease and hair cortisol: A novel biomarker of chronic stress. Current Cardiology Reports. 2019;**21**(10):1-11

[8] Stalder T, Kirschbaum C. Analysis of cortisol in hair–state of the art and future directions. Brain, Behavior, and Immunity. 2012;**26**(7):1019-1029

[9] Russell E et al. Toward standardization of hair cortisol measurement: Results of the first international interlaboratory round robin. Therapeutic Drug Monitoring. 2015;**37**(1):71-75

[10] Gray N et al. Determinants of hair cortisol concentration in children: A systematic review. Psychoneuroendocrinology. 2018;**87**:204-214

[11] Russell E, et al. Toward standardization of hair cortisol measurement: Results of the first international interlaboratory round robin. Therapeutic drug monitoring. 1 Feb 2015;**37**(1):71-75

[12] Guilliams TG, Edwards L. Chronic stress and the HPA axis. The Standard. 2010;**9**(2):1-12

[13] Manenschijn L et al. High long-term cortisol levels, measured in scalp hair, are associated with a history of cardiovascular disease. The Journal of Clinical Endocrinology & Metabolism. 2013;**98**(5):2078-2083

[14] Girod JP, Brotman DJ. Does altered glucocorticoid homeostasis increase cardiovascular risk? Cardiovascular Research. 2004;**64**(2):217-226

[15] Whitworth JA et al. Cardiovascular consequences of cortisol excess. Vascular Health and Risk Management. 2005;**1**(4):291

[16] Manenschijn L et al. Evaluation of a method to measure long term cortisol levels. Steroids. 2011;**76**(10):1032-1036

[17] Russell E et al. Hair cortisol as a biological marker of chronic stress: Current status, future directions and unanswered questions. Psychoneuroendocrinology. 2012;**37**(5):589-601

[18] Stalder T et al. Cortisol in hair and the metabolic syndrome. The Journal of Clinical Endocrinology & Metabolism. 2013;**98**(6):2573-2580

[19] Wester VL et al. Long-term cortisol levels measured in scalp hair of obese patients. Obesity. 2014;**22**(9):1956-1958

[20] Fuchs FD, Whelton PK. High blood pressure and cardiovascular disease. Hypertension. 2020;**75**(2):285-292

[21] Bautista LE et al. The relationship between chronic stress, hair cortisol and hypertension. International Journal of Cardiology Hypertension. 2019;**2**:100012

[22] Flack JM, Ferdinand KC, Nasser SA. Epidemiology of hypertension and cardiovascular disease in African Americans. The Journal of Clinical Hypertension. 2003;**5**(1):5-11

[23] Kjeldsen SE. Hypertension and cardiovascular risk: General aspects. Pharmacological Research. 2018;**129**:95-99

[24] Kelly J et al. Cortisol and hypertension. Clinical and Experimental Pharmacology and Physiology. 1998;**25**(S1):S51-S56

[25] Collaboration PS. Age-specific relevance of usual blood pressure to vascular mortality: A meta-analysis of individual data for one million adults in 61 prospective studies. The Lancet. 2002;**360**(9349):1903-1913

[26] Koliaki C, Liatis S, Kokkinos A. Obesity and cardiovascular disease: Revisiting an old relationship. Metabolism. 2019;**92**:98-107

[27] Poirier P, Eckel RH. Obesity and cardiovascular disease. Current Atherosclerosis Reports. 2002;**4**(6):448-453

[28] Lee CMY et al. Indices of abdominal obesity are better discriminators of cardiovascular risk factors than BMI: A meta-analysis. Journal of Clinical Epidemiology. 2008;**61**(7):646-653

[29] Seravalle G, Grassi G. Obesity and hypertension. Pharmacological Research. 2017;**122**:1-7

[30] Verma S, Hussain ME. Obesity and diabetes: An update. Diabetes & Metabolic Syndrome: Clinical Research & Reviews. 2017;**11**(1):73-79

[31] Jackson SE, Kirschbaum C, Steptoe A. Perceived weight discrimination and chronic biochemical stress: A population-based study using cortisol in scalp hair. Obesity. 2016;**24**(12):2515-2521

[32] Fodor G. Primary prevention of CVD: Treating dyslipidemia. American Family Physician. 2011;**83**(10):1207

[33] Hedayatnia M et al. Dyslipidemia and cardiovascular disease risk among the MASHAD study population. Lipids in Health and Disease. 2020;**19**(1):1-11

[34] Howard BV, Ruotolo G, Robbins DC. Obesity and dyslipidemia. Endocrinology and Metabolism Clinics. 2003;**32**(4):855-867

[35] Kuehl LK et al. Hair cortisol and cortisol awakening response are associated with criteria of the metabolic syndrome in opposite directions. Psychoneuroendocrinology. 2015;**51**:365-370

[36] Matheus ASdM et al. Impact of diabetes on cardiovascular disease: An update. International Journal of Hypertension. 2013;**2013**:1-15

[37] Olokoba AB, Obateru OA, Olokoba LB. Type 2 diabetes mellitus: A review of current trends. Oman Medical Journal. 2012;**27**(4):269

[38] Stern MP. Diabetes and cardiovascular disease: The "common soil" hypothesis. Diabetes. 1995;**44**(4):369-374

[39] Mosenzon O et al. CAPTURE: A multinational, cross-sectional study of cardiovascular disease prevalence in adults with type 2 diabetes across 13 countries. Cardiovascular Diabetology. 2021;**20**(1):1-13

[40] Lehrer HM et al. Hair cortisol concentration and glycated hemoglobin in African American adults. Psychoneuroendocrinology. 2016;**72**:212-218

[41] Abell JG et al. Assessing cortisol from hair samples in a large observational cohort: The Whitehall II study. Psychoneuroendocrinology. 2016;**73**:148-156

[42] Feller S et al. Predictors of hair cortisol concentrations in older adults. Psychoneuroendocrinology. 2014;**39**:132-140

[43] Staufenbiel SM et al. Determinants of hair cortisol and hair cortisone concentrations in adults. Psychoneuroendocrinology. 2015;**60**:182-194

[44] Barbaresko J, Rienks J, Nöthlings U. Lifestyle indices and cardiovascular disease risk: A meta-analysis. American Journal of Preventive Medicine. 2018;**55**(4):555-564

Chapter 20

Use of Cardiac Troponin for the Diagnosis of Cardiac Pathology in Postmortem Samples Taken at Autopsy

David C. Gaze

Abstract

The diagnosis of acute cardiac pathology is a clinical challenge in both the living and in the postmortem setting. Cardiac troponin (cTn) T and cardiac troponin I released from the contractile apparatus of cardiomyocytes into the circulation can be detected by sensitive and specific immunoassays and are the gold standard biochemical test for diagnosis of acute coronary syndromes (ACS). Recently with the advent of more sensitive detection methods, elevation in non-ACS has become apparent causing clinical confusion. In most cases, these elevations are related to subclinical cardiac damage and often confer poor prognosis in cTn-positive patients. Biomarkers of cardiomyocyte damage may be of value in routine hospital and medico-legal autopsy. A significant body of evidence has emerged since the late 1990s, assessing the clinical utility of cardiac troponin in biological fluids or in immunohistochemical staining of cardiac tissue to aid in the diagnosis of acute cardiac pathology when standard microscopic evidence is inconclusive. This chapter reviews the extensive literature on the subject and details the disparity between pericardial fluid and serum for the use of cTn in the postmortem setting.

Keywords: cardiovascular disease, risk, diagnostics, therapeutic intervention, treatment, prediction

1. Introduction

Cardiac troponins (cTn) T (cTnT) and I (cTnI) are the gold standard biochemical markers used to identify acute cardiac pathologies in patients who present with typical and atypical chest pain to the emergency department. These muscle-associated proteins confer superior diagnostic and prognostic ability compared to conventional nonspecific muscle derived enzyme markers such as creatine kinase (CK), its MB isoform (CK-MB), or myoglobin. Cardiac troponin determination is central to the diagnosis of non-ST segment elevation acute myocardial infarction (NSTEMI), contributing to international guidelines for diagnosis and management of NSTEMI patients [1].

Recent advancement in laboratory technology driven both by clinical demand and the commercial *in vitro* diagnostic market has seen the emergence of highly analytically sensitive immunoassays for the termination of cTnT and cTnI in biological samples, mainly serum and plasma. The role out and increasing popularity of the sensitive methods have introduced new clinical challenges, notably defining acceptable reference intervals in the apparently healthy population, sex-specific cut-off values and novel clinical roles in non-acute cardiac diseases where often secondary underlying cardiac disease is present [2].

One area of interest has been the potential value of cTnT and cTnI in the postmortem setting and may provide insight into the cause of death. Troponin analysis in postmortem blood and pericardial fluid during autopsy investigations can potentially help medical examiners and forensic pathologists attribute what happened before, during, and after a death. This chapter will explore the use of cardiac troponin in the postmortem setting, from its application in routine hospital as well as medico-legal autopsy and forensics, assessing the usefulness in offering a clearer picture of an individual's final moments.

2. Clinical utility of cardiac troponin in myocardial damage

Cardiac-specific isoforms of the contractile protein complex troponin, namely cTnT and cTnI, are released into the bloodstream following damage to cardiomyocytes. The mechanism by which these structural proteins are released into the circulation has been debated significantly over many years. Initially, it was thought that cTn could only be released following overt cellular necrosis; however, recently it has been suggested that release can occur in ischemia without necrosis [3]. A review of the subject by Ragusa and colleagues suggest release mechanisms, including apoptosis, necroptosis, physiological cardiomyocyte renewal, and cellular wounding can contribute to cTn release as well as necrosis [4]. An immunohistochemical study using a canine model of coronary occlusion ranging from 30 minutes to 6 hours demonstrated variable loss of both cTnT and cTnI in paraffin-embedded left ventricular myocardial sections [5]. Loss was variable but more so for cTnT than for cTnI, and loss was greater at the periphery of the infarct area rather than the centralised region (**Figure 1**).

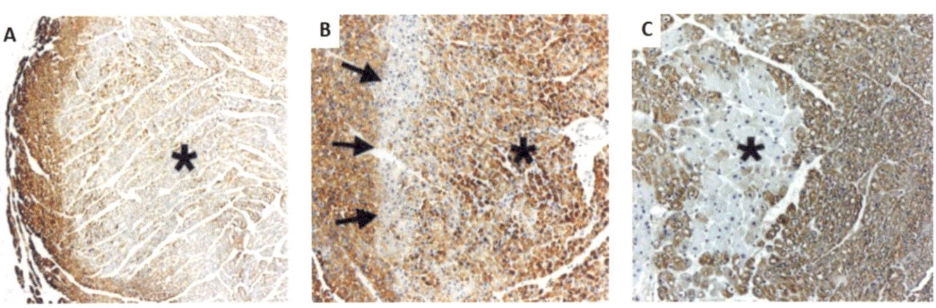

Figure 1.
Canine left ventricular myocardial tissue following 6 h of coronary artery occlusion. Immunohistochemical staining of (A) cTnI demonstrating decreased but non-uniform staining in the central necrotic area (asterisk); (B) cTnT demonstrating loss at edge of infarct zone (arrows) and (C) canine left ventricular myocardial tissue following 45 min of coronary artery occlusion demonstrating loss of cTnI in the zone of necrosis (asterisk) (source: Adapted from [5]).

Using monoclonal antibodies specific to the cardiac isoforms, immunoassay technologies can quantify the amount of cTnT or cTnI in a biological matrix [6]. Initially, early immunoassays utilised high clinical cut-off values (high specificity and low sensitivity) allowed the separation of patients with overt acute myocardial infarction (AMI) from apparently healthy persons who were deemed negative for cTn based on the equivalent cTnT or cTnI concentration to the then-used gold standard tests (CK or CK-MB). Subsequently, the large body of evidence demonstrating elevation of CK and CK-MB in the absence of an elevated cTn questioned the cardio-specificity of the enzyme markers, along with approximately 30% of patients ruled out with AMI

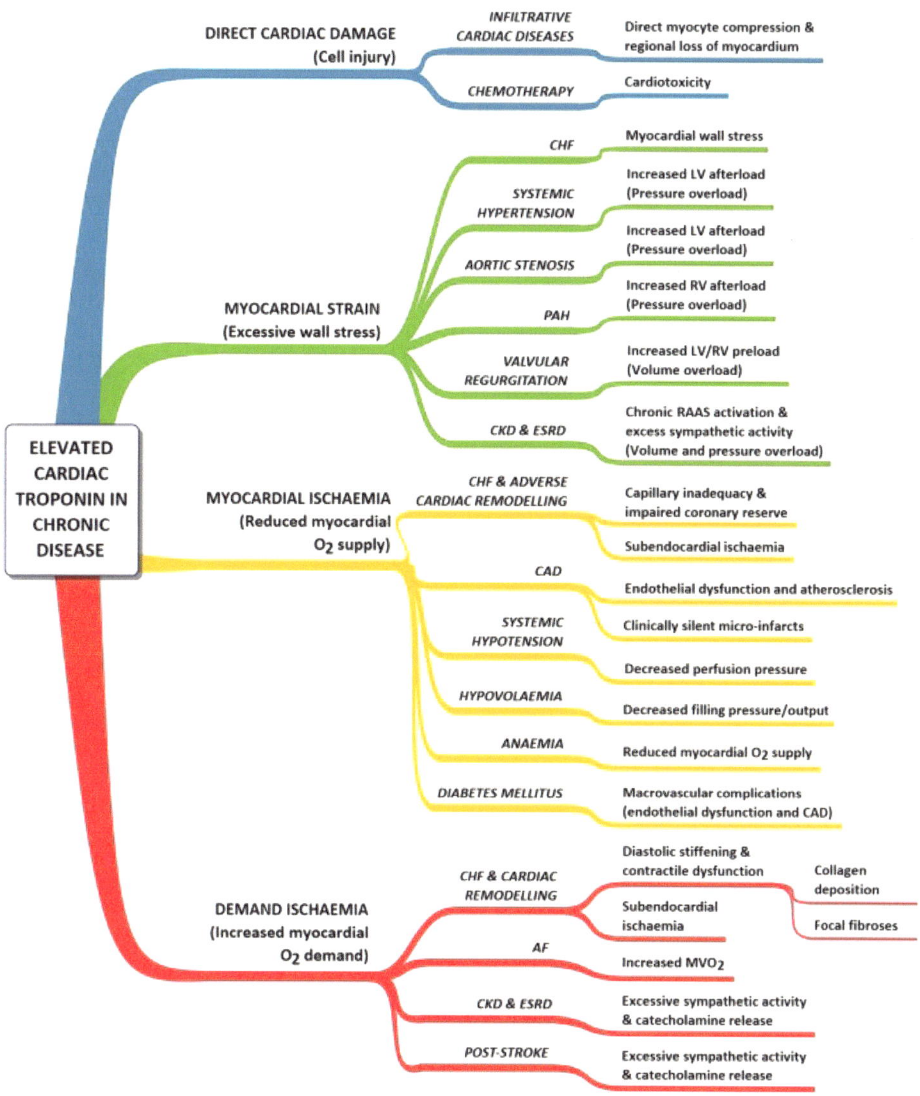

Figure 2.
Categories of cardiac troponin release in acute and chronic diseases. All conditions have documented evidence of elevated cTn. AF, atrial fibrillation; CAD, coronary artery disease; CHF, chronic heart failure; CKD, chronic kidney disease; ESRD end-stage renal disease; LV left ventricle; MVO2, myocardial oxygen consumption; PAH, pulmonary artery hypertension; RAAS, renin-angiotensin-aldosterone system; RV, right ventricle (source: [2], with authors permission).

demonstrating positive cTn which is associated with poor prognosis, resulted in the adoption of cTn as the gold standard test for diagnosis of AMI [6].

Integral to the adoption of cTn was the appropriate definition of cut-off to confer an abnormal concentration. This was subsequently defined as the 99th percentile value of an apparently healthy population. When adopted into routine clinical practice, this lowered the sensitivity of the assays allowing early diagnosis in the evolving infarction but at the cost of specificity. Initially, this caused clinical confusion with a larger number of patients presenting with low concentrations of cTn just above the AMI cut-off value, but further research of such patients found the presence of comorbid conditions (**Figure 2**) often with underlying cardiovascular pathophysiology [2].

3. Biochemical testing in assisting cause of death at postmortem

Biochemical testing in postmortem investigations (termed thanatochemistry, necrochemistry or the chemistry of death) was initially established in the early 1950s, and a great number of biochemical analytes have proved an adjunctive tool to assist the cause of death at postmortem [7]. Adoption of biochemical testing especially in the medico-legal forensic autopsy has often been limited. The determination of death may have significant impact on those directly or indirectly involved in the death of an individual and can carry a custodial sentence. Thus, the scientific evidence presented in court is intensely scrutinised both by the prosecution and defence counsels. Whilst no biochemical test is infallible, many are associated with the likelihood of a disease process rather than a definitive diagnosis of the disease. Often the barrier to use is the interpretation of results of biochemical assays from cadaveric sampling, hindered by the lack of reference normality in death; thus, results are compared to reference intervals generated in the living [7, 8] with few studies demonstrating corresponding histopathological findings to the biochemical results. Interpretation is further complicated by factors such as postmortem interference in the assay technology, appropriate sampling matrices, postmortem autolysis, microbial metabolism, fluid redistribution, and postmortem interval (PMI). Molecular biophysical properties such as molecular weight, structure, intracellular location, electrical charge, ionic strength, protein affinity, and cell membrane permeability may differ between life and death and can influence interpretation in both situations [7].

There are a number of fluid components which are suitable for cadaveric biochemical testing, namely vitreous humour from the posterior segment of the eye, cerebral spinal fluid (CSF), synovial fluid, pericardial fluid (PCF), venous femoral blood, venous jugular blood, peripheral blood sampling, urine, gastric contents and right ventricle heart whole blood [7–9]. Analytes and potential uses in postmortem samples are listed in **Table 1**.

4. Conventional cardiac biomarkers at postmortem

The importance of cardiac biomarkers assisting in postmortem diagnosis was highlighted in cases where a suspected myocardial lesion cannot be diagnosed by routine histological analysis. They were utilised initially for the determination of sudden cardiac death. Initially, CK and lactate dehydrogenase isoenzyme analysis of pericardial fluid was utilised [10, 11], followed by K:Na ratio [12]; CK isoenzymes,

Analyte	Sample matrix	Forensic utility
Adrenaline:Noradrenaline	Urine	Hypothermia
Acetone	Blood	Chronic alcohol abuse, hypothermia, diabetic ketoacidosis
Ammonia	Vitreous humour	Liver failure
Carbohydrate-deficient transferrin	Vitreous humour	Chronic alcohol abuse
Chloride	Vitreous humour	Saline poisoning, salt water drowning, dehydration
Chymase activity	Blood	Anaphylactic shock
Chromogranin A	Blood, CSF	Hypothermia
C-reactive protein	Blood	Recent infection, trauma, burns, ketoacidosis, malignancy, autoimmune diseases, inflammatory diseases, sepsis
Creatine Kinase & CK-MB	Blood	Cardiac pathology
Creatine Kinase-BB	CSF	Cerebral trauma, cerebral hypoxia
Creatinine	Vitreous humour	AKI, CKD, high-protein diet, large muscle mass (anabolic steroid abuse), heat shock
Ethyl glucuronide	Vitreous humour, Urine	Antemortem ethanol ingestion
Free fatty acids	Blood	Hypothermia
Fructoasmine	Vitreous humour	Diabetic ketoacidosis
Glucocortcoids	Blood	Hypothermia
Hypoxanthine	Vitreous humour	Time of death
Myoglobin	Blood, Urine	Hyperthermia, cardiac pathology
Neurone specific enolase	CSF	Cerebral traumatic injury, cerebral hypoxia
Potassium	Vitreous humour	Postmortem decomposition
S-100b	CSF	Cerebral injury
Thyroglobulin/fT3	Vitreous humour, Blood	Neck trauma, strangulation
Troponin	Pericardial fluid, Blood	Cardiac pathology
Tryptase	Blood	Anaphylactic shock
Urea	Vitreous humour	Renal dysfunction, upper GI haemorrhage

AKI, acute kidney injury; CKD, chronic kidney disease; CK-MB, creatine kinase-MB isoform, CK-BB; creatine kinase-BB isoform; CSF, cerebrospinal fluid.

Table 1.
Biochemical analytes, sample matrices, and potential forensic utility.

aspartate aminotransferase and hydroxybutyrate dehydrogenase [13] and myosin and cathepsin D, a lysosomal aspartyl protease that degrades proteins [14, 15].

5. Cardiac troponin analysis at postmortem

The first reported use of cTn analysis was in 1998 by Osuna and colleagues who studied 89 cadavers with a mean age of 51.38 ± 2.04y [16]. Subjects were assigned between four groups, MI (n = 25), asphyxia (n = 30), cranio/multiple trauma (n = 17), and other natural deaths (n = 17). MI was determined by H&E and acridine orange histological staining. The research group determined the concentration of myoglobin, myosin, CK-MB, and cTnI in femoral vein serum samples and PCF in each case. PCF concentrations for all makers were significantly different between each outcome group; however, only myoglobin and myosin demonstrated significance in serum. The PCF cTnI values were higher than serum samples when using the Sanofi Diagnostic Pasteur assay. Values in both matrices were higher in MI patients compared to the other three groups (mean (range) Pericardial cTnI [pg/L]): 2.4 (0.3–6.5); 1.7 (0.03–3.7); 1.1 (0.01–2.3); 0.4 (0.0–1.8) in each group, respectively.

Cina and colleagues [17] demonstrated the utility of cTnT using the then available commercial Cardiac Rapid T (cTnT) lateral flow test from Roche Diagnostics. This device allows testing in the autopsy suite at the time of postmortem with qualitative results (positive or negative test lines) at 15 minutes from sample application. In 40 autopsy cases, 20 were deemed cardiac deaths and 20 were controls (noncardiac related) deaths, diagnosed by gross pathology and histological analysis. 85% (n = 17) of subclavian or femoral blood samples in the cardiac death group were positive for cTnT which was significantly different to control group, where 30% (n = 6) of serum samples were positive for cTnT. The authors deemed these as false-positive results. In subjects aged over 50 years, sensitivity and specificity of cTnT for diagnosis of AMI were 91% and 86%, respectively. The authors noted however the assay was ineffective in frozen blood samples or those with significant haemolysis which was evident at a PMI of >24 h. A similar study of 100 autopsy cases of sudden unexplained death (SUD) was carried out in Chaing Mai, Thailand, and utilised the same rapid cTnT assay [18]. Fifty-two of the deaths were considered cardiac with 20 due to sudden MI and 32 with evidence of old infarction or arrhythmic fibrosis (n = 22), coronary atherosclerosis, >75% luminal without evidence of fibrosis or thrombosis (n = 3), cardiomegaly, and heart weight > 400 g (n = 7) or related to cardiac injury as a result of toxic substances. Thus, subjects were assigned to other cardiac death (SCD), non-cardiac natural death (NCD) or non-natural death (NND). The percentage positivity rate was higher in subclavian blood than femoral blood samples in all three groups. Subclavian blood sensitivity and specificity for SUD were 87.5% and 47%, respectively. Similar to the findings of Cina and colleagues, false-positive rates were associated with increasing PMI.

Davies and colleagues were the first to compare antemortem (<48 h before death) and postmortem concentrations of cTnT (Roche Elecsys 3rd generation electrochemiluminescent assay) and cTnI (Stratus CS fluorometric assay, Dade-Behring [now Siemens healthineers]) in five hospital-based autopsies [19]. One patient suffered cardiac death (myocarditis) with the remaining four were non-cardiac, but moribund before death. Results obtained between antemortem and postmortem samples were erratic. Four of the five subjects (n = 80%) had elevated antemortem cTnT and cTnI samples. The authors concluded postmortem cTn analysis in blood was not suitable due to lack of correlation of cause of death; however, they suggested that elevated antemortem cTn was related to all-cause mortality in those at end of life. A similar conclusion was made by Rahimi and colleagues in 2018 after studying 140 natural and unnatural deaths in Malaysia [20]. Subjects were classified into five groups: cardiovascular death, sudden unexplained death, thoracic trauma, non-thoracic trauma, and other diseases. Median jugular/subclavian/femoral blood cTnT (Roche Elecsys 3rd generation electrochemiluminescent assay) concentrations were 0.51, 0.17, 0.62, 0.90, and 0.51 μg/L, respectively, with no significant difference (p= > 0.05) in relation to cause of death. The authors concluded cTnT lacked specificity in postmortem sampling and is therefore not a useful tool.

Lai and colleagues also compared antemortem and postmortem blood sampling. Demonstrating in four cases, a marked proportionate rise in cTnT in postmortem samples compared to antemortem samples. Interestingly, the authors found cTnT values were higher (mean cTnT 5.32 μg/L) in non-cardiac deaths compared to 4.91 μg/L in cardiac-related deaths [21].

In 2006, Zhu and co-workers published two seminal papers in *Legal Medicine* examining the value of postmortem cTnT in cardiac, peripheral blood and PCF in relation to traumatic causes of death [22] and sudden cardiac death pathology [23] in medicolegal autopsies. In traumatic death (n = 405) due to blunt/sharp instrument injury, asphyxiation, drowning, fatal fire, hyper and hypothermia, and toxic poisoning are due to metamphetamine or carbon monoxide. Cardiac blood and PCF cTnT values were lower where PMI was <12 h compared cases where PMI ranged from 12 to 48 h. Elevated cTnT was associated, however, with histological evidence of advanced myocardial damage involving swelling and liquefactive necrosis [22]. In their cohort of sudden cardiac death autopsies (n = 96), 35% were due to AMI, 24% due to recurrent MI, 25% ischemic heart disease without infarction and 16% due to other cardiac causes. The comparative control group (n = 75) consisted of 47% asphyxiation, 36% drowning and 17% cerebrovascular diseases. In agreement with their first study, pericardial cTnT concentrations were higher than blood samples. Differences in cTnT concentrations related to pathological evidence of cardiac damage differed between early (<12 h) and late (12–48 h) postmortem period, concluding that elevations in blood and PCF are dependent not only on the severity of myocardial damage (determined by infarct size, intensity of lesions, interstitial haemorrhage and necrosis) but also by the PMI [22].

Remmer and colleagues [24] focused on postmortem serum and PCF cTnT in relation to PMI from 101 forensic autopsy cases in Estonia. PMI ranged from 8 h to 141 h. Although differences in cTnT were observed between five groups of cause of death (cardiovascular disease; other disease; poisoning; asphyxia; drowning; hypothermia; thoracic trauma, other trauma and fatal fires), significant attention to PMI (**Figure 3**) is important rather than comorbid cardiovascular disease.

In addition to the effects of PMI as demonstrated above, Kumar et al. used SDS-PAGE and Western blotting of cardiac tissue extracts from 10 medicolegal autopsies of burns cases [25]. The authors demonstrated a pattern of cTnT degradation in a time-dependent manner at room temperature (7.3 h, 18.2 h, 30.3 h, 41.2 h, 41.4 h, 54.3 h, 65.2 h and 88.4 h), demonstrating the disappearance of intact cTnT protein and the increasing presence of low-molecular-weight bands related to time (**Figure 4a**). Furthermore, the groups have examined degradation patterns according to the cause of death (**Figure 4b–d**) [26].

A study of 20 autopsies of sudden cardiac death and 8 controls (violent non-cardiac deaths) demonstrated significantly higher cTnT and cTnI concentrations in pulmonary venous blood. Mean ± SD cTnT were 1826 ± 363 μg/L versus 65 ± 11 μg/L, respectively, and for cTnI were 28 ± 3 mg/L versus 0.14 ± 0.02 μg/L; however, it should be noted that the PMI in all cases was 8 h [27].

The value of cTn as a biochemical marker in relation to sudden cardiac death has been the subject of a systematic review [28] and formal meta-analysis [29]. Whilst both reviews demonstrate the elevation of cTn to be higher in pericardial fluid compared to blood sampling in the postmortem setting (**Figure 5**), blood is

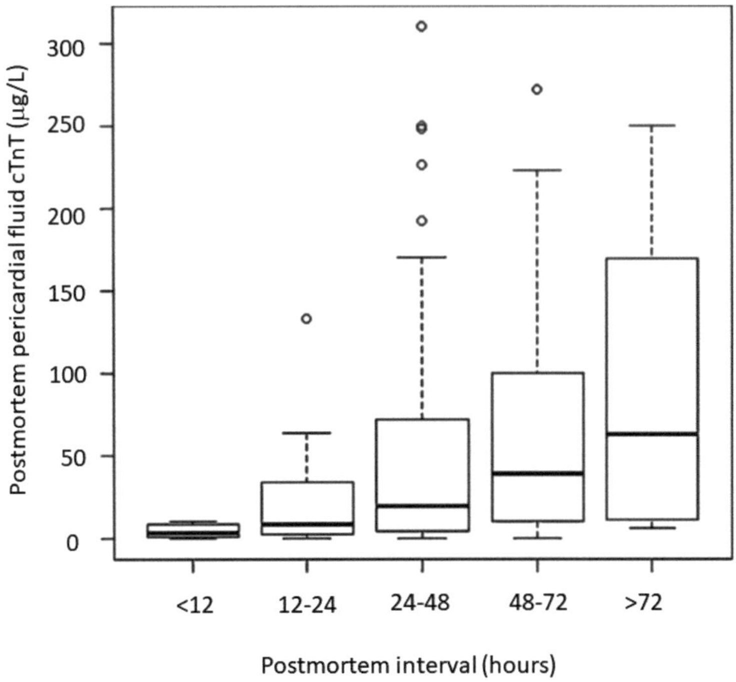

Figure 3.
Cardiac troponin T (cTnT) concentration in relation to postmortem interval in 101 medicolegal autopsies. Cause of death were due to cardiovascular disease, other disease, poisoning, asphyxia, drowning, hypothermia, thoracic and non-thoracic trauma and fatal fires. (source: Adapted from [24]).

susceptible to the effects of haemolysis, postmortem interval, autolysis, and potential bacterial interferences. Pericardial fluid is therefore the preferred sample of choice.

Both reviews also address the issue of cut-off values demonstrating significant difference to cut-off values in the living. Non-cardiac deaths often demonstrate significantly positive cTn values in PCF and blood, thus questioning the sensitivity and specificity at postmortem. Barberi and van den Hondel suggest that more work is required to determine the appropriate cut-off values at postmortem [28].

6. Correlation between postmortem cardiac troponin and histological evidence of cardiomyocyte necrosis

At postmortem, the diagnosis of myocardial infarction is typically assessed by gross macroscopic anatomy further confirmed by microscopic histology and immunohistochemical analysis. Defining AMI in a medico-legal autopsy is a clinical challenge for the forensic pathologist as detection can only be made 4–6 hours after the onset of cardiac ischemia. Histological changes indicative of AMI include oedema, congestion, haemorrhage, inflammation cytoplasmic vacuoles, contraction band alterations, fibrosis and necrosis. Immunohistochemical analysis at postmortem has focused on a number of markers of cellular damage, including C5b-9, myoglobin, CK-MB, fibronectin myosin heart-type fatty acid binding protein and desmin [30].

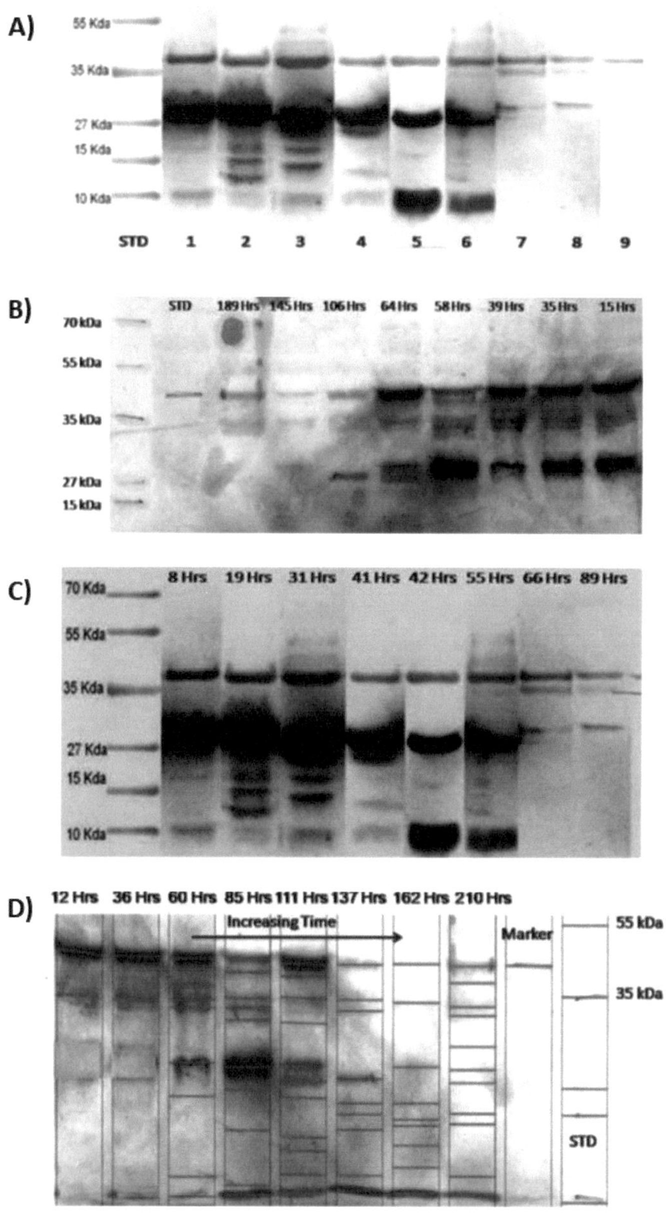

Figure 4.
Cardiac troponin T (cTnT) degradation patterns (Western blotting) in (a) fatal burn; (b) myocardial infarction; (c) electrocution; (d) asphyxiation (source: Adapted from (a) [25]; b–d [26]).

A number of studies have evaluated postmortem cTn concentrations in relation to evidence of cardiomyocyte necrosis (**Figure 6**). Ortmann and colleagues identified antigen depletion in the detection of early ischemic cardiac lesions in 8 cases of AMI, 8 cases of sudden cardiac death and 12 cases of acute exogenic hypoxia due to hanging or carbon monoxide poisoning. Strong evidence of immunohistochemical depletion

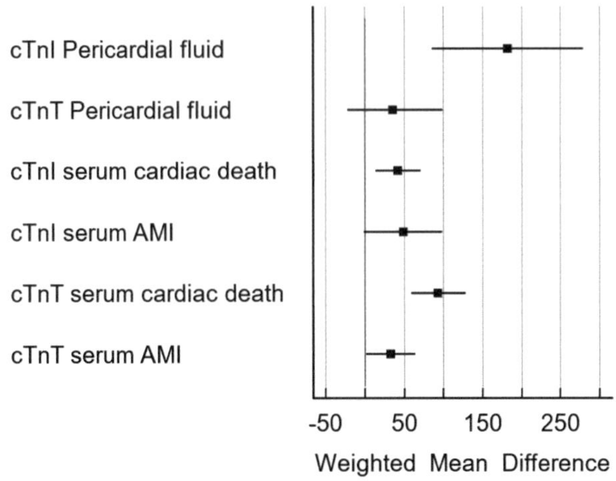

Figure 5.
Meta-analysis of pericardial fluid and serum cardiac troponin I, cTnI; or cardiac troponin T, cTnT; in the investigation of cardiac death and acute myocardial infarction, AMI (source: data extracted from [28]).

of cTnT was evident in all eight cases of AMI, in 50% of sudden cardiac death and in 1 (8%) of acute exogenic hypoxia, with 42% demonstrating weak loss and 50% demonstrating negative results (no loss of cTnT staining) [30].

Martinez Diaz and colleagues have demonstrated immunohistological changes in cTn in AMI or multiple trauma compared to other causes of death. PCF cTnI, myoglobin and CKMB were all significantly higher in AMI or multiple trauma cases compared to other causes of death. Serum concentrations of cTnI myoglobin and CKMB were not significantly different between the two groups [31]. Immunohistological analysis was performed by the authors with the analysis of troponin C and cTnT staining. 86% of cases demonstrated strong positive TnC with expression differing in isolated cells demonstrating contraction band necrosis but with significantly less intensity in the area of the infarction. cTnT staining was less evident in only 46% of cases in focal areas of the tissue.

Campobasso et al. [34] compared 4 immunohistochemical markers as early indicators of myocardial ischemia in 18 sudden cardiac deaths (4 AMI,4 coronary deaths, 8 acute cardiac deaths compared to 6 cases of acute traumatic death gunshot wounds with immediate lethal head injury). The authors stained paraffin-embedded myocardial tissue and immunohistochemically stained the tissue for C5b-9, fibronectin, myoglobin and cTnI. Diffuse depletion of cTnI was evident in all AMI deaths, in 75% of acute cardiac deaths, with 50% of coronary deaths demonstrating limited cellular foci depletion and normal distribution in all six cases of acute traumatic death. Whilst the staining patterns were significantly different between the cardiac and non-cardiac deaths, the authors concluded that no single marker was able to detect early myocardial ischemia and the combination of all four markers was useful in demonstrating evidence of myocardial ischemia and/or necrosis [34].

More recently, Amin and co-workers stained histological sections from ischemic and non-ischemic cardiac tissue for cTnT, myoglobin and caspase-3, demonstrating cTnT detection in normal myocardium and loss in necrotic tissue. The loss of cTnT was non-uniform with greater loss at the periphery compared to the central regions of infarcted tissue [35].

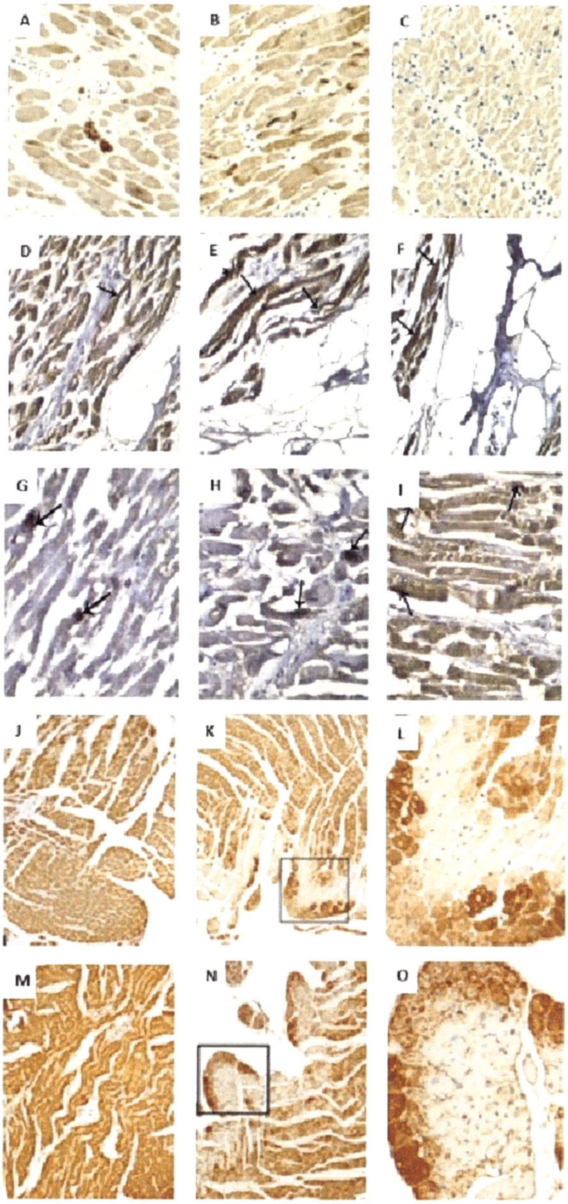

Figure 6
Immunohistochemical staining of cardiac troponin: (A) TnC in isolated cells with evidence of necrosis ×325; (B) TnC in contraction band necrosis ×300; (C) TnC in infarction zone ×200; (D–F) TnC in myocardium from sudden cardiac death due to coronary atherosclerosis. Brown expression (arrow) increases with PMI where (D) 1st PMI, (E) 2nd PMI, (F) 3rd PMI; (G–I) TnC in myocardium from sudden cardiac death due to myocardial infarction. Brown expression (arrow) increases with PMI where (G) 1st PMI, (H) 2nd PMI, (I) 3rd PMI; (J–L) cTnI immunohistochemical staining of the anteriolateral right ventricle in (J) non-ischemic cardiac tissue demonstrating no depletion in cTnI ×10; (K) 1 hour of LAD ligation demonstrating cTnI depletion in the subendocardial region [square box] ×10; (L) magnified box area from section K ×40. (M–O) cTnT immunohistochemical staining of the anteriolateral right ventricle in (M) non-ischemic cardiac tissue demonstrating no depletion in cTnT ×10; (N) 1 hour of LAD ligation demonstrating cTnT depletion in the subendocardial region [square box] ×10; (O) magnified box area from section N ×40 (sources: adapted from (A–C) [31]; (D–I) [32]; (J–O) [33]).

7. Conclusions

This chapter summarises the extensive literature base examining the clinical utility of cardiac troponin when tested in the postmortem setting. Whilst there is overwhelming evidence to support the superior value of pericardial fluid cTn rather than blood sampling due to significant interferences with the latter, there remains the issue of clinically validated cut-off concentrations in postmortem sampling. The effect of autolysis and increasing concentrations of cTn in fluid analysis correlated with increasing postmortem interval of significance. These features therefore suggest that cTn analysis is more suited as a rule out of cardiac involvement in sudden death rather than a rule in diagnostic aid. The diagnostic utility should be limited to the hospital autopsy rather than the medico-legal postmortem where these factors and interferences could provide scope for counter arguments by the defence counsel. Further work is required in the medico-legal setting to establish appropriate diagnostic cut-off values for cTnT and cTnI in postmortem samples, and clinical pathological guidelines should be written to provide support to the forensic teams to correctly interpret the evidence from this large selection of published literature.

Author details

David C. Gaze
Chemical Pathology, University of Westminster, London, United Kingdom

*Address all correspondence to: d.gaze@westminster.ac.uk

References

[1] Thygesen K et al. Fourth universal definition of myocardial infarction (2018). European Heart Journal. 2019;**40**(3):237-269

[2] Park KC et al. Cardiac troponins: From myocardial infarction to chronic disease. Cardiovascular Research. 2017;**113**(14):1708-1718

[3] Hickman PE et al. Cardiac troponin may be released by ischemia alone, without necrosis. Clinica Chimica Acta; International Journal of Clinical Chemistry. 2010;**411**(5-6):318-323

[4] Ragusa R et al. Cardiac troponins: Mechanisms of release and role in healthy and diseased subjects. BioFactors (Oxford, England). 2023;**49**:251-264

[5] Fishbein MC et al. Myocardial tissue troponins T and I. An immunohistochemical study in experimental models of myocardial ischemia. Cardiovascular Pathology: The Official Journal of the Society for Cardiovascular Pathology. 2003;**12**(2):65-71

[6] Collinson PO et al. Measurement of cardiac troponins. Annals of Clinical Biochemistry. 2001;**38**(Pt 5):423-449

[7] Luna A. Is postmortem biochemistry really useful? Why is it not widely used in forensic pathology? Legal Medicine (Tokyo, Japan). 2009;**11**(Suppl 1):27

[8] Belsey SL, Flanagan RJ. Postmortem biochemistry: Current applications. Journal of Forensic and Legal Medicine. 2016;**41**:49-57

[9] Madea B, Musshoff F. Postmortem biochemistry. Forensic Science International. 2007;**165**(2-3):165-171

[10] Luna A et al. The determination of CK, LDH and its isoenzymes in pericardial fluid and its application to the post-mortem diagnosis of myocardial infarction. Forensic Science International. 1982;**19**(1):85-91

[11] Stewart RV et al. Postmortem diagnosis of myocardial disease by enzyme analysis of pericardial fluid. American Journal of Clinical Pathology. 1984;**82**(4):411-417. [Accessed: February 22, 2023]

[12] Lachica E et al. Comparison of different techniques for the postmortem diagnosis of myocardial infarction. Forensic Science International. 1988;**38**(1):21-26

[13] Burns J et al. Necropsy study of association between sudden death and cardiac enzymes. Journal of Clinical Pathology. 1992;**45**(3):217-220

[14] Perez-Cárceles MD et al. Biochemical assessment of acute myocardial ischaemia. Journal of Clinical Pathology. 1995;**48**(2):124-128. [Accessed: February 22, 2023]

[15] Pérez-Cárceles MD et al. Usefulness of myosin in the postmortem diagnosis of myocardial damage. International Journal of Legal Medicine. 1995;**108**(1):14-18. [Accessed: February 22, 2023]

[16] Osuna E et al. Cardiac troponin I (cTn I) and the postmortem diagnosis of myocardial infarction. International Journal of Legal Medicine. 1998;**111**(4):173-176

[17] Cina SJ et al. A rapid postmortem cardiac troponin T assay: Laboratory evidence of sudden cardiac death. The

American Journal of Forensic Medicine and Pathology. 2001;**22**(2):173-176

[18] Kluakamkao G et al. Diagnosis of acute myocardia infarction in sudden unexplained death by a troponin T sensitive rapid assay. Chiang Mai Medical Bulletin. 2004;**43**(2):57-65

[19] Davies SJ et al. Investigation of cardiac troponins in postmortem subjects: Comparing antemortem and postmortem levels. The American Journal of Forensic Medicine and Pathology. 2005;**26**(3):213-215

[20] Rahimi R et al. Post mortem troponin T analysis in sudden death: Is it useful? The Malaysian Journal of Pathology. 2018;**40**(2):143-148

[21] Lai PS et al. Comparison between ante-mortem and post-mortem troponin T. Romanian Journal of Legal Medicine. 2018;**26**:359-362

[22] Zhu B et al. Postmortem cardiac troponin T levels in the blood and pericardial fluid. Part 1. Analysis with special regard to traumatic causes of death. Legal Medicine (Tokyo, Japan). 2006a;**8**(2):86-93

[23] Zhu B et al. Postmortem cardiac troponin T levels in the blood and pericardial fluid. Part 2: Analysis for application in the diagnosis of sudden cardiac death with regard to pathology. Legal Medicine (Tokyo, Japan). 2006b;**8**(2):94-101

[24] Remmer S et al. Cardiac troponin T in forensic autopsy cases. Forensic Science International. 2013;**233**(1-3):154-157

[25] Kumar S et al. The effect of elapsed time on cardiac troponin-T (cTnT) degradation and its relation to postmortem interval in cases of electrocution. Journal of Forensic and Legal Medicine. 2015;**34**:45-49

[26] Kumar S et al. Temperature-dependent postmortem changes in human cardiac troponin-T (cTnT): An approach in estimation of time since death. Journal of Forensic Sciences. 2016;**61**(Suppl. 1):241

[27] Carvajal-Zarrabal O et al. Use of cardiac injury markers in the postmortem diagnosis of sudden cardiac death. Journal of Forensic Sciences. 2017;**62**(5):1332-1335

[28] Barberi C, van den Hondel KE. The use of cardiac troponin T (cTnT) in the postmortem diagnosis of acute myocardial infarction and sudden cardiac death: A systematic review. Forensic Science International. 2018;**292**:27-38

[29] Cao Z et al. Diagnostic roles of postmortem cTn I and cTn T in cardiac death with special regard to myocardial infarction: A systematic literature review and Meta-analysis. International Journal of Molecular Sciences. 2019;**20**(13):3351

[30] Ortmann C et al. A comparative study on the immunohistochemical detection of early myocardial damage. International Journal of Legal Medicine. 2000;**113**(4):215-220. [Accessed: March 7, 2023]

[31] Martinez Diaz F et al. Biochemical analysis and immunohistochemical determination of cardiac troponin for the postmortem diagnosis of myocardial damage. Histology and Histopathology. 2005;**20**(2):475-481

[32] Abdel-Azeem E et al. Medicolegal use of troponin C expression to identify different causes of cardiac deaths at different postmortem intervals. Zagazig Journal of Forensic Medical and Toxicology. 2019;**17**(1):1-9

[33] Sabatasso S, Mangin P, Francasso T, Moretti Mx, Docquier M, Djonov V. Early markers of myocardial ischemia and sudden cardiac death. International Journal of Legal Medicine. 2016;**130**:1265-1280

[34] Campobasso CP et al. Sudden cardiac death and myocardial ischemia indicators: A comparative study of four immunohistochemical markers. The American Journal of Forensic Medicine and Pathology. 2008;**29**(2):154-161

[35] Amin HAA et al. Immuno-histochemistry in the detection of early myocardial infarction (a post mortem study). Egyptian Journal of Forensic Sciences. 2011;**1**:5-12

Section 3
Cardiovascular Treatments

Chapter 21

Moving beyond Cardio: The Value of Resistance Exercise Training for Cardiovascular Disease

Brandon S. Shaw, Gavin R.H. Sandercock, Anneke Van Biljon and Ina Shaw

Abstract

Cardiovascular disease (CVD) continues to be the leading cause of death and continuous efforts are needed to reduce CVD risk and established CVD. Most exercise training guidelines do not recommend RT as an integral component of an overall CVD prevention and/or rehabilitation programme. This is notwithstanding the increasing evidence of RT's orthopaedic and hemodynamic safety, its cardioprotective effects and positive effects on mortality, and even its unique role on improving the comorbidities associated with CVD. As with cardiorespiratory fitness, muscular fitness is increasingly being demonstrated to be related to the integrated function of numerous physiological systems and as a reflection of whole-body health and function. As such, '"counting reps'" should be as important as '"counting steps'" in any CVD prevention and management programme. While many current international recommendations and guidelines are based on the fact that not all health benefits can be achieved through a single type of exercise, emphasis is still placed on aerobic training over RT. This chapter will not only discuss the importance of RT in overall CVD prevention and/or rehabilitation, but will directly inform recommendations and provide guidelines on practical exercise as a safe and foundational component of CVD programmes.

Keywords: cardiac rehabilitation, exercise, non-communicable disease, physical fitness, strength training, weight training

1. Introduction

Cardiovascular disease (CVD) continues to be the number one cause of death worldwide [1] and accounts for approximately 50% percent of all deaths in high-income countries (HICs) and approximately 28% of deaths in low- and middle-income countries (LMICs), with figures increasing exponentially [2]. Problematically, the emergence of COVID-19, officially known as Severe Acute Respiratory Syndrome-Coronavirus-2 (SARS-CoV-2), presents an unparalleled challenge for people with CVD. This is because individuals with pre-existing CVD are more likely to develop COVID-19 are more likely to present with more severe symptoms and have worse clinical outcomes [3, 4]. Recent findings are also demonstrating that COVID-19 is responsible for both the development of new and exacerbation of pre-existing CVD due to a variety of factors, such as resultant myocardial injury and the development of new-onset cardiac dysfunction from the infection [3] and long-term consequences arising from infection, such as possible continued abnormalities of lipid metabolism [5].

2. Exercise training and the primary, secondary and tertiary prevention of cardiovascular disease

Although more than 200 risk factors have now been identified that can give rise to CVD, the major risk factors of smoking, hypertension, dyslipidemia and physical inactivity have been recognised for over 50 years [6, 7]. Problematically, the 200 or so risk factors often perform complex interactions and may act synergistically acting to amplify the damage caused by any one risk factor alone [8]. Despite the existence of proven strategies for the prevention and management of CVD risk, millions of individuals worldwide continue to develop and display behaviours and characteristics that increase the risk for developing CVD.

In this regard, physical inactivity, while listed as the fourth leading cause of death worldwide [6], is modifiable with an overwhelming body of evidence demonstrating the benefits of physical activity for cardiovascular health. Physical activity can both modify individual risk factors, but it also reduces overall risk of CVD [9]. As such, evidence supports the inclusion of exercise training in a) the primary prevention (preventing the onset of CVD) [10], b) secondary prevention (reducing the impact of CVD prior to any critical or permanent damage to health) [11] and c) tertiary prevention of CVD (slowing, arresting, or reversing CVD to prevent further deterioration, and reduce the risk of subsequent events) [12]. In addition, physical exercise can be employed in low, middle or high income countries [13].

3. Rationale for resistance training exercise training and the primary, secondary and tertiary prevention of cardiovascular disease as cardiovascular therapy

3.1 Moving beyond cardio and cardiorespiratory fitness: the value of resistance training in cardiovascular disease prevention and management

Many health organisations, such as the American Heart Association (AHA), provide exercise guidelines and recommendations for CVD, which tend to focus on aerobic exercise prescription [14]. While the health benefits of aerobic exercise are well established there is sufficient evidence from experimental studies, reviews and meta-analyses to justify the inclusion of RT, either alone, or at least in equal combination to aerobic training, not only in apparently healthy populations [15] but also for the attenuating of several risk factors of CVD [16] and in comprehensive cardiovascular therapy programmes [17]. Recently, in fact, a low volume, single-set RT exercise programme has proven sufficient to reduce CVD risk in untrained older women [18].

Further, evidence is mounting that RT plays a significant role in morbidity. This is because muscular fitness (a general term that describes the general health, endurance, power and strength of muscles) is increasingly being correlated to many types of mortality, including cardiovascular mortality [19]. As with cardiorespiratory fitness, muscular fitness may also be directly related to the integrated function of numerous physiological systems, including the cardiorespiratory and musculoskeletal systems, and could be utilised to provide a reflection of whole-body health and function. Research on the relationship between morbidity and muscular strength, and specifically handgrip strength [20, 21], quadriceps testing [21, 22] and bench press testing [22] suggest that muscular strength should be viewed as an independent CVD risk factor [23]. This is because these proxies of overall strength have been proven to have significant inverse relationships with all-cause mortality, even after controlling for other risk factors, including level of cardiorespiratory fitness [19, 24]. With regards to muscular endurance, research has shown an inverse association between the number of sit-ups in one minute and mortality [25]. Research has also demonstrated that death rates of 30 per 10,000 in individuals with low muscular fitness, compared with just 12 per 10,000 in individuals with high muscular fitness [26]. As with cardiorespiratory fitness, there may be many health benefits directly and indirectly associated with muscular fitness, for example, high levels of muscular fitness may indirectly improve cardiovascular health profiles, through its beneficial effects on hypertension [27], dyslipemia [8], body composition [28, 29], diet [30], aerobic performance [31] and functional capacity [19]. Given the prognostic power of muscular fitness (and specifically muscular endurance and muscular strength) as a predictor of all-cause mortality, muscular fitness assessments should be highly considered to improve the efficacy of individualised CVD patient risk assessment and resultant clinical decisions.

3.2 The rise of home-based exercise training

Many governments adopted hardened nationwide quarantine or implemented forms of lockdowns in attempts to reduce the spread of COVID-19. Lockdowns present a major problem in terms of physical activity. Lockdowns promote inactivity through direct personal restrictions, shutting down gymnasiums and fitness centers, and through suspension or cessation of many outdoor activities [32, 33]. These COVID-19 restriction attempts rapidly accelerated the uptake of home-based exercise training [34], a trend which has been building, albeit slowly, for decades [35]. As gymnasiums and fitness centers closed due to COVID-19 restrictions, individuals and health professionals were forced to exercise differently using limited equipment in limited space. While COVID-19 restrictions are being lifted worldwide, and even as gymnasiums and fitness centers begin to open, home-based exercise training may become a new mainstay, whether due to their ease of use, or even due to economic downturns. Already, the American College of Sports Medicine (ACSM) ranks home exercise gymnasiums, strength training with free weights and body weight training at 2, 4 and 8, respectively in their Worldwide Survey of Fitness Trends for 2022 [34]. Notwithstanding the COVID-19 crisis, many individuals chose to and will continue to choose home-based exercise training as it is more convenient and flexible. Importantly, home-based exercise training can be as effective as facility-based exercise training, in clinically stable low- to moderate-risk patients with CVD [36].

4. Cardiovascular disease and resistance training across the lifespan

While the focus of much CVD studies is on adults, it is important to recognise that CVD risk factors may develop and even begin to detrimentally affect health during in childhood and adolescence [37]. The arteriosclerotic process can begin and rapidly accelerate at an early age [38]. As with adults, CVD risk factors, and especially composite CVD scores, are strongly associated with physical fitness in children [39, 40]. This has led to several recent changes having occurred in international recommendations for children's participation in physical activity for health [39]. Research, evidence and subsequent guidelines predominantly promote the benefits of aerobic activity for children and adolescents. Again, RT has proven to be a safe exercise modality able to promote improved cardiovascular health in children. Despite some research indicating that the beneficial effects from RT interventions are sometime modest [39], RT can supply additional, unique benefits to the health and functional capacity of children in particular. These benefits can be realised over and above those from aerobic exercise [40]. In this regard, low muscle strength has been independently associated with a poorer metabolic profile during adolescence [41]. In addition, increasing evidence is arising indicating that concurrent training programmes utilising both aerobic and RT components display additive or crossover effects of both modes of training when compared to a single mode of exercise alone, even in children [40]. It is for this reason that the promotion of physical activity, including RT, should be a critical element in public health policy to prevent the onset of CVD later in life [39, 42]. This is because childhood provides an excellent window of opportunity to educate children about healthy lifestyle habits and cardiovascular health, rather than to attempt to re-programme well-established unhealthy behaviours in adults.

Despite some developed countries, such as the United Sates of America, seeing an overall reduction in CVD mortality, CVD mortality is on the rise in younger women [43]. This is because in addition to an increasing prevalence of CVD risk factors, women display several clinical conditions or sex-specific CVD risk factors, such as pre-eclampsia, gestational diabetes, polycystic ovary syndrome, early menopause and autoimmune diseases that have been shown to increase the development of CVD [43, 44]. Although great strides have been made regarding CVD mortality in women, not all women are benefitting equally from CVD-related mortality reduction. In this regard, women could gain significant cardioprotective benefits from engaging in RT. This is because RT has been proven safe for use in women and has a unique ability to maintain or increase muscle mass [45, 46] and may offset their lower muscle mass and higher fat mass when compared to men [47]. Individuals with high muscle mass, especially when combined with low fat mass display the lowest mortality risk compared with other body composition subtypes [48, 49]. Women's lower muscle mass when combined with their average 40% less upper-body strength and 33% less lower-body muscle strength and their effect on mortality [50], calls for the specific inclusion of RT as part of any guideline-directed, evidence-based, and sex-specific management and treatment recommendations aimed at improving CVD outcomes in women.

Age also plays a critical role in the deterioration of cardiovascular function, and it is for this reason that risk and prevalence of CVD both increase with age [51, 52]. Increases in CVD in older adults can be linked to functional changes in the ageing heart (i.e. diastolic and systolic dysfunction) and/or electrical dysfunction (i.e. arrhythmias) and other CVD risk factors, such as inflammation, oxidative stress, apoptosis and degeneration [52, 53]. This degeneration is as a result of a significant loss of muscle mass or sarcopenia that is one of the hallmarks of ageing. Without intervention, sarcopenia may eventually lead to physical disability and loss of independence [54]. Thankfully, older adults can gain the health benefits of physical activity, regardless of age, provided that the threshold for irreversible frailty has not been reached [54, 55]. While the optimal health benefits of exercise are best realised from a combination of aerobic and resistance exercise training, most older adults do not meet minimum guidelines for exercise or when they do, they do not engage in RT [56]. This is problematic in that RT remains the most consistent and effective method of promoting global muscular adaptations [56] and for promoting increases in muscle mass [46]. It is for this reason that RT, especially in the form of strengthening- and hypertrophic-exercise is even more critical for older adults and should be emphasised in future guidelines, as it may be the most effective standalone exercise strategy for improving health of older adults [57, 58]. Failing this, RT should be highlighted as an essential component in multimodal exercise training programmes in older adults, and especially frail adults [59, 60]. Problematically, even when RT training is recommended as equally important to aerobic exercise as in the UK PA Guidelines, guidelines regarding RT appear to be interpreted as secondary to the primary message of achieving 150 minutes of aerobic training, and there is some evidence that the strength guideline is both less well known and less often achieved. Given the importance of maintaining or increasing muscle strength, particularly for adults at the upper end of the 19–64 age range, this guideline should be given equal emphasis.

5. Practical resistance training Programme design for CVD prevention and management

RT, sometimes referred to as weight training or erroneously as strength training, involves the performance of physical exercise against resistance or weight. While RT is commonly associated with lifting of dumbbells and barbells in a gymnasium setting, it can also incorporate a variety of training techniques, such as callisthenics, Pilates, yoga, free weights, weight machines, resistance bands, isometrics, high-intensity interval training (HITT) and plyometrics [17]. It is this plethora of RT exercise types and programme design iterations (i.e. frequency, intensity, muscle groups, single–/multi-joint exercise, sets, repetition, rest intervals, etc.) that provides much consternation for many health organisations and health professionals, leading to guidelines

Frequency	Intensity	Repetitions	Sets	Type
RT Programme Design for Apparently Healthy Individuals/Low to Moderate CVD Risk				
2 or more sessions per week	Moderate to high 50–70% 1-RM	8–12 reps	3–4 sets per exercise; with short rest intervals (30–60 s)	8–10 different RT exercises using multi-joint or compound movements involving >1 muscle group
RT Programme Design for Individuals with High CVD Risk and existing CVD				
3 days per week	Low intensity >30% 1-RM	10–12 reps	1–3 sets per exercise; medium to long rest intervals (60–90 s)	8–10 different exercises including multi-joint or compound movements involving >1 muscle group

Table 1.
Guidelines for resistance training programme design based on CVD risk/presence of CVD (adapted from Shaw, Brown & Shaw, 2021 [17]).

or position statements for each CVD [17]. While it is these same design considerations that can be fine-tuned, by advanced exercise scientists in cardiovascular therapy, to exact a similar plethora of physiological changes and adaptions that are well suited to CVD prevention and management, practical and easy-to-follow RT regimes do exist for prevention and management of CVD (**Table 1**) [17].

6. Conclusions

The available evidence continues to support the recommendation that all adults should undertake activities which increase or maintain muscle strength at least twice a week. A credible amount of research exists demonstrating that RT, even when performed in isolation, does contribute to prevention [59], management and rehabilitation of CVD. Further, the historical idea that the benefits of RT and aerobic exercise training are independent of one another, with minimal crossover, is no longer supported by the evidence. This is because, at present, sufficient evidence exists to challenge existing exercise guidelines and recommendations that call for aerobic exercise training to be considered as the gold standard in CVD prevention and management, with RT, at best, being assigned a minor role in a comprehensive exercise therapy programme. In this regard, the available data clearly indicates that when RT is combined aerobic training, the impact in terms of reduction in CVD risk from this combination is greater than the sum of its parts. This is likely caused by the synergistic benefits realised through positive transference by modality - or crossover effect.

Acknowledgements

The authors would like to acknowledge the contributions made by the Non-Communicable Disease Intervention Research Unit (NCDIRU).

Conflict of interest

The authors declare no conflict of interest.

Author details

Brandon S. Shaw[1*], Gavin R.H. Sandercock[1], Anneke Van Biljon[2] and Ina Shaw[1]

1 School of Sport, Rehabilitation and Exercise Sciences, University of Essex, Wivenhoe Park, Colchester, Essex, United Kingdom

2 Department of Human Movement Science, University of Zululand, Kwadlangezwa, South Africa

*Address all correspondence to: b.shaw@essex.ac.za

References

[1] World Health Organization (WHO). Cardiovascular diseases. Available from: https://www.who.int/health-topics/cardiovascular-diseases#tab=tab_1

[2] Mathers CD, Lopez AD, Murray CJL. Chapter 3. The burden of disease and mortality by condition: Data, methods, and results for 2001. In: Lopez AD, Mathers CD, Ezzati M, Jamison DJ, Murray CJL, editors. Global Burden of Disease and Risk Factors. Washington (DC), USA: The International Bank for Reconstruction and Development/The World Bank; 2006

[3] Clerkin KJ, Fried JA, Radiohelia J, Sayer G, Griffin JM, Masoumi A, et al. COVID-19 and cardiovascular disease. Circulation. 2020;**141**:1648-1655. DOI: 10.1161/CIRCULATIONAHA.120.046941

[4] Wu Z, McGoogan JM. Characteristics of and important lessons from the coronavirus disease 2019 (COVID-19) outbreak in China: Summary of a report of 72314 cases from the Chinese Center for Disease Control and prevention. Journal of the American Medical Association. 2020;**323**(13):1239-1242. DOI: 10.1001/jama.2020.2648

[5] Bansal M. Cardiovascular disease and COVID-19. Diabetes & Metabolic Syndrome: Clinical Research & Reviews. 2020;**14**(3):247-250. DOI: 10.1016/j.dsx.2020.03.013

[6] Kohl HW 3rd, Craig CL, Lambert EV, Inoue S, Alkandari JR, Leetongin G, et al. Lancet physical activity series working group. The pandemic of physical inactivity: Global action for public health. Lancet. 2012;**380**(9838):294-305. DOI: 10.1016/S0140-6736(12)60898-8

[7] Lawrence KE, Shaw I, Shaw BS. Hemodynamic changes in normotensive overweight and obese individuals following home-based calisthenics training. African Journal for Physical, Health Education, Recreation and Dance. 2014;**Supplement 2**(September):82-90

[8] Shaw I, Shaw BS. Relationship between resistance training and lipoprotein profiles in sedentary male smokers. Cardiovascular Journal of Africa. 2008;**19**(4):194-197

[9] Pinckard K, Baskin KK, Stanford KI. Effects of exercise to improve cardiovascular health. Frontiers in Cardiovascular Medicine. 2019;**4**(6):69. DOI: 10.3389/fcvm.2019.00069

[10] Shaw BS, Shaw I, Brown GA. Resistance exercise is medicine: Strength training in health promotion and rehabilitation. International Journal of Therapy and Rehabilitation. 2015;**22**(8):385-389

[11] Geevar Z, Anoop GA. Exercise for prevention of cardiovascular disease: Evidence-based recommendations. Journal of Clinical and Preventative Cardiology. 2017;**6**(3):109-114. DOI: 10.4103/JCPC.JCPC_9_17

[12] Almody M, Ingle L, Sandercock GRH. Effects of exercise-based cardiac rehabilitation on cardiorespiratory fitness: A meta-analysis of UK studies. International Journal of Cardiology. 2016;**221**:644-651. DOI: 10.1016/j.ijcard.2016.06.101

[13] Shaw BS, Shaw I. Resistance training as a countermeasure for key non-communicable diseases in low-resource settings: A review. Asian. Journal of Sports Medicine. 2021;**12**(1):1-8, e106588. DOI: 10.5812/asjsm.106588

[14] Shaw BS, Dullabh M, Forbes G, Brandkamp J, Shaw I. Analysis of

physiological determinants during a single bout of Crossfit. International Journal of Performance Analysis in Sport. 2015;**15**:809-815. DOI: 10.1080/24748668.2015.11868832

[15] Shaw BS, Shaw I, Brown GA. Comparison of resistance and concurrent resistance and endurance training regimes in the development of strength. Journal of Strength and Conditioning Research. 2009;**23**(9):2507-2514. DOI: 10.1519/JSC.0b013e3181bc191e

[16] Carbone S, Kirkman DL, Garten RS, Rodriguez-Miguelez P, Artero EG, Lee D, et al. Muscular strength and cardiovascular disease: An updated state-of-the-art narrative review. Journal of Cardiopulmonary Rehabilitation and Prevention. 2020;**40**(5):302-309. DOI: 10.1097/HCR.0000000000000525

[17] Shaw BS, Brown GA, Shaw I. Importance of resistance training in the management of cardiovascular disease risk. In: Chahine J, editor. Cardiovascular Risk Factors. London, United Kingdom: IntechOpen Publishers; 2021

[18] Cunha PM, Ribeiro AS, Nunes JP, Tomeleri CM, Nascimento MA, Moraes GK, et al. Resistance training performed with single-set is sufficient to reduce cardiovascular risk factors in untrained older women: The randomized clinical trial. Archives of Gerontology and Geriatrics. 2019;**81**:171-175. DOI: 10.1016/j.archger.2018.12.012

[19] Volaklis KA, Halle M, Meisinger C. Muscular strength as a strong predictor of mortality: A narrative review. European Journal of Internal Medicine. 2015;**26**(5):303-310. DOI: 10.1016/j.ejim.2015.04.013

[20] Cheung CL, Nguyen US, Au E, Tan K, Kung A. Association of handgrip strength with chronic diseases and multimorbidity: A cross-sectional study. Age. 2013;**35**(3):929-941. DOI: 10.1007/s11357-012-9385-y

[21] McDermott MM, Liu K, Tian L, Guralnik JM, Criqui MH, Liao Y, et al. Calf muscle characteristics, strength measures and mortality in peripheral arterial disease: A longitudinal study. Journal of the American College of Cardiology. 2021;**59**(13):1159-1167. DOI: 10.1016/j.jacc.2011.12.019

[22] Artero EG, Lee D, Ruiz J, Sui X, Ortega FB, Church TS, et al. A prospective study of muscular strength and all-cause mortality in men with hypertension. Journal of the American College of Cardiology. 2011;**57**(18):1831-1837. DOI: 10.1016/j.jacc.2010.12.025

[23] Fourie M, Gildenhuys GM, Shaw I, Shaw BS, Toriola AL, Goon DT. Effects of a mat Pilates programme on muscular strength and endurance in elderly women. African Journal for Physical, Health Education, Recreation and Dance. 2012;**18**(2):296-304

[24] Metter EJ, Talbot LA, Schrager M, Conwit R. Skeletal muscle strength as a predictor of all-cause mortality in healthy men. Journals of Gerontology, Series A: Biological Sciences and Medical Sciences. 2002;**57**:B359-B365. DOI: 10.1093/gerona/57.10.B359

[25] Katzmarzyk PT, Craig CL. Musculoskeletal fitness and risk of mortality. Medicine and Science in ports and Exercise. 2002;**34**:740-744. DOI: 10.1097/00005768-200205000-00002

[26] FitzGerald SJ, Barlow CE, Kampert JB, Morrow JR Jr, Jackson AW, Blair SN. Muscular fitness and all-cause mortality: Prospective observations. Journal of Physical Activity and Health. 2004;**1**(1):7-18. DOI: 10.1123/jpah.1.1.7

[27] Shaw BS, Turner S, Shaw I. Comparison of muscle endurance and hypertrophy resistance training on cardiovascular disease risk in smokers. Asian. Journal of Sports Medicine. 2021;**12**(1):1-6: e106589. DOI: 10.5812/asjsm.106589

[28] Shaw BS, Shaw I, Brown GA. Resistance training and its effect on total, central and abdominal adiposity. South African Journal for Research in Sport, Physical Education and Recreation. 2009;**31**(2):97-108. DOI: 10.4314/sajrs.v31i2.46331

[29] Wanderley FAC, Moreira A, Sokhatska O, Palmares C, Moreira P, Sandercock G, et al. Differential responses of adiposity, inflammation and autonomic function to aerobic versus resistance training in older adults. Experimental Gerontology. 2013;**48**(3):326-333. DOI: 10.1016/j.exger.2013.01.002

[30] Shaw BS, Shaw I, Brown GA. Self-reported dietary intake following endurance, resistance and concurrent endurance and resistance training. Journal of Sports Science and Medicine. 2008;**7**(2):255-259

[31] Shaw BS, Shaw I. Effect of resistance training on cardiorespiratory endurance and coronary artery disease risk. Cardiovascular Journal of South Africa. 2005;**16**(5):200-204

[32] Fearnbach SN, Flanagan EW, Höchsmann C, Beyl RA, Altazan AD, Martin CK, et al. Factors protecting against a decline in physical activity during the COVID-19 pandemic. Medicine and Science in Sports and Exercise. 2021;**53**(7):1391-1399. DOI: 10.1249/mss.0000000000002602

[33] Lippi G, Henry BM, Sanchis-Gomar F. Physical inactivity and cardiovascular disease at the time of coronavirus disease 2019 (COVID-19). European Journal of Prevenative Cardiology. 2020;**27**(9):906-908. DOI: 10.1177/2047487320916823

[34] Thompson WR. Worldwide survey of fitness trends for 2022. Health & Fitness Journal. 2022;**26**(1):11-20. DOI: 10.1249/FIT.0000000000000732

[35] Billson JH, Cilliers JF, Pieterse JJ, Shaw BS, Shaw I, Toriola AL. Home versus gymnasium resistance training and flexibility performance in the elderly. South African Journal for Research in Sport, Physical Education and Recreation. 2011;**33**(3):1-9

[36] Thomas RJ, Beatty AL, Beckie TM, Brewer LC, Brown TM, Forman DE, et al. Home-based cardiac rehabilitation: A scientific statement from the American Association of Cardiovascular and Pulmonary Rehabilitation, the American Heart Association, and the American College of Cardiology. Circulation. 2019;**140**(1):e69-e89. DOI: 10.1161/CIR.0000000000000663

[37] King A, Fuster V. Children are key to CVD prevention. Nature Reviews Cardiology. 2010;7:297. DOI: /10.1038/nrcardio.2010.66

[38] Tanha T, Wollmer P, Thorsson O, Karlsson MK, Lindén C, Andersen LB, et al. Lack of physical activity in young children is related to higher composite risk factor score for cardiovascular disease. Acta Paediatrica. 2011;**100**(5):717-721. DOI: 10.1111/j.1651-2227.2011.02226.x

[39] Andersen LB, Riddoch C, Kriemler S, Hills AP, Hills A. Physical activity and cardiovascular risk factors in children. British Journal of Sports Medicine. 2011;**45**(11):1063-1063. DOI: 10.1136/bjsports-2011-090333

[40] Ogunleye AA, Sandercock GR, Voss C, Eisenmann JC, Reed K. Prevalence

of elevated mean arterial pressure and how fitness moderates its association with BMI in youth. Public Health Nutrition. 2013;**16**(11):2046-2054. DOI: 10.1017/S1368980012004466

[41] Faigenbaum AD, Geisler S. The promise of youth resistance training. B&G Bewegungstherapie und Gesundheitssport. 2021;**37**(02):47-51. DOI: 10.1055/a-1378-3385

[42] Ortega FB, Ruiz JR, Castillo MJ, Sjostrom M. Physical fitness in childhood and adolescence: A powerful marker of health. International Journal of Obesity. 2008;**32**:1-11. DOI: 10.1038/sj.ijo.0803774

[43] Shaw I, Boshoff VE, Coetzee S, Shaw BS. Efficacy of home-based callisthenic resistance training on cardiovascular disease risk in overweight compared to normal weight preadolescents. Asian Journal of Sports Medicine. 2021;**12**(1):1-5, e106591. DOI: 10.5812/asjsm.106591

[44] Young L, Cho L. Unique cardiovascular risk factors in women. Heart. 2019;**105**:1656-1660. DOI: 10.1136/heartjnl-2018-314268

[45] Maffei S, Guiducci L, Cugusi L, Cadeddu C, Deidda M, Gallina S, et al. Working group on "gender difference in cardiovascular disease" of the Italian Society of Cardiology. Women-specific predictors of cardiovascular disease risk - new paradigms. International Journal of Cardiology. 2019;**286**:190-197. DOI: 10.1016/j.ijcard.2019.02.005

[46] Shaw BS, Shaw I, Mamen A. Contrasting effects in body composition following endurance, resistance and concurrent endurance and resistance training. Journal of Sports Medicine and Physical Fitness. 2010;**50**(2):207-213

[47] Shaw I, Triplett NT, Shaw BS. Resistance training and weight management: Rationale and efficacy. In: Heshmati HM, editor. Weight Management - Challenges and Opportunities. London, United Kingdom: IntechOpen Publishers; 2022

[48] Schorr M, Dichtel LE, Gerweck AV, Valera RD, Torriani M, Miller KK, et al. Sex differences in body composition and association with cardiometabolic risk. Biology of Sex Differences. 2018;**9**:28. DOI: 10.1186/s13293-018-0189-3

[49] Srikanthan P, Horwich TB, Tseng CH. Relation of muscle mass and fat mass to cardiovascular disease mortality. The American Journal of Cardiology. 2016;**117**(8):1355-1360. DOI: 10.1016/j.amjcard.2016.01.033

[50] Tyrovolas S, Panagiotakos X, Georgousopoulou E, Chrysohoou C, Tousoulis D, Haro JM, et al. Skeletal muscle mass in relation to 10 year cardiovascular disease incidence among middle aged and older adults: The ATTICA study. Journal of Epidemiology and Community Health. 2020;**74**:26-31. DOI: 10.1136/jech-2019-212268

[51] Janssen I, Heymsfield SB, Wang ZM, Ross R. Skeletal muscle mass and distribution in 468 men and women aged 18-88 yr. Journal of Applied Physiology. 2000;**89**(1):81-88. DOI: 10.1152/jappl.2000.89.1.81

[52] Rodgers JL, Jones J, Bolleddu SI, Vanthenapalli S, Rodgers LE, Shah K, et al. Cardiovascular risks associated with gender and aging. Journal of Cardiovascular Development and Disease. 2019;**6**(2):19. DOI: 10.3390/jcdd6020019

[53] World Health Organization (WHO). Cardiovascular diseases (CVDs). Geneva: World Health Organization; 2017 Available from: http://www.who.int/cardiovascular_diseases/en/

[54] Steenman M, Lande G. Cardiac aging and heart disease in humans. Biophysical Reviews. 2017;**9**:131-137. DOI: 10.1007/s12551-017-0255-9

[55] Cadore EL, Casas-Herrero A, Zambom-Ferraresi F, Idoate F, Millor N, Gómez M, et al. Multicomponent exercises including muscle power training enhance muscle mass, power output, and functional outcomes in institutionalized frail nonagenarians. Age. 2014;**36**:773-785. DOI: 10.1007/s11357-013-9586-z

[56] Shaw I, Shaw BS, Brown GA. Concurrent training and pulmonary function in smokers. International Journal of Sports Medicine. 2011;**32**:776-780. DOI: 10.1055/s-0031-1277214

[57] Tavoian D, Russ DW, Consitt LA, Clark BC. Pragmatic exercise recommendations for older adults: The case for emphasizing resistance training. Frontiers in Physiology. 2020;**11**:799. DOI: 10.3389/fphys.2020.00799

[58] Miszko TA, Cress ME, Slade JM, Covey CJ, Agrawal SK, Doerr CE. Effect of strength and power training on physical function in community-dwelling older adults. Journals of Gerontology, Series A: Biological Sciences and Medical Sciences. 2003;**58**:M171-M175

[59] Liu C, Latham NK. Progressive resistance strength training for improving physical function in older adults. Cochrane Database Systematic Review. 2009;**6**:CD002759. DOI: 10.1002/14651858.CD002759.pub2

[60] Lopez P, Pinto RS, Radaelli R, Rech A, Grazioli R, Izquierdo M, et al. Benefits of resistance training in physically frail elderly: A systematic review. Aging Clinical and Experimental Research. 2018;**30**:889-899. DOI: 10.1007/s40520-017-0863-z

Chapter 22

Medication Adherence in Cardiovascular Diseases

Suol Thanh Pham, Thi Anh Nguyen, Nghia Minh Tran, Hoang Thi Kim Cao, Khanh Kim Le, Chu Xuan Duong, Thao Huong Nguyen, Katja Taxis, Khanh Duy Dang and Thang Nguyen

Abstract

Cardiovascular disease is a significant cause of death globally. While effective long-term medications that reduce the risk of morbidity and mortality related to cardiovascular disease are readily available, nonadherence to prescribed medications remains a significant reason for suboptimal management. Consequently, this might lead to increased morbidity and mortality and healthcare costs. Medication nonadherence causes are myriad and complicated, with factors at the patient, healthcare provider, and health system levels. Many clinical trials have investigated interventions to target these factors for improving medication adherence, including improving patient education, testing behavioral interventions, implementing medication reminder tools, reducing medication costs, utilizing social support, utilizing healthcare team members, and simplifying medication dosing regimens. This book chapter describes factors influencing medication adherence and highlights the impact of varying levels of adherence on patients' clinical and economic outcomes. We also summarize interventions for improving medication adherence in cardiovascular disease.

Keywords: cardiovascular disease, medication adherence, factors, health outcomes, economic outcomes, interventions

1. Introduction

Cardiovascular disease (CVD) is illnesses affecting the heart and blood vessels, including coronary heart diseases, cerebrovascular diseases, peripheral arterial diseases, rheumatic and congenital heart diseases, and venous thromboembolism [1]. CVD is a leading cause of death and disability worldwide [2]. According to the Global Burden of Diseases in 2019, CVD accounts for 15.52% of disability-adjusted life years (DALYs) and 32.84% of deaths [3].

Given the adverse health outcomes of CVD, if left untreated, long-term prevention and/or treatment of this disease is recommended. Treatment for CVD depends on its type and severity and can be divided into three main categories: lifestyle changes, medications, and surgical procedures. Overall, lifestyle changes and medications are often recommended for chronic CVD conditions, while surgical procedures are sometimes required to treat acute CVD events such as heart attack or stroke. In recognition of the vital role of medications in CVD management, this chapter is focused on medications for treating this disease.

Despite the availability of effective CVD medications, medication nonadherence remains pervasive globally [4]. A 27% nonadherence rate in patients with acute coronary syndrome (ACS) was reported only 1 week after discharge [5]. At 1 month following ACS, 34% of patients did not fill all prescriptions [6]. At 1–2 years following ACS, the nonadherence rate reaches 55–60% [7]. Medication adherence is how patients take medication(s) as prescribed by their healthcare providers [8]. Whereas nonadherence is defined as different behaviors: not initiating a new prescription, discontinuing medication(s) early, or not taking medication(s) as scheduled (e.g. less frequently) [9]. The rate of adherence for an individual patient is usually reported as the proportion of days covered (PDC) by the prescribed medication(s) over a specific time [10]. Methods for measuring adherence include direct and indirect methods, each of which has advantages and disadvantages. Direct methods, such as observed administration or measuring the concentration of medication in the blood, are more accurate but expensive and time-consuming. Indirect methods for measuring adherence, such as patient self-reporting or pill counting, are easier to conduct but less accurate. No measurement method is gold standard, and researchers should select a method based on their targeted nonadherence behavior(s) [11].

Past studies illustrated that nonadherence to cardiovascular medications negatively influences clinical and economic cardiovascular outcomes [12, 13]. Medication adherence in CVD is challenging to manage in routine practice due to multiple factors simultaneously affecting it [4]. These factors are classified into five interactive dimensions: patient, socioeconomic, healthcare system, therapy, and condition. Various interventions have been investigated to target these factors, and some appear promising. With accumulating studies on medication adherence in CVD in recent years, the chapter thus aims to update on common factors influencing medication adherence, clinical and economic outcomes of medications (non) adherence, and interventions targeting the identified factors to improve medication adherence in CVD.

2. Identification of nonadherence in clinical practice

The first and foremost issue for improving adherence is identifying nonadherence in all patients who do not respond to treatment. A simple and pragmatic solution for clinicians is to ask patients nonjudgmentally the frequency of their missed doses. Patients generally want to please their clinicians, thus avoiding declaring their missed doses. A few questions clinicians might ask their patients to feel more comfortable telling the truth were suggested: "I know it must be difficult to take all your medications regularly. How often do you miss taking them?" [8]. Other indirect questions should be asked to assess the likelihood of nonadherence, including how severe their disease is, what the benefits of taking medications are, whether they have any side effects from their medications and whether they have any troubles related to taking their medications (e.g. high medication costs or complex regimens).

3. Factors influencing adherence

After nonadherence is identified, there is a need to identify the underlying cause(s) to which intervention(s) might be tailored. According to World Health Organization (WHO), factors influencing medication adherence in CVD are classified into five different groups: patient-, socioeconomic-, healthcare system-, therapy-, and condition-related factors [14]. Based on the multidimensional nature of adherence, this classification accounts for all relevant factors influencing adherence. This corrects the traditional misconception that only patients are responsible for taking their medication(s) [14].

3.1 Patient-related factors

This aspect refers to the unique characteristics of each patient, not related to their illnesses or treatment, for example, age, gender, personal beliefs, education level, and understanding of their disease and treatment (see **Table 1** for details) [4, 15].

3.2 Socioeconomic-related factors

This aspect included influences originating from the patient's socioeconomic status (SES), not from the patient themselves nor the healthcare providers, for example, living conditions, financial situation, limited access to healthcare, and social support [4, 15]. Higher SES appeared to influence adherence positively, as detailed in **Table 2**.

3.3 Healthcare system-related factors

The relationship between patient and healthcare providers, or within the healthcare system itself, might influence medication adherence. This extended to communication problems and healthcare system requirements, making it difficult for patients to comprehend or follow treatment [4, 15].

The support from healthcare professionals played a vital role in improving patients' adherence, particularly during follow-ups. Inadequate communication between healthcare providers led to insufficient communication with patients, leading to nonadherence [4].

Insurance or other healthcare cost assistance was positively associated with medication adherence [29, 30]. Cost assistance helped patients to receive medications they would not afford otherwise. However, not all medications were covered [29, 30]. The ARTEMIS trial and the MI FREEE trial concluded that reducing the financial burden of treatment through full coverage prescription or copayment vouchers improved adherence [4]. One study reported increased adherence when providing a financial incentive to patients [31], while another reported that adherence only improved significantly when financial incentives were provided to both physicians and patients [4].

3.4 Therapy-related factors

This aspect included factors related to medication taking, such as medication class, side effects, dosing regimens, and polypharmacy [4]. The effects and complexity of the therapy might affect adherence.

Factor	Influence on medication adherence
Age	The correlation between age and medication adherence was controversial in the literature. While some found that increased age is positively correlated with adherence [16–20], and some found the inverse [16]. Patients aged 50–70 years had better adherence than those aged 18–50 years or over 70 years [15]. It was hypothesized that elderly patients had more comorbidities and, as such, were more concerned with their health and treatment [16].
Gender	The association between gender and adherence to cardiovascular medication remains inconsistent [15]. Some reported that the female gender was negatively correlated with adherence [19, 21–23]; one found that females have more adhered to medication than males [24]. In a systematic review, Bowry et al. found no association [25].
Ethnicity and linguistic proficiency	An American study reported Hispanic people have higher adherence rates than non-Hispanic people. Among native Spanish-speaking Hispanic people, those with better English skills showed lower adherence rates [26].
Forgetfulness	For more than one-third of all cases of nonadherence, forgetfulness was a common cause of nonadherence [4].
Education	Illiteracy or lower education level was associated with lower adherence [19, 27]. Understanding disease and treatment, especially the risk of nonadherence, increases the likelihood of adherence to treatment [15, 28].
Others	Alcohol use, stress, anxiety, impaired level of cognitive capabilities, and lack of time for medical appointments each separately had a negative impact on adherence [4, 15].

Table 1.
Patient-related factors that may influence medication adherence in CVD.

Factor	Influence on medication adherence
Living conditions	Living in areas with higher education rates or higher income positively impacted adherence [19].
Financial situation	One of eight patients with CVD had cost-related nonadherence [4]. People with higher income were inconsistently more likely to adhere to treatment, with some studies reporting correlation while others reporting none [15, 24]. The medication cost seemed to be inhibitive to adherence, and the unavailability of cheaper generic medications was also a factor in reducing adherence [29].
Access to healthcare	Geographical barriers preventing access to healthcare negatively affected adherence [27, 29]. The cost of travel to seek specific medications also impeded patients from following their treatment [29].
Social support	Culture inducing a distrust in medical treatment or problems with family relations may lead to nonadherence [27]. However, social support plays an important role in reinforcing adherence. Emotional support enabled people to voice their fears and ask for information as needed. Social support in the form of encouragement, prayers, and monetary aid helped keep patients motivated to follow treatment and maintain a healthy lifestyle [29].

Table 2.
Socioeconomic-related factors that may influence medication adherence in CVD.

Medication class consistently influenced adherence. Angiotensin II receptor blockers (ARBs) had the highest rate of adherence (~30–33% better than other classes), while diuretics showed the lowest rate [15]. Certain medications were reported to be hard to swallow [29]. Different packaging or brand names might cause some patients to dislike the medications, fearing fake medications [29]. Side effects might explain why different drug classes had different rates of adherence. At standard dose, thiazides were more likely to cause a side effect compared with beta-blockers (BBs), calcium-channel blockers, and angiotensin-converting enzyme inhibitors (ACEIs), while ARBs were not associated with any side effects [15, 32].

Complex dosing regimens (e.g. a large number of daily doses) might negatively influence adherence [15]. The once-daily dosing regimen was associated with better adherence as opposed to twice-daily in patients with atrial fibrillation receiving oral anticoagulants [33]. Adherence was decreased in patients taking many medications to treat their comorbidities, contributing to the forgetfulness of taking medications [4]. Frequent changes in regimens also affected adherence negatively [29].

3.5 Condition-related factors

This aspect was related to the patient's illnesses and comorbidities [15]. Factors in this aspect influenced medication adherence differently; certain comorbidities increased adherence, while others decreased it [15]. Generally, comorbidities were associated with lower adherence [34].

Severe chronic illnesses with significant symptoms hampered adherence, as were chronic diseases with little to no symptoms [27]. Patients receiving primary prevention were less likely to adhere than patients receiving secondary prevention [15]. The impact of comorbidity on adherence varied. While diabetes was reported to improve adherence in CVD patients [15, 27], depression affected adherence negatively [15, 32, 35, 36]. Persistent depression decreased adherence more than remittent depression, and severe depression came with a 3.7 times higher risk of nonadherence than no depression [35].

4. Medication adherence-related outcomes

4.1 Clinical outcomes

Many observational studies have assessed the relationship between medication adherence and outcomes in CVD. Past evidence shows the broad impact of untreated or inadequately treated CVD ranging from major cardiovascular events (MACEs) to mortality. This might be caused by suboptimal adherence to effective medications. Nonadherence to statins in post-myocardial infarction (MI) patients was associated with up to 25% increased hazard of death [37]. In chronic coronary artery disease, nonadherence to cardioprotective medications (antihypertensive and antihypercholesterolemic medications) was associated with up to 40% increase in the risk of hospitalizations for cardiovascular events and up to 80% increase in the risk of death [38]. Conversely, optimal adherence was associated with significantly reducing cardiovascular events and mortality. A recent meta-analysis indicated that each incremental 20% increase in adherence level of cardiovascular medication reduced the risk of cardiovascular events by 9%, stroke by 16%, and all-cause mortality by 10% [39]. Several clinical studies highlighted the benefits of cardiovascular medications and the importance of adherence to prescribed medications to optimize health outcomes. This can raise awareness of the importance of medication adherence in CVD among clinicians, patients, healthcare insurers, and policymakers. The potential of overestimating the adverse outcomes of suboptimal adherence should be noted. Nonadherent patients are less likely to follow health recommendations (e.g. flu vaccination) and more likely to engage in harmful behaviors (e.g. smoking), impacting health outcomes. Yet, these confounders can be minimized by (1) a well-designed study (i.e. using randomization, placebo, and double-blind) or (2) an appropriate statistical analysis. However, statistical analysis is less pronounced than study design, because a statistical analysis can be re-processed, but a poorly designed study can never be recovered. Medication adherence-related outcomes for specific diseases are detailed as follows:

4.1.1 Hypertension

Suboptimal adherence to antihypertensive drugs was associated with multiple adverse cardiovascular events from acute to chronic conditions (e.g. chronic heart failure) to death [32]. Suboptimal medication adherence was also associated with various organ disorders, including chronic kidney disease, cognitive dysfunction, and dementia [32]. A study including 155,597 patients with hypertension showed that highly adherent patients (≥80% PDC with antihypertensive medication) had less than half the risk of experiencing a cardiovascular event compared with lower adherent ones over a median duration of 5.8 years (adjusted hazard ratio [aHR] 0.44; 95% CI 0.42–0.45) [40].

In elderly diabetic patients having multiple comorbidities, a retrospective cohort study found that ≥80% adherence to ACEIs/ARBs was not associated with BP < 140/90 mmHg in those ≥85 years (risk ratio [RR] 1.01, 95% CI 0.96–1.07) or with multiple comorbid diseases (e.g. RR = 1.04, 95% CI 0.99–1.08) [41]. Reasons for uncontrolled BP despite optimal adherence might be (1) age-related physiological changes and (2) pathological changes by comorbidities (e.g. chronic kidney disease).

4.1.2 Myocardial infarction (MI)

Among post-MI patients, ≥80% adherence to both statins and ACEIs was associated with decreased risk of long-term MACEs (i.e. all-cause mortality, nonfatal MI hospitalization, stroke, or coronary revascularization) than <40% adherence (18.9% vs. 26.3%, HR 0.73, $P = 0.0004$) and 40–79% adherence (18.9% vs. 24.7%, HR 0.81; $P = 0.02$) at 2 years [42]. Another study across China in 4001 post-MI patients found that optimal adherence (≥90%) to cardiovascular medications was associated with a 39% reduction in the risk of 1-year cardiovascular events (aHR 0.61, 95% CI 0.49–0.77) [43].

4.1.3 Atherosclerotic cardiovascular disease (ASCVD)

In 12,976 patients with ASCVD from the American health insurance database, ≥80% adherence to both statins and ACEIs reduced the risk of long-term MACEs than <40% adherence (8.42% vs. 17.17%, HR 0.56, $P < 0.0001$) and 40–79% adherence (8.42% vs. 12.18%, HR 0.76, $P < 0.0001$) at 2 years [42]. Consistent with this finding, another study in 185,252 patients with ASCVD from the Taiwan National Health Insurance database found that ≥80% adherence to statins reduced the risk of ASCVD-related secondary rehospitalization (aHR 0.90, 95% CI 0.87–0.92, $P < 0.05$) and in-hospital death (aHR 0.59, 95% CI 0.53–0.65, $P < 0.05$) [44].

4.1.4 Heart failure (HF)

An analysis of 55,312 patients with HF indicated that each 10% increase in PDC by cardiovascular medications reduced all-cause mortality risk by 9% (odds ratio [OR]

0.91, 95% CI 0.90–0.92), emergency admissions by 11% (RR 0.89, 95% CI 0.89–0.89), hospital admissions by 6% (RR 0.94, 95% CI 0.94–0.94), and length of hospitalization by 1% (RR 0.99, 95% CI 0.99–1.00) (all $P < 0.0001$) [45].

4.1.5 Hypercholesterolaemia

Among 11,320 newly diagnosed patients with hypercholesterolemia initiated with statins, late statin initiation increased the risk of CVD events compared with early statin initiation (HR 1.24, 95% CI 1.02–2.51). Among early initiators, statin discontinuation was associated with increased risk for CVD (HR 1.71, 95% CI 1.10–2.67), but statin reinitiation was associated with decreased risk (HR 1.34, 95% CI 0.79–2.30) [46]. Another study in China with 99,655 adult patients indicated a 37% reduced risk of MACEs in those with ≥50% adherence with a statin (aHR 0.63, 95% CI, 0.41–0.98). Unlike primary prevention, no relationship between secondary prevention and statin adherence (PDC ≥ 50%) was detected in this study [47]. Previous studies, however, found statin adherence benefits in reducing the risk of adverse health outcomes for secondary prevention [48–51]. These discrepancies might be due to different baseline patient characteristics (CVD and its severity) and PDC cutoff points (50% in the Chinese study vs. 80% in others' studies). Secondary prevention seems to require ≥80% adherence to reduce cardiovascular risk.

In the elderly, a study on 29,047 patients aged ≥65 receiving polypharmacy found that those who discontinued statins while maintaining other medications had an increased risk of hospital admissions for any cardiovascular outcome (HR 1.14, 95% CI 1.03–1.26), HF (HR 1.24, 95% CI, 1.07–1.43), all-cause mortality (HR 1.15, 95% CI 1.02–1.30), and emergency admissions (HR 1.12, 95% CI 1.05–1.19) (all $P < 0.05$) [52]. In diabetic patients aged ≥65 with comorbidities, those adhering optimally to statins (PDC ≥ 80) had a decreased LDLc (<100 mg/dl) across all age groups (e.g., ≥85: RR 1.13, 95% CI 1.09–1.16, $P < 0.05$) and in all comorbid levels (e.g. ≥4: RR 1.13, 95% CI 1.12–1.15, $P < 0.05$) [41]. The LDLc target of <100 mg/dl was associated with a lower risk of adverse cardiac outcomes [53].

4.1.6 Acute coronary syndrome (ACS)

A study in 7152 post-ACS patients showed that optimal adherents (PDC ≥ 75%) to any combination of antiplatelets, statins, BBs, and ACEIs/ARBs led to a significant reduction in cardiovascular risks (HR 0.80, 95% CI 0.73–0.88) than suboptimal adherents for all medications, except BBs alone [54]. Adherence to 2 or 1 drug significantly increased mortality risk compared with adherents to 4 or 3 (for two drugs: HR 1.2, 95% CI 1.0–1.3, $P < 0.05$; for 1 drug: HR 1.5, 95% CI 1.2–1.8, $P < 0.05$) [54].

4.1.7 Chronic coronary syndrome

Optimal adherence to guideline-directed medication therapy (i.e. a combination of antiplatelet drugs, ACEIs/ARBs, BBs, and statins) that reduced the risk of MACEs (HR 0.41, 95% CI 0.18–0.92, $P = 0.03$) was reported [55].

4.1.8 Symptomatic peripheral artery disease (PAD)

Patients with PAD being never on statins had a significantly higher mortality rate (31%) than those being continuous on statins (13%) or being new on statins (8%;

$P < 0.0001$) or on intensified statins (9%). Those who terminated statin medication or reduced statin dosage had higher mortality (34% and 20%, respectively; $P < 0.0001$) [56].

4.2 Economic outcomes

The cost-effectiveness of optimal adherence to the guidelines was commonly assessed by calculating the incremental cost-effectiveness ratio (ICER), representing the discrepancies in costs between the intervention and control groups divided by the discrepancies in effectiveness between both groups (Eq. (1)) [57]. Effectiveness is commonly expressed as quality-adjusted life years (QALY), combining quality and quantity of life. Whether optimal adherence can be considered cost-effective relies on a community's affordability for one QALY. The lower the ICER, the more the cost-effectiveness. To define the ICER cutoff point, the WHO proposed using the per capita gross domestic product (GDP) [58]. An intervention must cost less than once the national annual GDP per capita per QALY to be highly cost-effective. An intervention must cost less than three times the national annual GDP per capita per QALY to be considered cost-effective:

$$\text{ICER} = \frac{\text{Cost}_{\text{intervention}} - \text{Cost}_{\text{control}}}{\text{Effectiveness}_{\text{intervention}} - \text{Effectiveness}_{\text{control}}} \quad (1)$$

For primary prevention, adherence was predicted to be more cost-effective in patients with a higher 10-year risk for a cardiovascular event in a study across 13 European countries. The risk was calculated from a risk score tool and included males, age >65 years, smoking, HTN, diabetes, hypercholesterolemia, and history of CVD. Adherence to the European guidelines on CVD prevention (e.g. smoking cessation medication, BP-lowering medication, and cholesterol-lowering medication) was used as an intervention. A base case ICER of 52,968€/QALY over 10 years was estimated for patients with an average baseline risk of 20%. Considering high-risk patients (≥20%), the ICER was reduced to 29,093€/QALY with decreasing ICERs in higher-risk patients. Patients with higher-risk reductions (≥0.5%) were also associated with lower ICERs [59]. Another study evaluating the cost-effectiveness of enhancing adherence to antihypertension medications indicated that enhancing adherence from 52% (the baseline) to 70% and 80% resulted in a reduced ICER from €76,484 (95% CI €74,807–€78,152) to €75,055 (95% CI €73,490–€76,623) and €73,605 (95% CI €72,180–€75,157), respectively, for each hospitalization for a MACE prevented. This aligns with the previous findings based on a large database (n = 625,620). Mean annual healthcare costs were estimated to be lower for patients with 80–100% adherence to antihypertensive medications ($7182) than for those with 60–79% adherence ($7560) and <60% adherence ($7995) ($P < 0.001$ for both) [57].

For secondary prevention, in the post-MI population, optimal adherence (≥80%) had lower per-patient annual medical costs for hospitalizations of $369 and $440 compared with suboptimal adherence (≥40–≤79%), and nonadherence (<40%), respectively. In the ASCVD subgroup, optimal adherence had lower per-patient annual medical costs for hospitalizations of $371 and $907 than suboptimal adherence and nonadherence [42]. Another study in India found positive findings that adherence (80% or lower) to aspirin and BBs was highly cost-effective. The additional

ACEIs were cost-effective, based on Indian gross domestic product per capita [60]. In patients discharged with ACS, those adhering to medications, outpatient controls, and rehabilitation had lower costs for medications (€199 per year) and higher costs for outpatient controls and rehabilitation (€292 and €1024) compared with those who did not [61]. An Australian secondary prevention program for CVD (i.e. optimizing medication use and lifestyle modification) was found to produce an ICER of AUD 8081 per disability-adjusted life year (DALY) prevented, which is well below the acceptable benchmark of AUD 50,000 per DALY within the Australian healthcare system [13].

In chronic vascular diseases, enhancing medication adherence increased medication costs but produced medical savings by reducing hospitalization. An American study in 224,231 patients with risk for CVD indicated that adherents' average annual medication costs were $1058 more for those with congestive HF, $429 more for HTN, $656 more for diabetes, and $601 more for hypercholesterolemia as compared with non-adherents. In contrast, adherence lowered mean annual medical costs by $8881 in congestive HF, $4337 in HTN, $4413 in diabetes, and $1860 in hypercholesterolemia [62].

In sum, higher adherence to medications to treat CVD was associated with higher medication costs but lower nonmedication medical costs, reducing overall healthcare costs. Health economic models were estimates based on available evidence and several assumptions. Interpreting the results thus needs to be cautious when applying these models in the health policy decision-making process.

5. Interventions to improve adherence and clinical outcomes

Given multiple factors influencing medication adherence in CVD, interventions addressing these factors to improve adherence have received rising interest (**Table 3**). They were classified partly or wholly into several categories of intervention: patient education, behavioral interventions, using reminder tools, cost reduction, and financial aid, using a healthcare team, and using fixed-dose therapy (polypill). Multifaceted interventions appeared more effective than single ones [63, 64]. This can partly be explained by the multifaceted nature of factors influencing medication adherence. Due to differences in healthcare resources and patient characteristics between high- and middle- or low-income countries, the interventions should be appropriately adapted to the local context. As most effective interventions on adherence improvement demand greater resources, the healthcare system needs to be supported. In waiting for support, some simple strategies for improving adherence to CVD medication were proposed (**Table 4**) [8]. An initial intervention might not be effective when applied in other settings. Thus, the healthcare team should continuously assess the effectiveness and feasibility of the intervention.

5.1 Patient education

The mode and frequency of the delivery of educational material may impact its effectiveness. Providing a few episodes of educational mails and/or phone calls did not improve adherence to secondary prevention medications in patients with MI (OR 1.03, 95% CI 0.77–1.36) [65] or with obstructive coronary artery disease (mail only vs. usual care, OR 0.98, 95% CI 0.81–1.19; mail and phone call vs. routine care, OR 0.99, 95% CI 0.82–1.20) [80]. However, tailored and interactive educational programs

Intervention	Population description	Outcome	Reference
Educational reminders	Myocardial infarction	Improved medication adherence	[65]
Physician-led intensive follow-ups	Unstable angina	1. Improved medication adherence 2. Lower MACEs: recurrence of angina, recurrence of myocardial ischemia, cardiac death, all-cause death, and revascularization	[66]
Physician-led education during hospitalization and telephone follow-ups	ACS	1. Lower all-cause death, cardiac death, and MACEs 2. Increased survival, cardiac death-free survival, and MACE-free survival	[67]
Nurse-led counseling	Statin user for primary or secondary prevention	1. Improved statin adherence 2. Lower LDLc	[68]
Live and web-based counseling	Risk for CVD	Reduced 10-year Framingham Risk Score at both 4 and 12-month follow-up for both formats	[69]
Motivational interviewing	New coronary stent	Improved medication adherence	[70]
Short message service (SMS) and structured telephone support (STS)	Chronic HF	1. Improved medication adherence 2. Lower 180-day all-cause mortality or readmission	[71]
Phone calls	Post-ACS	Improved adherence to aspirin and clopidogrel	[72]
Phone calls and reminder letters	New statins users	Improved statin adherence	[73]
Phone calls, reminder letters	≥40 years with diabetes or ASCVD	1. Improved adherence to statin and ACEIs/ARBs 2. Reduced LDLc	[74]
Smartphone apps	Elderly patients with atrial fibrillation	Improved medication adherence	[75]
Social support	Heart failure	Improved medication adherence	[76]
Pharmacist-led intervention	New users of cardiovascular medications	Improved medication adherence	[77]
Multifacet (education and regular follow-up)	CVD	1. Improved medication adherence	[63]
Multifacet (patient's pill count, family support, and education)	≥50 years and hypertension with 10-year cardiovascular risk >30%	1. Improved medication adherence at 6 months 2. Decreased SBP at 6 months 3. Reduced cardiovascular events at 5 years	[78]

Intervention	Population description	Outcome	Reference
Multifacet	ASCVD	1. Improved medication adherence for all interventions 2. Improved both adherence and BP and LDLc control for SMS, community health worker-led intervention, and polypills	[79]

Abbreviations: ACEIs/ARBs, angiotensin-converting enzyme inhibitors and angiotensin receptor blockers; ACS, acute coronary syndrome; ASCVD, atherosclerotic cardiovascular disease; BP, blood pressure; CI, confidence interval; CVD, cardiovascular disease; HR, hazard ratio; LDLc, low-density lipoprotein cholesterol; NA, not available; OR, odds ratio; RCT, randomized controlled trial; RR, risk ratio; SBP, systolic blood pressure; SMS, short message service; STS, structured telephone support.

Table 3.
Interventions that may improve medication adherence and clinical outcomes in CVD.

Identify nonadherence
• Assess predictors of nonadherence: nonresponse to medication missed appointments.
• Ask nonjudgmentally about missed doses and barriers to adherence
Emphasize the benefits of the regimen and the outcomes of adherence
Simplify the regimen as much as possible and provide simple, clear instructions
Assess patient's readiness to follow the regimen and provide advice on how to do it when needed
Involve multidisciplinary healthcare team members (e.g. nurse, pharmacist, and primary care staff)
Customize the regimen according to the patient's wishes
Obtain support from family, friends, and social services when needed
Follow up on the patient's progress at every appointment

Table 4.
Strategies for improving medication adherence in CVD.

with reinforcements improved CVD medication adherence. Earlier and more regular health checks with clinicians have improved adherence to cardiovascular medications [43, 81]. Intensive follow-up phone calls and regular consultations with cardiologists for patients with ACS were associated with higher adherence (58% intervention vs. 40% control, $P < 0.001$) and lower MACEs (19% intervention vs. 29% control, $P < 0.001$) at 36 months follow-up [67]. Face-to-face education by a nurse also significantly improved adherence to statin therapy ($P < 0.01$) and significantly lowered LDLc levels for primary prevention (2.66 vs. 3.00 mmol/l, $P = 0.024$) [68].

Regular educational information formats besides in-person also indicated an improvement in medication adherence. Both web-based and counselor-delivered formats improved adherence to medications in moderate-to-high risk patients with coronary heart disease (18% improvement in the web-based group and 21% improvement in the counselor group) [69]. Structured text messages and phone calls regularly made by a nurse positively affected medication adherence (78.9% message vs. 81.4% call vs. 69.5% control, $P = 0.011$) and reduced mortality or readmission (50.4% message vs. 41.3% call vs. 36.5% control, both $P < 0.05$) in patients hospitalized for acute HF [48]. A series of educational phone calls from nurses over 9 months improved

12-month medication adherence to dual antiplatelet therapy among patients with recent drug-eluting stent placement (87.2% call vs. 43.1% control ($P < 0.001$)) [72].

Patient education might improve medication adherence in CVD patients who do not fully understand the severity of their disease and the benefits of cardiovascular medication(s). The educational programs with reinforcements have improved adherence in most studies.

5.2 Behavioral interventions

A meta-analysis evaluating the impact of motivational interviewing over a year demonstrated a modest increase in medication adherence in patients with stroke (pooled RR 1.13, 95% CI 1.01–1.28) [70]. Promising results were again demonstrated in another RCT in which motivational interviewing improved both adherence (OR 1.91, 95% CI 1.19–3.05) and reduced rates of uncontrolled SBP (OR 0.62, 95% CI 0.50–0.78) compared with the control group [78]. Other counseling techniques such as providing patient feedback regarding medication adherence and enhancing family involvement showed a beneficial but negligible effect on medication adherence [82, 83].

Improving patient motivation and behaviors has not shown significant improvements in adherence outcomes. These interventions should be tailored to patients who are less motivated to take medication.

5.3 Reminder tools

Mobile phone-delivered interventions seemed to increase adherence to medication prescribed for the primary prevention of CVD, according to a Cochrane review of 14 trials with 25,633 randomized participants. Trials of BP self-monitoring with mobile phone telemedicine support modest benefits. One trial reported modest reductions in LDLc but no benefits for BP [84]. In a randomized trial of 5216 initiators of statin, those who received automated phone calls had significantly increased adherence (42.3% intervention vs. 26.0% control; absolute difference = 16.3%, $P < 0.001$; RR 1.63, 95% CI 1.50–1.76) [73]. Utilizing text message reminders also improved medication adherence in CVD in recent meta-analyses [85, 86].

Smartphone apps providing reminder alerts, adherence reports, and optional peer support significantly improved medication adherence (between-group difference 0.4; 95% CI 0.1–0.7, $P = 0.01$). However, this difference in adherence did not produce a significant difference in BP control between the groups (between-group difference −0.5, 95% CI −3.7–2.7, $P = 0.78$) [87]. A smartphone app integrating education, automatic reminder, and patient engagement strategies improved medication adherence among elderly patients with atrial fibrillation. Approximately 78% (14/18) of the patients in the high-adherence group at baseline remained in the same state, 45% (24/53) of the patients in the medium-adherence group at baseline moved to the high-adherence group, and 72% (18/25) of the patients in the low-adherence group moved to either the medium- or high-adherence group [75]. A meta-analysis of nineRCTs evaluating the impact of apps on medication adherence showed an improvement in SBP, DBP, total cholesterol, and LDLc levels in the intervention arm. Apps have an acceptable degree of usability, yet the app characteristics conferring usability and effectiveness are ill defined [88].

Mobile phone calls, text messages, and applications can improve adherence and clinical outcomes. Patients who often forget to take medications and use technology can try these techniques.

5.4 Social support

Frequent seeing friends and relatives in a structural manner were modestly associated with greater adherence in 17,113 patients with CVD or CVD risk factors [89]. In hypertensive patients, structural social support improved adherence in two prior meta-analyses [90, 91]. In patients with severe mental diseases (e.g. schizophrenia and bipolar disorder), perceived social support improved adherence to CVD medication. There was a 4.2% increase in medication adherence for each 1% increase in social support (OR 1.04, 95% CI 1.02–1.07, $P = 0.002$) [92]. In an HF setting, a prospective cohort study in Taiwan showed an intimate relationship with a spouse or caregiver was associated with a lower risk of 18-month all-cause readmission and cardiac readmission. The intimate partners will likely enhance HF patients' profound physical and psychological well-being [93]. In a Japanese study, poor adherence to medication in super-aged patients with HF is associated with poor clinical outcomes. Multivariable analysis revealed that not receiving assisted living at least once a week was independently associated with hospitalization, mainly due to poor medication adherence. The analysis also revealed that assisted living was particularly effective for patients affected by dementia [76].

Social support can significantly facilitate medication adherence in CVD, especially in frail populations such as the elderly and comorbid patients.

5.5 Cost reduction and financial aid

Current evidence suggests that reducing medication costs improves patient adherence and clinical outcomes. A trial randomized 10,102 hospitalized patients with acute MI to a group of copayment vouchers for P2Y12 inhibitors or no vouchers. At 1 year, patient adherence was reported to be higher in the intervention group than in the control group (aOR 1.19, 95% CI 1.02–1.40), but no significant difference was observed in MACEs (aHR 1.07, 95% CI 0.93–1.25) [94]. Another positive result was found in the MI FREEE trial randomized 5855 hospitalized patients with AMI to full prescription coverage vs. usual coverage for BBs, statins, and ACEIs/ARBs over about 1 year. Adherence rates were increased in the full-coverage group compared with the usual coverage group by 5.6% for ACEI/ARBs (95% CI 3.4–7.7), by 4.4% for BBs (95% CI 2.3–6.5), by 6.2% for statins (95% CI 3.9–8.5), and by 5.4% for all three medication groups (95% CI 3.6–7.2). A significant reduction was observed in total MACEs in the full-coverage group (HR 0.89, 95% CI 0.90–0.99; $P = 0.03$) was observed, despite no significant differences in the first MACEs (HR 0.93; 95% CI 0.82–1.04; $P = 0.21$) [95].

Cost reduction strategies using either copayment reduction or financial incentives have shown modest changes in medication adherence, although further research is needed to determine the sustainability of these interventions. Another possible cost reduction solution is replacing brand-name medications with well-proven, equally effective, and less costly generic ones. In a study of over 300,000 privately insured adults aged ≥18, generic drug therapy improved adherence [96].

5.6 Healthcare team

Community health workers (e.g. community pharmacists) often regularly interact with patients and provide access, education, and support regarding medication use. Enhanced community health workers' involvement has been explored to improve medication adherence. Recent systematic reviews evaluating community health worker-led intervention demonstrate improvement in adherence and reduction in secondary ASCVD (97% intervention vs. 92% control; OR 2.62, 95% CI 1.32–5.19) [79].

Pharmacist-led consultations improved medication adherence in CVD patients compared with usual care (4.5% difference, 95% CI 0.8–8.2, $P = 0.017$) [77]. Another standardized counseling intervention by pharmacists at hospital discharge of ACS patients showed (1) an increased medication adherence at 1 year (11.9% non-counseling receivers vs. 18.4% counseling receivers, $P = 0.19$) and (2) decreased cardiovascular readmission and all-cause mortality (17.6% intervention vs. 22.3% usual care, $P = 0.42$; and 3.4% intervention vs. 4.2% usual care, $P > 0.99$, respectively) [97].

The healthcare team plays an important role in patients' adherence by identifying medication nonadherence and adherence barriers and providing interventions that address these barriers. One of the consistent features of successful interventions has been regular follow-up with the healthcare team [98].

5.7 Fixed-dose therapy (polypill)

The relationship between polypill therapy and CVD outcomes was studied enormously, and most studies found positive findings. A systematic review and meta-analysis of eight studies involving 25,584 patients demonstrated that the use of polypills (1) significantly enhanced drug adherence (RR 1.31, 95% CI 1.11–1.55, (2) significantly reduced CVD risk factors (hypertension) and the risk of all-cause mortality (RR 0.90, 95% CI 0.81–1.00, $P < 0.05$) and MACEs (RR 0.85, 95% CI 0.70–1.02, $P > 0.05$) [99]. Another systematic review indicated that polypills improved adherence and reduced secondary ASCVD (86% intervention vs. 65% control, OR 1.33, 95% CI 1.26–1.41) [79]. A meta-analysis demonstrated significant improvement in adherence with the use of polypill of two or more antihypertensive drugs (OR 1.21, 95% CI 1.03–1.43, $P = 0.02$), but beneficial trends in BP and adverse effects [100]. Challenges can explain this in matching patients to a specific polypill and adjusting the dose of a component in a polypill.

In summary, since nonadherence factors are patient-specific, personalized interventions are required to enhance the impact of an intervention to improve medication adherence in CVD [98]. Evidence demonstrated that simple strategies requiring low healthcare resources such as simplifying the regimen, organizing medications in pillboxes, obtaining family and social support, using motivational interviewing, and educating patients on the importance of medication adherence appear cost-effective.

6. Conclusions

Adherence to cardiovascular medication reduces substantial morbidity and mortality and reduces healthcare costs. Despite these advantages, medication nonadherence remains common due to multiple barriers from patients, providers, and system levels. Various interventions have been tested to overcome these barriers, and most of them have illustrated positive findings. A combination of interventions is more likely to be effective as several factors simultaneously influence adherence. The heterogeneity of effect within each intervention may result from the inappropriate matching of intervention and factors influencing adherence. Thus, after identifying medication nonadherence, clinicians should consider potential factor(s) influencing adherence to select intervention(s) targeting the identified factor(s).

Author details

Suol Thanh Pham[1], Thi Anh Nguyen[1,2], Nghia Minh Tran[3], Hoang Thi Kim Cao[1], Khanh Kim Le[1], Chu Xuan Duong[1], Thao Huong Nguyen[4], Katja Taxis[5], Khanh Duy Dang[1*] and Thang Nguyen[1*]

1 Department of Pharmacology and Clinical Pharmacy, Can Tho University of Medicine and Pharmacy, Can Tho, Vietnam

2 School of Pharmacy, Faculty of Medicine and Health, The University of Sydney, Sydney, Australia

3 Faculty of Medicine, Can Tho University of Medicine and Pharmacy, Can Tho, Vietnam

4 Department of Clinical Pharmacy, University of Medicine and Pharmacy at Ho Chi Minh City, Ho Chi Minh City, Vietnam

5 Groningen Research Institute of Pharmacy, University of Groningen, Groningen, The Netherlands

*Address all correspondence to: ddkhanh@ctump.edu.vn and nthang@ctump.edu.vn

References

[1] Stewart J, Manmathan G, Wilkinson P. Primary prevention of cardiovascular disease: A review of contemporary guidance and literature. JRSM Cardiovascular Disease. 2017;**6**:204800401668721

[2] Roth GA, Abate D, Abate KH, Abay SM, Abbafati C, Abbasi N, et al. Global, regional, and national age-sex-specific mortality for 282 causes of death in 195 countries and territories, 1980-2017: A systematic analysis for the global burden of disease study 2017. The Lancet. 2018;**392**(10159):1736-1788

[3] Vos T, Lim SS, Abbafati C, Abbas KM, Abbasi M, Abbasifard M, et al. Global burden of 369 diseases and injuries in 204 countries and territories, 1990-2019: A systematic analysis for the global burden of disease study 2019. The Lancet. 2020;**396**(10258):1204-1222

[4] Simon ST, Kini V, Levy AE, Ho PM. Medication adherence in cardiovascular medicine. British Medical Journal. 2021;**374**:n1493

[5] Jackevicius CA, Li P, Tu JV. Prevalence, predictors, and outcomes of primary nonadherence after acute myocardial infarction. Circulation. 2008;**117**(8):1028-1036

[6] Rudd P, Byyny RL, Zachary V, LoVerde ME, Mitchell WD, Titus C, et al. Pill count measures of compliance in a drug trial: Variability and suitability. American Journal of Hypertension. 1988;**1**(3 Pt 1):309-312

[7] Jackevicius CA. Adherence with statin therapy in elderly patients with and without acute coronary syndromes. Journal of the American Medical Association. 2002;**288**(4):462

[8] Osterberg L, Blaschke T. Adherence to medication. The New England Journal of Medicine. 2005;**353**(5):487-497

[9] Cramer JA, Roy A, Burrell A, Fairchild CJ, Fuldeore MJ, Ollendorf DA, et al. Medication compliance and persistence: Terminology and definitions. Value in Health. 2008;**11**(1):44-47

[10] Choudhry NK, Kronish IM, Vongpatanasin W, Ferdinand KC, Pavlik VN, Egan BM, et al. Medication adherence and blood pressure control: A scientific statement from the American Heart Association. Hypertension. 2022;**79**(1):1-14

[11] Kronish IM, Thorpe CT, Voils CI. Measuring the multiple domains of medication nonadherence: Findings from a Delphi survey of adherence experts. Translational Behavioral Medicine. 2021;**11**(1):104-113

[12] Faridi KF, Peterson ED, McCoy LA, Thomas L, Enriquez J, Wang TY. Timing of first Postdischarge follow-up and medication adherence after acute myocardial infarction. JAMA Cardiology. 2016;**1**(2):147

[13] Chew DP, Carter R, Rankin B, Boyden A, Egan H. Cost-effectiveness of a general practice chronic disease management plan for coronary heart disease in Australia. Australian Health Review. 2010;**34**(2):162

[14] Sabaté E, Bender B, Boulet LP, Chaustre I, Rand C, Weinstein A, et al. Adherence to Long-Term Therapies: Evidence for Action [Internet]. World Health Organization - Institutional Repository for Information Sharing; 2003. Available from: https://apps.who.int/iris/handle/10665/42682

[15] Leslie KH, McCowan C, Pell JP. Adherence to cardiovascular medication: A review of systematic reviews. Journal of Public Health. 2019;**41**(1):e84-e94

[16] Lee GKY, Wang HHX, Liu KQL, Cheung Y, Morisky DE, Wong MCS. Determinants of medication adherence to antihypertensive medications among a Chinese population using morisky medication adherence scale. Cameron DW, editor. PLoS ONE. 2013;**8**(4):e62775

[17] Hashmi SK, Afridi MB, Abbas K, Sajwani RA, Saleheen D, Frossard PM, et al. Factors associated with adherence to anti-hypertensive treatment in Pakistan. Baune B, editor. PLoS ONE. 2007;**2**(3):e280

[18] Wong MCS, Jiang JY, Griffiths SM. Factors associated with antihypertensive drug compliance in 83 884 Chinese patients: A cohort study. Journal of Epidemiology & Community Health. 2010;**64**(10):895-901

[19] Rolnick SJ, Pawloski PA, Hedblom BD, Asche SE, Bruzek RJ. Patient characteristics associated with medication adherence. Clinical Medicine & Research. 2013;**11**(2):54-65

[20] Assawasuwannakit P, Braund R, Duffull SB. A model-based meta-analysis of the influence of factors that impact adherence to medications. Journal of Clinical Pharmacy and Therapeutics. 2015;**40**(1):24-31

[21] Mann DM, Woodward M, Muntner P, Falzon L, Kronish I. Predictors of nonadherence to statins: A systematic review and meta-analysis. The Annals of Pharmacotherapy. 2010;**44**(9):1410-1421

[22] Nordstrom BL, Simeone JC, Zhao Z, Molife C, McCollam PL, Ye X, et al. Adherence and persistence with prasugrel following acute coronary syndrome with percutaneous coronary intervention. American Journal of Cardiovascular Drugs. 2013;**13**(4):263-271

[23] Bots SH, Inia JA, Peters SAE. Medication adherence after acute coronary syndrome in women compared with men: A systematic review and Meta-analysis. Front Glob Womens Health. 2021;**2**:637398

[24] Lima PRG, Gonçalves GMS, Rodrigues RCM, Oliveira-Kumakura AR d S. Factors related to patient adherence to the use of new oral anticoagulants. Revista da Escola de Enfermagem da U.S.P. 2022;**56**:e20210191

[25] Bowry ADK, Shrank WH, Lee JL, Stedman M, Choudhry NK. A systematic review of adherence to cardiovascular medications in resource-limited settings. Journal of General Internal Medicine. 2011;**26**(12):1479-1491

[26] Liyanage-Don NA, Cornelius T, Romero EK, Alcántara C, Kronish IM. Association of Hispanic ethnicity and linguistic acculturation with cardiovascular medication adherence in patients with suspected acute coronary syndrome. Preventive Medicine Reports. 2021;**23**:101455

[27] Ferdinand KC, Yadav K, Nasser SA, Clayton-Jeter HD, Lewin J, Cryer DR, et al. Disparities in hypertension and cardiovascular disease in blacks: The critical role of medication adherence. Journal of Clinical Hypertension. 2017;**19**(10):1015-1024

[28] Nielsen JØ, Shrestha AD, Neupane D, Kallestrup P. Nonadherence to anti-hypertensive medication in low- and middle-income countries: A systematic review and meta-analysis

of 92443 subjects. Journal of Human Hypertension. 2017;**31**(1):14-21

[29] Mishra P, Vamadevan AS, Roy A, Bhatia R, Naik N, Singh S, et al. Exploring barriers to medication adherence using COM-B model of behaviour among patients with cardiovascular diseases in low- and middle-income countries: A qualitative study. Power Purchase Agreement. 2021;**15**:1359-1371

[30] Schneider APH, Gaedke MÂ, Garcez A, Barcellos NT, Paniz VMV. Effect of characteristics of pharmacotherapy on nonadherence in chronic cardiovascular disease: A systematic review and meta-analysis of observational studies. International Journal of Clinical Practice. 2018;**72**(1):e13044

[31] Barankay I, Reese PP, Putt ME, Russell LB, Loewenstein G, Pagnotti D, et al. Effect of patient financial incentives on statin adherence and lipid control: A randomized clinical trial. JAMA Network Open. 2020;**3**(10):e2019429

[32] Burnier M, Egan BM. Adherence in hypertension: A review of prevalence, risk factors, impact, and management. Circulation Research. 2019;**124**(7):1124-1140

[33] Smits E, Andreotti F, Houben E, Crijns HJGM, Haas S, Spentzouris G, et al. Adherence and persistence with once-daily vs twice-daily direct Oral anticoagulants among patients with atrial fibrillation: Real-world analyses from the Netherlands, Italy and Germany. Drugs—Real World Outcomes. 2022;**9**:199-209 [Internet]. Available from: https://link.springer.com/10.1007/s40801-021-00289-w.s. [Accessed: February 24, 2022]

[34] Abegaz TM, Shehab A, Gebreyohannes EA, Bhagavathula AS, Elnour AA. Nonadherence to antihypertensive drugs: A systematic review and meta-analysis. Medicine. Jan 2017;**96**(4):e5641

[35] Goldstein CM, Gathright EC, Garcia S. Relationship between depression and medication adherence in cardiovascular disease: The perfect challenge for the integrated care team. Power Purchase Agreement. 2017;**11**:547-559

[36] Hennein R, Hwang SJ, Au R, Levy D, Muntner P, Fox CS, et al. Barriers to medication adherence and links to cardiovascular disease risk factor control: The Framingham heart study: Medication adherence and CVD risk. Internal Medicine Journal. 2018;**48**(4):414-421

[37] Rasmussen JN, Chong A, Alter DA. Relationship between adherence to evidence-based pharmacotherapy and long-term mortality after acute myocardial infarction. Journal of the American Medical Association. 2007;**297**(2):177

[38] Ho PM, Bryson CL, Rumsfeld JS. Medication adherence: Its importance in cardiovascular outcomes. Circulation. 2009;**119**(23):3028-3035

[39] Liu M, Zheng G, Cao X, Chang X, Zhang N, Liang G, et al. Better medications adherence lowers cardiovascular events, stroke, and all-cause mortality risk: A dose-response meta-analysis. Journal of Cardiovascular Development and Disease. 2021;**8**(11):146

[40] Yang Q, Chang A, Ritchey MD, Loustalot F. Antihypertensive medication adherence and risk of cardiovascular disease among older adults: A population-based cohort study. Journal of the American Heart Association. 2017;**6**(6):e006056 [Internet]. Available

from: https://www.ahajournals.org/doi/10.1161/JAHA.117.006056. [Accessed: February 23, 2022]

[41] Raebel MA, Dyer W, Nichols GA, Goodrich GK, Schmittdiel JA. Relationships between medication adherence and cardiovascular disease risk factor control in elderly patients with diabetes. Pharmacotherapy. 2017;**37**(10):1204-1214

[42] Bansilal S, Castellano JM, Garrido E, Wei HG, Freeman A, Spettell C, et al. Assessing the impact of medication adherence on long-term cardiovascular outcomes. Journal of the American College of Cardiology. 2016;**68**(8):789-801

[43] Shang P, Liu GG, Zheng X, Ho PM, Hu S, Li J, et al. Association between medication adherence and 1-year major cardiovascular adverse events after acute myocardial infarction in China. Journal of the American Heart Association. 2019;**8**(9):e011793 [Internet]. Available from: https://www.ahajournals.org/doi/10.1161/JAHA.118.011793. [Accessed: February 23, 2022]

[44] Shau WY, Lai CL, Huang ST, Chen ST, Li JZ, Fung S, et al. Statin adherence and persistence on secondary prevention of cardiovascular disease in Taiwan. Heart Asia. 2019;**11**(2):e011176

[45] Hood SR, Giazzon AJ, Seamon G, Lane KA, Wang J, Eckert GJ, et al. Association between medication adherence and the outcomes of heart failure. Pharmacotherapy. 2018;**38**(5):539-545

[46] Ryou IS, Chang J, Son JS, Ko A, Choi S, Kim K, et al. Association between CVDs and initiation and adherence to statin treatment in patients with newly diagnosed hypercholesterolaemia: A retrospective cohort study. BMJ Open. 2021;**11**(4):e045375

[47] Zhao B, He X, Wu J, Yan S. Adherence to statins and its impact on clinical outcomes: A retrospective population-based study in China. BMC Cardiovascular Disorders. 2020;**20**(1):282

[48] Chen PS, Cheng CL, Kao Yang YH, Li YH. Statin adherence after ischemic stroke or transient ischemic attack is associated with clinical outcome. Circulation Journal. 2016;**80**(3):731-737

[49] Wei L. Adherence to statin treatment and readmission of patients after myocardial infarction: A six year follow up study. Heart. 2002;**88**(3):229-233

[50] Xie G, Sun Y, Myint PK, Patel A, Yang X, Li M, et al. Six-month adherence to statin use and subsequent risk of major adverse cardiovascular events (MACE) in patients discharged with acute coronary syndromes. Lipids in Health and Disease. 2017;**16**(1):155

[51] Korhonen MJ, Ruokoniemi P, Ilomäki J, Meretoja A, Helin-Salmivaara A, Huupponen R. Adherence to statin therapy and the incidence of ischemic stroke in patients with diabetes. Pharmacoepidemiology and Drug Safety. 2016;**25**(2):161-169

[52] Rea F, Biffi A, Ronco R, Franchi M, Cammarota S, Citarella A, et al. Cardiovascular outcomes and mortality associated with discontinuing statins in older patients receiving polypharmacy. JAMA Network Open. 2021;**4**(6):e2113186

[53] Leibowitz M, Karpati T, Cohen-Stavi CJ, Feldman BS, Hoshen M, Bitterman H, et al. Association between achieved low-density lipoprotein levels and major adverse cardiac events in

patients with stable ischemic heart disease taking statin treatment. JAMA Internal Medicine. 2016;**176**(8):1105

[54] Sotorra-Figuerola G, Ouchi D, Giner-Soriano M, Morros R. Impact of adherence to drugs for secondary prevention on mortality and cardiovascular morbidity: A population-based cohort study. IMPACT study. Pharmacoepidemiology & Drug Safety. 2021;**30**(9):1250-1257

[55] Ishii M, Kuramitsu S, Yamanaga K, Matsuo H, Horie K, Takashima H, et al. Association of guideline-directed medical therapy adherence with outcomes after fractional flow reserve-based deferral of revascularization. The European Heart Journal—Cardiovascular Pharmacotherapy. 2022;**8**(6):600-608

[56] Dopheide JF, Veit J, Ramadani H, Adam L, Papac L, Vonbank A, et al. Adherence to statin therapy favours survival of patients with symptomatic peripheral artery disease. European Heart Journal—Cardiovascular Pharmacotherapy. 2021;**7**(4):263-270

[57] Pittman DG, Tao Z, Chen W, Stettin GD. Antihypertensive medication adherence and subsequent healthcare utilization and costs. The American Journal of Managed Care. 2010;**16**(8):568-576

[58] Marseille E, Larson B, Kazi DS, Kahn JG, Rosen S. Thresholds for the cost–effectiveness of interventions: Alternative approaches. Bulletin of the World Health Organization. 2015;**93**(2):118-124

[59] De Smedt D, Annemans L, De Backer G, Kotseva K, Rydèn L, Wood D, et al. Cost-effectiveness of optimized adherence to prevention guidelines in European patients with coronary heart disease: Results from the EUROASPIRE IV survey. International Journal of Cardiology. 2018;**272**:20-25

[60] Megiddo I, Chatterjee S, Nandi A, Laxminarayan R. Cost-effectiveness of treatment and secondary prevention of acute myocardial infarction in India: A modeling study. Global Heart. 2014;**9**(4):391

[61] Rea F, Ronco R, Martini N, Maggioni AP, Corrao G. Cost-effectiveness of posthospital management of acute coronary syndrome: A real-world investigation from Italy. Value in Health. 2022;**25**(2):185-193

[62] Roebuck MC, Liberman JN, Gemmill-Toyama M, Brennan TA. Medication adherence leads to lower health care use and costs despite increased drug spending. Health Affairs. 2011;**30**(1):91-99

[63] Fitzpatrick C, Gillies C, Seidu S, Kar D, Ioannidou E, Davies MJ, et al. Effect of pragmatic versus explanatory interventions on medication adherence in people with cardiometabolic conditions: A systematic review and meta-analysis. BMJ Open. 2020;**10**(7):e036575

[64] Ogungbe O, Byiringiro S, Adedokun-Afolayan A, Seal SM, Dennison Himmelfarb CR, Davidson PM, et al. Medication adherence interventions for cardiovascular disease in low- and middle-income countries: A systematic review. Power Purchase Agreement. 2021;**15**:885-897

[65] Schwalm JD, Ivers NM, Natarajan MK, Taljaard M, Rao-Melacini P, Witteman HO, et al. Cluster randomized controlled trial of delayed educational reminders for long-term medication adherence in ST-elevation myocardial infarction (DERLA-STEMI). American Heart Journal. 2015;**170**(5):903-913

[66] Jia JJ, Dong PS, Du LJ, Li ZG, Lai LH, Yang XM, et al. Impact of physician-coordinated intensive follow-up on long-term medical costs in patients with unstable angina undergoing percutaneous coronary intervention. Acta Cardiologica Sinica. 2017;**33**(2):173-181

[67] Du L, Dong P, Jia J, Li Z, Lai L, Yang X, et al. Impacts of intensive follow-up on the long-term prognosis of percutaneous coronary intervention in acute coronary syndrome patients—A single center prospective randomized controlled study in a Chinese population. European Journal of Preventive Cardiology. 2016;**23**(10):1077-1085

[68] Nieuwkerk PT, Nierman MC, Vissers MN, Locadia M, Greggers-Peusch P, Knape LPM, et al. Intervention to improve adherence to lipid-lowering medication and lipid-levels in patients with an increased cardiovascular risk. The American Journal of Cardiology. 2012;**110**(5):666-672

[69] Keyserling TC, Sheridan SL, Draeger LB, Finkelstein EA, Gizlice Z, Kruger E, et al. A comparison of live Counseling with a web-based lifestyle and medication intervention to reduce coronary heart disease risk: A randomized clinical trial. JAMA Internal Medicine. 2014;**174**(7):1144

[70] Palacio AM, Uribe C, Hazel-Fernandez L, Li H, Tamariz LJ, Garay SD, et al. Can phone-based motivational interviewing improve medication adherence to antiplatelet medications after a coronary stent among racial minorities? A randomized trial. Journal of General Internal Medicine. 2015;**30**(4):469-475

[71] Chen C, Li X, Sun L, Cao S, Kang Y, Hong L, et al. Post-discharge short message service improves short-term clinical outcome and self-care behaviour in chronic heart failure: Post-discharge SMS in short-term clinical outcome and self-care behaviour. ESC Heart Failure. 2019;**6**(1):164-173

[72] Rinfret S, Rodés-Cabau J, Bagur R, Déry JP, Dorais M, Larose É, et al. Telephone contact to improve adherence to dual antiplatelet therapy after drug-eluting stent implantation. Heart. 2013;**99**(8):562-569

[73] Derose SF, Green K, Marrett E, Tunceli K, Cheetham TC, Chiu VY, et al. Automated outreach to increase primary adherence to cholesterol-lowering medications. JAMA Internal Medicine. 2013;**173**(1):38

[74] Vollmer WM, Owen-Smith AA, Tom JO, Laws R, Ditmer DG, Smith DH, et al. Improving adherence to cardiovascular disease medications with information technology. The American Journal of Managed Care. 2014;**20**(11 Spec No 17):SP502-SP510

[75] Senoo K, Miki T, Ohkura T, Iwakoshi H, Nishimura T, Shiraishi H, et al. A smartphone app to improve oral anticoagulation adherence in patients with atrial fibrillation: Prospective observational study. JMIR mHealth and uHealth. 2022;**10**(1):e30807

[76] Kawada K, Kubo T, Ishida T, Jobu K, Morisawa S, Hamada T, et al. Assisted living and medication adherence in super-aged patients with heart failure in the Japanese population. Journal of Cardiovascular Pharmacology. 2021; Publish Ahead of Print [Internet]. Available from: https://journals.lww.com/10.1097/FJC.0000000000001212. [Accessed: March 2, 2022]

[77] Hovland R, Bremer S, Frigaard C, Henjum S, Faksvåg PK, Sæther EM, et al.

Effect of a pharmacist-led intervention on adherence among patients with a first-time prescription for a cardiovascular medicine: A randomized controlled trial in Norwegian pharmacies†. International Journal of Pharmacy Practice. 2020;**28**(4):337-345

[78] Pladevall M, Brotons C, Gabriel R, Arnau A, Suarez C, de la Figuera M, et al. Multicenter cluster-randomized trial of a multifactorial intervention to improve antihypertensive medication adherence and blood pressure control among patients at high cardiovascular risk (the COM99 study). Circulation. 2010;**122**(12):1183-1191

[79] Fuller RH, Perel P, Navarro-Ruan T, Nieuwlaat R, Haynes RB, Huffman MD. Improving medication adherence in patients with cardiovascular disease: A systematic review. Heart. 2018;**104**(15):1238-1243

[80] Ivers NM, Schwalm JD, Bouck Z, McCready T, Taljaard M, Grace SL, et al. Interventions supporting long term adherence and decreasing cardiovascular events after myocardial infarction (ISLAND): Pragmatic randomised controlled trial. British Medical Journal. 2020;**369**:m1731

[81] Faridi KF. Medication adherence and cardiovascular outcomes. Journal of the American College of Cardiology. 2017;**69**(5):598-599

[82] Reddy A, Huseman TL, Canamucio A, Marcus SC, Asch DA, Volpp K, et al. Patient and partner feedback reports to improve statin medication adherence: A randomized control trial. Journal of General Internal Medicine. 2017;**32**(3):256-261

[83] Wu JR, Mark B, Knafl GJ, Dunbar SB, Chang PP, DeWalt DA. A multi-component, family-focused and literacy-sensitive intervention to improve medication adherence in patients with heart failure—a randomized controlled trial. Heart & Lung. 2019;**48**(6):507-514

[84] Palmer MJ, Machiyama K, Woodd S, Gubijev A, Barnard S, Russell S, et al. Mobile phone-based interventions for improving adherence to medication prescribed for the primary prevention of cardiovascular disease in adults. Cochrane Heart Group, editor. Cochrane Database of Systematic Reviews. 2018;**6**(6):CD012675 [Internet]. Available from: http://doi.wiley.com/10.1002/14651858.CD012675.pub3. [Accessed: March 2, 2022]

[85] Adler AJ, Martin N, Mariani J, Tajer CD, Serrano NC, Casas JP, et al. Mobile phone text messaging to improve adherence to cardiovascular disease secondary prevention interventions. In: The Cochrane Collaboration, editor. Cochrane Database of Systematic Reviews [Internet]. Chichester, UK: John Wiley & Sons, Ltd; 2015. p. CD011851. Available from: https://doi.wiley.com/10.1002/14651858.CD011851. [Accessed: March 13, 2022]

[86] Thakkar J, Kurup R, Laba TL, Santo K, Thiagalingam A, Rodgers A, et al. Mobile telephone text messaging for medication adherence in chronic disease: A meta-analysis. JAMA Internal Medicine. 2016;**176**(3):340

[87] Morawski K, Ghazinouri R, Krumme A, Lauffenburger JC, Lu Z, Durfee E, et al. Association of a smartphone application with medication adherence and blood pressure control: The MedISAFE-BP randomized clinical trial. JAMA Internal Medicine. 2018;**178**(6):802

[88] Al-Arkee S, Mason J, Lane DA, Fabritz L, Chua W, Haque MS, et al. Mobile apps to improve medication

adherence in cardiovascular disease: Systematic review and Meta-analysis. Journal of Medical Internet Research. 2021;**23**(5):e24190

[89] Mondesir FL, Carson AP, Durant RW, Lewis MW, Safford MM, Levitan EB. Association of functional and structural social support with medication adherence among individuals treated for coronary heart disease risk factors: Findings from the REasons for Geographic and Racial Differences in Stroke (REGARDS) study. Akinyemiju TF, editor. PLoS ONE. 2018;**13**(6):e0198578

[90] DiMatteo MR. Social support and patient adherence to medical treatment: A meta-analysis. Health Psychology. 2004;**23**(2):207-218

[91] Magrin ME, D'Addario M, Greco A, Miglioretti M, Sarini M, Scrignaro M, et al. Social support and adherence to treatment in hypertensive patients: A meta-analysis. Annals of Behavioral Medicine. 2015;**49**(3):307-318

[92] Burton A, Walters K, Marston L, Osborn D. Is there an association between perceived social support and cardiovascular health behaviours in people with severe mental illnesses? Social Psychiatry and Psychiatric Epidemiology. 2020;**55**(12):1659-1669

[93] Lin TK, Hsu BC, Li YD, Chen CH, Lin JW, Chien CY, et al. The impact of sources of perceived social support on readmissions in patients with heart failure. Journal of Psychosomatic Research. 2022;**154**:110723

[94] Wang TY, Kaltenbach LA, Cannon CP, Fonarow GC, Choudhry NK, Henry TD, et al. Effect of medication co-payment vouchers on P2Y 12 inhibitor use and major adverse cardiovascular events among patients with myocardial infarction: The ARTEMIS randomized clinical trial. Journal of the American Medical Association. 2019;**321**(1):44

[95] Choudhry NK, Avorn J, Glynn RJ, Antman EM, Schneeweiss S, Toscano M, et al. Full coverage for preventive medications after myocardial infarction. The New England Journal of Medicine. 2011;**365**(22):2088-2097

[96] Sokol MC, McGuigan KA, Verbrugge RR, Epstein RS. Impact of medication adherence on hospitalization risk and healthcare cost. Medical Care. 2005;**43**(6):521-530

[97] Neville HL, Mann K, Killen J, Callaghan M. Pharmacist intervention to improve medication adherence in patients with acute coronary syndrome: The PRIMA-ACS study. Canadian Journal of Hospital Pharmacy. 2021;**74**(4):350-360 [Internet]. Available from: https://www.cjhp-online.ca/index.php/cjhp/article/view/3198. [Accessed: March 2, 2022]

[98] Xu HY, Yu YJ, Zhang QH, Hu HY, Li M. Tailored interventions to improve medication adherence for cardiovascular diseases. Frontiers in Pharmacology. 2020;**11**:510339

[99] Rao S, Jamal T, Khan MS, Michos E, Navar AM, Wang TJ, et al. Association of polypill therapy with cardiovascular outcomes, mortality, and adherence: A systematic review and meta-analysis of randomized controlled trials. Progress in Cardiovascular Diseases. 2022;**73**:48-55. S0033062022000056

[100] Gupta AK, Arshad S, Poulter NR. Compliance, safety, and effectiveness of fixed-dose combinations of antihypertensive agents: A meta-analysis. Hypertension. 2010;**55**(2):399-407

Chapter 23

Treating Type 2 Diabetes with Therapeutic Carbohydrate Restriction

Joshua Chadwick, Lokesh Shanmugam and Balasubramanian Ganesh

Abstract

This chapter gives clinicians the tools to use therapeutic carbohydrate restriction as a dietary intervention for type 2 diabetes patients. The chapter is divided into three section, each addressing a different aspect of therapeutic carbohydrate restriction (TCR). Section 1 delves into the background of carbohydrate restriction, nutrition physiology, the three levels of therapeutic carbohydrate restriction physiological, and metabolic rationale for using TCR to treat the symptoms of type 2 diabetes. Section two explains how to start TCR in a patient population. It goes over which patients are good candidates for TCR and which ones should be approached with caution when implementing this dietary change and explains the importance of baseline assessments. Section three spells out how to administer and manage TCR in a clinical setting. It covers behavior change support, patient education on TCR principles, medication adjustments during the early stages of the intervention, and anticipating and treating common side effects.

Keywords: type 2 diabetes, obesity, therapeutic carbohydrate restriction, low carbohydrate diet, diabetes remission

1. Introduction

For the past 50 years, global rates of metabolic syndrome, diabetes, and obesity have been steadily rising [1]. While pharmaceutical interventions can assist patients in managing their conditions, and nutritional therapy is also important. Increased use of certain medications, such as insulin or sulfonylureas, can exacerbate the underlying insulin resistance, potentially leading to poorer glycaemic control over time [2]. Medications can help, but only to a certain extent. However, as we will see later in this course, nutritional therapy enhances their benefit and even helps lower the required dosage or allows for elimination. High quality evidence supports the efficacy of therapeutic carbohydrate restriction can be an important component for diabetes treatment, whether used alone or in combination with medications [3].

Therapeutic carbohydrate restriction is not a "cure-all, "and it's not the right treatment for everyone. It is, however, a successful clinical intervention that is tailored to specific conditions and patient groups.

In the early nineteenth century, therapeutic carbohydrate restriction for diabetes treatment was fairly common [4]. Its use in the treatment of epilepsy began in the early twentieth century. Physicians and nutritionists commonly recommended carbohydrate restriction for weight loss in the 1960s and 1970s [5].

1.1 The evidence of a low GI diet for type 2 diabetes

2021 systematic review and meta-analysis of published and unpublished randomized trial data

- A 2021 systematic review looked at 23 trials and found that those who followed a low carbohydrate diet achieved higher rates of diabetes remission (**Table 1**) compared to those who followed a low-fat diet without adverse events [7].
- Low-carbohydrate diets were also associated with a reduction in triglycerides, insulin sensitivity and weight loss at six months compared to the low-fat diets.

The Prospective Urban Rural Epidemiology (PURE) study.

- Epidemiological cohort study published in 2017 [8].
- 135,335 patients in high, medium and low-income countries with a median follow-up of 7.4 years.
- Recorded dietary intake using validated questionnaires; 52% were those whose carbohydrate calorie intake was over 60%.
- Patients with diabetes were not excluded from the study.
- 1230 patients (0.9%) dropped out, and 7369 (5.4%) were excluded from the final analysis due to pre-existing cardiovascular disease.
- Higher carbohydrate intake was associated with increased overall mortality (hazard ratio 1.28), and higher fat intake was associated with reduced overall

Type 2 diabetes outcome	Criteria and cut-offs used
Reversal	HbA1c below 6.5% (7.8 mmol/L; 47.4 mmol/mol) without any diabetes medication, except metformin
Partial remission	Two HbA1c measurements 5.7–6.5% (6.5–7.8 mmol/L; 38.8–47.4 mmol/mol) Over the course of 1 year No medications
Complete remission	Two HbA1c measurements below 5.7% (6.5 mmol/L; 38.8 mmol/mol) Over the course of 1 year No medications

Table 1.
Type 2 diabetes reversal and remission definition defined by the American diabetic association as follows [6].

mortality (hazard ratio 0.77)- both of these were statistically significant. There was, however, no statistically significant link with cardiovascular disease.

- Saturated fat intake was associated with an increased risk of stroke, but mono-unsaturated fat intake was associated with reduced total mortality, and polyunsaturated fat intake was associated with reduced total mortality and reduced risk of stroke.

- There were some possible confounders in this study, for example, the fact that many who had a high carbohydrate diet lived in poorer areas, and it is difficult to separate the effects of the diet from the general impact of poverty on mortality. There was also no assessment of intake of trans fats and no analysis of the different types of carbohydrates that were eaten.

1.1.1 Effect on lipids

- A 2019 meta-analysis of 8 studies have shown improvements in HDL and triglyceride levels associated with a lowcarbohydrate diet [9].

- They conclude that 'dietary guidelines should consider carbohydrate restriction as an alternative dietary strategy for the prevention/management of dyslipidemia for populations with cardiometabolic risk'.

1.1.2 American Diabetes Association

- In 2019, the American Diabetes Association (ADA) published a consensus review regarding diet for patients with diabetes or pre-diabetes [3].

- This includes the statement that 'reducing overall carbohydrate intake for individuals with diabetes is associated with the most evidence for improving glycemia and may be applied in a variety of eating patterns.

- The review also states that 'a low-carbohydrate diet is a viable approach to a patient who is not meeting their diabetes targets or wants to reduce their diabetic medication'.

1.1.3 2017 National Institute for health and care excellence (NICE) guidance

The 2017 NICE guidance has several points which support a low GI diet. A low GI diet can be an effective way to consider, as many patients prefer to trial weight loss and lifestyle change before medication [10].

1.2 Carbohydrate

Unlike amino acids, fatty acids, and many micronutrients, dietary carbohydrate is not required for survival. Although some cells, such as red blood cells, white blood cells, and some parts of the kidney, require glucose, the body can produce enough glucose to meet those needs. Despite the widespread belief that the brain can only run on glucose, the brain can run on both glucose and ketones [11]. When we do not eat a lot of carbs, our bodies have three options for getting energy:

- We synthesize glucose from the liver through glycogenolysis. When the body requires energy, this provides a quick source of glucose.

- Gluconeogenesis is a process that allows us to make glucose from proteins and fatty acids. "Gluconeogenesis" literally means "the production of new glucose." It's a demand-driven process in which our livers convert fatty acids and amino acids into glucose to keep blood sugar levels from dropping too low.

- Fatty acids can be converted to ketone bodies. The brain and all glucose-dependent tissues get enough fuel naturally on a TCR diet [12].

Carbohydrate-restricted diets usually include some carbohydrates, but even if we eat no carbohydrates, our bodies will provide us with all the glucose and energy we require as long as we eat enough fat and protein. As a result, a well-planned, carbohydrate-restricted diet will provide all the nutrients needed.

1.3 What is the difference between a glycemic index and a glycemic load?

The ability of dietary carbohydrates to raise blood glucose levels varies greatly [13]. However, the carbohydrate density of each food is also a factor [14]. The glycemic index (GI) and glycemic load (GL) are terms used to describe these concepts.

When 50 grams of carbohydrate in watermelon are compared to 50 grams of carbohydrate in bananas, the carbohydrate in watermelon metabolizes quickly, resulting in a higher blood glucose response. As you can see, this indicates that its GI is higher. On the other hand, a banana has a much higher carbohydrate density than a watermelon. When similar serving sizes (120 grams of watermelon vs. 120 grams of banana) are compared, the serving of watermelon has a lower impact on blood sugar and thus has a lower GL.

The glycemic index response to food varies from person to person. The glycemic index of any given food can be influenced by the glycemic index of other foods eaten simultaneously [15]. The glycemic index is a good general guide, but the essential information is understanding how people react to specific foods (**Figure 1**).

1.4 Different carbohydrate restriction levels

Any dietary intervention that uses less than 130 grams of dietary carbohydrate per day is referred to as therapeutic carbohydrate restriction. The Dietary Reference Intake for the United States recommends this as the "minimum" level [11]. There are, however, various levels of carbohydrate restriction. The following definitions are used for better understanding:

- Ketogenic diets that are very low in carbohydrate — or keto diets — recommend no more than 20 grams of net dietary carbohydrate per day. The principles outlined in Dr. Atkins' New Diet Revolution are usually followed [17]. Other studies and protocols, such as those conducted by Virta Health, which you may have heard of, limit total dietary carbohydrates to 30 grams per day [18]. These two approaches will end up being very similar in practice. Almost everyone will experience a metabolic shift into nutritional ketosis due to both. The majority of patients find these diets to be incredibly filling. We advise patients to eat until they are satisfied rather than restricting or counting calories.

DOI: http://dx.doi.org/10.5772/intechopen.107184

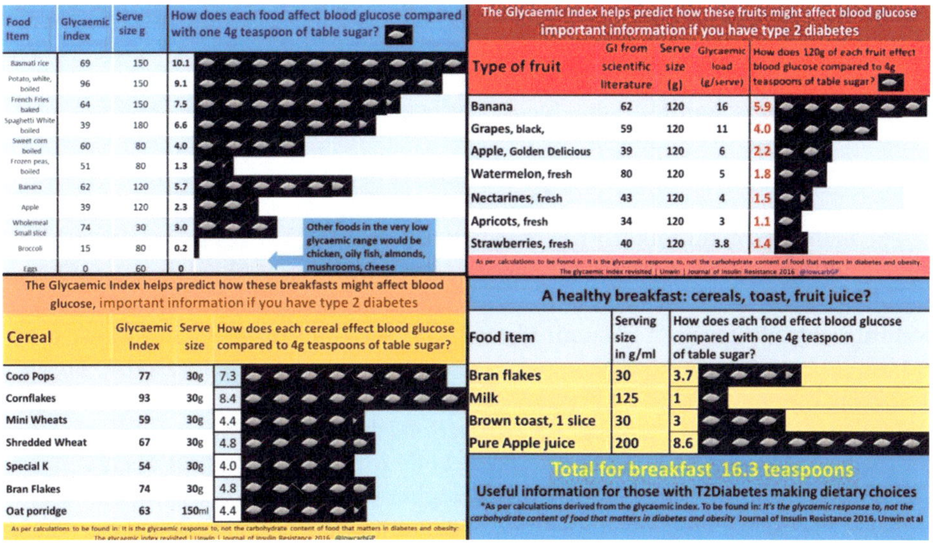

Figure 1.
An infographic to show how the glycemic index helps inform dietary choices [16].

- Low-carbohydrate diets with a moderate carbohydrate content recommend 20 to 50 grams of carbohydrate per day [19]. Nutritional ketosis may or may not occur at this carbohydrate restriction level. However, at this carbohydrate intake, most people will lose weight and improve their metabolic markers [19]. On a moderately low-carb diet, deliberate calorie restriction is not typically recommended, as it is on very low-carb ketogenic diets.

- Low-carbohydrate diets with a liberal carbohydrate intake typically recommend 50–100 grams per day. This carbohydrate intake is higher than most low-carb diets but lower than the US Daily Recommended Intake of 130 grams (DRI). Calorie and carbohydrate restrictions may or may not be used at this level. For some people, this level of carbohydrate restriction may not lead to nutritional ketosis or weight loss. However, studies have shown that even moderate carbohydrate restriction can improve metabolic markers such as blood sugar, HDL, and triglycerides [20].

2. Restricted carbohydrate diet and its physiological and metabolic effects

2.1 Therapeutic restricted carbohydrate

Therapeutic carbohydrate restriction lowers fasting and postprandial blood glucose and insulin levels while also reducing insulin resistance. All of these changes can improve metabolic syndrome markers [21]. In insulin resistance, it is harder for the body to maintain normal blood glucose leading to type 2 diabetes. Thus, it is counterproductive to consume carbohydrates that digest down into significant amounts of glucose [16].

As predicted by the glycemic index, restricting any foods that break down into glucose lowers blood glucose levels and insulin secretion. This includes whole-grain starches and high-sugar fruits. A glucometer can easily track blood glucose levels at home or in a clinical setting. A glucometer is an essential tool for identifying foods that raise blood glucose levels, even for people who do not have diabetes. We recommend that patients monitor their glucose levels when starting TCR if possible.

2.2 Insulin

The main reason for monitoring blood glucose levels may have less to do with glucose and more with insulin. Carbohydrates in the diet raise blood sugar levels and stimulate insulin secretion. While this is a normal physiological response, it can negatively affect health. Insulin maintains homeostasis by transporting glucose into cells and inhibiting glucose production in the liver when blood glucose levels rise. This is a life-saving response because it prevents dangerously high glucose levels in the blood.

On the other hand, insulin has other functions that we, as clinicians, frequently overlook. Insulin, for example, prevents the body from burning fat for energy instead of encouraging fat storage [22]. As a result, higher insulin levels can be a problem for people trying to lose weight. Giving insulin to people with type 2 diabetes can set off a vicious cycle of weight gain and insulin resistance.

Genetics, environment, and lifestyle all play a role in how well someone manages their dietary carbohydrate intake. Insulin levels rise and can remain chronically elevated when people consume more carbohydrates than their bodies can handle, known as hyperinsulinemia [23]. When this happens, the body's response to insulin signals becomes ineffective. Insulin resistance is the term used to describe this condition [24].

The development of the metabolic syndrome and an increased risk of heart disease are strongly linked to hyperinsulinemia and insulin resistance [25]. Insulin resistance is thought to be a common underlying mechanism for various chronic diseases, including type 2 diabetes, hypertension, atherogenic dyslipidemia, and chronic inflammation [26].

We tend to use glucose levels as a proxy for insulin levels because point-of-care insulin meters are unavailable. However, it's important to note that just because glucose levels are normal does not mean insulin levels are as well. Glucose levels may be normal in the early stages of diabetes and metabolic syndrome because high insulin levels keep them there.

Restriction of carbohydrate intake, fortunately, is an effective way of addressing the root cause of hyperinsulinemia and insulin resistance.

3. Getting the intervention started for metabolic diseases

This section covers which patients are good candidates for TCR and which patients should be approached with caution when implementing this dietary change. It also explains the importance of baseline assessments and briefly covers pre-diet evaluation and counseling.

3.1 Selection of patients

Patients with any metabolic syndrome symptoms are ideal candidates for therapeutic carbohydrate restriction. Patients with hypertension, mixed dyslipidemia, hyperglycemia, including type 2 diabetes, or obesity, particularly abdominal obesity, fall into this category.

3.2 Exclusion criteria

- Acute, decompensated medical condition
- Advanced renal insufficiency not on hemodialysis
- Pyruvate carboxylase deficiency
- Hyperchylomicronemia

3.3 The necessity for caution

It's uncommon to come across someone completely against therapeutic carbohydrate restriction. You'll often come across a patient who will benefit from TCR but who will require more attention and caution from you.

3.4 Risks associated with a low carbohydrate diet

A study published in May 2018 followed over 2000 men for over 20 years and found that higher protein intake was slightly associated with a higher risk of heart failure [27]. However, not all associations reached statistical significance, and some confidence intervals crossed zero. The long-term effects of a low carbohydrate diet are largely unknown. There has been a concern raised by some studies about a high protein intake increasing the risk of renal stones. However, a low carbohydrate diet only needs to contain a normal amount of protein. Thus a low carbohydrate diet is not known to worsen renal function, and some studies have shown an association with an improvement in eGFR.

In August 2018, a paper was published suggesting an increase in mortality for those who ate a low carbohydrate diet, in which carbohydrates were replaced with animal proteins, in contrast to those who replaced carbohydrates with plant-derived protein [28]. Those who developed diabetes during the study were excluded from follow-up, which may limit the applicability of this study to the diabetic patients at whom this chapter is aimed. If patients ask about this study (which has been extensively covered in the media), it would be reasonable to suggest that their diet remains balanced even when carbohydrates are reduced with proteins coming from plant and animal sources.

3.4.1 Diabetes type 2

As evidence shows, therapeutic carbohydrate restriction is a valuable intervention for patients with type 2 diabetes. Patients with diabetes, particularly those taking glucose-lowering medications, must be able to use a blood glucose meter and communicate their results to their health care team quickly [29].

To avoid hypoglycemic episodes and ensure patient safety, you as a healthcare provider must be more vigilant with patients with type 2 diabetes.

3.4.2 Hypertension

For patients with hypertension, therapeutic carbohydrate restriction is also an effective intervention. On the other hand, these patients must be able to monitor their blood pressure at home and communicate with their healthcare providers quickly to adjust antihypertensive medications appropriately. Remember that your team is critical in assisting the patient in avoiding symptomatic hypotension.

3.4.3 Gallbladder removal

Therapeutic carbohydrate restriction may still be a promising intervention for patients with gallbladders removed. When teaching these patients what foods to eat, tell them to gradually increase the amount of fat in their diet to avoid diarrhea. However, most patients without a gallbladder can successfully follow TCR after a slow transition period.

3.4.4 Chronic kidney disease

Due to the misconception that these diets are "high protein diets," there is often concern about using therapeutic carbohydrate reduction in patients with decreased kidney function. In reality, protein accounts for no more than 30% of calories in TCR diets. Except for those with pre-existing, advanced renal failure, this level is likely safe.

There is no evidence that protein intake at levels commonly consumed during TCR is harmful to people with mildly or moderately reduced kidney function [30], and plenty of evidence demonstrates its safety.

3.4.5 Kidney stones

When starting TCR, patients predisposed to kidney stones may increase their risk. In particular, uric acid levels in the blood can rise, increasing the risk of uric acid kidney stones in susceptible people. Patients with kidney stones should stay hydrated by following general guidelines. Experienced clinicians have discovered that encouraging adequate amounts of sodium, potassium, and, most importantly, magnesium can help reduce the risk of kidney stones. We should advise patients who have had calcium oxalate stones, the most common type of kidney stone, to avoid high oxalate foods like spinach, almonds, and cashews. TCR is completely safe in patients who have had kidney stones.

3.4.6 Gout

Patients prone to gout have the same concerns as those prone to uric acid kidney stones. As previously mentioned, uric acid levels can rise in the early stages of TCR. This can trigger a gout flare-up in susceptible individuals, though gout may improve over time on a carbohydrate-restricted diet [31]. These patients should drink plenty of water and get plenty of sodium, potassium, and magnesium. Another option for those prone to frequent attacks is to use prophylactic allopurinol during the early stages of the intervention.

3.4.7 Breastfeeding and pregnancy

When it comes to TCR, pregnancy and breastfeeding must be considered. Although moderate carbohydrate restriction has long been used to treat pregnant women with gestational diabetes [32], carbohydrates are rarely restricted to the very low levels used for weight loss or type 2 diabetes treatment. The amount of carbohydrate restriction should be individualized for the patient based on her medical history, but it should usually be at least 50 grams per day. According to a few case reports in the medical literature, more aggressive carbohydrate restriction during pregnancy or breastfeeding may increase the risk of ketoacidosis [33]. Fresh vegetables, meat, fish, eggs, dairy, nuts, seeds, and a small amount of fruit, on the other hand, provide adequate essential nutrition for both mother and baby.

3.5 Baseline tests

All TCR patients should have baseline and follow-up assessments to screen for potential harm and document successful progress.

To begin, keep track of each patient's starting weight. Even though it provides less detailed information, waist circumference is the simplest method. Furthermore, it is simple for patients to notice if their pants have suddenly become looser. Another critical vital sign, especially for those taking antihypertensives, is baseline blood pressure. Keep in mind that medications will almost certainly need to be adjusted once a patient begins TCR.

3.6 Lab tests

We recommend running the following baseline lab tests when starting a patient on TCR.

- **Comprehensive metabolic panel (CMP)**: This test includes fasting glucose, kidney, and liver function, as well as basic electrolytes, which are all important to track on TCR. We must ensure that patients' baseline GFR is less than 30 ml/min because severe renal dysfunction is potentially contraindicated to TCR. Also, if the patient has fatty liver with elevated transaminases, we must document and monitor this, as it frequently improves with TCR.

- **HbA1c**: This is a three-month average glucose level measurement. This is critical to establish a baseline and track it over time as one of the main indicators of TCR success. HbA1c levels of 5.7 to 6.4% (6.5 to 7.6 mmol/L) are considered prediabetes, while 6.5% (7.8 mmol/L) or higher are considered diabetes.

- **Fasting insulin**: Homeostatic Model Assessment of Insulin Resistance (HOMA-IR) can be calculated using fasting insulin and fasting glucose. We recommend checking insulin resistance at baseline because it is a major focus of TCR. On the other hand, fasting insulin is not a common test for most doctors. We recommend that you practice ordering and interpreting this test. While fasting insulin levels vary naturally [34], tracking the trend over time is an excellent way to track TCR progress.

Although there is no universally accepted reference range for fasting insulin, we can use the literature to help us develop useful ranges.

One study [35] found that levels above 25 micro IU/ml were associated with a very high risk of developing prediabetes, and levels above 12 were associated with a moderate risk, confirming an earlier study. In a later study, it was discovered that insulin levels above 8 micro IU/ml c orrectly predicted prediabetes in 80% of the people tested [35].

Furthermore, one study claimed that a HOMA-IR of less than 1.6 was a normal values [36].

- **Fasting lipid profile**: A baseline fasting lipid panel is recommended for everyone because mixed dyslipidemia is common in metabolic syndrome. We expect high-density lipids (HDL) to rise and triglycerides to fall due to TCR. We also need to keep an eye on LDL-C levels, as this is likely the first area of concern with TCR. While some guidelines recommend non-fasting panels to improve compliance, this makes interpreting triglycerides more difficult because their value is dependent on the content and timing of the most recent meal. As a result, fasting lipid panels are recommended for consistency.

3.7 Additional tests

- **Complete blood count**: Although significant changes in the CBC are uncommon, it's important to know that the patient does not have any baseline abnormalities like anemia or cytopenia.

- **Uric acid**: A baseline uric acid level is recommended for those prone to gout attacks or who have a history of uric acid kidney stones. The results may influence whether or not prophylactic allopurinol should be started for those with elevated levels.

- **TSH**: Because severe hypothyroidism affects weight loss, we recommend that everyone get a baseline TSH before starting TCR.

4. Carbohydrate restriction for therapeutic purposes

We'll go over the basics of patient education when starting TCR and how to support patients' lifestyle behavior changes in this section. We'll go over the initial medication adjustments that need to be made and potential side effects and how to deal with them.

4.1 Assisting with behavior change

A patient education and support component should be included in therapeutic carbohydrate restriction. Maintaining a simple initiation with as much support as possible will aid adherence and success.

The first step is to talk to patients about their current diet, diet history, and health goals to help them prepare for this nutritional change. If patients have a history of weight loss and regain, this is an opportunity to address their fears of failure and explain how this could be different.

Next, determine the patient's familiarity with carbohydrate restriction and provide education tailored to their level of understanding. Patients may be unsure if therapeutic carbohydrate restriction is the right treatment option. As discussed in previous sections, addressing these concerns is an opportunity to educate patients about the approach's safety and efficacy.

At the same time, the healthcare provider should inform patients about any possible side effects. Patients should be taught how to handle the most common problems and when to seek medical help.

4.2 Education of the patient

Therapeutic carbohydrate restriction usually entails eating a diet rich in whole foods that have been minimally or traditionally processed. Although meal replacement shakes or kits can be used to administer this diet, we will focus on using whole foods readily available in most grocery stores in this course.

The three principles of therapeutic carbohydrate restriction are as follows:

- To begin, keep carbs to a minimum.
- Second, make sure you are getting enough protein.
- Third, as needed, add or subtract fat to achieve satiety or weight loss goals.

Patients are encouraged to eat only when they are hungry and stop eating when they are satisfied. Because TCR makes patients feel fuller, they no longer need to eat on a regular 3-meal-per-day schedule and can instead rely on their hunger cues.

Based on their preference, your patients can be encouraged to eat meat, fish, poultry, eggs, above-ground vegetables, nuts, cheese, and fatty "fruits" like olives and avocados. They can also use olive oil, avocado oil, coconut oil, butter, and ghee as fat sources. Patients should avoid sugary foods that would be restricted on any weight-loss diet, including cake, cookies, ice cream, and other desserts, as well as pancakes, potato chips, fries, and soda and other sweetened beverages. You should also teach your patients why and how to avoid foods that are commonly portrayed as healthy, such as whole-grain bread and cereals, rice, beans, pasta, low-fat milk and dairy products with added sugar, and a variety of fruits. Because these foods are broken down into glucose, they may have unfavorable effects on blood sugar and insulin levels in those who are susceptible. These foods should be avoided when using therapeutic carbohydrate restriction to treat obesity, metabolic syndrome, or diabetes.

This usually results in a diet where carbohydrates account for less than 10% of total calories, protein accounts for 20–25% of total calories, and fat accounts for more than 65% of total calories. However, because we rarely ask patients to track their calories during TCR, data based on percentages of total calories is usually useless.

Furthermore, rather than a macronutrient ratio, the levels at which carbohydrates and protein exert metabolic effects appear to reflect absolute thresholds in grams consumed (Accurso et al., 2008; Layman, 2009). Instead of focusing on macronutrient percentages when educating your patients, you should focus on making food choices that limit carbohydrate intake, provide adequate-protein, and allow enough fat for satiety and flavor.

4.3 Low carbohydrate diet and medication changes

The issues that should be considered when patients taking diabetic medications decide to start a low GI diet. Particular care should be taken with sulfonylureas due to the risk of hypoglycaemia and SGL T-2 inhibitors due to the risk of euglycaemic ketoacidosis. Insulin requirements will often drop, and the healthcare provider should supervise this. The following are the points to consider while using diabetic medications in type 2 when on a low carbohydrate diet [37].

- Risk for hypoglycemia?

- Degree of adherence to carbohydrate restriction?
- Benefit of using the medication and/or any adverse effects or risks outweigh the benefits? (**Table 2**).

4.4 Medication for diabetes

The most important medications to reduce or eliminate first are those that lower blood glucose. The most serious concern we have with TCR in patients with blood sugar problems is that it will cause symptomatic hypoglycemia. As a result, the most important point to emphasize is the importance of blood glucose monitoring regularly. This means that insulin users must test several times throughout the day, including fasting and pre-meal tests. If you are only taking oral medications, you might have to test once or twice a day.

The degree to which we reduce or discontinue medications is determined by the wishes and concerns of our patients. For example, if avoiding hypoglycemia is more important, we can quickly lower drugs and temporarily allow higher blood glucose levels. We would adjust medications more slowly if the patient is more concerned about maintaining strict glucose control. The most important thing is to teach the patient about hypoglycemia symptoms and the importance of testing their blood glucose multiple times per day, especially in the first few weeks.

4.4.1 Metformin

We recommend continuing metformin with no dose adjustments when starting TCR because it does not cause hypoglycemia.

Class of antidiabetic medication#	Action	Hypo risk?	Suggested action (to continue/stop)
Biguanides	Reduce hepatic gluconeogenesis, and reduce peripheral insulin resistance	No	Optional, consider clinical pros/cons.
Insulins	Exogenous insulin	Yes	Reduce/Stop (see under insulin section)
Sulfonylureas	Increase pancreatic insulin secretion	Yes	Stop (or if gradual carbohydrate restriction, then wean by e.g. halving dose successively)
DPP-4 inhibitors	Inhibit DPP-4 enzyme	No	Stop. No significant risk, but no benefit in most cases.
Thiazolidinediones	Reduce peripheral insulin resistance	No	Usually stop. Concern over risks usually outweighs benefits.
GLP-1 agonists	Slow gastric emptying. Glucose dependent pancreatic insulin secretion.	No	Optional, consider clinical pros/cons.
Alpha-glucosidase inhibitors	Delay digestion of starch and sucrose	No	Stop. No benefit on a low carbohydrate diet.

#*Arranged as per Most Commonly Prescribed Diabetes Medications (data from 2020 [38]).*

Table 2.
A summary of low carbohydrate diet and diabetic medication changes.

4.4.2 Insulin

Insulin, as the most potent glucose-lowering medication, should be adjusted first. When starting TCR, we should discontinue the use of short-acting insulin given before meals. The patients will likely not require the pre-meal, short-acting insulin because their meals are now much lower in carbohydrates. You can reintroduce short-acting insulin if their postprandial glucose levels are consistently above 200 mg/dL (11 mmol/L) despite TCR compliance.

Patients should also cut back on their long-acting insulin. If the patient is more concerned about hypoglycemic episodes, the long-acting insulin should be reduced by half when TCR begins. It should be reduced by one-third if they are more concerned with strict glucose control. This, however, assumes that their fasting blood glucose is less than 200 mg/dL (11 mmol/L) and that they have had adequate control. If their blood sugars are poorly controlled, and their lowest recent fasting glucose is greater than 200 mg/dL (11 mmol/L), hold off on lowering the long-acting insulin until their blood sugars improve. Finally, mixed insulins, which are a mix of long and short-acting insulins, are difficult to adjust accurately and should be avoided entirely. Only long-acting insulin should be given to the patient.

The one caveat to lowering insulin dosage is that we must be aware of adults with latent autoimmune diabetes (LADA). Although uncommon, these people are more insulin-dependent and will not be able to reduce or stop their dose as quickly or completely as others. TCR is still beneficial for them, but it should be done with caution and at a slower pace when reducing medication dosages. LADA should be considered if someone has a history of DKA or hospitalizations for severe hyperglycemia.

4.4.3 Sulfonylureas

We recommend stopping sulfonylureas when starting TCR because they can cause significant hypoglycemia. Continue sulfonylureas until sugars are below 200 mg/dL (11 mmol/L) if someone has poorly controlled sugars at baseline, with fasting glucose above 200 mg/dL (11 mmol/L).

4.4.4 GLP-1 agonists and DPP-4 inhibitors

These can also be continued until excellent glucose control is shown. We can then cut their doses in half to completely stop them once their blood sugars are under control.

4.4.5 Inhibitors of SGLT-2

These medications are beneficial for people with diabetes because they have been shown to reduce cardiovascular mortality. However, they have been linked to an increased risk of DKA, which could be amplified if you are on a carbohydrate-restricted diet. SGLT-2 inhibitors, in particular, increase the risk of euglycemic ketoacidosis, which occurs when blood glucose remains normal despite significantly elevated ketones, to the point where the blood becomes dangerously acidic. As a result, if we aren't looking for it specifically, we may miss it. Check a beta-hydroxybutyrate level as well as a metabolic panel for acid–base status if you suspect euglycemic DKA. Because of this risk, we advise all patients starting TCR to stop taking SGLT-2 inhibitors one or two days before reducing carbohydrate intake.

4.4.6 GLP-1 agonists and DPP-4 inhibitors

These can also be continued until excellent glucose control is shown. We can then cut their doses in half to completely stop them once their blood sugars are under control.

4.5 Antihypertensive medications

Because TCR is an effective blood pressure (BP)-lowering treatment, many people taking antihypertensive medications may experience symptomatic hypotension. The first step is to inform your patients about low blood pressure symptoms such as dizziness, orthostasis, and fatigue. Ascertain that patients can monitor their blood pressure at home and quickly communicate the results to you or your healthcare team.

When starting TCR, we do not recommend stopping BP medications automatically unless the baseline BP is consistently below 110/70. However, if patients develop symptomatic hypotension, we advise discontinuing or reducing medicines as needed to alleviate symptoms.

4.6 Additional medications

Although this is not necessarily a TCR target, we have found that many people's gastroesophageal reflux disease (GERD) symptoms improve, allowing them to reduce or eliminate the use of proton pump inhibitors (PPIs) or H2 blockers. Patients may experience a rebound effect if treatment is abruptly stopped. Consider switching from a PPI to an H2 blocker for a few weeks before stopping or switching from every other day dosing to every other day dosing before stopping.

4.7 Treatment and side-effects

Preparing our patients for possible side effects is an integral part of increasing carbohydrate reduction compliance. Although TCR's side effects are usually mild and short-lived, they can be quite unpleasant when the patient is ready for them.

5. Conclusion

Physiological necessary glucose can be provided by gluconeogenesis. Starchy foods that are sometimes considered healthy, such as cereals, are broken down into glucose. It is possible to improve type 2 diabetes without drugs by following a low GI diet.

Author details

Joshua Chadwick[1]*, Lokesh Shanmugam[1] and Balasubramanian Ganesh[2]

1 Indian Council of Medical Research, National Institute of Epidemiology, Ministry of Health and Family Welfare, Government of India, Chennai, India

2 Laboratory Division, ICMR-National Institute of Epidemiology (ICMR-NIE), Chennai, India

*Address all correspondence to: joshuachadwick89@gmail.com

References

[1] Saklayen MG. The global epidemic of the metabolic syndrome. Current Hypertension Reports. 2018;**20**(2):12

[2] Marín-Peñalver JJ, Martín-Timón I, Sevillano-Collantes C, del Cañizo-Gómez FJ. Update on the treatment of type 2 diabetes mellitus. World Journal of Diabetes. 2016;**7**(17): 354

[3] Evert AB, Dennison M, Gardner CD, Timothy Garvey W, Karen Lau KH, Mac Leod J, et al. Nutrition therapy for adults with diabetes or prediabetes: A consensus report. Diabetes Care. 2019;**42**(5):731-754

[4] Westman EC, Yancy WS, Humphreys M. Dietary treatment of diabetes mellitus in the pre-insulin era (1914-1922). Perspectives in Biology and Medicine. 2006;**49**(1):77-83

[5] Mackarness R. Eat Fat and Grow Slim: Mackarness. Hawthorne, CA: Books-Amazon; 2017

[6] Riddle MC, Cefalu WT, Evans PH, Gerstein HC, Nauck MA, Oh WK, et al. Consensus report: Definition and interpretation of remission in type 2 diabetes. Diabetes Care. 2021;**44**(10):2438-2444

[7] Goldenberg JZ, Johnston BC. Low and very low carbohydrate diets for diabetes remission. The BMJ. 2021;**373**:m 4743

[8] Teo K, Chow CK, Vaz M, Rangarajan S, Yusuf S, Islam S, et al. The prospective urban rural epidemiology (PURE) study: Examining the impact of societal influences on chronic noncommunicable diseases in low-, middle-, and high-income countries. American Heart Journal. 2009;**158**(1):7.e1

[9] Gjuladin-Hellon T, Davies IG, Penson P, Baghbadorani RA. Effects of carbohydrate-restricted diets on low-density lipoprotein cholesterol levels in overweight and obese adults: A systematic review and meta-analysis. Nutrition Reviews. 2019;**77**(3):161-180

[10] Feinman RD, Pogozelski WK, Astrup A, Bernstein RK, Fine EJ, Westman EC, et al. Dietary carbohydrate restriction as the first approach in diabetes management: Critical review and evidence base. Nutrition. 2015;**31**(1):1-13

[11] Trumbo P, Schlicker S, Yates AA, Poos M. Dietary reference intakes for energy, carbohydrate, fiber, fat, fatty acids, cholesterol, protein and amino acids. Journal of the American Dietetic Association. 2002;**102**(11):1621-1630

[12] Westman EC, Feinman RD, Mavropoulos JC, Vernon MC, Volek JS, Wortman JA, et al. Low-carbohydrate nutrition and metabolism. The American Journal of Clinical Nutrition. 2007;**86**(2):276-284

[13] Atkinson FS, Foster-Powell K, Brand-Miller JC. International tables of glycemic index and glycemic load values: 2008. Diabetes Care. 2008;**31**(12):2281-2283

[14] Unwin D, Haslam D, Livesey G. It is the glycaemic response to, not the carbohydrate content of food that matters in diabetes and obesity: The glycaemic index revisited. Journal of Insulin Resistance. 2016;**1**(1):a8

[15] Meng H, Matthan NR, Ausman LM, Lichtenstein AH. Effect of macronutrients and fiber on postprandial glycemic responses and meal glycemic

index and glycemic load value determinations. The American Journal of Clinical Nutrition. 2017;**105**(4):842

[16] Unwin D, Haslam D, Livesey G. It is the glycaemic response to, not the carbohydrate content of food that matters in diabetes and obesity: The glycaemic index revisited. Journal of Insulin Resistance. 2016;**1**(1)

[17] Atkins RC. Dr. Atkins' New Diet Revolution. London, United Kingdom: Penguin Random House; 1998. p. 417

[18] Hallberg SJ, McKenzie AL, Williams PT, Bhanpuri NH, Peters AL, Campbell WW, et al. Effectiveness and safety of a novel care model for the Management of Type 2 diabetes at 1 year: An open-label, non-randomized. Controlled Study. Diabetes Ther. 2018;**9**(2):583-612

[19] Saslow LR, Daubenmier JJ, Moskowitz JT, Kim S, Murphy EJ, Phinney SD, et al. Twelve-month outcomes of a randomized trial of a moderate-carbohydrate versus very low-carbohydrate diet in overweight adults with type 2 diabetes mellitus or prediabetes. Nutrition and Diabetes. 2017;7(12):1-6

[20] Krauss RM, Blanche PJ, Rawlings RS, Fernstrom HS, Williams PT. Separate effects of reduced carbohydrate intake and weight loss on atherogenic dyslipidemia. The American Journal of Clinical Nutrition. 2006;**83**(5):1025-1031

[21] Volek JS, Feinman RD. Carbohydrate restriction improves the features of metabolic syndrome. Metabolic syndrome may be defined by the response to carbohydrate restriction. Nutrition and Metabolism. 2005;**2**:31

[22] Wilcox G. Insulin and insulin resistance. Clinical Biochemist Reviews. 2005;**26**(2):19

[23] Corkey BE. Diabetes: Have we got it all wrong? Insulin hypersecretion and food additives: Cause of obesity and diabetes? Diabetes Care. 2012;**35**(12):2432

[24] Templeman NM, Skovsø S, Page MM, Lim GE, Johnson JD. A causal role for hyperinsulinemia in obesity. Journal of Endocrinology. 2017;**232**(3):R173-R183

[25] Hyde PN, Sapper TN, Crabtree CD, LaFountain RA, Bowling ML, Buga A, et al. Dietary carbohydrate restriction improves metabolic syndrome independent of weight loss. JCI Insight. 2019;**4**(12):e128308

[26] Reaven GM. Effect of dietary carbohydrate on the metabolism of patients with non-insulin dependent diabetes mellitus. Nutrition Review. 1986;**44**(2):65-73

[27] Virtanen HEK, Voutilainen S, Koskinen TT, Mursu J, Tuomainen TP, Virtanen JK. Intake of different dietary proteins and risk of heart failure in men: The Kuopio Ischaemic heart disease risk factor study. Circulation Heart Failure. 2018;**11**(6):e004531

[28] Seidelmann SB, Claggett B, Cheng S, Henglin M, Shah A, Steffen LM, et al. Dietary carbohydrate intake and mortality: A prospective cohort study and meta-analysis. The Lancet Public Health. 2018;**3**(9):e419-e428

[29] Cucuzzella M, Hite A, Patterson K, Saslow L, Heath R. A clinician's guide to inpatient low carbohydrate diets for remission of type 2 diabetes: Toward a standard of care protocol. Diabetes Management. 2019;**9**(1):7-19

[30] Brinkworth GD, Wycherley TP, Noakes M, Buckley JD, Clifton PM. Long-term effects of a very-low-carbohydrate weight-loss diet and an isocaloric low-fat

diet on bone health in obese adults. Nutrition. 2016;**32**(9):1033-1036

[31] Steelman M. From Obesity: Evaluation and Treatment Essentials. Second ed. Florida, United States: Taylor & Francis; 2016

[32] Mulla WR. Carbohydrate content in the GDM diet: Two views: View 2: Low-carbohydrate diets should remain the initial therapy for gestational diabetes. Diabetes Spectrum. 2016;**29**(2):89-91

[33] Nnodum BN, Oduah E, Albert D, Pettus M. Ketogenic diet-induced severe ketoacidosis in a lactating woman: A case report and review of the literature. Case Reports in Nephrology. 2019;**2019**:1214208

[34] Wallace TM, Matthews DR. The assessment of insulin resistance in man. Diabetic Medicine. 2002;**19**(7):527-534

[35] Johnson JL, Duick DS, Chui MA, Aldasouqi SA. Identifying prediabetes using fasting insulin levels. Endocrine Practice. 2010;**16**(1):47-52

[36] Shashaj B, Luciano R, Contoli B, Morino GS, Spreghini MR, Rustico C, et al. Reference ranges of HOMA-IR in normal-weight and obese young Caucasians. Acta Diabetologica. 2016;**53**(2):251-260

[37] Cucuzzella M, Riley K, Isaacs D. Adapting medication for type 2 diabetes to a low carbohydrate diet. Frontiers in Nutrition. 2021;**8**:486

[38] InformedHealth.org [Internet]. Cologne, Germany: Institute for Quality and Efficiency in Health Care (IQWiG); 2006-. Medication for type 2 diabetes. [Updated 2020 Oct 22]. Available from: https://www.ncbi.nlm.nih.gov/books/NBK279506/

Chapter 24

Diagnosis and Management of Acute Ischemic Stroke

Anwer Zohaib Siddiqi, Angela Young and Ankur Wadhwa

Abstract

This chapter will review updates in the various imaging modalities used to diagnose acute ischemic stroke (AIS), how these are used to select patients for intervention, and the different interventions used for management of AIS. The backbone of the AIS diagnostic algorithm remains the computed tomography scan (CT) given its speed of use and sensitivity. CT-angiography (CTA) is crucial in diagnosing large-vessel occlusions (LVOs) and multiphase CTA and CT-perfusion (CTP) can demonstrate the number of collaterals in the area and remaining salvageable tissue. MRI can be used to select patients presenting in an unknown time window for thrombolysis. The primary goal of AIS management is to rescue the ischemic penumbra and the approach to treating AIS has gone from a time-based to tissue-based approach. While tPA is still the agent of choice for thrombolysis in patients with AIS, tenecteplase (TNK) may be just as effective and more efficient to use. Endovascular thrombectomy (EVT) has shown considerable efficacy for alleviating LVOs and using CTP, patients can be selected for hours after symptom-onset if viable tissue remains. It remains unclear if an "EVT-alone" strategy is superior to "tPA + EVT" strategy but this may be dependent on clot, patient, and geographical characteristics.

Keywords: stroke, ischemia, neuroimaging, thrombolysis, thrombectomy

1. Introduction

Globally, stroke remains the second leading cause of death and the third leading cause of death and disability (as expressed by disability-adjusted life-years lost—DALYs) [1]. 88% of all acute strokes are ischemic strokes, caused by reduced blood flow and of the remaining, 10% are intracerebral hemorrhages, due to rupture of cerebral arteries and 2% subarachnoid hemorrhages, due to trauma or rupture of aneurysm [2]. This chapter will focus on acute ischemic strokes (AIS). Among AIS, 22% are cardioembolic (thrombus originally formed in the heart), 23% due to large artery atherosclerosis, 22% due to small vessel occlusion or lacunar infarct (2–20 mm in size and occur deep in the brain), and 29% are other causes [3, 4].

The typical presentation of AIS is abrupt focal neurological deficit that is due to a lack of blood flow [5, 6]. As neurological dysfunctions caused by focal brain, retinal or spinal cord ischemia may be reversible if presented early and treated promptly, acute stroke care at the hospital setting should begin with prompt history taking, neurological exam, emergent neuroimaging and pertinent investigations to establish a plan of management [7].

IntechOpen

The TOAST (Trial of Org 10,172 in Acute Stroke Treatment), classification categorizes ischemic stroke etiologies into five major subtypes [8]: large artery sclerosis, cardioembolism, small artery occlusion, stroke of other determined cause, and stroke of undetermined cause. Newer classification criteria such as the Causative Classification System further stratifies high and low risk cardiac sources of embolism. In this system, the 'stroke of undetermined cause' category is divided into unknown, incomplete evaluation, unclassified stroke with more than one etiology, and cryptogenic embolism, where there is evidence of embolism in otherwise normal looking artery or subsequent complete recanalization [9].

Other disorders may masquerade as ischemic strokes (**Table 1**). Between 15 and 25% stroke suspects presented to the emergency room are stroke mimics [2, 5]. Patients who have seizures often present with post-ictal hemiparesis, also known as Todd's Paresis. This is a transient weakness that usually resolves within 24 hours [10]. Migraine auras may present as motor weakness, aphasia, sensory disturbances, and visual auras, that potentially resemble stroke symptoms. Focal neurological deficits are frequently the sequalae of severe hypoglycemia, necessitating blood glucose measurements. Tumors can cause seizures, may directly compress surrounding vessels, and can be easily ruled out with MR brain. Other stroke mimics include hyponatremia, conversion disorder, and positional vertigo [11]. The key to ruling out the mimics is through heightened clinical suspicion and tailored investigations.

2. Diagnosis of acute ischemic stroke

2.1 Last known normal time (LKNT)

The ECASS III trial has established that thrombolysis efficacy was significant up to 4.5 hours post stroke [12]. The precise onset of stroke allows a clear decision on whether to provide thrombolysis. However, 1 in 7 strokes are a wake-up stroke, and oftentimes patients and their families were vague about the time onset [13]. A key piece of information in the history of present illnesses is the LKN, which establishes the maximal duration from onset to presentation for those without a precisely known onset.

Seizures
Migraine with aura
Infection: encephalitis, brain abscess
Metabolic: Hypo/hyperglycemia, hyponatremia, Wernicke's encephalopathy
Neoplasia: CNS tumor, CNS metastasis
Drug toxicity
Hypertensive encephalopathy
Positional vertigo
Conversion disorder

Table 1.
Differential diagnosis to stroke.

2.2 Rapid acquisition of medical and surgical history

Pertinent history and neurological exam are essential to establish a stroke diagnosis and guide subsequent treatment. History not only provide clues for potential stroke etiologies, but also detects contraindications for thrombolysis (discussed in detail later) and guide stroke prevention. Of particular importance in medical history are vascular risk factors, including modifiable conditions such as obesity, diabetes, hypertension, dyslipidemia, metabolic syndrome, chronic obstructive pulmonary disease, previous ischemic or hemorrhagic strokes, ischemic heart disease, congestive heart failure, atrial fibrillation, smoking, and excessive alcohol use [14]. The presence of some or many of these factors increase the likelihood of AIS.

2.3 Focused neurological exam and use of NIHSS score

After history is obtained, the clinician should perform a focused neurological exam, calculating National Institutes of Health Stroke Scale (NIHSS) score, originally used for the NINDS Trial [15]. The NIHSS is a standardized scale ranging from 0 to 42 that grades patient's level of consciousness, language, visual fields, facial weakness, limb weakness, sensation, and incoordination [16]. Each category has a different score and a higher score for a component would indicate a worse deficit (for example, when testing left arm weakness, a score of 0 would mean no weakness, and 4 would indicate flaccid paralysis of the arm).

The NIHSS score strongly correlates with post-stroke modified Rankin scale (mRS) score[1] at discharge from stroke stay [17, 18]. An NIHSS <5 is predictive of better outcomes with an mRS generally less than 3, and an NIHSS >22 predictive for poorer outcomes with an mRS greater than 3 or death. NIHSS scores between 5 and 22 inclusive on the other hand had a weaker correlation with mRS scores [19]. However, on the NIHSS, left hemispheric deficits are more heavily rated than those of the right [20]. Further the scores do not reliably detect posterior circulation findings, for example, vertigo and dizziness [21]. Nevertheless, the NIHSS is known as a reliable predictor for stroke severity, informing treatment decisions and post-thrombolysis prognosis. Of note, neurological exams should not be entirely limited to the items of the NIHSS, as the signs outside of those of NIHSS may inform alternate explanations. For example, a new vertical gaze palsy points to a midbrain localization and an acute onset dysphagia with saliva pooling may be caused by posterior circulation infarct. These are examples of signs separate from the NIHSS, and a rapid and focused neurological exam should not miss.

2.4 Emergent acquisition and interpretation of brain imaging

2.4.1 Non-contrast computed tomography (NCCT) brain

Ideally, within 25 minutes after presenting at the hospital, a non-contrast CT (NCCT) brain with an axial section thickness no more than 5 mm may detect the

[1] The MRS is a scale that measures disability from stroke that is scored from 0 to 5 with a higher score indicating higher disability. A score of 0 means no disability, 1 means mild symptoms, 2 means inability to carry out previous activities, 3 means requiring help but able to walk, 4 means inability to walk without assistance, and 5 means, bedridden.

following: acute hemorrhage which is an absolute contraindication to IV tPA, early ischemic changes, chronic infarcts, and dense artery sign [7, 22]. NCCT has a sensitivity and specificity exceeding 95–98% for the detection of intracranial hemorrhage [23]. Hypoattenuation (dark on NCCT) of gray matter, in forms of the insular ribbon sign defined by loss of gray-white distinction, obscured outline and partial disappearance of the lentiform nucleus, and loss of gray-white matter differentiation, tend to be subtle when patients present early [24, 25]. The hyperdense artery sign (**Figure 1**) can be seen within 90 minutes of an MCA stroke and is usually caused by thromboembolic material in the lumen of the MCA [24] but can also commonly seen in the anterior cerebral artery (ACA), posterior cerebral artery (PCA), and basilar artery [26].

2.4.2 The Alberta stroke program early CT score (ASPECTS), a treatment and prognosis tool

NCCT allows computing the ASPECTS, which assesses early ischemic changes *in the anterior circulation* using 10 anatomically defined regions: 1 point for subcortical structures such as the caudate, lentiform, internal capsule, insular ribbon, and 6 for cortical MCA territories designated M1 to M6 [27, 28]. Therefore, an ASPECTS of 10 indicates no ischemic change in the above territories but does not eliminate infarcts in posterior circulation territories, and an ASPECTS of 0 is tantamount to very large infarcts that involves all the above anterior circulation territories. ASPECTS has a sensitivity of 78% and specificity of 96% for predicting functional outcome [27]. As the score predicts functional independence after thrombolysis, one generally requires a cut off score of 6 or more, age older than 18, an NIHSS score of 6 or more, and a

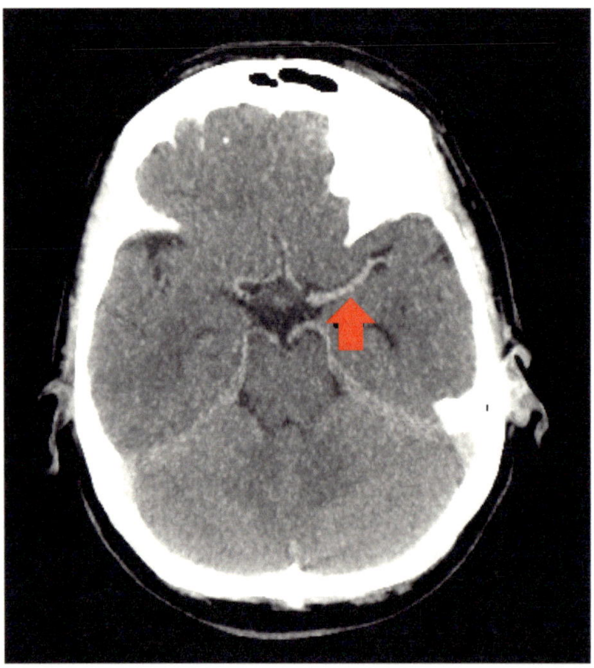

Figure 1.
Non-contrast CT scan demonstrating hyperdense left middle cerebral artery sign (arrow). It is evident that the vessel shows up as brighter or hyperdense, compared to the contralateral vessel. A clot in the artery is more dense as it contains more red blood cells and therefore, more iron.

reasonable pre-stroke functional baseline to be eligible for thrombectomy, as will be discussed later [29]. There are however drawbacks to the ASPECTS. First, it is not helpful for strokes in the posterior circulation. Second, there is significant variation in interrater reliability. Finally, ASPECTS can be affected by the quality of the NCCT as well as bone and metal artifacts [24].

2.4.3 CT angiography

CT angiography (CTA) requires administering iodinated contrast material through an 18–20 gauge needle, and it is not necessary to obtain the results of renal function prior to CTA [30]. Ehrlich et al. studied safety of CTA in evaluation of patients with acute stroke [31]. Within 24 to 48 hours after CTA, they found no statistical difference in both renal function and changes in creatinine. They drew the conclusion that CTA should not be delayed for testing for creatinine in AIS. CTA is performed immediately after the NCCT, with the aim to visualize occlusions in both extracranial and intracranial vasculature from the aortic arch to vertex [24] and may be performed as a single, delayed, or multiphase study (**Figure 2**). Evidence suggests that performing CTA is all individuals presenting within 24 hours improved detection of LVO, increased the population of AIS patients treated with endovascular thrombectomy, and was associated with better outcome [32].

Thus, CTA may reliably discover locations of stenosis and occlusions, providing clues to etiologies and allowing further assessments for the eligibility of thrombectomy. As an example, an occlusion in the internal carotid (ICA) with ipsilateral infarct may sway the etiology towards thromboembolism originated from a large vessel, while stenosis of the ICA with bilateral embolic showers is more commonly caused by an embolism from a proximal source such as the heart of aortic arch.

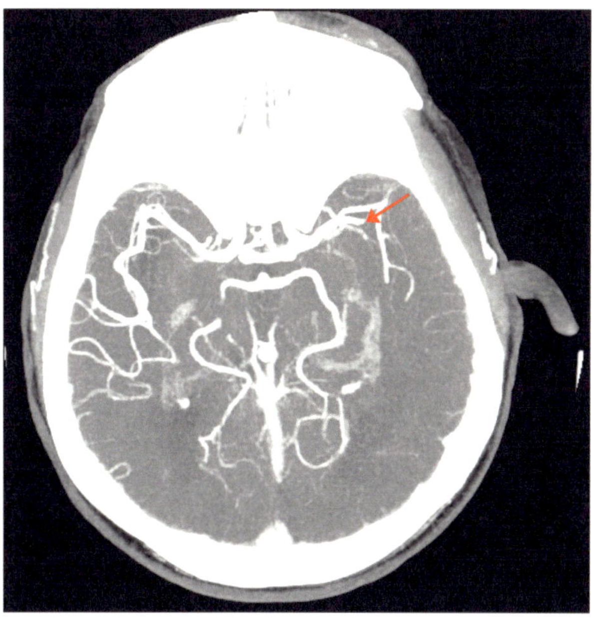

Figure 2.
CT angiogram with circle of Willis reconstruction. After the region marked by the red arrow, there is no contrast filling the artery indicating an occlusion in the distal M1 branch of the left middle cerebral artery.

Multiphase CTA (mCTA) is an imaging tool that provides three time-resolved images of pial arterial filling in the whole brain and is superior to conventional single-phase CT angiography (sCTA) [33]. After injection of contrast bolus, the first phase, also known as the peak arterial phase, scans from the aortic arch through the vertex. The second phase, the peak venous phase, scans the skull base through the vertex, and is performed 4 seconds after completion of the peak arterial phase scan. The third phase, the late venous phase, scans from the skull base through the vertex performed 4 seconds after completion of the second phase. Multiphase CTA (mCTA) is especially useful in assessing collateral vasculature. Collaterals are connections between cerebral blood vessels; when an artery is occluded, these collaterals reroute blood flow to maintain perfusion to the ischemic tissue [24]. Patients with diminished or absent collateral vessels in the symptomatic hemisphere experienced markedly higher risk for further deterioration. Compared to sCTA, mCTA improves detection of large-vessel occlusion (LVO; occlusion of large artery in brain such as terminus of the ICA, M1/M2 branch of MCA,, ACA, and basilar artery), improved characterization of collateral status, improved tolerance of patient motion and poor hemodynamics, and higher interrater reliability [34]. Therefore, the mCTA is incredibly useful in determining prognosis and guiding treatment decisions [24, 35, 36].

2.4.4 The concept of the ischemic penumbra and mismatch

In a patient presenting with AIS, there exists an ischemic "penumbra" [37]. This is the region which receives greater than 10% of its baseline blood flow but less than 30% [38]. This tissue has not irreversibly infarcted yet, but the neurons are electrically silent (i.e. not conducting action potentials) and causing the patient's acute clinical deficits. The tissue that is already infarcted and cannot be recovered, even after reperfusion is called the ischemic "core". **Figure 3** depicts a rat model of the effect of decreased blood flow on neuronal physiology. In humans, estimates of the ischemic penumbra have been best achieved using CT-perfusion (CTP) and MRI. Using imaging modalities, we can determine which tissue is being hypoperfused, the volume of tissue being hypoperfused, and the volume of tissue that is already infarcted. The ratio between the total volume of tissue being hypoperfused and the volume of tissue that is already infarcted, the core, is known as the mismatch ratio (MMR). To define the specifics of the MMR, it is important to discuss CTP parameters.

2.4.4.1 The parameters of CTP

CTP is the accepted modality for selecting patients with AIS within 6 to 24 hours of LKNT, as it is can determine how much salvageable tissue remains [24]. There are four primary parameters that CTP uses to determine if tissue is hypoperfused and if so, if can be saved. Cerebral blood flow (CBF) is the volume of blood flowing in a unit (100 g) of brain tissue during a unit of time (1 minute). Time-to-maximum (Tmax) is the time delay between the contrast arriving in the large vessels to when it arrives in brain tissue. Cerebral blood volume (CBV) is the volume of blood/contrast in mL per 100 g of brain tissue. Finally, mean-transit-time (MTT) is the average time required for the blood/contrast to traverse the 100 g of brain tissue. Automated software computes these qualitative and quantitative maps of ischemic lesion tissue [39]. **Table 2** presents a visual comparison of CTP parameters distinguishing core from penumbra.

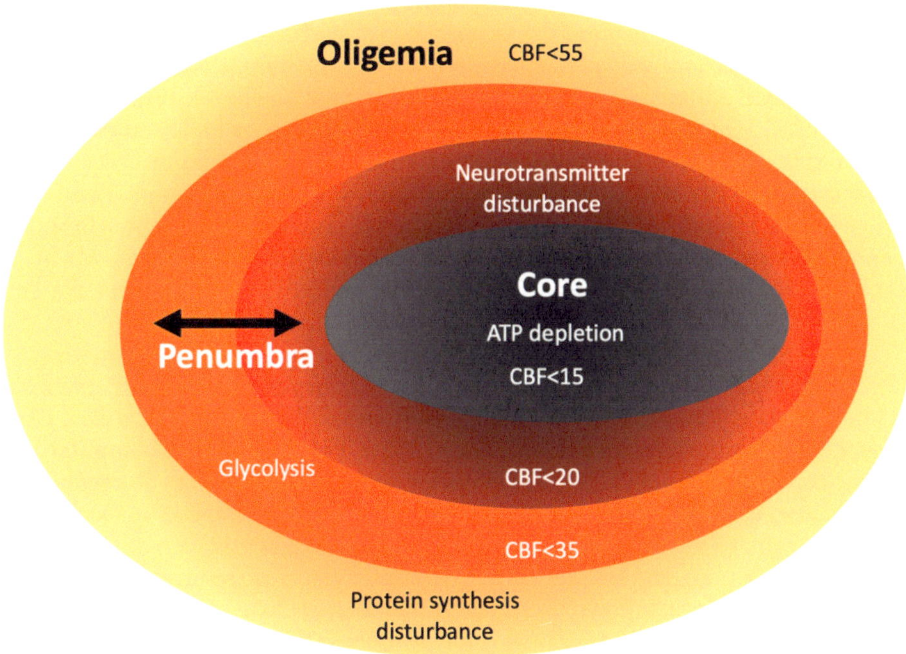

Figure 3.
A rat model of the effect of decreased cerebral blood flow (CBF; measured in mL/100 g/min) on neuronal physiology and brain tissue. Below 15 mL/100 g/min, ATP is depleted, Na/K pumps fail, and cells die, forming the ischemic core. Below 35 mL/100 g/min, there is a change in neuronal metabolism and the neuron is not conducting action potentials. The tissue is non-functional but has not infarcted yet. This is the ischemic penumbra, the region that is still salvageable by intervention and "doomed to die" without it. Below 55 mL/100 g/min, the tissue is "at risk" but will not necessarily die, even without intervention. Adapted from lieu et al. 2020.

Measurement parameter	Core	Penumbra
Mean Transit Time (MTT)	↑	↑
T Max	↑	↑
Cerebral Blood Flow (CBF)	↓	↓
Cerebral Blood Volume (CBV)	↓	↔ ↑

Table 2.
CT perfusion measurements for core and penumbra. In both the core and the penumbra, due to blockage of the artery, there is less flow of blood to the tissue, leading to decreased CBF. The blood is also taking longer to fill and to leave the tissue and therefore, MTT and T max are increased. In the core infarct, cerebral blood volume is decreased as blood is no longer filling the dead tissue.

The penumbra can be determined by subtracting the ischemic core from the tissue at risk There have been multiple methods of estimating the tissue-at-risk or the perfusion deficit as well as estimating the ischemic core. Visually, comparing MTT maps to CBV maps gives a qualitative estimate of the penumbra (**Figure 4**). The most useful quantitative measurements are Tmax>6 s, which best estimates tissue-at-risk and CBF < 30 ml/100 g/min, which best estimates core [40]. One can also calculate the MMR, which is the ratio between the core volume and perfusion deficit volume. These numbers are crucial as they determine eligibility for endovascular thrombectomy. To be eligible for the intervention, the MMR must be greater than 1.8, the penumbra must be greater than 15 mL, and the Tmax >10 seconds [41].

There are caveats pertaining to potential inaccuracy of the above parameters. CTP parameters may be affected by reduced cardiac output, carotid artery stenosis, and injection rate. Technical factors such as motion artifacts, and erroneous CTP protocol, for example wrong contrast injection rate, can also bias the computation of ischemic core and penumbra [39]. A perfusion protocol shorter than 60 seconds, as a further example, is known to overestimate the infarct core volume [30]. Occasionally CTP results can be entirely misleading when a non-stroke hemisphere is labeled as ischemic due to recanalization and luxury hyperperfusion of the stroked hemisphere [42]. Stroke mimics causing vascular dysregulation, such as seizures, hypertensive encephalopathy, hemiplegic migraines, may produce false images of penumbra, and so can vascular anatomical variations [39]. Although CTP has become standard in assessing anterior circulation stroke, there is to date insufficient evidence for its application in posterior circulation strokes. In particular, the CBF cut off of 30%, a defining feature of the ischemic core, can only be applied to anterior circulation strokes. MRI on the other hand is considered the gold standard for assessing posterior circulation infarcts [43].

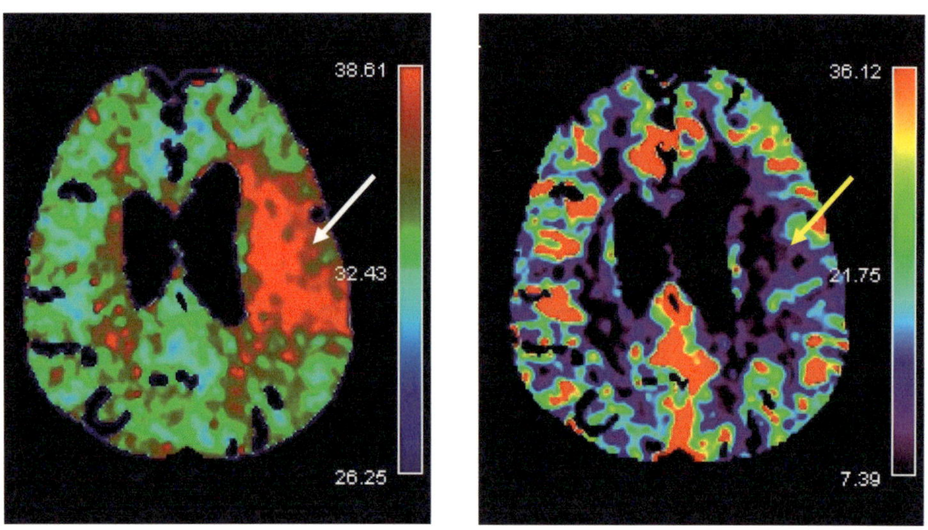

Figure 4.
CT perfusion map of a patient with acute left MCA occlusion with mean transit time map (MTT; left) and cerebral blood volume map (CBV; right) demonstrating acute occlusion of left MCA. In the MTT map, increased time is indicated by a color higher on the spectrum with the longest time being red. It can be seen that the region marked by the white arrow has a prolonged MTT versus the right hemisphere. On the CBV map, the color lower on the spectrum demonstrates lower CBV.

2.4.4.2 Magnetic resonance imaging (MRI) and diffusion weighted imaging (DWI)-fluid attenuated inversion recovery (FLAIR) mismatch

Another method of determining mismatch is by using magnetic resonance imaging (MRI). This is a newer, more sensitive form of imaging compared to CT. Its primary advantages are its high spatial resolution and versatility in use. Its main disadvantages are that the images take longer than CT to acquire and the scanners are not nearly as common or accessible as for CT. Nevertheless, specific MRI sequences can provide crucial information for the diagnosis of AIS. A diffusion-weighted imaging (DWI) measures the diffusion of water molecules across the cellular membrane [44]. In patients with AIS, due to disruption of the electrochemical gradient, this diffusion is disrupted. This shows up at hyperintense or bright on imaging. This bright signal can be detected for at least 2 weeks after the initial event [45]. The apparent diffusion coefficient (ADC) image is the inverse of the DWI and has low intensity during this period. The DWI and ADC image are useful in demonstrating whether there is any ischemia to a region, reversible or irreversible. The T2 fluid attenuated inversion recovery (FLAIR) image is the sequence that is used to see the structure and anatomy of the brain tissue. In the hyperacute phase, the FLAIR has variable intensity and increases in intensity after 6 hours. The FLAIR image demonstrates structural damage and irreversible infarcted tissue [44]. To be a candidate for endovascular thrombectomy, the DWI volume must be greater than 70 mL [40]. In situations of uncertain onset, positive DWI with negative FLAIR, known as a DWI-FLAIR mismatch, strongly suggest that the stroke is hyperacute and there is significant mismatch (**Figure 4**). Using DWI-FLAIR mismatch, once can predict if an AIS is presenting within 4·5 h of LKNT with 62% (95% CI: 57–67) sensitivity, 78% (95% CI: 72–84) specificity, 83% (95% CI: 79–88) positive predictive value, and 54% (95% CI: 48–60) negative predictive value [46]. Therefore, in patients in whom LKNT is unknown, MRI DWI-FLAIR mismatch can be used to identify patients who would still remain candidates for thrombolysis, which will be discussed in detail later [47].

There are a plethora of other MR sequences and techniques that can be used in the diagnosis and management of AIS. Susceptibility weighted imaging (SWI) is a sequence that is sensitive to products that especially distort the magnetic field like iron. Given blood breakdown products contain iron, SWI provides information about the existence of possible hemorrhagic transformation has occurred within the first 12 hours [25, 48]. MR angiography without contrast (time-of-flight) is an alternative to CT angiography [49]. And MR perfusion has obtained 90% concordance between CT-based and MR-based mismatch status [40], and is a highly reliable alternative for patients not amenable to NCCT and CTA.

2.5 Emergent bloodwork

Emergent laboratory investigations should include complete blood count, electrolytes, aPTT, INR, creatinine, and glucose [7]. It is not necessary to wait for all the results before thrombolysis, as blood glucose can be reliably given by a finger stick test, and as mentioned, creatinine values are not needed prior to performing CTA. Other labs such as an INR > 1.7, platelets <100,000/mm^3, and blood glucose <50 mg/dL, are also helpful as they are part of the relative contraindications for tPA, discussed in further detail later. Patients suspected of having ischemic strokes should have a 12-lead EKG and initiate telemetry. This may assess cardiac rhythm and uncover atrial fibrillation [50].

3. Treatment of acute ischemic stroke

3.1 Introduction

As discussed in the previous section, the prompt recognition of AIS using physical exam and its diagnosis using non-contrast CT (NCCT), CT-angiography (CTA), and CT Perfusion (CTP) is the first step in the efficient and effective management. In the last two decades, we have learned much about the treatment of AIS beginning with the concept of the “ischemic penumbra” to the use of thrombolysis in AIS and finally, to the revolutionary procedure of mechanical thrombectomy.

3.2 Principles of treatment

As mentioned previously, there exists an ischemic penumbra in patients with AIS, tissue that is at risk but that has not yet infarcted. The primary goal of AIS management is to use interventions to recanalize the occluded artery and restore perfusion to the penumbra [38]. These interventions and these patients must be selected carefully to maximize benefit and avoid harm. In the following section, these interventions and the selection process will be discussed.

3.3 Thrombolysis

One of the methods of recanalizing the occluded artery is by breaking up the thrombus using intravenous pharmacotherapy. Thrombi that occlude intracerebral arteries are created when the protein *fibrin* creates strands of protein that are long and insoluble [51]. The insoluble protein binds to platelets and the cross-linked fibrin forms a mesh over the platelet-protein complex forming a plug. Thrombolytic/fibrinolytic drugs such as alteplase, or tissue-plasminogen activator (tPA) cleave the inactive protein plasminogen into its active form plasmin. Plasmin degrades the fibrin matrix that was reinforcing the thrombus, thereby allowing clot break down and recanalization. In 1995, the landmark NINDS trial [15] demonstrated that patients with AIS that received tPA within 3 hours of patient LKNT had a significantly higher likelihood of favorable outcome (39%) at 3 month follow-up compared to those who received placebo (26%) as measured by the Modified Rankin Scale (Odds ratio: 1.7). However, there was also a significantly higher risk of symptomatic intracerebral hemorrhage (ICH; **Table 3**) in the tPA group (6.4%) versus the placebo group (0.6%). It was not until 2008 “European Cooperative Acute Stroke Study” (ECASS) III trial [52], that the tPA window was extended to 4.5 hours. A subsequent systematic review of four clinical trials investigating thrombolysis [55] determined that, as the time to symptom onset increases, the benefit from tPA declines and the risk of mortality increases. Beyond the 4.5 hour window, the risk of tPA outweighs the benefits (**Figure 4**). In a metanalysis of 6756 patients from nine studies [56], the authors found that patients who received tPA and a 5.55% increase in absolute risk of parenchymal type II hematoma [54] (Odds ratio: 5.55), 3.1% increase in absolute risk of SITS-MOST ICH (Odds ratio: 6.67), and 2.3% increase in absolute risk of fatal ICH (Odds ratio: 7.14). One of the main caveats of thrombolysis is that the clinician *must know* the patient’s LKNT. There are a significant proportion of patients that in whom the time of symptom onset is unknown. Traditionally, these patients would not be candidates for thrombolysis as the benefit-to-risk ratio would not be known. However, the landmark WAKE-UP trial, investigated the use of thrombolysis in this

Study	Definition of symptomatic ICH
NINDS	Any new ICH on NCCT associated with any neurologic deterioration [15]
ECASS III	If associated with neurological decline of an increase of ≥4 points on the NIHSS [52]
SITS-MOST	Parenchymal hematoma type 2* on imaging 22–36 hours after intervention with neurological deterioration of ≥4 points on NIHSS [53]

**A hematoma which occupies 30% or more of the infarcted tissue and is accompanied with obvious mass effect on adjacent tissue [54].*

Table 3.
Different definitions of symptomatic ICH depending on clinical trial [47]. The NINDS trial used the most liberal definition, explaining the higher estimates of ICH compared to what was reported in subsequent studies.

group of patients [47]. The authors used MRI with diffusion to determine if there was still a significant volume of penumbra and mismatch, and in carefully selected patients, thrombolysis was administered. There was a greater likelihood of favorable outcome in patients administered tPA (53.3%) versus those who received placebo (41.8%) at 3 months (Odds ratio: 1.61). In the DIAS trial, the authors used a highly fibrin-specific thrombolytic agent, desmoteplase, in patients presenting with AIS [57]. The patients presented between 3 and 9 hours from LKNT and were carefully selected by use of MRI to determine who would be a good candidate for thrombolysis. A higher rate of reperfusion and favorable outcome was seen in patients who were given thrombolysis (71.4% and 60.0%) compared with those who received placebo (19.2% and 22.2%). Therefore, if a center does have MRI capabilities, carefully selected patients with AIS with unknown time of symptom onset may be candidates for thrombolysis.

Table 4 shows the indications and contraindications for thrombolysis for patients presenting with AIS [7]. The only *absolute* contraindication to administration of thrombolysis is demonstration of ICH on NCCT. The other criteria listed are relative and are dependent on the clinical situation. For a patient to be a candidate for thrombolysis, the stroke should be classified as clinically disabling, usually referring to a NIHSS>5[2]. The "Phase IIIB, Double-Blind, Multicenter Study to Evaluate the Efficacy and Safety of Alteplase in Patients With Mild Stroke: Rapidly Improving Symptoms and Minor Neurologic Deficits" (PRISMS) trial compared administration of tPA to aspirin in patients with AIS presenting with a NIHSS≤5 and determined that there was no significant difference in favorable outcome at 3 months [58].

Once it is determined that a patient is a candidate for thrombolysis, the dosing should be calculated, and formulation prepared. The dose that is primarily used for AIS is 0.9 mg/kg of patient's ideal body weight, with a maximum dose of 90 mg [7]. Of the total dose, 10% is administered as a bolus over 1 minute and the remainder as an infusion over 60 minutes. The ENCHANTED trial investigated a lower dose of tPA, 0.6 mg/kg in a cohort of Asian patients presenting with AIS and although they demonstrated a lower risk of ICH compared to standard dose (1% vs. 2.1%), the trial was not able to show noninferiority of the lower dose with respect to death or disability at 3 months [59]. While alteplase is standard of care for thrombolysis in AIS, in the last 10 years, there is evidence suggesting that tenecteplase (TNK) the

[2] While NIHSS >5 is usually used as the standard for clinically disabling, there are exceptions to this. For example, a patient presenting with AIHS who demonstrates global aphasia would have a NIHSS of 4. However, this would be significantly disabling for the patient and therefore, he would likely qualify for thrombolysis.

Indications
Clinically disabling AIS (NIHSS>5) with *known* time of onset ≤4.5 hours
BP <185/110 mmHg
Blood glucose >50 mg/dL
Contraindications
Intracerebral Hemorrhage on CT
Anticoagulation (thrombin or factor Xa inhibtors)
History of intracranial hemorrhage
Ischemic stroke within 3 months
Intracerebral neoplasm
Infective endocarditis
Coagulopathy (Platelets 1.7, aPTT >40s, PT > 15 s)

Table 4.
Indications and contraindications for tPA [7]. Importantly, the only absolute contraindication to tPA use is intracerebral hemorrhage on noncontrast CT. The rest are dependent on the clinical scenario.

medication used in thrombolysis for acute myocardial infarctions, is as safe and at least as effective as tPA [60–62]. The primary advantages to TNK would be its longer half-life, eliminating the need for a 60 minute infusion, and its greater specificity for fibrin, which could mean more effective thrombolysis [2]. There are currently large-scale clinical trials underway to determine the non-inferiority of TNK compared to tPA (NOR-TEST) and efficacy and safety of TNK in patients presenting more than 4.5 hours since LKNT (TIMELESS), and in patients with basilar artery occlusions (POST-ETERNAL). In the next 10 years, TNK may indeed be the standard of practice.

There are two primary complications that can occur from thrombolysis administration in the acute phase. The first is angioedema and this might occur minutes to hours after administration of tPA [51]. As mentioned earlier, tPA cleaves plasminogen into its active form plasmin. Plasmin activates complement as well as the kinin pathways which leads to an inflammatory response and an increase in systemic cytokines. Therefore, it should not be surprising that one of the consequences of tPA administration is angioedema, an acute albeit transient swelling of deeper layers of the skin and mucosa. The swelling is red and well-circumscribed and usually involves the orolingual, periorbital, and pharyngeal regions. Angioedema is seen in approximately 5% of patients who receive tPA and is usually mild and patients who are on ACE inhibitors are at higher risk [63]. These patients require careful monitoring as if the swelling becomes severe and involves the airway, the patient may need intubation. Usually the angioedema is mild and self-resolves after the tPA infusion is complete. The signs and symptoms of the reaction can be managed by IV diphenhydramine and/or ranitidine histamine (H1) receptor antagonists [64].

The second major complication of tPA administration, which was alluded to earlier, is ICH. ICH can occur in up to 7% of tPA administrations and can be associated with up to 83% mortality [65]. Patients must be counseled about this increased risk to make an informed decision about receiving tPA and clinicians should be aware of the risk of ICH to recognize and manage it promptly. The factors associated with a higher risk of ICH include larger volume of hypoperfused tissue, larger established infarct, higher NIHSS, and higher glucose and/or blood pressure at the time of tPA administration [64, 66]. Therefore, patients who receive tPA must have their systolic blood pressure kept below 185mmg and be euglycemic. In *all* patients who receive tPA, a NCCT should be repeated 24 hours post-administration. Even if a patient does not have a hemorrhage large enough to cause clinical deficits or change in level of consciousness, the size and location of the ICH will influence future decisions about secondary stroke prevention. The clinician should have a low threshold to order a stat repeat NCCT earlier than 24 hours if there is a clinical deterioration of the patient.

In summary, tPA is an effective tool in the management of AIS in carefully selected patients in whom the benefits of thrombolysis outweigh the risk of hemorrhage. Unfortunately, a significant number of patients present with AIS outside of the 4.5 hour window or meeting another contraindication to tPA. In 2015, a new hope of treatment emerged for these patients.

3.4 Endovascular thrombectomy

While thrombolysis is effective for a select group of patients, it is accompanied by several limitations. First, given that this is a systemic fibrinolytic medication, it is accompanied with the risk of bleeding anywhere in the body, especially in the brain. Second, only select patients qualify for its administration. Third, the rate of recanalization for proximal, large-vessel occlusions (LVOs) is poor, ranging from 13–50% [2, 67]. These are dense clots that are in the major arteries in the brain (the terminus of the internal carotid artery, the early branches of middle cerebral artery (MCA; M1, M2), and the basilar artery), even though these occlusions make up at least one-third of strokes [67] and can cause significant disability.

These three disadvantages are not shared by the endovascular thrombectomy (EVT) procedure. In this procedure, a patient is taken to interventional neuroradiology suite, IV contrast is administered to the patient which sequential x-rays of the head and neck are obtained. An occlusion is localized when it is evident that there an abrupt

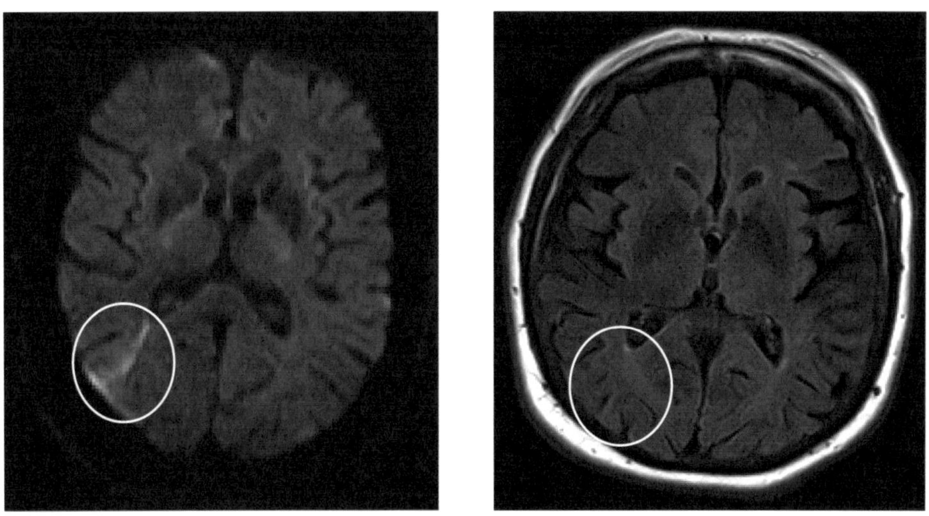

Figure 5.
MRI of patient with acute right middle cerebral artery stroke with DWI on the left and FLAIR on the right. In the DWI image, the white circle marks an area of diffusion restriction indicating acute ischemia. However, there are minimal to no changes in the corresponding FLAIR image. This indicates that a significant core has not yet formed yet and mismatch exists.

halt of contrast filling the artery. A catheter attached to a wire is inserted into the femoral artery and advanced until it reaches the clot, which can then be aspirated or retrieved using a stent (**Figure 5**). The first trials to examine the benefit of EVT were performed in 2013 and did not show the procedure to be clinically efficacious [2]. This changed with the advent of new methods of imaging and better catheters and in 2015, the "Multicenter Randomized Clinical Trial of Endovascular Treatment for Acute Ischemic Stroke in the Netherlands" (MR CLEAN) trial demonstrated that patients that received EVT within 6 hours of symptom onset were more likely to achieve functional independence at 3 months (32.6%) compared to those who received placebo (19.1%) [68]. Other trials confirmed the findings of MR CLEAN and thus emerged new guidelines for the eligibility for EVT: **1) patients ≥ 18** who presented **2) within 6 hours of symptom onset** with a **3) LVO**, a **4) NIHSS ≥ 6** and an **5) ASPECTS score of CT ≥ 6 on NCCT** [7]. With the introduction of CTP, clinicians could identify core and penumbra in patients with AIS and determine which patients could still benefit from intervention. In the subsequent AURORA, DEFUSE 3 and DAWN trials, it was determined that EVT could be safe and effective in patients presenting up to 24 hours post symptom onset [69–71]. However, if a patient presents outside of the initial six-hour window, they must receive a CT perfusion or MRI with DWI to determine the volume of core infarct that exists and if there is still mismatch; otherwise it will be impossible to determine if the patient could benefit from the procedure. As mentioned earlier, there are specific CTP criteria that allow a patient to be eligible for EVT if they present outside of the initial 6 hour window. The MMR must be greater than 1.8, the penumbra must be greater than 15 mL, and the Tmax >10 seconds [41]. The HERMES meta-analysis of five EVT trials found that patients who received standard of care without EVT had a 14% higher absolute risk of not having a favorable outcome compared to those who received EVT. There was no significant difference in symptomatic hemorrhage between groups. Therefore, it is now standard of care to consider each patient who presents within 24 hours with a proximal LVO for EVT [72].

Unfortunately, not all AIS patients are eligible for EVT. The patient must have a proximal LVO to be accessible by the current clot-retrieval tools. As clots become more distal, there is a lower likelihood of successful procedure and higher likelihood of complications. While experienced interventionalists may go after clots in the basilar artery, anterior cerebral arteries, and distal middle cerebral arteries, there is little evidence to suggest the efficacy of these procedures. Second, not all AIS patients have access to EVT. The intervention is only offered at major, tertiary care centers. While thrombolysis can be done even in remote settings with neurologists guiding the treatment via "telestroke", for EVT a patient needs to be transferred, often over hundreds of kilometers, to obtain the procedure and by the time they reach the EVT site, there may be no penumbra left [2].

EVT is also accompanied by its own risks [73]. While ICH is more common with tPA, there is still a risk of hemorrhagic transformation with EVT as causing reperfusion to already infarcted tissue can cause injury, edema, and resulting hemorrhage. As this is an interventional procedure, there is always the risk of infection or clot developing at the site of entry. When the interventionalist is trying to access the occlusion, pieces of the clot can break off and move distally creating occlusions not accessible by the catheter. In rare cases, arteries can be damaged or even ruptured from the catheter itself.

Despite the disadvantages to EVT, it remains at the forefront of AIS therapy. The advent of EVT has revolutionized stroke protocols and care across the world with the acute stroke window being extended from a mere 4.5 to an entire day.

Reperfusion advantages	**Complications with tPA**	**Geographic factors**
Longer clots	Full basal ganglia infarction	Fast local workflow
Tandem Occlusions	Severe hyperglycemia	High costs of tPA
Longer times from LKNT	Higher age of patient	Thrombectomy team available
Proximal Occlusions	Severe microangiopathy	
Reperfusion advantages	**Delays with EVT**	**Geographic factors**
Shorter clots	Unfavorable vascular anatomy	Prolonged local workflow
Good Collaterals	Delays with anesthesia	Low costs of tPA
Earlier presentation		EVT team not readily available
Distal thrombus location		

Adapted from Nogueira et al. [79].

Table 5.
Factors that would favor EVT alone (top) vs. factors that favor tPA and EVT strategy (bottom).

Given the advantages of EVT, the question arises of whether patients with LVO should go straight for EVT or if they would benefit from tPA administration first. There have been multiple trials that have compared the use of EVT alone to EVT combined with thrombolysis and have yielded mixed results. The "Multicenter Randomized Clinical trial of Endovascular treatment for Acute ischemic stroke in the Netherlands-NO IV" (MR-CLEAN-NO IV) [74] and "Randomized study of endovascular therapy with versus without intravenous tissue plasminogen activator in acute stroke with ICA and M1 occlusion" (SKIP) trials [75] did not demonstrate noninferiority of EVT alone compared to EVT and tPA whereas the DIRECT MT [76] and DEVT trials [77] demonstrated that EVT alone was indeed noninferior. The different results of the studies may have been due to different characteristics of the study population or of the study design itself. For example, in the DEVT trial, the population had a higher proportion of patients with intracranial atherosclerosis which can change the benefit obtained with thrombolysis. There is currently not enough evidence to suggest a strategy of EVT alone for patients presenting with AIS who have LVOs. It is necessary to determine if there is a particular subgroup that would benefit from EVT alone [78]. For example, according to DIRECT MT and MR-CLEAN-NOIV, patients with tandem occlusions (simultaneous blockage of both internal carotid artery and middle cerebral artery) may benefit from EVT alone. Patients with large ischemic cores who receive EVT alone may also have decreased likelihood of symptomatic ICH as per all of the trials except MR-CLEAN-NOIV. At the same time, taking the time to select these patient subgroups in a clinical scenario may be detrimental to those who would benefit from both EVT and tPA. **Table 5** illustrates the specific factors that could favor an EVT alone strategy as well as factors that would favor a thrombolysis and EVT strategy [79]. As per current guidelines, patients presenting with LVO not meeting the contraindications to thrombolysis should receive thrombolysis as long as it *does not delay the patient receiving EVT* (**Figures 6** and 7) [7].

3.5 Post-acute care

In the acute window, in patients who receive intervention or have a very large infarct, it is essential to monitor heart rate and blood pressure every 15 minutes for

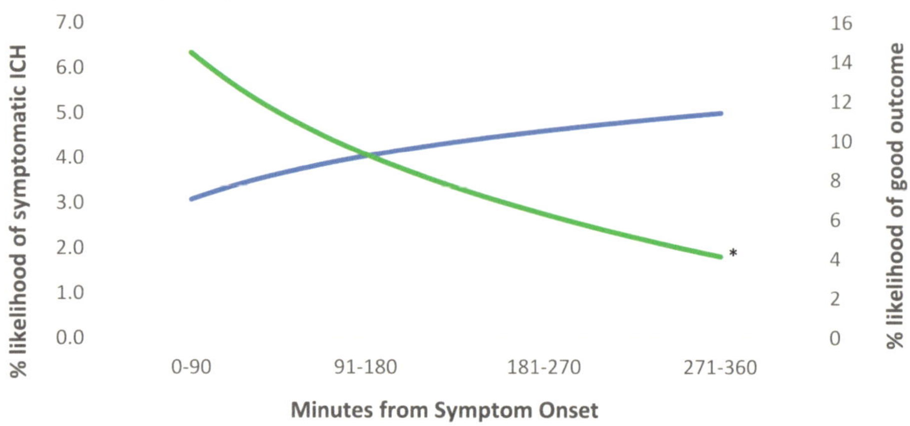

Figure 6.
*Relationship between time of symptom onset to tPA administration to likelihood of symptomatic ICH (blue line; left axis) and likelihood of good outcome (green line; right axis). As is evident, with increasing time, the risk of symptomatic ICH increases and the likelihood of good outcome decreases. Importantly, beyond 270 minutes there is still a higher likelihood of ICH but no significant difference in good outcome. *no significant difference between treatment and placebo. (adapted from Lees et al. [55]).*

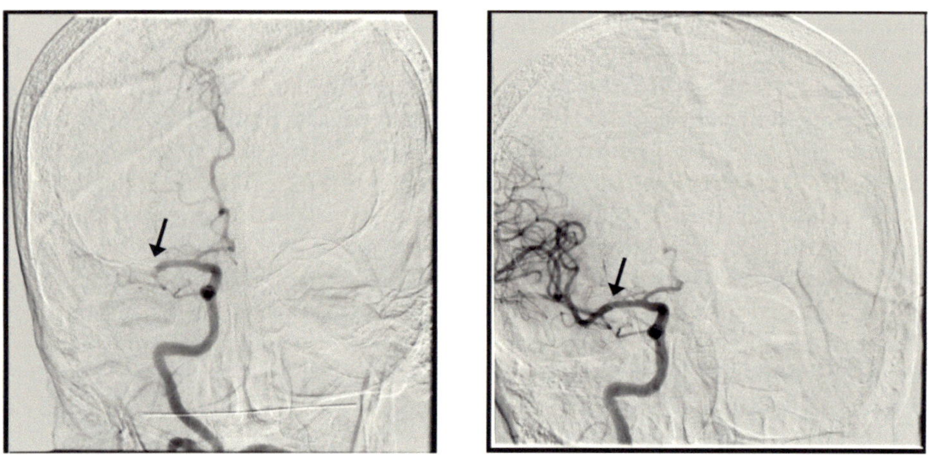

Figure 7.
Radiograph of proximal M1 occlusion pre (left) and post (right) EVT procedure. An 81 year old female presented with acute left sided weakness and complete neglect of the left side of space. Her CT angiogram demonstrated an occlusion on the proximal M1 branch of the MCA and she was sent to the interventional neuroradiology suite. The figure on the left demonstrates no contrast filling the branches of the MCA distal to the clot (arrow). After thrombectomy, the artery is recanalized and there is anterograde flow (right).

2 hours, every 30 minutes for 6 hours, and every 60 minutes until 24 hours after starting treatment [80]. It is also pertinent to monitor the patients "neurovitals" their level of consciousness, strength, and language to ensure their clinical status is not deteriorating. As previously discussed, there should be a low threshold for repeating a NCCT in the acute period. Patients with AIS should also be kept NPO until their swallowing is assessed formally as their decreased level of consciousness and facial weakness can increase the likelihood of aspiration. All stroke patients who receive tPA, EVT, or who present with significant deficits, should be admitted to a dedicated stroke unit where

they can be monitored closely by stroke specialists and an interdisciplinary team of nurses, physiotherapists, speech and language pathologists, and dieticians to ensure favorable functional outcome. Evidence suggests that patients that are cared for at an acute stroke unit have less likelihood of disability and mortality compared to those that are admitted to a general ward [81]. Early rehabilitation is crucial in preventing long-term disability and early management of blood pressure, diabetes, cholesterol, and antiplatelet/anticoagulant therapy is crucial in the secondary prevention of stroke.

4. Conclusion

Gone are the days in which AIS was thought to be a terminal disease. Since The National Institutes of Neurological Disorders and Stroke rt-PA Stroke Study Group (NINDS) trial in 1995 there have been numerous advances which have prevented patients from long-term disability. Both thrombolysis and EVT are potential treatments for carefully selected patients presenting with AIS and each has its benefits as well as disadvantages. However, there still exist a major proportion of the stroke population that does not qualify for either therapy, either because they have presented out of the window or because there is no LVO. There are numerous trials underway and show promise to cover a wider population. For example, the trial TEMPO II is examining the use of thrombolysis in patients presenting with minor stroke, NIHSS<6. The TIMELESS trial is investigating the use of thrombolysis in patients presenting outside of the 4.5 hour window who would still be a candidate for EVT. Finally, better catheters and stent-retrievers are being developed to reach more distal clots without increasing complications. There are also trials underway investigating methods of improving neuroprotection and reducing cell death after AIS. Nerinetide, a drug that showed promise in pre-clinical models of ischemia and reperfusion was recently investigated and humans [82]. The drug did not seem to improve functioning in those patients who had received tPA but did show a mild treatment effect in those who did not, opening doors for future possibilities for the use of neuroprotection. While stroke creates a tremendous healthcare burden across the world, the plethora of trials currently underway provide hope that this burden will continue to decrease over the next decade.

Author details

Anwer Zohaib Siddiqi*, Angela Young and Ankur Wadhwa
University of Manitoba Max Rady College of Medicine, Winnipeg, Canada

*Address all correspondence to: siddiqia@myumanitoba.ca

References

[1] Roth GA et al. Global burden of cardiovascular diseases and risk factors, 1990-2019: Update from the GBD 2019 study. Journal of the American College of Cardiology. 2020;**76**(25):2982-3021

[2] Campbell BCV, Khatri P. Stroke. Lancet. 2020;**396**(10244):129-142

[3] Wardlaw JM. What causes lacunar stroke? Journal of Neurology, Neurosurgery & Psychiatry. 2005;**76**(5):617

[4] Saini V, Guada L, Yavagal DR. Global epidemiology of stroke and access to acute ischemic stroke interventions. Neurology. 2021;**97**(20 Supplement 2):S6-S16

[5] Moulin S, Leys D. Stroke mimics and chameleons. Current Opinion in Neurology. 2019;**32**(1):54-59

[6] Caplan LR. Caplan's Stroke. Cambridge: Cambridge University Press; 2016

[7] Powers WJ et al. Guidelines for the early Management of Patients with Acute Ischemic Stroke: 2019 update to the 2018 guidelines for the early Management of Acute Ischemic Stroke: A guideline for healthcare professionals from the American Heart Association/ American Stroke Association. Stroke. 2019;**50**(12):e344-e418

[8] Adams HP Jr et al. Classification of subtype of acute ischemic stroke. Definitions for use in a multicenter clinical trial. TOAST. Trial of org 10172 in acute stroke treatment. Stroke. 1993;**24**(1):35-41

[9] Chen PH et al. Classifying ischemic stroke, from TOAST to CISS. CNS Neuroscience & Therapeutics. 2012;**18**(6):452-456

[10] Mastriana J et al. Todd Paresis, in StatPearls. Treasure Island (FL): StatPearls Publishing LLC.; 2022, StatPearls Publishing Copyright © 2022

[11] Mokin M et al, editors. Acute Stroke Management in the First 24 Hours: A Practical Guide for Clinicians. Online ed. New York: Oxford Academic; June 1, 2018. DOI: 10.1093/med/9780190856519.001.0001 [Accessed: August 3, 2022]

[12] Davis SM, Donnan GA. 4.5 hours: The new time window for tissue plasminogen activator in stroke. Stroke. 2009;**40**(6):2266-2267

[13] Mackey J et al. Population-based study of wake-up strokes. Neurology. 2011;**76**(19):1662-1667

[14] Arboix A. Cardiovascular risk factors for acute stroke: Risk profiles in the different subtypes of ischemic stroke. World Journal of Clinical Cases. 2015;**3**(5):418-429

[15] The National Institute of Neurological Disorders and Stroke rt-PA Stroke Study Group. Tissue plasminogen activator for acute ischemic stroke. The New England Journal of Medicine. 1995;**333**(24):1581-1587

[16] Brott T et al. Measurements of acute cerebral infarction: A clinical examination scale. Stroke. 1989;**20**(7):864-870

[17] Rost NS et al. Stroke severity is a crucial predictor of outcome: An international prospective validation study. Journal of the American Heart Association. 2016;**5**(1):1-7

[18] Wilson JT et al. Improving the assessment of outcomes in stroke: Use of a structured interview to assign grades on the modified Rankin scale. Stroke. 2002;**33**(9):2243-2246

[19] Sablot D et al. Predicting acute ischaemic stroke outcome using clinical and temporal thresholds. ISRN Neurology. 2011;**2011**:354642

[20] Fischer U et al. NIHSS score and arteriographic findings in acute ischemic stroke. Stroke. 2005;**36**(10):2121-2125

[21] Meyer BC, Lyden PD. The modified National Institutes of Health stroke scale: Its time has come. International Journal of Stroke. 2009;**4**(4):267-273

[22] Southerland AM. Clinical evaluation of the patient with acute stroke. Continuum (Minneap Minn). 2017;**23** (1, Cerebrovascular Disease):40-61

[23] Perry JJ et al. Sensitivity of computed tomography performed within six hours of onset of headache for diagnosis of subarachnoid haemorrhage: Prospective cohort study. BMJ. 2011;**343**:d4277

[24] Menon BK. Neuroimaging in acute stroke. Continuum (Minneap Minn). 2020;**26**(2):287-309

[25] Sohn C-H. Radiological assessment of ischemic stroke. In: Park J, editor. Acute Ischemic Stroke: Medical, Endovascular, and Surgical Techniques. Singapore: Springer Singapore; 2017. pp. 35-58

[26] Jensen-Kondering U, Riedel C, Jansen O. Hyperdense artery sign on computed tomography in acute ischemic stroke. World Journal of Radiology. 2010;**2**(9):354-357

[27] Barber PA et al. Validity and reliability of a quantitative computed tomography score in predicting outcome of hyperacute stroke before thrombolytic therapy. ASPECTS study group. Alberta stroke programme early CT score. Lancet. 2000;**355**(9216):1670-1674

[28] Schröder J, Thomalla G. A critical review of Alberta stroke program early CT score for evaluation of acute stroke imaging. Frontiers in Neurology. 2016;**7**:245

[29] Rabinstein AA. Treatment of acute ischemic stroke. Continuum (Minneap Minn). 2017;**23**(1, Cerebrovascular Disease):62-81

[30] Potter CA et al. CT for treatment selection in acute ischemic stroke: A code stroke primer. Radiographics. 2019;**39**(6):1717-1738

[31] Ehrlich ME et al. Safety of computed tomographic angiography in the evaluation of patients with acute stroke: A single-Center experience. Stroke. 2016;**47**(8):2045-2050

[32] Mayer SA et al. CTA-for-all: Impact of emergency computed tomographic angiography for all patients with stroke presenting within 24 hours of onset. Stroke. 2020;**51**(1):331-334

[33] Menon BK et al. Multiphase CT angiography: A new tool for the imaging triage of patients with acute ischemic stroke. Radiology. 2015;**275**(2):510-520

[34] Dundamadappa S et al. Multiphase CT angiography: A useful technique in acute stroke imaging—Collaterals and beyond. American Journal of Neuroradiology. 2020;**42**(2):221-227

[35] Maas MB et al. Collateral vessels on CT angiography predict outcome in acute ischemic stroke. Stroke. 2009;**40**(9):3001-3005

[36] Yu AY et al. Multiphase CT angiography increases detection of anterior circulation intracranial occlusion. Neurology. 2016;**87**(6):609-616

[37] Liu S, Levine SR, Winn HR. Targeting ischemic penumbra: Part I - from pathophysiology to therapeutic strategy. Journal of Experimental Stroke & Translational Medicine. 2010;**3**(1):47-55

[38] Ramos-Cabrer P et al. Targeting the ischemic penumbra. Stroke. 2011;**42** (1 Suppl):S7-S11

[39] Vagal A et al. Automated CT perfusion imaging for acute ischemic stroke: Pearls and pitfalls for real-world use. Neurology. 2019;**93**(20):888-898

[40] Demeestere J et al. Review of perfusion imaging in acute ischemic stroke: From time to tissue. Stroke. 2020;**51**(3):1017-1024

[41] Lansberg MG et al. MRI profile and response to endovascular reperfusion after stroke (DEFUSE 2): A prospective cohort study. Lancet Neurology. 2012;**11**(10):860-867

[42] Sotoudeh H et al. Luxury perfusion: A paradoxical finding and pitfall of CT perfusion in subacute infarction of brain. Radiology Case Reports. 2019;**14**(1):6-9

[43] Lin SF et al. Predicting functional outcomes of posterior circulation acute ischemic stroke in first 36 h of stroke onset. Journal of Neurology. 2018;**265**(4):926-932

[44] Srinivasan A et al. State-of-the-art imaging of acute stroke. Radiographics. 2006;**26**(Suppl. 1):S75-S95

[45] Lansberg MG et al. Evolution of apparent diffusion coefficient, diffusion-weighted, and T2-weighted signal intensity of acute stroke. AJNR. American Journal of Neuroradiology. 2001;**22**(4):637-644

[46] Thomalla G et al. DWI-FLAIR mismatch for the identification of patients with acute ischaemic stroke within 4·5 h of symptom onset (PRE-FLAIR): A multicentre observational study. Lancet Neurology. 2011;**10**(11):978-986

[47] Thomalla G et al. MRI-guided thrombolysis for stroke with unknown time of onset. The New England Journal of Medicine. 2018;**379**(7):611-622

[48] Allen LM et al. Sequence-specific MR imaging findings that are useful in dating ischemic stroke. Radiographics. 2012;**32**(5):1285-1297 discussion 1297-9

[49] Nael K et al. Imaging-based selection for endovascular treatment in stroke. Radiographics. 2019;**39**(6):1696-1713

[50] Boulanger JM et al. Canadian stroke best practice recommendations for acute stroke management: Prehospital, emergency department, and acute inpatient stroke care, 6th edition, update 2018. International Journal of Stroke. 2018;**13**(9):949-984

[51] Alakbarzade V, O'Kane D, Pereira AC. Hypersensitivity reactions to recombinant tissue plasminogen activator. Practical Neurology. 2020;**20**(1):75-79

[52] Hacke W et al. Thrombolysis with alteplase 3 to 4.5 hours after acute ischemic stroke. The New England Journal of Medicine. 2008;**359**(13):1317-1329

[53] Wahlgren N et al. Thrombolysis with alteplase for acute ischaemic stroke in the safe implementation of thrombolysis in stroke-monitoring study (SITS-MOST): An observational study. Lancet. 2007;**369**(9558):275-282

[54] von Kummer R et al. The Heidelberg bleeding classification: Classification of bleeding events after ischemic stroke and reperfusion therapy. Stroke. 2015;**46**(10):2981-2986

[55] Lees KR et al. Time to treatment with intravenous alteplase and outcome in stroke: An updated pooled analysis of ECASS, ATLANTIS, NINDS, and EPITHET trials. Lancet. 2010;**375**(9727):1695-1703

[56] Whiteley WN et al. Risk of intracerebral haemorrhage with alteplase after acute ischaemic stroke: A secondary analysis of an individual patient data meta-analysis. Lancet Neurology. 2016;**15**(9):925-933

[57] Hacke W et al. The Desmoteplase in acute ischemic stroke trial (DIAS): A phase II MRI-based 9-hour window acute stroke thrombolysis trial with intravenous desmoteplase. Stroke. 2005;**36**(1):66-73

[58] Khatri P et al. Effect of Alteplase vs aspirin on functional outcome for patients with acute ischemic stroke and minor nondisabling neurologic deficits: The PRISMS randomized clinical trial. JAMA. 2018;**320**(2):156-166

[59] Anderson CS et al. Low-dose versus standard-dose intravenous Alteplase in acute ischemic stroke. The New England Journal of Medicine. 2016;**374**(24):2313-2323

[60] Zhong CS et al. Routine use of Tenecteplase for thrombolysis in acute ischemic stroke. Stroke. 2021;**52**(3):1087-1090

[61] Campbell BCV et al. Tenecteplase versus Alteplase before Thrombectomy for ischemic stroke. The New England Journal of Medicine. 2018;**378**(17):1573-1582

[62] Logallo N et al. Tenecteplase versus alteplase for management of acute ischaemic stroke (NOR-TEST): A phase 3, randomised, open-label, blinded endpoint trial. Lancet Neurology. 2017;**16**(10):781-788

[63] Hill MD et al. Hemi-orolingual angioedema and ACE inhibition after alteplase treatment of stroke. Neurology. 2003;**60**(9):1525-1527

[64] O'Carroll CB, Aguilar MI. Management of Postthrombolysis Hemorrhagic and Orolingual Angioedema Complications. Neurohospitalist. 2015;**5**(3):133-141

[65] Flick MJ. Mechanism of ICH with tPA thrombolysis. Blood. 2021;**138**(1):8-9

[66] Lansberg MG et al. Risk factors of symptomatic intracerebral hemorrhage after tPA therapy for acute stroke. Stroke. 2007;**38**(8):2275-2278

[67] Sweid A et al. Acute ischaemic stroke interventions: Large vessel occlusion and beyond. Stroke and Vascular Neurology. 2019;**5**(1):80-85

[68] Berkhemer OA et al. A randomized trial of intraarterial treatment for acute ischemic stroke. The New England Journal of Medicine. 2015;**372**(1):11-20

[69] Jovin TG et al. Thrombectomy for anterior circulation stroke beyond 6 h from time last known well (AURORA): A systematic review and individual patient data meta-analysis. Lancet. 2022;**399**(10321):249-258

[70] Nogueira RG et al. Thrombectomy 6 to 24 hours after stroke with a mismatch between deficit and infarct. The New England Journal of Medicine. 2018;**378**(1):11-21

[71] Albers GW et al. Thrombectomy for stroke at 6 to 16 hours with selection by perfusion imaging. The New England Journal of Medicine. 2018;**378**(8):708-718

[72] Goyal M et al. Endovascular thrombectomy after large-vessel ischaemic stroke: A meta-analysis

of individual patient data from five randomised trials. Lancet. 2016;**387**(10029):1723-1731

[73] Krishnan R, Mays W, Elijovich L. Complications of mechanical Thrombectomy in acute ischemic stroke. Neurology. 2021;**97**(20 Suppl. 2): S115-s125

[74] LeCouffe NE et al. A randomized trial of intravenous Alteplase before endovascular treatment for stroke. The New England Journal of Medicine. 2021;**385**(20):1833-1844

[75] Suzuki K et al. Effect of mechanical Thrombectomy without vs with intravenous thrombolysis on functional outcome among patients with acute ischemic stroke: The SKIP randomized clinical trial. JAMA. 2021;**325**(3):244-253

[76] Yang P et al. Endovascular Thrombectomy with or without intravenous Alteplase in acute stroke. The New England Journal of Medicine. 2020;**382**(21):1981-1993

[77] Zi W et al. Effect of endovascular treatment alone vs intravenous Alteplase plus endovascular treatment on functional Independence in patients with acute ischemic stroke: The DEVT randomized clinical trial. JAMA. 2021;**325**(3):234-243

[78] Campbell BCV, Kappelhof M, Fischer U. Role of intravenous Thrombolytics prior to endovascular Thrombectomy. Stroke. 2022;**53**:2085-2092. DOI: 10.1161/STROKEAHA.122.036929

[79] Nogueira RG, Tsivgoulis G. Large vessel occlusion strokes after the DIRECT-MT and SKIP trials: Is the Alteplase syringe half empty or half full? Stroke. 2020;**51**(10):3182-3186

[80] Aiyagari V et al. Hourly blood pressure monitoring after intravenous tissue plasminogen activator for ischemic stroke. Stroke. 2004;**35**(10):2326-2330

[81] Indredavik B et al. Benefit of a stroke unit: A randomized controlled trial. Stroke. 1991;**22**(8):1026-1031

[82] Hill MD et al. Efficacy and safety of nerinetide for the treatment of acute ischaemic stroke (ESCAPE-NA1): A multicentre, double-blind, randomised controlled trial. Lancet. 2020;**395**(10227):878-887

Chapter 25

Cost-Effective Interventions to Curb Cardiovascular Diseases in Africa

Mabitsela Hezekiel 'Pitso' Mphasha

Abstract

Cardiovascular diseases (CVDs) are the leading cause of death globally and in Africa, and the cost of care is expensive. Finances of the state may need to be re-channeled to CVDs leading to delay in the development of the country and that of the family since the cost of care also burdens the family. Cost-effective interventions to curb the prevalence and incidences of CVDs are required. A comprehensive literature search was conducted. The risk factors include unhealthy diet, physical inactivity, tobacco use, and harmful use of alcohol. On that background, the CVD can be prevented through behavioral interventions aimed at addressing these risk factors. Moreover, behavioral interventions could be helpful in minimizing costs of care and curb prevalence of cardiovascular diseases. Behavioral interventions have been found to be cost-effective and assist in the management of cardiovascular diseases. Therefore, healthcare providers must at each consultation sessions with patients emphasize more on behavioural change. They must help patients visualize the do's and dont's for the successful attainment of their health goals. In doing so, healthcare providers must collaborate among themselves and also collaborate with communities and families of patients. At the same time, it is significant to alter false perceptions and attitudes toward cardiovascular diseases to help individuals develop positive attitudes.

Keywords: cardiovascular diseases, cost-effectiveness, behavioral changes, factors, healthcare providers

1. Introduction

Cardiovascular diseases (CVDs) are regarded as a broader concept describing diseases of the heart or blood vessels, including coronary heart disease, cerebrovascular disease, rheumatic heart disease, and other conditions [1]. The development of CVD is linked with build-up of fatty deposits in the arteries resulting in a condition called atherosclerosis, increased risk of blood clots, and damage to arteries in organs such as the brain, heart, kidneys, and eyes [2]. Detection of cardiovascular diseases at an early age permits possible management before the development of adverse effects, which may be costly to manage. The risk for the development of CVD includes behaviors such as unhealthy diet, physical inactivity, tobacco use, and harmful use of alcohol [3]. The effects of these behaviors may present in the form of increased blood pressure, glucose, and lipids, including overweight and obesity. On that background, the CVD can be prevented through behavioral interventions aimed at addressing these risk factors [3]. Moreover, behavioral interventions could be helpful in minimizing costs of care and also curb prevalence of cardiovascular diseases.

The care of cardiovascular disease is expensive and requires more state resources leading to delay in the development of the country due to increased healthcare expenditure and diminished productivity from disability, premature death, and absenteeism [4]. It has been reported that patients diagnosed with cardiovascular diseases incur more than double the medical costs as compared to a patient without CVD of the same age and sex [5]. Patients living with cardiovascular diseases and requiring medical treatment are unable to receive such due to financial constraints. These financial implications manifest themselves in the form of physical barriers (transportation to the healthcare facility), and system barriers (lack of medication at the healthcare facilities) [6]. It has been discovered that patients experience financial barriers related to payment of medical costs and visit to health care which may require transportation costs [7]. In addition, in the event of long queues at the healthcare facilities, patients may need lunch money. Furthermore, it has been found that there are also indirect financial barriers, which may occur when a certain patient who has a child may need to pay for someone to look after the child while visiting the healthcare facilities [6]. Various studies have indicated that patients experiencing financial barriers are likely not to adhere to medical therapies or health behavior change due to direct or indirect financial costs [8, 9]. On that basis, patients' outcomes are impacted by financial barriers and cost-related non-adherence, leading to deterioration in the quality of life, poor health status, and general well-being, and may also increase the rates of hospitalization [6]. Moreover, CVDs do not only impact the health, quality of life, and general well-being of patients, but also burden the individual and his/her family financially [4]. These may also lead to the underdevelopment of the family and consequently lead to financial burden and re-channeling of state resources. This may result in financial toxicity. Financial toxicity can be described as healthcare-related at the patient level and state expenditure related to provision of medical care and improving quality of life of patients. State experiences more financial costs due to rising medication costs [10]. The primary healthcare facilities which provide care to outpatients must emphasize more on these behavioral interventions as cost-effective strategy to curb cardiovascular diseases.

2. Cardiovascular diseases as public health concern

World Health Organization (WHO) reported that CVDs are the leading cause of death globally. In 2019 alone, approximately 17.9 million deaths associated with CVDs were reported, which constitute 32% of all global deaths. Around 85% or four in five CVDs deaths are due to heart attack and stroke [1]. However, in high-income countries, 80% of cardiovascular deaths are due to myocardial infarctions and strokes [11]. One-third of these deaths occur prematurely in patients diagnosed with CVDs and are under the age of 70 years. Many cases of cardiovascular diseases (about 80%) are mainly reported in low- and middle-income countries with higher mortality [1]. The burden and prevalence of CVDs are expected to increase considering the lifestyle and urbanization.

One million deaths due to CVDs were sub-Saharan Africa alone, resulting in 5.5% of all global and 11.3% of all CVDs deaths in the world and Africa, respectively [12]. Cardiovascular diseases are the leading cause of death among non-communicable diseases, with about 38% of all non-communicable disease-related deaths in Africa due to CVDs. These are approximately twofold increase of CVD deaths since 1990, with over 10% difference in mortality among women compared with men [13]. Moreover, in South Africa, 215 persons die daily due to heart diseases or strokes, while every hour 5 and 10 persons die due to heart attacks and stroke, respectively [14].

3. Urbanization

Urbanization involves the mass migration of persons from rural to urban area and/or urbanization. Historically, urbanization was associated with human development and progress; however, recently it is associated with significant inequalities and health problems [15]. Some of the major health problems resulting from urbanization include poor nutrition, pollution-related health conditions and communicable diseases, poor sanitation and housing conditions, and related health conditions. All these challenges have an impact on quality of life, health status, and overall well-being resulting in the necessity for more cost of care burdening the public purse [15, 16]. Conversely, rural areas have been progressively urbanized and realizing similar health challenges. In Africa, the rural people have due to urbanization abandoned the traditional way of living including healthy eating and physical activity [17]. Reports show that incidences of cardiovascular diseases began to increase with increasing urbanization in Africa [17]. As such, there is a need to encourage communities to embrace urbanization, emulate good things it brings, and at the same time restore the way of life which was more beneficial to their health.

Obesity is most prevalent in urban areas and has become public health problem, particularly because obesity is associated with CVDs [18]. However, obesity is also increasing in rural areas due to urbanization, hence the increase of prevalence of CVDs and its death rates. Obesity threat is increasing because of unhealthy behaviors such as increased physical inactivity, and consumption of fatty food, and sugar intake [15].

4. Primary healthcare facilities

The Primary Health Care (PHC) facilities as the first health service visited by patients/public with a health concern and serves mainly outpatients [19]. The PHC intends to promote attainment by all people of a level of health that will permit them to live socially and economically productive lives. Accordingly, PHC is essential, scientifically sound, ethical, accessible, equitable, affordable, and accountable to the community [20]. Therefore, it is important that a clear collaboration with communities and family of patients is established for improved health outcomes and curbing of cardiovascular diseases. Healthcare providers at primary healthcare facilities are therefore expected to provide cardiovascular diseases awareness, treatment, and preventative care [20]. Preventative healthcare is cost-effective; therefore, it is necessary for PHC providers to be well-equipped through in-service training with preventative healthcare to minimize the cost of care and improve health outcomes of patients [21]. Moreover, healthcare providers must at each consultation sessions with patients emphasize more on behavioural change in relation to physical activity, healthy eating, and alcohol and tobacco use [22]. These interventions have been found to be cost-effective and assist in the management of cardiovascular diseases.

5. Collaborations with family and communities

Collaboration is about working together to achieve a particular purpose; in this context working together to achieve improved health outcomes using cost-effective interventions. The components of collaborations include openness, focus, accountability, and knowledge sharing [23]. Collaboration in health care is defined as professionals assuming complementary roles and cooperatively working together, sharing responsibility for problem-solving and making decisions to formulate and carry out plans for patient care [23]. Collaboration is about teamwork, which when applied in health care implies interdisciplinary approach. Unlike a multidisciplinary approach, in which each team member is responsible only for the improved healthcare collaboration has been cited as a key strategy for healthcare reform [24]. So far, collaboration in health care improved patient outcomes such as reducing preventable adverse drug reactions, decreasing morbidity and mortality rates, and optimizing medication dosages [23]. In addition, teamwork is beneficial to healthcare providers by reducing extra work and increasing job satisfaction [23]. Most of the care of outpatients takes place where they reside; therefore, there is a need for health care to collaborate with family members and communities for improved outcomes using cost-effective strategies.

Figure 1 shows the collaboration of communities and families of patients in providing an appropriate care.

5.1 Collaboration with families

Family is regarded as the most important source of social support and is tightly related with self-care activities and improved health outcomes [25]. Since most of the patients with heart failure live with other family members at home, participation and support of family members can play a key role in self-care behaviors and efficiency of disease control, as shown in **Figure 1**. Therefore, family can influence a patient's

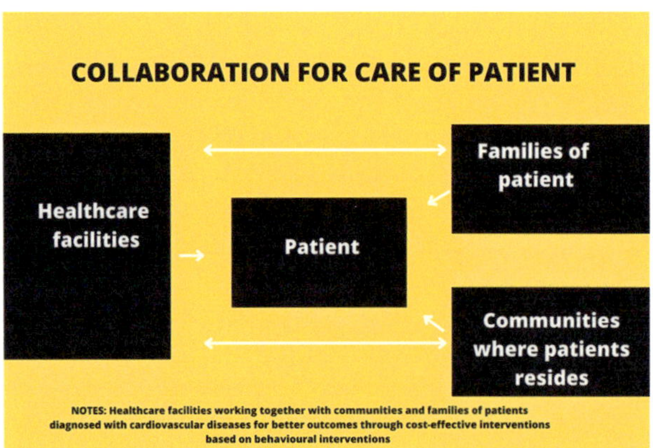

Figure 1.
Collaborating in the care of patient.

success and stability of their behavior change in self-care programs. Several studies revealed the association between family support and heart failure patients' self-care [26, 27]. Earlier studies showed that patients with more support had better compliance of self-care health behaviors. Adherence to self-care behaviors such as restricting fluid intake, regular medication, and exercise are associated with patients with social or family support [28]. It has been found that the level of family support was directly associated with adherence to dietary modification and other dimensions of self-care in heart failure patients [29].

Family members, who provide support at home, were found to have inadequate knowledge regarding management of disease, its signs and treatment [29]. In addition, they were found not to have knowledge on how best to support and encourage patients to follow self-care behaviors [29]. Therefore, the support from families with inadequate knowledge may be harmful and lead to poor health outcomes [30]. Hence, collaboration of primary healthcare providers with family in the care of patients is significant [31] and can close identified knowledge gap. In addition, the primary healthcare providers could play a significant role in support, education, counseling, and taking care of patients diagnosed with cardiovascular diseases and their caregivers or family members [32]. The collaboration can help in familiarizing family members of patients' necessary behavioral changes to equip them to act as a knowledgeable and capable source of family-focused nursing at home where most care happen [32]. It has been reported that effective behavioral changes require baseline line analysis to gain insight into family dynamics and mutual interdependence of the family system [33]. Interventions which target family members, caregivers, and children, encourage communication among family unit, and address the structural and environmental conditions in which families live and operate, are likely to be the most effective approach to promote cardiovascular health [33]. Therefore, there is a need for the adoption of the family-centered care approach.

Family-centered care (FCC) is considered as an approach of responding to the needs, values, and cultural needs of the patient and their families [32] and begins from consultation at the healthcare facility involving healthcare professionals, patients, and family members, being involved in decision-making and shared leadership [31]. Family members are often asked to share responsibility in support of the person living with diabetes; this responsibility includes driving patients to appointments, and social and emotional support, among others. The FCC has so far produced better outcomes in younger children who are usually cared for by their parents or families, since younger children are unable to perform certain tasks related to self-care [34]. The aim of the FCC is to maintain and strengthen family bond and roles so as to provide healthy family functioning, and at the same time improving the quality of life (QoL) of patients, as well as minimizing new cases involving family members who are already at risk due to family history [35].

5.2 Collaboration with communities

Collaboration with communities was found to be essential and cornerstones of efforts to improve public health [36]. A community can be regarded as the social and political networks that link individuals, community organizations, and leaders [37]. Therefore, it is critical to understand these networks in planning engagements with communities. The purpose of community engagement is to build trust, enlist new resources and allies, create better communication, and improve overall health outcomes [37, 38]. The importance of collaboration with communities derives from acknowledgment that lifestyle, behaviors, and the incidence of illness are all shaped by social and physical environments [38]. Community engagement and mobilization have been critical in addressing smoking cessation, obesity, cancer, heart disease, and other health concerns [37, 38]. Community awareness campaigns or intervention which involves communities during planning were essential in identification of most pertinent health issues as well as to design the most effective and appropriate strategies to solve them [39]. **Figure 1** indicates that working together with all stakeholders within communities is required to effectively change environmental and organizational conditions that promote rather that inhibit healthy lifestyles [36].

A community collaboration that considers the behavioral risks of associated with increased chances of development of CVD has the potential to improve access to health checks [37]. These could be an effective strategy for improved implementation and uptake of health checks leading to early detection and management of CVDs. Community engagement is defined as the process of working collaboratively with and through groups of people affiliated by geographic proximity, special interest, or similar situations, to address issues affecting the well-being of those people [37]. A review on community engagement interventions was conducted and the findings showed that it is effective in improving health behaviors, health consequences, and psychological outcomes [40].

It has been found that a healthy community has well-connected, interdependent sectors that share responsibility for recognizing and resolving problems, including enhancing its well-being [40]. Effective and successful community interventions are based on integration, collaboration, and coordination of resources from all parts [40]. Health can be impacted by social factors; therefore, it is significant to engage stakeholders within the communities who can bring their own perspectives and understandings of community life and health issues to help in developing an intervention [38].

6. Behavioral change

Behavioral change is the process of altering habits and behaviors for particular purpose [41]. Behaviors can be highly ingrained and turn into habits which are done without thinking. It has been found that little changes in behavior can lead to significant health improvement and life expectancy of patients by decreasing the negative impact of unhealthy behaviors [42]. Behavior change is influenced by number of factors including knowledge and attitudes which are important determinants of behavior change [43]. It has been found that education programs that contain behavior change approaches are extra effective in changing behavior [44]. Behavior change is a complex process which requires theoretical foundation during planning any behavioral intervention program [45]. Theory enables greater understanding of the relationships among factors that influence behavior change [46].

They must work jointly with patients in designing health goals, eliminating barriers to adopting a healthy lifestyle, and tracking their own behavior can be beneficial [46]. Healthcare providers regularly see patients who engage in unhealthy lifestyle behaviors; therefore, healthcare providers particularly at the primary healthcare facilities must be equipped with skills to encourage patients change their behaviors [45].

6.1 Goal setting for health

Goal setting is regarded as an essential intervention for patients intending to change behaviors [44]. Healthcare providers particularly at primary healthcare facilities should help patients visualize the does and do not for the successful attainment of their health goals [44]. In doing so, they must work together with patients in designing health goals and eliminating barriers to adopting a healthy lifestyle. Identification of barriers will enable development of possible solutions and ultimately in achieving improved clinical outcomes. The healthcare providers can use "SMART' acronym goal setting strategy to encourage patients to realize their goal setting; the acronym stands for [44]:

Specific: Encourage patients to get as specific as possible about their goals. For instance, if patients want to lose weight, he/she must indicate how much weight he/she wants to lose.

Measurable: Ensure that the goal set is measurable. For example, exercise for 30 minutes, 3 days a week.

Attainable: Make sure patients' goals are feasible; for example, the patients wanting to exercise daily but working far from home can be encouraged to wake up early for exercise or late after coming from work.

Relevant: Ensure that the goal is relevant to the patient. Why does the person want to make this change? How will this change improve his or her life?

Timely: Help patients define a specific timeline for the goal. When do they want to reach their goal? When will you follow-up with them? For instance, helping patients set a goal to lose 10 kilograms (kg) in the next month may feel less overwhelming than a goal of losing 5 kg in the next year.

7. Attitude of patients

Attitudes of patients are significant to behavioral change and assumes an enormous importance with positivity in attitude becoming an absolute necessity [31]. Attitude is regarded as positive/negative behaviors an individual acquires through experience. It is significant to alter false perceptions and attitudes toward cardiovascular diseases to help individuals develop positive attitudes [47]. It has been found that individuals' perception and attitudes toward the disease influence how they deal with it [47]. According to Muchiri, Gericke, and Rheeder [48], attitudes are considered as the most important determinants of behavior change among patients. It is therefore important that patients must have positive attitudes toward cardiovascular diseases, particularly behavioral change interventions.

8. Self-monitoring of behavior change program

Self-monitoring refers to regular keeping or tracking of components of behavior; for example, patients who intend to lose weight could keep track of daily minutes of exercise undertaken [49]. It is important to encourage patients to keep diaries of their behaviors so that they could relay progress in the subsequent or follow-up consultation [44]. It may be difficult for patients to remember their activities or behavior during follow-up visit if they are not recorded leading to inaccurate and invaluable. The moment patients agree to be on behavioral intervention and monitor their behavior, it becomes essential for healthcare providers to emphasize on the specifics of the plan. For example, the patient wants to monitor the physical activity behavioral intervention and discuss when during the day he/she can exercise. How will the patient remember to observe and record the behavior? Recording the behavior soon after its occurrence led to accurate data [44]. Although patients may be tempted to omit unhealthy behaviors or exaggerate healthy ones, healthcare providers should encourage patients to be completely honest to maximize the usefulness of their self-monitoring program. For self-monitoring to be most effective, healthcare providers should ask patients to bring their self-monitoring book to follow-up visits. These will help in reviewing the behavior together with patients celebrate successes, discuss challenges, and co-create plans for next steps. The process of consistently tracking one's behavior is sometimes an intervention itself, with patients often sharing that it created self-reflection and resulted in some changes [50].

9. Conclusion

This study acknowledges that cardiovascular diseases are costly to manage and that its prevalence is increasing daily and threatening the health budget. Therefore, the cost-effective interventions target behaviors such as: (1) cessation of tobacco use, (2) avoidance of alcohol abuse, (3) regular physical activity, (4) healthy eating, and (5) reduction of salt. The adoption of these behavioral interventions is associated with reduced costs burden and improved outcomes among patients diagnosed with cardiovascular diseases. Health policies that create conducive environments for making healthy choices affordable and available are essential for motivating people to adopt and sustain healthy behaviors. In the implementation of cost-effective behavioral change interventions, it is important that primary healthcare providers help patients through SMART acronym and also help patients visualize what they need to do to reach their goals through the use of SMART acronym strategy. Attitudes of patients toward the behavior change and the self-monitoring program are crucial for better outcomes of cost-effective interventions to curb cardiovascular diseases.

Author details

Mabitsela Hezekiel 'Pitso' Mphasha
Department of Human Nutrition and Dietetics, University of Limpopo, Polokwane, South Africa

*Address all correspondence to: pitso85@gmail.com

References

[1] World Health Organization. Primary health care Online. www.who.int [published April 1, 2021]

[2] Villarruz-Sulit MV, Forster R, Dans AL, Tan FN, Sulit DV. Chelation therapy for atherosclerotic cardiovascular disease. Cochrane Database of Systematic Reviews. 2020;**5**:1-3. DOI: 10.1002/14651858.CD002785.pub2

[3] Yusuf S, Joseph P, Rangarajan S, et al. Modifiable risk factors, cardiovascular disease, and mortality in 155 722 individuals from 21 high-income, middle-income, and low-income countries (PURE): A prospective cohort study. Lancet. 2020;**395**(10226):795-808. DOI: 10.1016/S0140-6736(19)32008-2

[4] Kumar A, Siddharth V, Singh SI, Narang R. Cost analysis of treating cardiovascular diseases in a super-specialty hospital. PLoS One. 2022;**17**(1):1-11. DOI: 10.1371/journal.pone.0262190

[5] Nichols GA, Brown JB. The impact of cardiovascular disease on medical care costs in subjects with and without type 2 diabetes. Diabetes Care. 2002;**25**(3):482-486

[6] Dhaliwal KK, King-Shier K, Manns BJ, Hemmelgarn BR, Stone JA, Campbell DJ. Exploring the impact of financial barriers on secondary prevention of heart disease. BMC Cardiovascular Disorders. 2017;**17**(61):1-8

[7] Campbell DJT, King-Shier K, Hemmelgarn BR, Sanmartin C, Ronksley PE, Weaver RG, et al. Self-reported financial barriers to care among patients with cardiovascular related chronic conditions. Statistics Canada Health Reports. 2014;**25**:3-12

[8] Kennedy J, Morgan S. Cost-related prescription nonadherence in the United States and Canada: A system-level comparison using the 2007 international health policy survey in seven countries. Clinical Therapeutics. 2009;**31**:213-219

[9] Law MR, Cheng L, Dhalla IA, Heard D, Morgan SG. The effect of cost on adherence to prescription medications in Canada. CMAJ. 2012;**184**:297-302

[10] Warraich HJ, Ali HJR, Nasir K. Financial toxicity with cardiovascular disease management: A balancing act for patients. Circulation. Cardiovascular Quality and Outcomes. 2020;**13**(12):978-980. DOI: 10.1161/circoutcomes.120.007449

[11] Mensah GA, Roth GA, Sampson UK, Moran AE, Feigin VL, Forouzanfar MH, et al. Mortality from cardiovascular diseases in sub-Saharan Africa, 1990-2013: A systematic analysis of data from the global burden of disease study 2013. Cardiovascular Journal of Africa. 2015;**26**:S6-S10

[12] Keates AK, Mocumbi AO, Ntsekhe M, Sliwa K, Stewart S. Cardiovascular disease in Africa: Epidemiological profile and challenges. Nature Reviews. Cardiology. 2017;**14**(5):273-293

[13] Msemburi W, Pillay-van Wyk V, Dorrington RE, Neethling I, Nannan N, Groenewald P, et al. Second National Burden of Disease Study for South Africa: Cause-of-Death Profile for South Africa, 1997 2010. Cape Town: South African Medical Research Council; 2014 ISBN: 978-1-920618-34-6

[14] Statistics South Africa. Mortality and Causes of Death in South Africa, 2014: Findings from Death Notification/

Statistics South Africa. Pretoria: Statistics South Africa, 2015; 2014

[15] Li X, Stringer LC, Chapman S, Dallimer M. How urbanisation alters the intensity of the urban heat island in a tropical African city. PLoS One. 2021;**16**(7):1-18. DOI: 10.1371/journal.pone.0254371

[16] Kuddus MA, Tynan E, McBryde E. Urbanization: A problem for the rich and the poor? Public Health Reviews. 2020;**41**(1):1-4. DOI: 10.1186/s40985-019-0116-0

[17] Eckert S, Kohler S. Urbanization and health in developing countries: A systematic review. World Health & Population. 2014;**15**(1):7-20

[18] World Health Organization. Overweight and obesity. 2016. www.who.int [Published June 9, 2021]

[19] Dookie S, Singh S. Primary health services at district level in South Africa: A critique of the primary health care approach. BMC Family Practice, 2012. 2012;**13**(67):1-4. DOI: 10.1186/1471-2296-13-67

[20] World Health Organization: Technical Paper: Primary Health Care: 25 Years after Alma-Ata. Regional Committee for the Eastern Mediterranean. Fiftieth Session, EM/RC50/8. 2003, 1-21. [http://gis.emro.who.int/HealthSystemObservatory/.../TechnicalandDiscussionPapers]

[21] Bhatia M, Rifkin S. A renewed focus on primary health care: Revitalize or reframe. Globalization and Health. 2010;**6**:13 Website address: [http://www.globalisationandhealth.com/content/6/1/13

[22] Swann C, Carmona C, Ryan M, Raynor M, Baris E, Dunsdon S, et al. Health systems and health-related behaviour change: A review of primary and secondary evidence. National Institute for Health and Clinical Excellence. 2010

[23] Gillies P. Effectiveness of alliances and partnerships for health promotion. Health Promotion International. 1998;**13**(2):99-120. DOI: 10.1093/heapro/13.2.99

[24] Wheelan SA, Burchill BN, Tilin F. The link between teamwork and patients' outcomes in intensive care units. American Journal of Critical Care. 2003;**12**:527-534

[25] Carman KL, Dardess P, Maurer M, et al. Patient and family engagement: A framework for understanding the elements and developing interventions and policies. Health Affirmation (Millwood) [Internet]. Project HOPE - The People-to-People Health Foundation, Inc. 2013;**32**(2):223-231. Available from: http://www.ncbi.nlm.nih.gov/pubmed/23381514

[26] Dunbar SB, Clark P, Quinn C, Gary R. Family influences on heart failure self-care and outcomes. The Journal of Cardiovascular Nursing. 2008;**23**:258-265

[27] Shahriari M, Ahmadi M, Babaee S, Mehrabi T, Sadeghi M. Effects of a family support program on self-care behaviors in patients with congestive heart failure. Iranian Journal of Nursing and Midwifery Research. 2013;**18**(2):152-157

[28] Gallager R, Luttik ML, Jaarsma T. Social support and self-care in heart failure. The Journal of Cardiovascular Nursing. 2011:1-7

[29] Sayers SL, Riegel B, Pawlowsk IS, Coyne J. Social support and self-care of

patients with heart failure. Annals of Behavioral Medicine. 2008;**35**:70-79

[30] Masoodi R, Alhani F, Moghadassi J, Ghorbani M. The effect of family-centered empowerment model on skill, attitude, and knowledge of multiple sclerosis caregivers. Journal of Birjand University of Medical Sciences. 2010;**17**:87-97

[31] Mphasha MH, Mothiba TM. Family-centered diabetes Care for Better Glycemic Outcomes of outpatients in rural areas. In: Monyeki KD, Kemper HC, editors. Lifestyle and Epidemiology - the Double Burden of Poverty and Cardiovascular Diseases in African Populations. London, UK: IntechOpen; 2021. DOI: 10.5772/intechopen.96223

[32] Mphasha MH, Mothiba TM, Skaal L. Assessment of diabetes dietary knowledge and its impact on intake of patients in Senwabarwana, Limpopo, South Africa. Journal of Endocrinology, Metabolism and Diabetes of South Africa. 2021;**26**(3):89-95. DOI: 10.1080/16089677.2021.1927584

[33] Vedanthan R, Bansilal S, Soto AV, Kovacic JC, Latina J, Jaslow R, et al. Family-based approaches to cardiovascular health promotion. Journal of the American College of Cardiology. 2016;**67**(14):1725-1737. DOI: 10.1016/j.jacc.2016.01.036

[34] Mayberry LS, Rothman RL, Osborn CY. Family members' obstructive behaviors appear to be more harmful among adults with type 2 diabetes and limited health literacy. Journal of Health Communication. 2014;**19**(2):132-143. DOI: 10.1080/10810730.2014.938840

[35] Kuo DZ, Houtrow AJ, Arango P, Kuhlthau KA, Simmons JM, Neff JM. Family-centered care: Current applications and future directions in pediatric health care. Maternal and Child Health Journal. 2012;**16**(2):297-305. Available from: http://www.ncbi.nlm.nih.gov/pubmed/21318293

[36] Baig AA, Benitez A, Quinn MT, Burnet DL. Family interventions to improve diabetes outcomes for adults. Annals of the New York Academy of Sciences. 2015;**1353**(1):89-112. Available in PMC 2016 September 01

[37] Butterfoss FD, Kegler M. Toward a comprehensive understanding of community coalitions: Moving from practice to theory. In: DiClemente R, Crosby R, Kegler M, editors. Emerging Theories of Health Promotion Practice and Research. San Francisco, CA: Jossey-Bass; 2002. pp. 157-193

[38] Center for Disease Control and Prevention (CDC). Principles of Community Engagement. 2nd ed. 2011. http://www.atsdr.cdc.gov/communityengagement/pdf/PCE_Report_508_FINAL.pdf

[39] Pennington K, Harwood E, Sick B. Characterizing the community collaborations of a community-based student-run clinic. Journal of Primary Care & Community Health. 2020;**11**:1-7. DOI: 10.1177/2150132720984400

[40] Glik DC, Sharif MZ, Tucker KL, Tejada SA, Prelip ML, Ammerman AS, et al. Community-engagement to support cardiovascular disease prevention in disparities populations: Three case studies. Journal of Health Disparities Research and Practice. 2016;**9**(1):90-108

[41] O'Mara-Eves A, Brunton G, Oliver S, Kavanagh J, Jamal F, Thomas J. The effectiveness of community engagement in public health interventions for disadvantaged groups: A meta-analysis. BMC Public

Health. 2015;**15**(129):1-23. DOI: 10.1186/s12889-015-1352-y

[42] Davis R, Campbell R, Hildon Z, Hobbs L, Michie S. Theories of behaviour and behaviour change across the social and behavioural sciences: A scoping review. Health Psychology Review. 2015;**9**(3):323-344

[43] Kwasnicka D, Dombrowski SU, White M, Sniehotta F. Theoretical explanations for maintenance of behaviour change: A systematic review of behaviour theories. Health Psychology Review. 2016;**10**(3):277-296. DOI: 10.1080/17437199.2016.1151372

[44] Dombrowski SU. Form of delivery as a key 'active ingredient' in behaviour change interventions. British Journal of Health Psychology. 2016;**21**(4):733-740

[45] Hooker S, Punjabi A, Justesen K, Boyle L, Sherman MD. Encouraging health behavior change: Eight evidence-based strategies. Family Practice Management. 2018;**25**(2):31-36 PMID: 29537244

[46] Cropsey KL, McClure LA, Jackson DO, Villalobos GC, Weaver MF, Stitzer ML. The impact of quitting smoking on weight among women prisoners participating in a smoking cessation intervention. American Journal of Public Health. 2010;**100**(8):1442-1448. DOI: 10.2105/AJPH.2009.172783

[47] Hajar R. Risk factors for coronary artery disease: Historical perspectives. Heart Views: the Official Journal of the Gulf Heart Association. 2017;**18**(3):109-114. DOI: 10.4103/HEARTVIEWS.HEARTVIEWS_106_17

[48] Al Mutair A, Plummer V, O'Brien AP, Clerehan R. Attitudes of healthcare providers towards family involvement and presence in adult critical care units in Saudi Arabia: A quantitative study. Journal of Clinical Nursing. 2014;**23**(5-6):744-575. DOI: 10.1111/jocn.12520 PMID: 24734275

[49] Muchiri J, Gericke GJ, Rheeder P. Impact of nutrition education on diabetes knowledge and attitudes of adults with type 2 diabetes living in a resource-limited setting in South Africa: A randomised controlled trial. Journal of Endocrinology, Metabolism and Diabetes of South Africa. 2016;**21**(2):26-34. DOI: 10.1080/16089677.2016.1200324

[50] Larsen RT, Wagner V, Korfitsen CB, Keller C, Juhl CB, Langberg H, et al. Effectiveness of physical activity monitors in adults: Systematic review and meta-analysis. BMJ. 2022;**376**

Chapter 26

Paravalvular Leaks: From Diagnosis to Management

Fathia Mghaieth Zghal, Abdeljelil Farhati and Mohamed Sami Mourali

Abstract

Paravalvular leaks (PVLs) are complications of a surgical or percutaneous valve replacement. They are persistent defects between the native annulus and the sewing ring, which result in a regurgitant prosthesis. They are observed in 2–18% of patients after a surgical valve replacement (SVR) and in 7–40% after a transcatheter aortic valve replacement (TAVR). Clinical manifestations are heart failure and hemolysis. They develop in 1–5% of PVL patients, and they have a poor prognosis. Surgery was the only available treatment to improve the patient's outcome. But it is a high-risk surgery in frail patients and PVL relapse is not rare. Percutaneous PVL closure has emerged as a promising technique. Nevertheless, it needs a careful assessment, demands high technical expertise, and still has limitations. This chapter focuses on the diagnosis of PVL after a SVR and transcatheter PVL closure (TPVL).

Keywords: surgical valve replacement, transcatheter aortic valve replacement, paravalvular leak, transesophageal echocardiography, 3D echocardiography

1. Introduction

Paravalvular leaks (PVLs) are complications of a surgical or percutaneous valve replacement. They are persistent defects between the native annulus and the sewing ring, which result in a regurgitant prosthesis. They are more frequent after a surgical replacement (SVR) of the mitral (SMVR) than the aortic valve (SAVR) (7–17% and 2–10%, respectively) [1–3]. They can be detected early or several decades after the index surgery [4]. PVL reemerged as a frequent and deleterious complication with transcatheter aortic valve replacement (TAVR) development. Where it was reported variably in 7–40% of patients, it decreased with prostheses and technical improvements. Only 1–5% of PVLs result in patent clinical effect [5]; hemolytic anemia or congestive heart failure. In patients with one or both clinical manifestations, spontaneous evolution is unfavorable, and an intervention is indicated. Percutaneous closure seems an optimal therapeutic solution, less invasive than surgery, and has promising results. Nevertheless, this technique demands high technical expertise, and it has its proper limitations and complications, hence indications should be carefully weighed.

2. Etiopathogenesis

PVL after SVR are several co-contributing factors, related to the anatomy of the valve, the surgical technique, the status of the patient, and/or to the surgeon's experience [6], they are depicted in **Table 1**. In TAVR, massive and asymmetrical calcifications and elliptical annulus shape as the main anatomical contributors, insufficient sizing and insufficient depth implantation as procedural predictors and functional c.

Lass and low left ventricular ejection fraction (LVEF) as patient condition factors [7, 8], the experience of the operator remains important to consider. Infective endocarditis (IE) is a main cause of valve disinsertion and can also be a consequence of a mechanical disinsertion with a secondary bacterial infection [9, 10].

3. Clinical and subclinical manifestations

The three main clinical manifestations of PVLs consist of congestive heart failure (HF), anemia, and IE [9].

Congestive HF occurs in the case of large or multiple PVLs with a severe valve regurgitation.

While *hemolytic anemia syndrome* occurs in small PVLs. They are more frequent in mitral valves with preserved LVEF [10], which results in a high velocity and turbulent systolic regurgitant jet. Hemolysis and anemia may be permanent or intermittent. Hence, a partial improvement during follow-up should not exclude the diagnosis nor lead to investigation cessation.

Infective endocarditis syndrome may be secondary to a previous mechanical known or unknown disinsertion or the cause of the valve disinsertion. It is important to detect IE for specific treatment. TPVL is contraindicated in this case.

Clinical tolerance is not directly correlated to the size of the PVL [9], it is influenced by several factors, including the compliance of cardiac chambers compliance, ventricular functions, the existence and degree of anemia, and the rapidity of installation. Symptomatic patients are at the tip of the iceberg.

Subclinical PVLs are more frequent, they can remain stable and or lead to progressive heart function deterioration, or they can be unmasked by an intercurrent event like IE.

Subclinical PVLs were reported to affect the patient's prognosis in SAVR and in TAVR [11, 12], they require a close follow-up and IE prevention. While symptomatic PVLs have a severe prognosis and an intervention, when feasible, is needed to improve their outcome [13].

Local anatomy	Intervention technique	Patient's status	Operator's/center's expertise
Infection Friability Calcifications Elliptical annulus	Supra-annular aortic valve implantation Continuous mitral valve sutures Annular reconstruction Difficult annular access	Advanced age Endocarditis Low body mass index Denutrition Previous valvular interventions and paravalvular leak relapses	Lack of experience and low activity volume

Table 1.
Factors contributing to paravalvular leak occurrence after a surgical valve replacement.

We should have a high index of PVL's suspicion when a patient presents with one of these figures even if first-line investigations, namely, transthoracic echocardiography (TTE) is negative. This is an essential step toward the diagnosis.

4. Cardiac imaging for paravalvular leak assessment and procedural guidance

Assessment of PVLs relay first on ultrasounds. Imaging modalities are complementary and multimodality imaging is usual.

4.1 Transthoracic Doppler echocardiography

TTE is performed as a first-line noninvasive test. It is essential for detection or suspicion of PVLs through direct or indirect signs. Indirect signs include chambers' enlargement and pulmonary pressure elevation. Direct signs consist of visualization of the defect between the annulus and the prosthetic sewing ring, which should be distinguished from an artifact by simultaneous application of color Doppler and identification of the regurgitant jet. The whole circumference of the annulus should be examined carefully, the number, size, and extension of defects are noticed.

TTE can be sufficient, particularly, in anterior aortic PVLs to determine PVL characteristics, however, its sensitivity and precision are weak in mitral PVLs that can be totally missed by TTE due to acoustic shadows.

TTE is fundamental for the assessment of prosthetic valve flows, left and right ventricles and atria sizes and functions, pulmonary pressures, and other valves' status [14–16].

TTE is usually the main test for periodic follow-up.

4.2 Transesophageal Doppler echocardiography

Two (2D) and Three (3D) dimensional TEE is the reference test for PVL assessment, it is performed after a comprehensive TTE, whether this latter was contributive or not.

TEE is essential for the investigation of mitral PVL, multiple PVLs, and complex ones [14–16] TEE permits to assess accurately the sites of the leaks by exploring the whole circumference of the sewing ring by 2D, 3D, and color Doppler modes. When using 3D imaging a careful gain setting and joint color Doppler imaging are important to eliminate gain dropouts [15].

A double opposite clock face is used to indicate the mitral and aortic PVLs sites. The mitral clock face is divided into septal, posterior, lateral, and anterior dials (**Figure 1**).

The number, shape, area, length, and height of PVLs are determined by 3D TEE [9, 14] which also indicates the defect distance from the ring and the PVL spatial position in relation to the mechanism of the prosthesis. Precise sizing using 3D multiplanar reconstruction is a key to choose an adequate device when a TPVL is indicated. Identification of calcifications and IE signs are important to discuss the feasibility and difficulty of a TPVL or surgical treatment (**Table 2**) [16, 17].

The quantification of the regurgitation is better evaluated by non-orifice-related parameters. In fact, vena contracta and proximal isovelocity methods, are

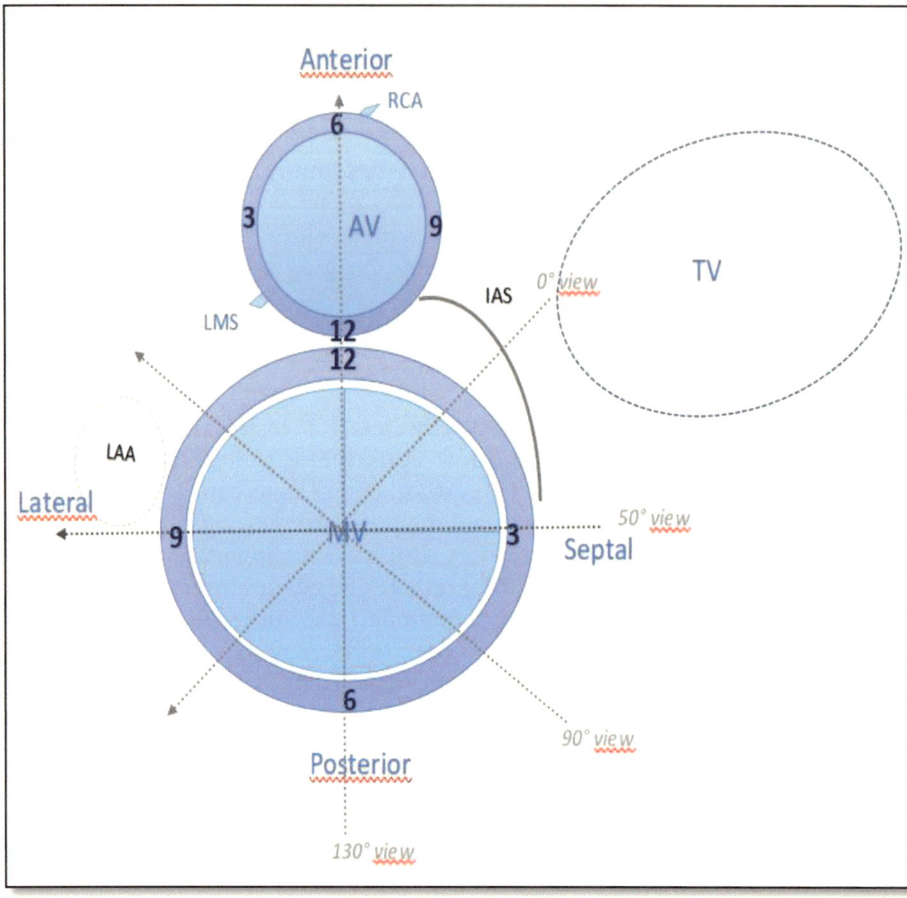

Figure 1.
Schematization of en face view by transesophageal three-dimensional echocardiography. 0, 50, 90, and 130° views: corresponding bidimensional transesophageal echocardiography plans, AV: Aortic valve, IAS: interatrial septum, LAA: left atrial appendage, LMS: left main stem, MV: mitral valve, RCA: right coronary artery, TV: tricuspid valve.

distorted by the irregular shape and location of the defect, they are rarely useful. The severity of the regurgitation is better appreciated by continuity equation, end-diastolic descending aorta velocity or reversal systolic pulmonary venous flow, cavities' dilatation, and pulmonary pressures. The circumferential extension of the defect is also a useful parameter for the severity of the regurgitation as well as the feasibility of TPVL. These parameters are to consider in parallel with the clinical status of the patient.

2D and 3D TEE are essential for TPVL guidance, especially in mitral PVLs, while TTE and fluoroscopy can be sufficient to guide aortic PVLs closure. The utility of per procedure TEE is depicted in **Table 2**. Septal puncture is guided by biplane (45 and 130°) imaging when an anterograde approach is chosen for a mitral PVL reduction, real-time 3D and zoom mode are used to localize the guides and orient the crossing of the PVL then the right positioning of the occluder device. At crucial time of the procedure, the deploying, orientation, and position of the device are to be verified as well as the mobility of the prosthetic valve and its flow (**Figure 2**). Before the release of the occluder

Pre intervention	Per TPVL guiding	Post intervention
Comprehensive cardiac assessment, including chamber sizes and functions, pulmonary pressure, all valves 'morphologies, and flows Research for infective endocarditis Assessment of local anatomy of PVLs: location, shape, number, size/extension, rocking, local, calcifications Gradation of the severity of the regurgitation Gradation of suitability for TPVL, relying on previous anatomical Planification of procedures; choice of the approach, devices and occluders	Septal puncture Spatial catheters and guides orientation Occluder positioning Normal function of prosthetic valve Immediate results Residual leak Complications (tamponade)	Position (migration) Function of prosthetic valve Residual leak/relapse of regurgitation Complications (infective endocarditis...) General cardiac assessment, chambers' size and function, pulmonary pressure.

PVL: paravalvular leak, TPVL: transcatheter paravalvular leak closure.

Table 2.
Role of Doppler transthoracic and transesophageal echocardiography in paravalvular leak management.

device, the residual leak is searched, qualified, and quantified. When significant, it leads to a change of the choice of the device or the indication of a complimentary ad hoc or differed procedure; residual leaks impact the prognosis (**Figure 2**) [16].

Permanent per-procedural monitoring detects at any time of the intervention the occurrence of complications like pericardial effusion or tamponade, embolization of the occluder, impinging, and blocking of the valve.

TEE is important to consider during follow-up if a complication is suspected (i.e., endocarditis, relapse, or extension of PVLs).

4.3 Fluoroscopy

Fluoroscopy is useful to detect rocking prosthetic valves when there is an extensive disinsertion, or an abnormal movement is seen in TTE or TEE. Fluoroscopy is important for TPVL guiding [16].

Fusion imaging combines echocardiography and fluoroscopy, is precious to guide the TPVL, it saves intervention time and increase the success rate [17, 18].

4.4 Intracardiac echocardiography

Intracardiac echocardiography is also an innovative mean to guide TPVL. Unlike TEE it allows to get free from general anesthesia. A series of 21 interventions in 18 patients with intracardiac echocardiography help was reported without any complication related to the imaging technique itself and with an acceptable rate of procedural success [19].

4.5 Magnetic resonance imaging and cardiac tomography imaging

Magnetic resonance imaging and cardiac tomography imaging are useful in a multimodality imaging approach, which is crucial for aortic post-SAVR or post-TAVR PVLs. *Cardiac tomography-fluoroscopy fusion imaging* was used in experienced teams to achieve more reproducible results, higher success, and better short and long terms

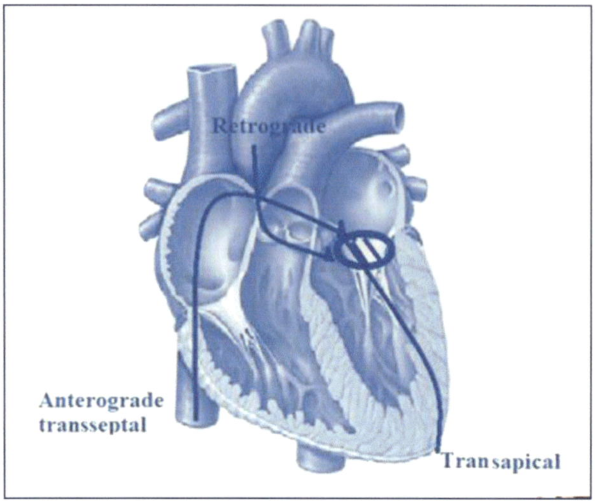

Figure 2.
Approaches for transcutaneous paravalvular leak closure.

outcomes. Also, the extension of indications and treatment with the confidence of complex, multiple PVLs (especially aortic PVLs) were allowed [20, 21].

4.6 Angiography and video-densitometry

Video-densitometric angiography is an emerging method, it was used in prospective trials as a reference tool for post-TAVR PVL assessment. It was reported to have high accuracy and allowed an objective comparison between different TAVR prostheses [22, 23]. For Kitamura M et al. it is helpful in litigious cases and intermediate degrees of regurgitation [24].

Accurate assessment of PVLs remains challenging. American and Japanese imaging and interventional societies collaboration resulted in a key guideline article dedicated to the evaluation of valvular regurgitation after percutaneous valve repair or replacement to help the development and result assessment of these interventions [25].

5. Indications for intervention

Intervention is needed when the patient with PVL is symptomatic or has evolving subclinical consequences, such as left ventricular enlargement and function impairment, significant pulmonary pressure elevation at rest or with exercise, significant hemolysis, and infective endocarditis. In certain situations, the PVL-symptoms causality relationship has to be assessed in case of comorbidities. In other situations, symptoms have to be unmasked by effort tests. TPVL is currently considered in first-line when expertise is available. The first step is to eliminate contraindications to TPVL: evolutive sepsis, extensive disinsertion greater than the third of the circumference, and rocking valves. When these figures are present surgery is chosen. Otherwise, TPVL offers a less invasive solution in generally operated and frail patients.

6. Transcatheter paravalvular leak closure

After a full assessment, defining *the objective* of the procedure is primordial; in the case of heart failure presentation, every PVL reduction is beneficial. When the TPVL is motivated by hemolytic anemia it is important to achieve a total closure of the PVL.

TPVL planification includes the choice of an adequate approach and devices. The procedure is usually performed in a catheter laboratory under general anesthesia and joint TEE and fluoroscopy guidance. Antibiotic prophylaxis is applied by administration of a cephalosporine or vancomycin in case of penicillin anaphylaxis. Nonfractioned heparin is administrated to obtain an active cephalin time between 250 and 300 and prevent catheter thrombosis. These are generally long procedures; the use of fluoroscopy is optimized to 7.5 images/second and the use of a higher image frame rate (15 images/second) is restricted to necessary (device delivery).

Approaches: For the mitral valve, the anterograde transeptal approach is the most used, however, an anterograde transaortic approach is more suitable for septal and posterior PVLs. The combination of both approaches forming an arteriovenous loop and transapical access are alternatives particularly for large or multiple PVLs necessitating the use of multiple devices [21]. The retrograde approach is not feasible in the case of mechanical aortic valve (**Figure 2**).

Device	Amplatzer Vascular plug III	Occlutech paravalvular leak device	
En face view	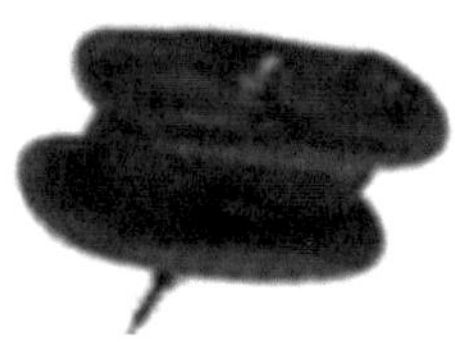	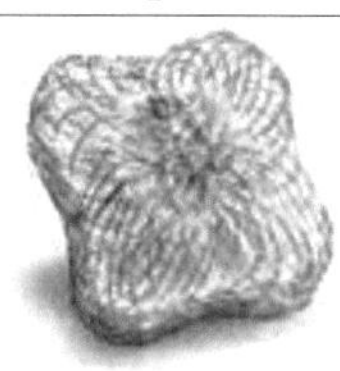 a1	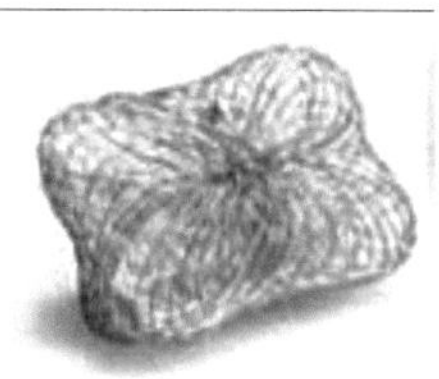 b1
Profile view	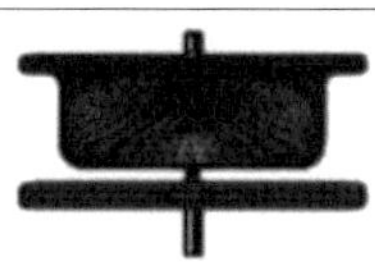	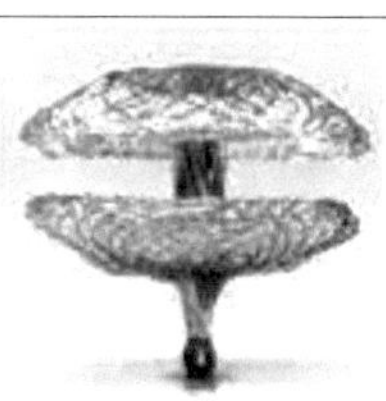 a2	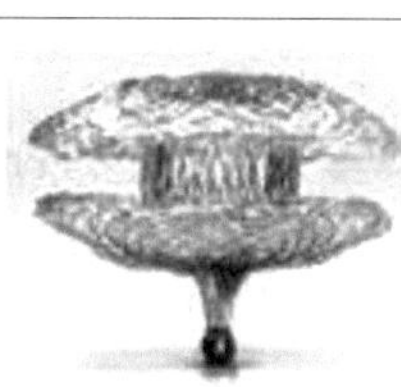 b2
Material	Multiple layer nitinol mesh	Nitinol braided wires	
Advantages	Accommodation to the shape of the channel Relative insusceptibility to deformation	Available in two shapes: square (a1) and rectangular (b1) Available in two types twist (a2) and waist (b2) Stable position in large Paravalvular leaks	
Risks	"overhanging" with larger sizes and multiple device implantation	"Dog bone" formation in case of oversizing with a leak across the device	

Table 3.
Characteristics of dedicated paravalvular leak devices.

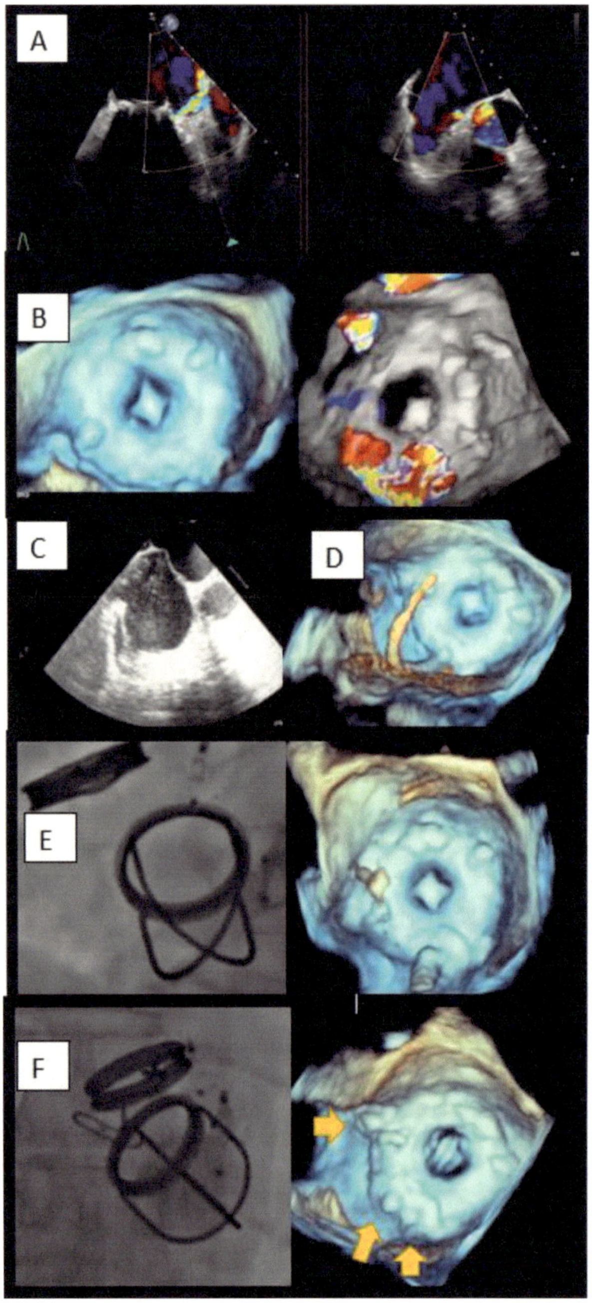

Figure 3.
Illustration of steps of a complex mitral lateral and posterior paravalvular leak transcutaneous closure in a 52-years-old female with an aortic valve prosthesis and a Starr mitral valve prosthesis. A: Paravalvular leak in color Doppler transesophageal echocardiography. B: Assessment of the defect by three-dimensional transesophageal echocardiography. C: The septal tenting. prior to the septal crossing by the wire. D: crossing of the paravalvular leak by the delivery catheter. E: assessment of the occluder device deploying by fluoroscopy and echocardiography and verification of the prosthetic valve flow. F: final result assessment by fluoroscopy and three-dimensional echography after delivery of one lateral and two posterior devices (arrows).

For the aortic valve is concerned, the retrograde approach is the most used, and transapical approach, which is useful for multiple and complex PVLs [26].

Devices: Rare dedicated devices were designed by manufacturers; Amplatzer vascular plug III (Abbott Vascular) and the paravalvular leak device (Occlutech), they are theoretically more suitable than non-dedicated devices. Their characteristics are summarized in **Table 3**.

Other non-dedicated devices were used for TPVL amplatzer vascular plug II and IV (Abbott Vascular), amplatzer duct occluder devices (Saint Jude Medical), atrial septal defect, and ventricular septal defect devices.

All devices are used off-label and do not have FDA approval [27].

The use of multiple devices can be necessary for large or multiple PVLs. This can be achieved one or more times [5].

Delivery sheaths: There is no dedicated delivery sheaths for PVL dedicated devices. Delivery sheaths for atrial septum, ventricular septum, or arterial duct devices adapted for PVL may have an insufficient length for aortic PVLs or nonoptimal diameters. Steerable sheaths facilitate the procedure and are imperative in mitral posteroseptal PVLs.

Figure 3 illustrates the main steps of a TEE-guided mitral TPVL.

6.1 Specific considerations for post-transcatheter aortic valve replacement paravalvular leaks

PVL after TAVR increases late mortality [28]. The assessment relies on a multimodality approach (ultrasounds, MSCT, hemodynamic, and angiography). The closure of TAVR-related PVLs can be considered during the TAVR procedure or subsequent follow-up. During the procedure, many techniques are available to reduce regurgitation. Oversized balloon post dilatation is effective to optimize the valve expansion and ensure a better seal but exposes to an over risk of cerebral embolic events. Snares are used when there is an inadequate depth of implantation. It is to consider with caution when there is heavy calcification as it can result also in their detachment and embolization. Valve-in-valve is used when the previous techniques are not feasible, especially when there is a nonoptimal first valve procedure. This technique can also be used later for surgical or transcatheter degenerated valves [29]. TAVR-related PVL can also be reduced by a TPVL as previously described.

7. Transcutaneous paravalvular leak closure results

Compared to surgery TPVL has lower technical success (about 90% vs. 70–86%) but less short-term adverse events and lower 30 days mortality (about 4 vs. 11%) [27, 30–32]. Mitral TPVL has higher adverse events and mortality rates than aortic TPVL [27]. Three years prognosis and survival are improved when the TPVL is successful without or with the only mild residual leak [33]. Indeed favorable result is obtained in case of the absence of significant residual regurgitation. After a first TPVL, repeated transcutaneous or surgical interventions can be needed during follow-up. The main adverse problems are worsening or new hemolysis in mitral PVLs, significant residual PVL, encroachment of the prosthetic valve, vascular injury, tamponade, hemothorax (transapical approach), device embolization, stroke, relapsing and new PVL, infective endocarditis, and death [3, 27].

8. Wrap-up

Essential steps forward TPVL achievement begin with a clinical suspicion that should include heart failure, anemia, infection, and equivalent syndromes. TTE should be very large. Multimodality imaging assessment is encouraged and facilitates the localization, anatomy evaluation, and measurement of the PVLs, and it prepares and guides the closure intervention. Full patient assessment is also needed, including comorbidities, frailty. Indication should be led by a structural valve specialized heart team. The patient's preferences are taken into account. The planification of intervention is precise and demands a large material set preparation to be able to adapt the technique and address complications, and can miss the diagnosis, particularly in the case of mitral PVL. The procedure is conducted in expertise centers. A long-term close follow-up is then needed as complications can occur at any time of the evolution.

9. Conclusion

Since its first description in 1992, TPVL has undergone an important evolution and become a confirmed technique. It is currently considered as a first-line and vital solution for PVLs reduction by many teams, even if surgery remains the reference technique in guidelines. It is important to note that it demands high expertise and is feasible only in Ref. centers with a multidisciplinary team contribution. It remains limited by dedicated devices availability and lack of financial support.

Author details

Fathia Mghaieth Zghal[1,2]*, Abdeljelil Farhati[2] and Mohamed Sami Mourali[1,2]

1 Faculty of Medicine of Tunis, Tunis El Manar University, Tunis, Tunisia

2 Rabta Hospital, Tunis, Tunisia

*Address all correspondence to: fathia.zghal@fmt.utm.tn; zghal.fathia@gmail.com

References

[1] Ionescu A, Fraser AG, Butchart EG. Prevalence and clinical significance of incidental paraprosthetic valvar regurgitation: A prospective study using transoesophageal echocardiography. Heart. 2003;**89**(11):1316-1321. DOI: 10.1136/heart.89.11.1316

[2] Saia F, Martinez C, Gafoor S, Singh V, Ciuca C, Hofmann I, et al. Long-term outcomes of percutaneous paravalvular regurgitation closure after transcatheter aortic valve replacement: A multicenter experience. JACC. Cardiovascular Interventions. 2015;**8**(5):681-688. DOI: 10.1016/j.jcin.2014.11.022

[3] Cruz-Gonzalez I, Rama-Merchan JC, Rodríguez-Collado J, Martín-Moreiras J, Diego-Nieto A, Barreiro-Pérez M, et al. Transcatheter closure of paravalvular leaks: State of the art. Netherlands Heart Journal. 2017;**25**(2):116-124. DOI: 10.1007/s12471-016-0918-3

[4] García E, Sandoval J, Unzue L, Hernandez-Antolin R, Almería C, Macaya C. Paravalvular leaks: Mechanisms, diagnosis and management. Euro Intervention. 2012;**8 Suppl Q**:Q41-Q52. DOI: 10.4244/EIJV8SQA9

[5] Bhushan S, Huang X, Li Y, He S, Mao L, Hong W, et al. Paravalvular leak after transcatheter aortic valve implantation its incidence, diagnosis, clinical implications, prevention, management, and future perspectives: A review article. Current Problems in Cardiology. 2021:100957. DOI: 10.1016/j.cpcardiol.2021

[6] Jilaihawi H, Kashif M, Fontana G, Furugen A, Shiota T, Friede G, et al. Cross-sectional computed tomographic assessment improves accuracy of aortic annular sizing for transcatheter aortic valve replacement and reduces the incidence of paravalvular aortic regurgitation. Journal of the American College of Cardiology. 2012;**59**(14):1275-1286. DOI: 10.1016/j.jacc.2011.11.045

[7] Milhorini Pio S, Bax J, Delgado V. How valvular calcification can affect the outcomes of transcatheter aortic valve implantation. Expert Review of Medical Devices. 2020;**17**(8):773-784. DOI: 10.1080/17434440.2020.1789456

[8] Nietlispach F, Maisano F, Sorajja P, Leon MB, Rihal C, Feldman T. Percutaneous paravalvular leak closure: Chasing the chameleon. European Heart Journal. 2016;**37**(47):3495-3502. DOI: 10.1093/eurheartj/ehw165

[9] Bernard S, Yucel E. Paravalvular leaks-from diagnosis to management. Current Treatment Options in Cardiovascular Medicine. 2019;**21**(11):67. DOI: 10.1007/s11936-019-0776-6

[10] Choi JY, Suh YJ, Seo J, Choi KU, Hong GR, Lee S, et al. Structural and functional characteristics of mitral paravalvular leakage identified by multimodal imaging and their implication on clinical presentation. Journal of Clinical Medicine. 2021;**10**(2):222. DOI: 10.3390/jcm10020222

[11] Kodali SK, Williams MR, Smith CR, Svensson LG, Webb JG, Makkar RR, et al. Two-year outcomes after transcatheter or surgical aortic-valve replacement. The New England Journal of Medicine. 2012;**366**(18):1686-1695. DOI: 10.1056/NEJMoa1200384

[12] Ando T, Briasoulis A, Telila T, Afonso L, Grines CL, Takagi H. Does

mild paravalvular regurgitation post transcatheter aortic valve implantation affect survival? A meta-analysis. Catheter Cardiovascular Intervention. 2018;**91**(1):135-147. DOI: 10.1002/ccd.27336

[13] Genoni M, Franzen D, Vogt P, Seifert B, Jenni R, Künzli A, et al. Paravalvular leakage after mitral valve replacement: Improved long-term survival with aggressive surgery? European Journal of Cardio-Thoracic Surgery. 2000;**17**(1):14-19. DOI: 10.1016/s1010-7940(99)00358-9

[14] Gafoor S, Franke J, Bertog S, Lam S, Vaskelyte L, Hofmann I, et al. A quick guide to paravalvular leak closure. Interventional Cardiology. 2015;**10**(2):112-117. DOI: 10.15420/ICR.2015.10.2.112

[15] Gürsoy MO, Güner A, Kalçık M, Bayam E, Özkan M. A comprehensive review of the diagnosis and management of mitral paravalvular leakage. Anatolian Journal of Cardiology. 2020;**24**(6):350-360. DOI: 10.14744/AnatolJCardiol.2020.10018

[16] Lázaro C, Hinojar R, Zamorano JL. Cardiac imaging in prosthetic paravalvular leaks. Cardiovascular Diagnostic Theraphy. 2014;**4**(4):307-313. DOI: 10.3978/j.issn.2223-3652.2014.07.01

[17] Pascual I, Pozzoli A, Taramasso M, Maisano F, Ho EC. Fusion imaging for transcatheter mitral and tricuspid interventions. Annals of Translational Medicine. 2020;**8**(15):965. DOI: 10.21037/atm.2020.02.169

[18] Kim BH, Koh YS, Lee KY, Chung WB. Three-dimensional Echo navigator system guided transcatheter closure of paravalvular leakage. Journal of Cardiovascular Imaging. 2019;**27**(3):227-229. DOI: 10.4250/jcvi.2019.27.e30

[19] Ruparelia N, Cao J, Newton JD, Wilson N, Daniels MJ, Ormerod OJ. Paravalvular leak closure under intracardiac echocardiographic guidance. Catheterization and Cardiovascular Interventions. 2018;**91**(5):958-965. DOI: 10.1002/ccd.27318

[20] Suh YJ, Hong GR, Han K, Im DJ, Chang S, Hong YJ, et al. Assessment of mitral paravalvular leakage after mitral valve replacement using cardiac computed tomography: Comparison with surgical findings. Circulation. Cardiovascular Imaging. 2016;**9**(6):e004153. DOI: 10.1161/CIRCIMAGING.115.004153

[21] Liu Y, Xu C, Ding P, et al. Transcatheter closure of mitral paravalvular leak via multiple approaches. Journal of Interventional Cardiology. 2021;**2021**:6630774. DOI: 10.1155/2021/6630774

[22] Crouch G, Tully PJ, Bennetts J, Sinhal A, Bradbrook C, Penhall AL, et al. Quantitative assessment of paravalvular regurgitation following transcatheter aortic valve replacement. Journal of Cardiovascular Magnetic Resonance. 2015;**17**(1):32. DOI: 10.1186/s12968-015-0134-0

[23] Asami M, Pilgrim T, Stortecky S, Heg D, Roost E, Windecker S, et al. Impact of valvular resistance on aortic regurgitation after transcatheter aortic valve replacement according to the type of prosthesis. Clinical Research in Cardiology. 2019;**108**(12):1343-1353. DOI: 10.1007/s00392-019-01469-z

[24] Kitamura M, Von Roeder M, Abdel-Wahab M. Quantitative assessment of aortic regurgitation following transcatheter aortic valve replacement. Expert Review of Cardiovascular Therapy. 2021;**19**(7):633-645. DOI: 10.1080/14779072.2021.1924675

[25] Zoghbi WA, Asch FM, Bruce C, Gillam LD, Grayburn PA, Hahn RT, et al. Guidelines for the evaluation of valvular regurgitation after percutaneous valve repair or replacement: A report from the American Society of Echocardiography developed in collaboration with the Society for Cardiovascular Angiography and Interventions, Japanese Society of Echocardiography, and Society for Cardiovascular Magnetic Resonance. Journal of the American Society of Echocardiography. 2019;**32**(4):431-475. DOI: 10.1016/j.echo.2019.01.003

[26] Joseph TA, Lane CE, Fender EA, Zack CJ, Rihal CS. Catheter-based closure of aortic and mitral paravalvular leaks: Existing techniques and new frontiers. Expert Review of Medical Devices. 2018;**15**(9):653-663. DOI: 10.1080/17434440.2018.1514257

[27] Giblett JP, Rana BS, Shapiro LM, Calvert PA. Percutaneous management of paravalvular leaks. Nature Reviews. Cardiology. 2019;**16**(5):275-285. DOI: 10.1038/s41569-018-0147-0

[28] Laakso T, Laine M, Moriyama N, et al. Impact of paravalvular regurgitation on the mid-term outcome after transcatheter and surgical aortic valve replacement. European Journal of Cardio-Thoracic Surgery. 2020;**58**:1145-1152. DOI: 10.1093/ejcts/ezaa254

[29] Stundl A, Rademacher MC, Descoups C, et al. Balloon post-dilation and valve-invalve implantation for the reduction of paravalvular leakage with use of the selfexpanding Core valve prosthesis. Euro Intervention. 2016;**11**:1140-1147. DOI: doi.org/10.4244/EIJY15M11_04

[30] Alkhouli M, Sarraf M, Maor E, Sanon S, Cabalka A, Eleid MF, et al. Techniques and outcomes of percutaneous aortic paravalvular leak closure. JACC. Cardiovascular Interventions. 2016;**9**(23):2416-2426. DOI: 10.1016/j.jcin.2016.08.038

[31] Alkhouli M, Rihal CS, Zack CJ, Eleid MF, Maor E, Sarraf M, et al. Transcatheter and surgical Management of Mitral Paravalvular Leak: Long-term outcomes. JACC. Cardiovascular Interventions. 2017;**10**(19):1946-1956. DOI: 10.1016/j.jcin.2017.07.046

[32] Choi JW, Hwang HY, Kim KH, Kim KB, Ahn H. Long-term results of surgical correction for mitral paravalvular leak: Repair versus re-replacement. The Journal of Heart Valve Disease. 2013;**22**(5):682-687

[33] Alkhouli M, Zack CJ, Sarraf M, Eleid MF, Cabalka AK, Reeder GS, et al. Successful percutaneous mitral paravalvular leak closure is associated with improved midterm survival. Circulation. Cardiovascular Interventions. 2017;**10**(12):e005730. DOI: 10.1161/CIRCINTERVENTIONS.117.005730

Chapter 27

Cryoablation: From Techniques to Tips and Tricks

Bruno Papelbaum, André Sbaraini Brambilla and Bruno Kioshi Kimura Numata

Abstract

In this chapter, readers will be able to know a better mechanism of lesion formation, the benefits of the technique for specific arrhythmias, practical uses, and tips and tricks on the procedure. The chapter will also contain the first trials that validated the technique showing recent trials comparing cryoablation of atrial fibrillation versus medical treatment. The main idea is to explore how it works for clinical cardiologists and to show electrophysiologists how to use it practically. Readers will see a comparison of cryoablation versus radiofrequency versus laser to decide which one to be used, comparing total procedure time, success rates, and clinical experience.

Keywords: cryoablation, mapping, lesion formation, tips and tricks, atrial fibrillation

1. Introduction

Cryoablation is a method of destroying tissue by freezing, and it was first used for cancer treatments by Dr. James Arnott. It can be performed via surgical or percutaneous approaches. In this chapter, the focus will be on catheter ablation for cardiac arrhythmia treatments, which means percutaneous ablation.

Cryoablation causes cellular damage, death, and tissue necrosis with direct injury to cells and indirect mechanisms. Tissue cooling forms ice crystals in the extracellular space, leading to hypertonicity of this space, osmotic tension taking water from inside the cells, and dehydrating them. The intracellular membrane is altered and damage to cytoplasmic enzymes occurs but warming still can reverse this process.

When the cooling process occurs rapidly, there is no time for cellular dehydration, and free water is trapped within cells during freezing. In this scenario, there is intracellular crystal formation, which is a stage just before cellular death.

During thawing, melting ice within the extracellular space results in cell swelling and the influx of free water into the intracellular space can result in ice crystal growth, which is maximized at −20° to −25°C [1].

The rapid expansion of nitric oxide causes a decrease in the temperature of the gas (Joule–Thompson effect), which is rapidly transferred by convection and conduction to the metallic walls of the cryoprobe. The cryoprobe consists of the hollow shaft, closed electrode tip, and integrated thermocouple for the distal temperature recording. The refrigerated fluid is delivered under high pressure to the distal electrode after the fluid goes through the tip, cooling occurs to −55 to −60°C and gas is aspirated through a separate return lumen. There is also the cryoablation balloon, specific for atrial fibrillation ablation with pulmonary veins isolation [2].

By 12 weeks, small full-thickness lesions disrupt local cellularity but preserve scaffolding. Damaged cells in the center are surrounded by fibrotic scar tissue.

The advantages of cryoablation over radiofrequency (RF) are the ability to monitor the ablation zone in real-time, less painful since cooling of tissues and nerves provide an anesthetic effect, low risk of thrombus formation, and ease of use, but care must be taken when performing right pulmonary vein isolation because phrenic nerve palsy may occur. Studies have found rates ranging from 3.5% to 10% of phrenic nerve injury with most cases being transient [3].

RF uses alternating current to produce electromagnetic energy at high frequency when it passes through the small probe, gives high density, the tissue is heated directly by a resistive effect and deeper tissues are heated by conduction. Tissue within 2–3 mm from the probe is heated to 50°C–60°C, leading to coagulation and permanent cell destruction, damaging the sarcoplasmic reticulum, and irreversibly

	Cryoablation	**Radiofrequency**	**Microwave**	**Laser**	**Ultrasound**
Linear lesions	With linear probes	Coil-tip and pen-tip	With coil tip device	With diffusion linear tips	With serial transducers
Transmural lesion	Good	Limited (requires optimal contact)	Marginal	Excellent	Excellent (epicardial only)
Width/ depth ratio	Moderate	High	Moderate	Low-moderate	Low
Duration of single ablation	Long	Moderate	Moderate	Low	Low-moderate
Endocardial application	+	+	+	+	–
Epicardial application	+	+	+	+	+
Endocardial damage	Low	Moderate	Low	Low	?
Risk for perforation	Low	Moderate	Possible at high energy	Low-high (wavelength dependent)	?
Char formation	N/A	+ (avoided with irrigation)	+	+/–	–
Flexible probe	+	+	+	+	+/–
Clinical experience	Extensive	Extensive	Moderate	Early	Early

Adapted from Recent Advances in Lesion Formation for Catheter Ablation of Atrial Fibrillation Circ Arrhythm Electrophysiol. 2016;9:e003299. Different energy sources and characteristics of lesion formation, areas of application, possible complications, and clinical experience.

Table 1.
Energy sources compared.

disrupting electrophysiological properties. Energy is dissipated by the convection of blood. Later, tissue is replaced by fibrin and collagen scar, and weeks more, an 8–10 mm scar remains.

Laser is another energy source recently available for cardiac ablation. It produces high-energy optical waves via an optical coupling fiber and radiating fiber tip. Power, time, and energy vary from 30 to 80W, 60–180 seconds, and from 1.5 to 9 kilojoules, respectively. Ablation occurs through controlled dielectric heating. Spectroscopic absorption of electromagnetic frequencies is converted into vibrational kinetic energy of water molecules manifested as direct heat, indirect lesions by shock waves, and blast effects that disturb myocyte elasticity. The light beam is collimated, heats the tissue without dispersion and lines are well-demarcated. Lesion length is between 2 and 5 cm, with a depth of 4 mm, and deeper lesions occur with heat conduction. At high power, laser energy causes protein denaturation and coagulation, leading to membrane destruction and loss of water. Experimentally, 30W for 180 seconds or 50W for 60 seconds can create lesions 5–7 mm deep. Excess heat can cause craters, and duration beyond 60–80 seconds, risk of perforation. Advantages are long uniform lesions during a single application with low temperature (50°C), the reduced area of ablated tissue preserves contractility, reduces the risk of thromboembolism, and minimizes perforation.

Choosing energy source must be done according to physician experience, availability of consoles, location of arrhythmias, and success rates of the technique based on multiple trials (**Table 1**).

2. Trials for cryoablation

The first-generation cryoballoon was evaluated in the cryoballoon ablation of pulmonary veins for paroxysmal atrial fibrillation [First Results of the North American Arctic Front (STOP-AF) Pivotal Trial] [4], which demonstrated an acute isolation rate of 97.6% and a relatively low rate of complications. However, long-term success rates varied from 62% with a single procedure and 77% after multiple procedures. The limitation of the first-generation balloon was a narrow zone of cooling around the equator of the balloon, the second-generation balloon has an extended cooling from the equator of the balloon to the tip, with more uniform lesions independent of balloon positioning.

A meta-analysis of 15 studies showed a success rate of 82% at 1 year in patients with paroxysmal AF and 70% in persistent AF [5]. Another meta-analysis comparing cryoablation versus radiofrequency ablation for paroxysmal AF (PAF) analyzed 16 studies including 7194 patients (2863 with cryo and 4332 with RF). There was no statistical difference between the two strategies ($p = 0.159$) as well as procedure-related adverse events, but procedure time was shorter with cryoablation [6].

The most impacting trial comparing these two energy sources was the FIRE and ICE Trial, with results presented in 2016. The trial compared RF ablation using a 3D mapping system with cryoablation guided by fluoroscopy in patients with paroxysmal atrial fibrillation and prior antiarrhythmic drug failure. A total of 762 patients were randomized and they found that procedure time was shorter with cryoablation but using more fluoroscopy when compared to radiofrequency. The trial conclusion was that cryoablation is non-inferior to radiofrequency when performing pulmonary vein isolation in paroxysmal atrial fibrillation in terms of efficacy and safety [7].

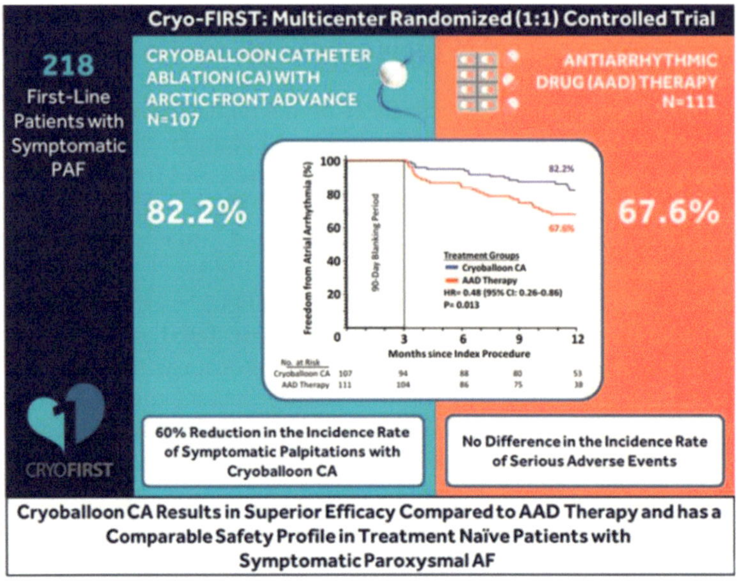

Figure 1.
Results showing the superiority of cryoablation in atrial fibrillation compared to the antiarrhythmic drug as first-line therapy. (Adapted from Cryoballoon ablation vs. antiarrhythmic drugs: first-line therapy for patients with paroxysmal atrial fibrillation. For the CRYO-First Investigators. Europace (2021) 23, 1033–1041. doi:10.1093/europace/euab029).

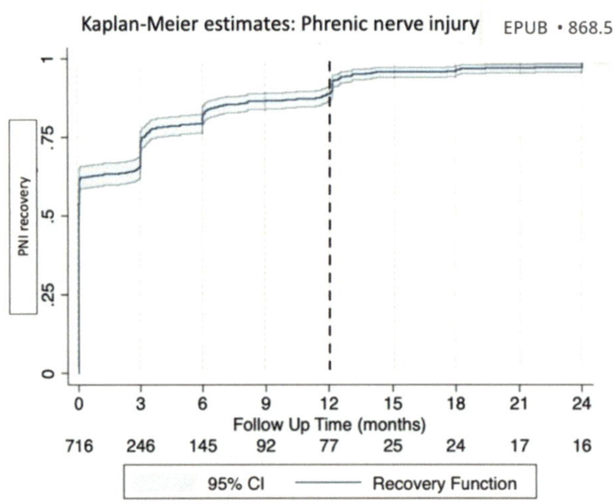

Figure 2.
Graphic showing percentual or phrenic nerve injury recovered after 12 months, and full recovery in 2 years. (Adapted from the Phrenic Nerve Injury During Cryoballoon-Based Pulmonary Vein Isolation: Results of the Worldwide YETI Registry. Circ Arrhythm Electrophysiol. 2022;15:e010516).

In 2021, Cryo-FIRST Trial [8] randomized 218 patients with paroxysmal atrial fibrillation to be treated with cryoablation as first-line therapy compared to antiarrhythmic drugs (AAD). The results were freedom from AAD after 12 months in 82.2% of subjects in the cryoballoon arm against 67.6% in the AAD arm, a 52% benefit with statistical significance (HR = 0.48, P = 0.013) (**Figure 1**). The conclusion was that the positive results demonstrate cryoablation being superior to AAD therapy in reducing AF recurrence in the first-line patient population.

Recently, the phrenic nerve injury during cryoballoon-based pulmonary vein isolation: Results of the worldwide YETI registry [9], a retrospective, multicenter, and multinational registry evaluated the incidence, characteristics, prognostic factors for phrenic nerve (PN) recovery and follow-up data during cryoablation. A total of 17356 patients underwent pulmonary vein isolation in 33 centers from 10 countries. Patients experiencing phrenic nerve injury was 4.2% (731), the mean time to occur was 127.7 ± 50.4 seconds, and the mean temperature at the time of injury was −49±8°C [9]. Recovery at 12 months was found in 97.0% (**Figure 2**), with only 0.06% showing symptomatic and permanent injury.

3. How to preform tips and tricks

Patient preparation must be as usual, with a 12-lead electrocardiogram monitoring system, vital parameters, such as heart rate, blood pressure, and oxygen saturation throughout the entire procedure, and external pads prepared, or adhesive pads put on the patient´s chest for electrical cardioversion as needed. If the procedure to be done is for supraventricular tachycardia (focal), the type of sedation can be the physician´s choice, cryoablation with a balloon can be easily performed with deep conscious sedation but, if general anesthesia is chosen, the anesthesiologist must know that curarization/neuromuscular blockade must be reversed when moving to right pulmonary vein ablation, in order not to interfere with phrenic nerve pacing/capture using a decapolar or quadripolar catheter.

For focal procedures, usually, three venous femoral access are done, one for decapolar catheter inside the coronary sinus, another for a quadripolar catheter positioned at the atrioventricular node level, capturing atrial, HIS bundle and ventricular electrograms, and the last one to be used with the cryoablation catheter, which is a 7F catheter 4 mm tipped and deflectable connected to a console and the electrophysiology (EP) system stimulator.

Ablation with a focal catheter can be performed transiently or definitely, the first one is a limited time and temperature to ensure that the chosen area isn´t going to cause any kind of damage, such as atrioventricular block (−30°C for 40–60 seconds), this technique is called cryomapping and can be divided into efficacy cryomapping when the exact site responsible for abolishing the arrhythmia is determined, or safety cryomapping when you search for unintended consequences during ablation. Definitive lesions occur at −50° to −75°C during 2–4 minutes, with the ice ball at the tip of the catheter producing good stability of the catheter. With cryomapping and good catheter adhesion, the risk of atrioventricular block for septal accessory pathways can be eliminated. The acute procedural success rate is around 84%, which is comparable to RF ablation, however, there is a high recurrence rate of approximately 29% [10].

When performing pulmonary vein isolation with cryoballoon only two venous femoral punctions can be done, one to be used with a pacing catheter (either a decapolar or quadripolar), and the other for transeptal access followed by the exchange to cryoballoon sheath. A manifold must be prepared with two connections, one for contrast injection and the other one with 1000 mL of heparinized saline in a compressed bag; another 1000 mL of heparinized saline must be prepared, with or without a second compressed bag, to be connected to the steerable sheath of the cryoballoon.

Transeptal puncture with fixed sheath (FS) must be performed according to physician's practice, either using only fluoroscopy, or complemented by transesophageal echocardiogram (TEE) or intracardiac echocardiogram (ICE); lower transeptal puncture helps a better approach and occlusion of the right inferior pulmonary vein (RIPV), usually the most chalenge vein.

After transeptal access with FS, if one wishes to make left atrial and pulmonary veins angiography, the best way to do it is to maintain the FS at left vein ostium and, during fast ventricular pacing (400 ms), rapidly injecting contrast and recording fluoroscopy, since less amount of contrast will be needed with the first sheath. The next step is exchanging sheaths from FS to the 15F deflectable sheath (DS), which is done by preferably keeping a wire inside the left superior pulmonary vein (LSPV), while removing FS before introducing the DS, deepening the site of puncture with a small blade is needed in order to best pass through it with the sheath, which has a more robust and harder tip. When the sheath is at the transeptal orifice, viewing in left anterior oblique (LAO) projection (30° or 40°), a deflection can be done pointing toward the LSPV so the wire doesn´t come off the left side, while advancing the sheath. With the sheath inside the vein, the wire and dilator can both be retracted, the sheath flushed with heparinized saline solution, and the saline solution connected with continuous slow flushing.

Preparing the cryoballon is crucial to avoid bubbles inside the plastic cap at the tip of the catheter, two fixed sizes are available but the 28 mm is the most used. There are two "dry" connections that must be done before any flushing, one for balloon inflation and deflation with nitric oxide gas (coaxial umbilical), and a second one to capture electrical signals from the cryoConsole, such as temperature, and to energize the catheter (electrical umbilical) this latter catheter has a box in-between that decodify possible catheter or balloon errors to stop ablation and prevent injuries. The manifold and Y-shape device are connected directly to the balloon and flushed; the Y connection is flushed backward then closed and flushed forwards until the solution passes through the balloon tip. In sequence, the tip of the cryoballoon is submerged into a saline solution and its plastic cap is moved in a back-and-forth manner to completely remove air.

The last step before passing the balloon is introducing the circular multipolar diagnostic catheter (called achieve) through the Y connection until the very tip of the system, then the plastic cap is necessarily used to open the DS valve permitting the balloon to get off the sheath.

Common pulmonary vein isolation suggested sequence is LSPV, left inferior pulmonary vein (LIPV), RIPV, and right superior pulmonary vein (RSPV), because the right side is where PN injury can occur, RIPV has a greater distance to PN, pulmonary vein isolation typically precedes PN injury in RSPV, and if RIPV ablation results into PN palsy, at least three veins were already isolated. In pulmonary vein isolation, cryomapping is not usually applied and freezing until, at least, −40°C is the goal.

Ablation time began with a 4-minute freeze using the first-generation balloon in STOP-AF Trial, and in the FIRE and ICE Trial, a 4-minute bonus freeze was applied; for the second-generation balloon, a 3-minute initial ablation time has been suggested. Investigators reported an 80% success rate with 3 minutes of freezing in 143 patients in a single-arm, non-controlled study [11].

During cryoablation some parameters must be observed to ensure good vein isolation—visual fluoroscopy of vein occlusion with the balloon plus contrast injection without leaks to the left atrium (**Figure 3**); once you find this position the operator must maintain it until, at least 30–35 seconds of freezing, enough time to secure the

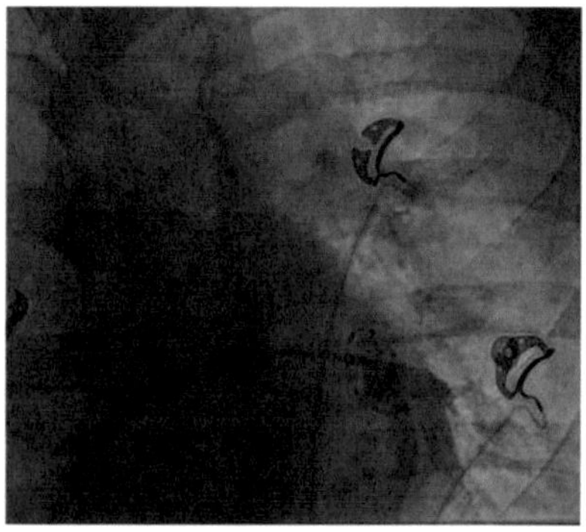

Figure 3.
Fluoroscopy showing cryoballoon catheter occluding left inferior pulmonary, and contrast is filling the vein without leaking to the left atrium. (From the authors).

system in a stable position. A good relationship between freezing time and temperature drop, which best occurs in a one-to-one fashion (e.g., −30°C at 30 seconds of freezing), graphically can be seen as a straight-line drop. Vein isolation in less than 30 seconds or 60 seconds of freezing time helps the physician to decide whether second freeze is to be performed or not, we usually take as practice one full 3 minutes ablation when isolation occurs in less or at 30 seconds, and a 2 or 3 minutes bonus freeze if isolate at or after 60 seconds.

Another parameter indicating good contact and occlusion within the vein is temperature reaching −40°C between 30 to 40 seconds at a maximum of −60°C to halt freezing. A steep and rapid drop in temperature (<−40°C within 30 seconds) and nadir of the temperature of −55°C to −65°C are potential indicators that the balloon is deep inside the vein and not at an antral position, and freezing should be terminated.

There are some techniques described for ablation—the direct approach, the hockey stick approach, and alone or combined with the pull-down maneuver. If the catheter direct occludes the vein ostium, it is called the direct approach (**Figure 4**) and is usually good for LSPV and RSPV.

The so-called hockey stick alone or in combination with a pulldown maneuver is commonly used in LIPV and RIPV. A careful PV angiogram can be used, and the most caudal branch of the inferior PV should be wired with the mapping catheter

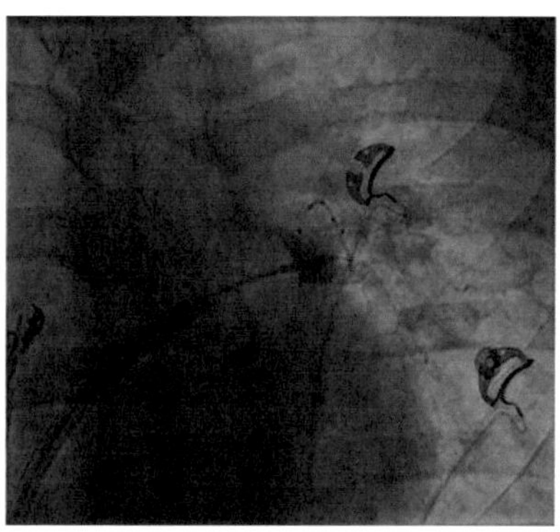

Figure 4.
Fluoroscopy showing cryoballoon catheter in a direct approach, only pushing at vein antrum, and the vein in the example is a left superior pulmonary vein. (From the authors).

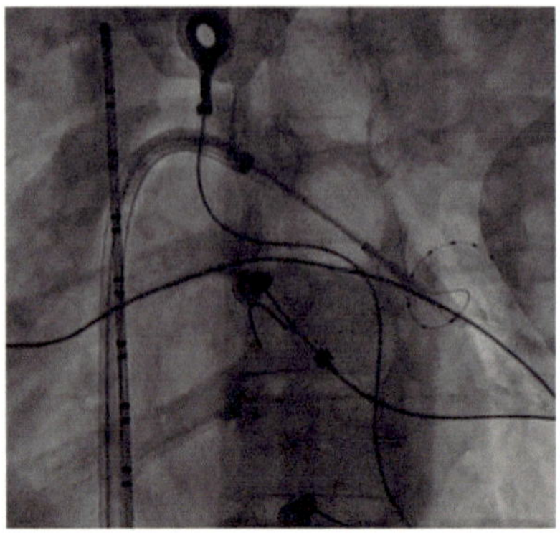

Figure 5.
Fluoroscopy showing the circular mapping catheter (achieve) in an inferior branch of the left inferior vein, and balloon and sheath in a "hockey stick" approach for better occlusion.

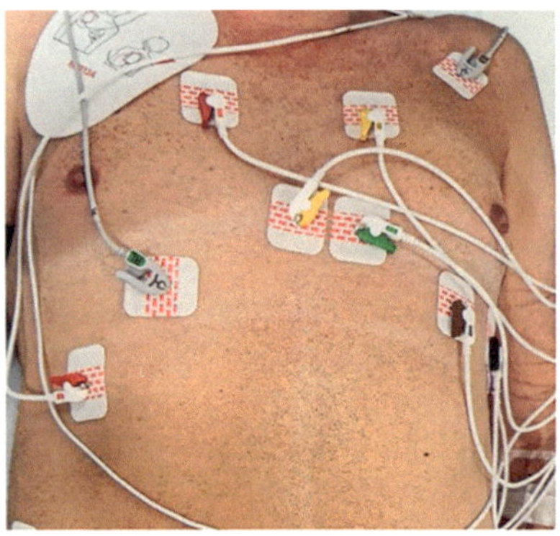

Figure 6.
Positioning polygraph electrodes (12-lead electrocardiogram) with the right arm placed 5 cm above the xiphoid, and left-arm surface ECG electrode placed 16 cm from the xiphoid along the costal margin to obtain the CMAP.

(achieve). After CB inflation, the sheath should be curved down and pushed up with the bending point at the LA roof. The CB should then be advanced to improve contact with the inferior aspect of the inferior PV, resulting in a hockey stick figure on fluoroscopy (**Figure 5**). If an inferior gap remains, we combine the hockey stick with a pulldown maneuver (CB and sheath) after 60 seconds. At this point in time, the CB is frozen to the superior aspect of the inferior PV and a typical response consists of an additional CB temperature drop and isolation in the next 20 seconds.

Before freezing right veins, PN should be paced at twice the capture threshold using a deflectable catheter, a good place for pacing is at the junction of the superior vena cava (SVC) and the right subclavian vein. Monitoring PN function can be done by direct manual palpation of the patient´s thorax or by monitoring de diaphragmatic compound motor action potential (CMAP) since the latter one alters first before PN palsy.

The CMAP is implemented using a modified ECG lead I technique. The right-arm surface ECG electrode is placed 5 cm above the xiphoid, and the left-arm surface ECG electrode is placed 16 cm from the xiphoid along the costal margin (**Figure 6**). Freezing is stopped in the event of a 30% reduction in the maximal diaphragmatic CMAP amplitude or any perceived reduction in the strength of diaphragmatic contraction.

DOI: http://dx.doi.org/10.5772/intechopen.105861

4. Conclusions

Cryoablation is a feasible technique for SVT procedures with a high acute success rate, but also higher rates of recurrence compared to RF ablation; it is suggested to use it in targets where the risks of the procedure are higher than the benefits if using RF as an energy source, such as in right septal accessory pathways.

Cryoablation with a balloon catheter to treat atrial fibrillation by pulmonary vein isolation is non-inferior to RF procedure and, to date has a unique trial of superiority to antiarrhythmic drugs as first-line therapy.

Conflict of interest

The authors declare no conflict of interest.

Thanks

I would like to thank Dr. Silvia Helena Cardoso Boghossian for the first cryoballoon procedures with high expertise and patience. My thanks to Sociedade Brasileira de Arritmias Cardíacas (SOBRAC) for encouraging physicians to novel techniques by performing continuous medical education. I also thank my colleagues who helped me in writing this chapter and Dr. David C. Gaze for the opportunity of this chapter.

Author details

Bruno Papelbaum[1]*, André Sbaraini Brambilla[2] and Bruno Kioshi Kimura Numata[3]

1 Beneficência Portuguesa Hospital, São Paulo, Brazil

2 Dom Alvarenga Hospital, São Paulo, Brazil

3 Bartira Hospital, Brazil

*Address all correspondence to: brpapel@gmail.com

References

[1] Joseph P, Clark TWI. Cryoablation: Mechanism of action and devices. Journal of Vascular and Interventional Radiology. 2010;**21**(8 Suppl):S187-S191

[2] Comas GM, Imren Y, Williams MR. An overview of energy sources in clinical use for the ablation of atrial fibrillation. Seminars in Thoracic and Cardiovascular Surgery. 2007;**19**:16-12

[3] Barnett AS, Bahnson TD, Piccini JP. Recent advances in lesion formation for catheter ablation of atrial fibrillation. Circulation: Arrhythmia and Electrophysiology. 2016;**9**:e003299

[4] Packer DL, Kowal RC, Wheelan KR, Irwin JM, Champagne J, Guerra PG, et al. Cryoballoon ablation of pulmonary veins for paroxysmal atrial fibrillation. Journal of the American College of Cardiology. 2013;**61**:1713-1723

[5] Xin HE, Chen Y, Zhou Y, Huang Y, He J. One-year clinical outcome of pulmonary vein isolation using the second-generation cryoballoon: A meta-analysis. Pace. 2016;**39**:182-189

[6] Chen Y-H, Lu Z-Y, Xiang Y, Hou J-W, Wang Q, Lin H, et al. Cryoablation vs. radiofrequency ablation for treatment of paroxysmal atrial fibrillation: A systematic review and meta-analysis. Europace. 2017;**19**:784-794

[7] Kuck K-H, Brugada J, Furnkranz A, Metzner A, Feifan O, Julian Chun KR, et al. Cryoballoon or radiofrequency ablation for paroxysmal atrial fibrillation. New England Journal of Medicine. 2016;**374**:2235-2245

[8] Kuniss M, Pavlovic N, Velagic V, Hermida JS, Healey S, Aren G, et al. Cryoballoon ablation vs. antiarrhythmic drugs: First-line therapy for patients with paroxysmal atrial fibrillation. Europace. 2021;**23**:1033-1041

[9] Heeger CH, Sohns C, Pott A, Metzner A, Inaba O, Straube F, et al. Phrenic nerve injury during cryoballoon-based pulmonary vein isolation: Results of the Worldwide YETI Registry. Circulation: Arrhythmia and Electrophysiology. 2022;**15**:e010516

[10] Chan N-Y. Catheter ablation of peri-nodal and pulmonary veno-atrial substrates: Should it be cool? Europace. 2015;**17**:ii19-ii30

[11] Ciconte G, Asmundis C, Sieira J, Conte G, DiGiovanni G, Mugnai G, et al. Single 3-minute freeze for second-generation cryoballoon ablation: One-year follow-up after pulmonary vein isolation. Heart Rhythm. 2015;**12**:673-680

Chapter 28

Transcatheter Treatment of Aortic Valve Disease Clinical and Technical Aspects

Francesco Gallo, Alberto Barolo, Enrico Forlin and Marco Barbierato

Abstract

Degenerative aortic valve disease is the most common heart valve disease in western countries. After the onset of symptoms, the prognosis of aortic stenosis is poor, despite optimal medical therapy. In recent years transcatheter aortic valve implantation has been affirmed as a viable treatment for patients with high to low surgical risk. Patient screening and procedural planning are crucial for minimizing complications and achieving procedural success. In the last decade, we have seen a progressive technological development in the percutaneous approach, allowing for expanding indications even in low-risk populations. Here we report a brief review summarizing patient screening and procedural planning in patients with aortic valve disease undergoing a transcatheter approach.

Keywords: aortic valve stenosis, aortic valve disease, transcatheter aortic valve implantation, transcatheter aortic valve replacement, interventional cardiology

1. Introduction

Alongside the progressive aging of the general population, aortic valve disease is currently one of the most common heart valve diseases worldwide, and its management is going to have a central role in public health, with an expected doubling of the cases in the next 50 years [1, 2]. This topic is particularly significant in developed countries, as in the United States, 4.2 to 5.6 million (approximately 2.5% of the population) are estimated to have a clinically relevant form of heart valve disease in which aortic valve diseases account for 35% of cases [3]. Notwithstanding worldwide primary etiology of aortic stenosis is rheumatic fever. In western countries, regular access to antibiotic therapy and the aging of the population made calcific aortic valve disease, its most common cause, giving account to the rise of aortic stenosis as the most significant heart valve disease in the elderly population [4].

Transcatheter aortic valve implantation (TAVI) has progressively emerged as a valid alternative and choice since 16 April 2002, the date of the world's first TAVI, performed by Alain Cribier in Lyon (France). In the European Society of Cardiology (ESC) 2012 Guidelines TAVI was limited to surgical high/prohibitive risk patients [5], mainly based on the results of the Placement of Aortic Transcatheter Valves I (PARTNER I; NCT005308944) trial. This trial investigated patients with severe aortic stenosis who were not suitable candidates for surgery; TAVI, as compared with standard therapy, significantly reduced the rates of death from any cause (71.8% vs. 93.6%, Hazard Ratio 0.50; 95% CI 0.39–0·65; $p < 0.0001$), cardiovascular death (57.3% vs. 85.9%; $p < 0.0001$), repeat hospitalizations (47.6% vs. 87.3%; $p < 0.0001$), and cardiac symptoms in terms of New York Heart Association (NYHA) class improvement (NYHA III-IV 14.3% vs. 40%; $p = 0.531$) [6]. In 2016 PARTNER II trial (NCT01314313), comparing SAVR and TAVI in a randomized trial considering intermediate-risk, patients concluded that TAVI had a similar rate of the primary endpoint (death and disabling stroke) at 2 years follow-up in the overall cohort (Hazard Ratio 0.87; 95% CI 0.71–1.07; $p = 0.18$) and lower in the transfemoral-access cohort (Hazard Ratio 0.78; 95% CI 0.61–0.99; $p = 0.04$). On the other hand, surgery demonstrated fewer major vascular complications and less paravalvular aortic regurgitation compared to transcatheter approach [7]. In 2019 results from PARTNER III trial (NCT02675114), comparing SAVR and TAVI in surgical low-risk, patients confirmed that the rate of the composite of death, stroke, or rehospitalization at 1 year was significantly lower with TAVI than with conventional surgery (8.5% vs. 15.1%) [8]. In parallel to PARTNER trials, based on a balloon-expandable prosthesis (Edwards Sapien valve), surgical replacement and transcatheter aortic valve implantation (SURTAVI - intermediate-risk; NCT01586910) and Evolut (low-risk; NCT02701283) trials were conducted, comparing standard surgical therapy to transcatheter implantation of a self-expandable aortic prosthesis (Medtronic Evolut valve). In both studies, TAVI was not inferior to surgery in reducing the primary endpoint of death from any cause or disabling stroke at 24 months [9, 10]. In 2019, based on the evidence generated by these clinical trials, the U.S. Food and Drug Administration (FDA) and the European Medicines Agency (EMA) approved TAVI for the treatment of symptomatic severe aortic stenosis in surgical low-risk patients (**Figure 1**) [11, 12].

2021 ESC/EACTS Guidelines (**Figure 2**) for the management of valvular heart disease have a more balanced approach, currently recommending TAVI for elderly (≥ 75 anni, STS-PROM/EuroSCORE II >8%) or patients unsuitable for surgery and

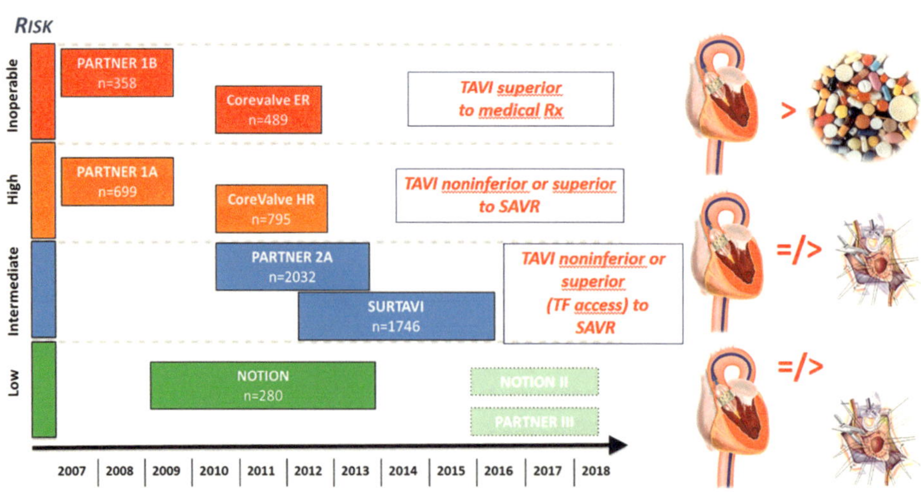

Figure 1.
Overview of the most important clinical trials, stratified according to surgical risk scores.

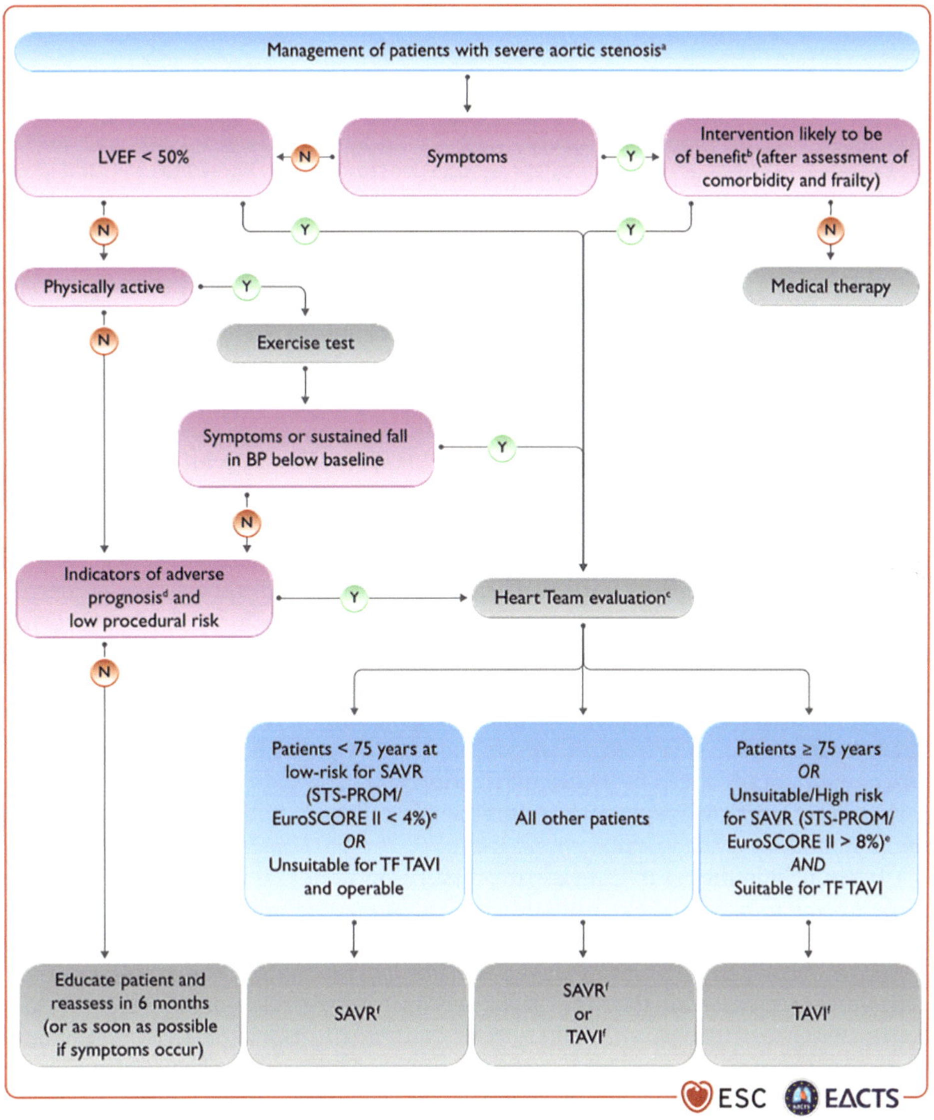

Figure 2.
Management of patients with aortic stenosis [13].

SAVR for younger patients who are low risk for surgery (<75 years and STS-PROM/ EuroSCORE II <4%) or in patients who are operable and unsuitable for transfemoral TAVI, leaving gray-zone context to the comprehensive evaluation of individual clinical, anatomical, and procedural factors by the Heart Team, which discussion is however recommended in every scenario [13].

2. Patients selection

Aortic stenosis is frequently associated with advanced age and numerous cardio-vascular non-cardiovascular diseases. Because of that, the treatment choice is based on a careful and 360° patient evaluation.

2.1 General screening: symptoms and prognostic impact

A typical benign course characterizes aortic valve stenosis during most of its natural history. At the same time, a drastic prognostic worsening occurs after symptoms onset, with an event-free survival of only 30–50% at two years and with an average survival of just 2–3 years without aortic valve replacement [14–17]. For that reason, looking for even vague symptoms and closer follow-up have a central role during the medical visit. Aortic stenosis typically manifests itself with effort angina, dyspnea, progressively evolving to congestive heart failure, pre-syncopal, and syncopal events. However, symptoms may be atypical, like fatigue or tiredness, especially in the elderly who, for concomitant reasons, are not able to perform relevant efforts. Usually, in western countries, the onset of the symptoms occurs between 7th and 9th decade of life as a consequence of progressive calcification of valvular cusps [18]. In elderly/complex patients, a critical effort should be to recognize the most likely cause of symptoms, especially in mild or moderate aortic stenosis, as symptoms normally occur in severe stenosis. Moreover, aortic stenosis shares the same risk factors and symptoms as other cardiac and noncardiac diseases. Dyspnea can be present in asthma, chronic obstructive pulmonary disease (COPD), anemia, renal failure, deconditioning, and coronary artery disease (CAD), which could also be manifest with angina and arrhythmias-related presyncope or syncope. In particular, CAD in aortic valve stenosis patients is highly-prevalent; it was found in 69.7% of patients addressed to TAVR in the PARTNER II trial and in 69.2% of patients assigned to SAVR in the SURTAVI trial [7, 9]. Coronary angiography is recommended in assessing each patient with severe aortic stenosis to identify patients that could benefit from contemporary coronary revascularization [13].

In general, aortic valve stenosis progression is constant, with an average annual reduction in the valvular aortic area of 0.03 ± 0.01 cm2/year and about 2.7 ± 0.1 mmHg in the mean transaortic pressure gradient [19]. To improve proper follow-up and identify the most suitable time to proceed to aortic valve replacement, In 2020, American Heart Association (AHA)/American College of Cardiology (ACC) guidelines classify patients into 4 stages according to the natural history phase of aortic valve stenosis: from those at risk of development aortic stenosis (Stage A), to progressive aortic stenosis with mild or moderate calcifications (Stage B), to asymptomatic severe aortic stenosis with normal or reduced left ventricular ejection fraction (LVEF) (Stage C), and to symptomatic aortic stenosis with normal or reduced LVEF (Stage D). This classification is useful in the management of patients because each stage is associated with a proper diagnostic-therapeutic iter; in particular, aortic valve replacement is recommended in all Stage D patients and in Stage C with reduced LVEF (< 50%) [20]. In fact, despite improving symptoms in the short term, medical therapy is not capable of changing the natural history of severe aortic stenosis; therefore, aortic valve replacement is the only effective therapy.

2.2 Risk stratification

According to 2021 ESC/EACTS guidelines for the management of valvular heart disease, aortic valve replacement is recommended for every symptomatic severe aortic stenosis (IB) and asymptomatic severe aortic stenosis with systolic left ventricular dysfunction (LVEF <50% IB; < 55% IIa B) without another cause, undergoing coronary artery bypass graft (CABG) or surgical intervention on the ascending aorta or another heart valve, demonstrable symptoms or sustained fall in blood pressure (> 20 mmHg) on exercise testing (IIa B-C), and/or procedural low-risk plus a risk parameter (very severe aortic stenosis, severe valve calcification and peak aortic valve velocity progression ≥0.3 m/sec/year, markedly elevated brain natriuretic peptide levels) [13].

Once indication to valve replacement is defined, the choice between surgical and transcatheter intervention lies on age, surgical hazard, previous cardiac surgery, a concomitant cardiac condition requiring intervention, technical parameters, comorbidities, and frailty. These parameters should be evaluated by a multidisciplinary heart team, whose role is predominant, especially in moderate-risk patients, in which cases guidelines provide less indications [13]. Aspects favoring SAVR are younger age (typically <75 years), low surgical risk, no previous thoracic surgery, coronary or heart valve disease requiring intervention, and nonrelevant comorbidities, while older age (≥ 75 years), high surgical risk, previous thoracic surgery, and comorbidities favor TAVR. The scores that are commonly used in the definition of the surgical risk are Society of Thoracic Surgeons Mortality (STS) score and EuroSCORE II. Although, these scores were born and developed for stratifying risk in patients undergoing cardiac surgery and not for those who are scheduled for transcatheter therapy. Moreover, they provide just only low correlation with 30-day mortality [21]. In a recent multicenter study performed on patients assigned to TAVI, STS score and EuroSCORE II demonstrated just a moderate correlation and a low accuracy for inhospital adverse events and for 30-day and medium-term mortality, pointing out the necessity of dedicated scores [22].

Technical aspects will be discussed in a separate section (see Anatomical assessment).

2.3 Futility

Transcatheter aortic valve implantation was developed to improve prognosis and has revolutionized the treatment of elderly patients affected by severe aortic stenosis. The expansion in indication and the spread among centers determined the increase of its demand. Consequently, adequate patients selection has become fundamental to avoid wasted resources. Currently, TAVI represents a highly expensive intervention and a relevant issue in a health system where economic resources are limited. However, cost/efficacy analysis had demonstrated a non-inferiority of TAVI respective to SAVR in the long run; in particular, Cohen *et al.* [23] demonstrated how, despite a higher procedural cost, TAVI allows significantly reduced follow-up costs, compared to SAVR. According to the 2017 American College of Cardiology (ACC) consensus, avoiding intervention on patients who are not going to benefit in survival or quality of life is appropriate. In particular, futility is defined for patients with a life expectancy inferior to 1 year and for those with expected survival with benefit of <25% at 2 years, as evaluated with NYHA class and/or Canadian Cardiovascular Society (CCS) angina grade improvement [24].

In the recent frailty in older adults undergoing aortic valve replacement (FRAILTY-AVR; NCT01845207) study, 646 TAVI patients have been stratified with several frailty scores. The one that had the major correlation with prognosis was the essential frailty toolset (ETF) score. This score is composed of 4 items: mobility (assessed by the time necessary to get up from a chair), cognitive function, hemoglobin value, and serum albumin value. It is interesting to notice that the highest (i.e. the worst) score (5) was associated with a mortality rate of 63% and a major disability rate of 16%. The persistence of a high ETF score value after interventions focused on its reduction could be a futility marker in this kind of patient [25].

In addition to the futility issue, the TAVI's outcome still has several possibilities of improvement; after implantation, there is a 30-days mortality rate of 7.8% and 2.2%, with old and new devices, respectively [26]. Moreover, considering 5 years of follow-up derived from major trials, the mortality rates exponentially increase. In the Core Valve US pivotal extreme and High-Risk trial (NCT01240902), a prospective, multicenter, and single-arm clinical trial of TAVI enrolling 639 patients with severe aortic stenosis at extreme surgical risk, with a mean age of 82.8 ± 8.4 years, a 5-year mortality rate of 71.6% was observed (with futility of 50.8%) [27]. The same behavior was confirmed in the PARTNER I and II trials, enrolling, respectively, inoperable and surgical intermediate-risk patients randomly assigned to TAVI or SAVR, reporting a 5-year mortality of 71.8% vs. 93.6% ($p < 0.0001$; PARTNER I) and of 47.9% and 43.4% ($p = 0.21$; PARTNER II) [6, 7]. It is interesting to notice that a rapid increase in mortality is observed after about 30 days from intervention [28]. Several studies have demonstrated that in patients undergoing TAVI, after an early phase of high cardiovascular risk, this drastically reduces but, in elderly, non-valvular heart failure and noncardiac diseases represent the main causes of death. According to Chen et al. metanalysis, main etiologies are: infections/sepsis (14%), cancer (7%), renal insufficiency (4%), multi-organ failure (3%), and other causes (23%) [29]. This scenario is easily understandable considering that TAVI patients are generally older and have more comorbidities, compared to patients addressed to conventional surgery, and despite valvular disease correction, advanced age and comorbidities still represent a heavy frailty burden [30, 31]. Although, age is not automatically a synonymous of frailty, the latter has demonstrated to significantly affect the outcome of patients undergoing TAVI even in the 90-years-old population [32].

Several factors are associated with increased morbidity and mortality at 1 year after aortic valve replacement among cardiac conditions, atrial fibrillation (AF), left ventricular systolic dysfunction, mitral regurgitation, pre-capillary pulmonary hypertension, and right ventricular dysfunction. Among extracardiac conditions, COPD and restrictive lung diseases, chronic kidney disease, cancer, advanced age, and frailty are the most impacting from a prognostic point of view [33]. In this context, a fundamental question concerns if aortic valve replacement may improve or resolve symptoms and associated conditions affecting prognosis. Indeed, left ventricular systolic dysfunction, when other potential causes are excluded, improves in about two-thirds of the patients from 48 hours to 1-year post aortic valve replacement [34], and mitral regurgitation, especially if functional, may be positively affected after TAVI [35]. Conversely, COPD (with poor exercise tolerance, oxygen-dependency or use of noninvasive ventilation), precapillary pulmonary hypertension (especially with systolic pulmonary artery pressure > 60 mmHg), primary mitral valve regurgitation, active cancer, and cognitive impairment are unlikely to get better after aortic valve replacement and are thus associated with a worse prognosis [36–38].

Considering the multidimensional phenotype and the discordance among the various tests and scores used in clinical practice, quantifying the impact of frailty could be challenging. Its assessment is however essential in patients' selection in order to improve extracardiac diseases and avoid vain invasive procedures.

2.3.1 Balloon aortic valvuloplasty (BAV)

Widely used in high surgical risk patients since it was first introduced by Cribier *et al*. in 1985, BAV is progressively gaining significance in patients' stratification, clinical stabilization, and forecasting the results of a definitive correction of the valve disease, as a "bridge to decision (medical therapy/TAVI/SAVR)" therapy. In particular, the evaluation of BAV's results provides prognostic information and is capable of identifying patients who are going to take advantage of aortic valve disease correction [39, 40]. In addition, performing BAV could improve mobility and general status of frailty patients, helping them to bear intensive rehabilitation courses that could be fundamental to face up to aortic valve intervention with the lowest frailty degree. In the end, in frailty patients, in which a judgment of futility has been made (especially for poor life expectancy), BAV may be used as a temporary palliative treatment, as a "destination therapy" [24]. A major limitation of BAV has always been the risk of vascular complications, as the most widespread vascular access site is the femoral venous and arterial access. This site is associated with a rate of major and minor vascular complications of, respectively, 2.7% and 6.6%, even with the use of advanced hemostasis systems (Angio-Seal and ProGlide) [41]. In recent years, there was an important effort in researching techniques to minimize periprocedural complications and, in this context, the Safety and Feasibility of Transradial Mini-invasive Balloon Aortic Valvuloplasty (SOFTLY; NCT03087552) study showed the feasibility and safety of a mini-invasive approach combining radial artery access and LV pacing through the wire (without implantation of a temporary pacemaker through venous access) [42]. The possibility of a mini-invasive approach able to significantly reduce access-related complications could be a great incentive for the use of BAV in order to improve frailty situations before an aortic valve disease definitive correction is performed.

3. Anatomical assessment

3.1 Echocardiography

Echocardiography is fundamental to diagnosis and to assess aortic stenosis severity, valve calcifications, LV systolic and diastolic function, and other cardiac pathologies. Current ESC guidelines underline the importance of echocardiographic evaluation when blood pressure is well controlled to reduce confounding flow effects of increased afterload [13].

Aortic stenosis severity assessment lies on the measurement of mean pressure transvalvular gradient, peak transvalvular velocity (Vmax), and aortic valve area (AVA). Based on these parameters, three categories of severe aortic stenosis may be identified and could benefit from aortic valve replacement [13]:

- High-gradient AS: characterized by mean gradient ≥40 mmHg, Vmax ≥4 m/s, AVA ≤ 1 cm2 (or AVAi ≤0.6 cm2/m2);

- "Classical" low-flow, low-gradient AS (LF-LG AS): characterized by mean gradient <40 mmHg, AVA ≤ 1 cm2 (or AVAi ≤0.6 cm2/m2), LVEF <50%, and as an additional variable, indexed stroke volume (SVi) ≤ 35 ml/m2; in these cases, dobutamine stress echocardiogram is recommended to identify true classical LF-LG AS, which presents increasing mean pressure (≥ 40 mmHg) and could benefit from AVR, form pseudo-severe AS. In particular, patients with true classical LF-LG AS have developed functional improvement one year after TAVI, but no significant LV function improvement [43].

- "Paradoxical" low-flow, low-gradient AS: characterized by mean gradient <40 mmHg, AVA ≤ 1 cm2 (or AVAi ≤0.6 cm2/m2), LVEF ≥50% and SVi ≤ 35 ml/m2. This condition is typical of patients with profound concentric LV hypertrophy with small cavities that are not able to generate enough SV to effectively open the aortic valve [44]. In this context, a computerized tomography (CT) assessment of valve calcification's degree helps to define the probability of true severe AS (highly likely with Agatston units >3000 for men and > 1600 for women).

In peculiar cases, especially with patients with poor echocardiographic transthoracic windows, transesophageal echocardiography could be a valid alternative (**Figure 3**).

3.2 Cardiac catheterization

Despite the evaluation of aortic valve stenosis is mainly based on echocardiography, there is a not negligible discrepancy between effective aortic valve area (AVA) derived from Doppler and from cardiac catheterization. According to Minners *et al.,* there are inconsistencies in grading aortic valve stenosis in patients with normal LV function, in particular with respect to AVA, while mean pressure gradient seems to be a more robust parameter [45]. In a prospective study on assessment of aortic stenosis severity between echocardiography and cardiac catheterization, AVA correlated poorly between the two techniques, with an average AVA difference of 0.25 cm2 (range 0–1.59) [46]. That is due to the fact transvalvular pressure gradient is maximal at the level of the vena contracta, the point in a fluid stream where the diameter of the stream is the least and fluid velocity is at its maximum, which occurs where all the layers of the stream converge, slightly downstream of anatomic aortic valve area. After the vena contracta, part of the jet kinetic energy is recovered in pressure but, during this process, there is some energetic dispersion as a result of flow separation and vortex formation. Echocardiography, measuring transvalvular pressure gradient at the vena contracta (where it is maximal), tends to overestimate pressure gradient and, therefore, underestimate aortic orifice area. Cardiac catheterization, instead, tends to measure a lower transvalvular pressure gradient because it samples it at some distance downstream to vena contracta, where conversely catheter would have trouble maintaining the position of the pressure sensor due to the instabilities secondary to flow-jet turbulence [46]. As assessed by Garcia *et al.*, effective orifice area calculated by catheterism (EOA_{cath}) may therefore be larger than the one calculated by echocardiography (EOA_{echo}). This overestimation becomes relevant as the ascending aorta diameter decreases, mostly when sino-tubular junction diameter is ≤30 mm [47]. Moreover, echocardiography could also overestimate EOA because of poor alignment of the ultrasound beam with the stenotic jet [48]. In the end, cardiac catheterization provides data about pulmonary pressures and resistances that, if elevated, could identify an advanced pathology grade that may not benefit from valve correction [37]. Nevertheless, current ESC/EACTS Guidelines for the management of valvular heart disease recommend LV catheterization only when there is a severe aortic stenosis clinic and noninvasive assessment is inconclusive [13]. Criteria for defining aortic valve stenosis severity and its prognosis are derived from catheter measurements, and nowadays the invasive assessment could be a valid ally in an accurate definition of aortic stenosis severity, although a proper selection is mandatory to limit unavoidable complications related to its invasiveness.

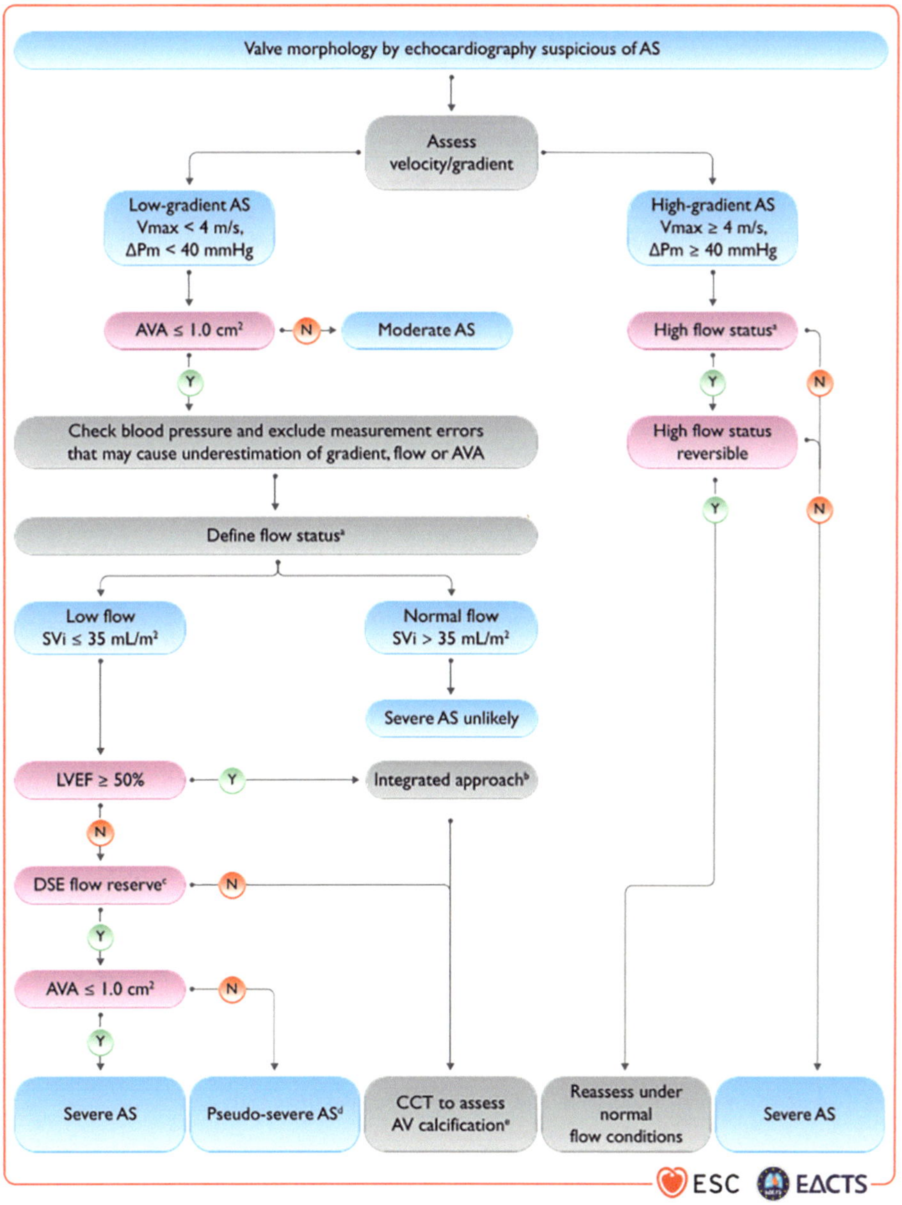

Figure 3.
Integrated assessment of patients with aortic valve stenosis [13].

3.3 Computerized tomography scan

Electrocardiogram-gated CT scan has a central role in the pre-procedural planning for TAVI. First of all, it is fundamental to evaluate annular valvular area and perimeter (essential to guide the choice of prosthesis' size), extent and distribution of calcifications, aortic root anatomy, and height of coronary ostia from aortic annulus and LV outflow tract dimension (**Figure 4**). All this information is pivotal to define prosthesis implantation. For example, an overestimation of the aortic annulus dimensions

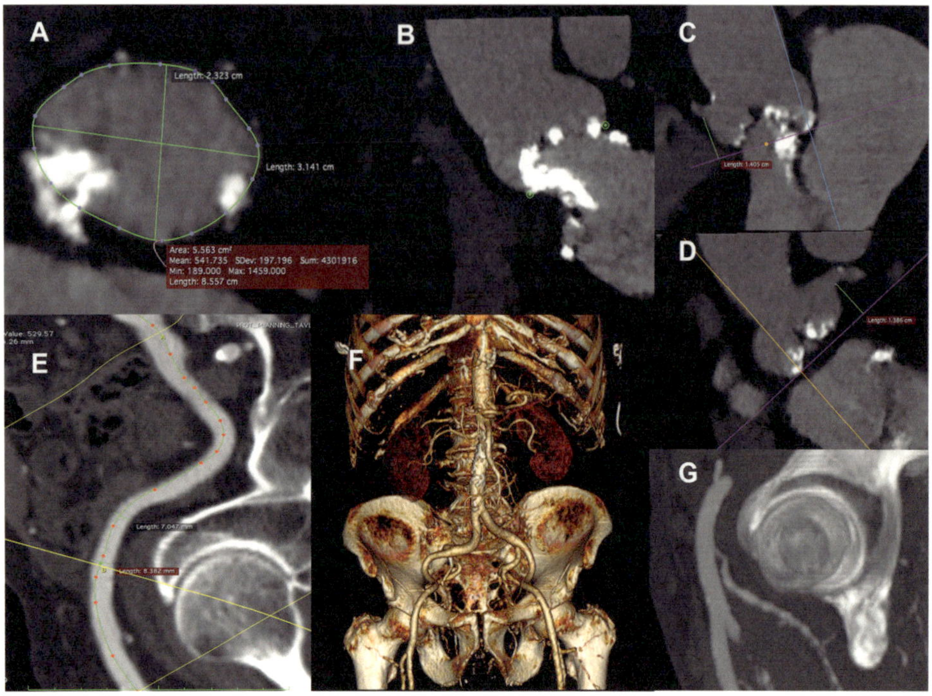

Figure 4.
Computed tomography evaluation for TAVI procedural planning. Aortic annulus measure (A) and calcium distribution (B). Coronary distance from virtual basal ring (C, D). Aorta and peripheral artery evaluation for a transfemoral access (E-G).

poses a significant risk for aortic root lesions or disruption during prosthesis release. On the other hand, underestimation increases the risk of paravalvular aortic regurgitation [49, 50]. Considering that aortic annulus dimensions vary throughout the cardiac cycle, they should be measured during systole, i.e., when they are larger.

Another main scope of CT scan concerns the planning of vascular access through imaging of aorta and iliofemoral vasculature. This assessment has become increasingly important and has led to a significant decrease of pre- and post-procedural major and minor vascular complications in TAVR patients [51].

4. Device

Transcatheter therapies for the treatment of aortic stenosis have seen a fast and progressive development in technology. Many platforms are nowadays available; it is possible to categorize the devices according to the deployment mechanism: balloon-expandable valves (BEV) and self-expandable valves (SEV). The third category of devices, mechanically expandable, is less widespread. They also differ in the leaflets' position and their relationship with the annular plane (**Figure 5**).

4.1 Balloon-expandable valves

The SAPIEN platform (Edwards Lifesciences, Irvine, USA) is one of the most diffuse BEVs. It is an intra-annular device, with bovine pericardial leaflets mounted on a

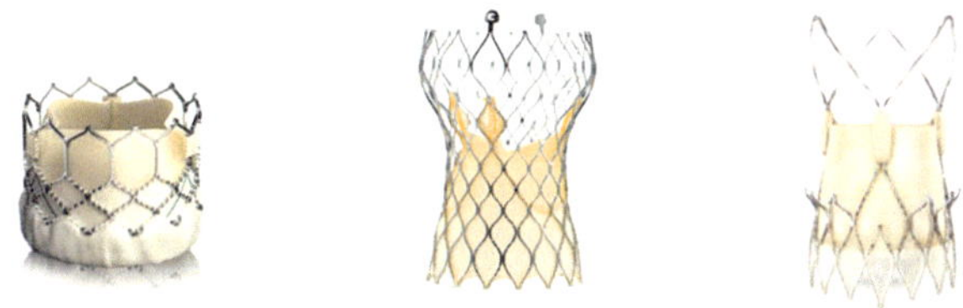

	SAPIEN 3	Evolut Pro	Acurate Neo2
Frame/Deployment	Balloon expandable cobalt chromium alloy	Self expanding nitinol	Self expanding nitinol
Valve	Bovine pericardium	Porcine pericardium	Porcine pericardium
Seal/skirt/cuff	Yes	Yes	Yes (Active PV sealing)
Access	TF - TA – Tao	TF	TF - TA
Anti calcification treatment	Thermafix Process	Alpha-amino Oleic Acid	Biofix

Figure 5.
Principal TAVI platforms and technical characteristics.

cobalt-chromium balloon-expandable frame. SAPIEN valves have a flexible delivery system that allows adapting the implantation in angulated aorta; the balloon expansion allows volumetric modification according to annular sizes, although it is not recapturable during the implantation. The fourth-generation SAPIEN 3 Ultra features an increased outer seal cuff to reduce paravalvular leak (PVL). There are 4 currently available sizes: 20, 23, 26, and 29 mm. The SAPIEN family valves have a lower stent frame profile, which makes easier the coronary catheterization after TAVI [52].

4.2 Self-expanding valves

The Evolut PRO+ (Medtronic, Minneapolis, USA) is the last generation prosthesis of the Evolut family of SEV. They have a supra-annular design and consists of three porcine pericardial leaflets attached to a self-expanding nitinol stent. The stent is a diamond-shaped cell and the valve has an hourglass shape, with a larger circumference at the proximal and distal anchoring points. The delivery system allows the device to recapture after partial deployment and repositioning. Four valve sizes are available (23, 26, 29 and 34 mm) [52].

The ACURATE Neo 2 valve (Boston Scientific, MA, USA) is a SEV with supra-annular design and porcine pericardial leaflets. Its design includes stabilizing arches to facilitate correct positioning. Its top-down deployment, with or without the need for ventricular pacing, does not allow any recapture. It has less radial force, so pre-dilatation is mandatory. The open-cell design and the short-stent body should ease coronary access after implantation. Furthermore, it has a superior crown designed to keep the native cusps away from the coronary ostia [53].

The Portico valve (Abbott Vascular, Santa Clara, CA, USA) comprises a bioprosthetic bovine pericardial aortic valve mounted upon a self-expandable nonflared nitinol frame. The leaflets are located at the annular level, ensuring valve function immediately upon deployment.

Allegra (Biosensors International, Morges, Switzerland) and HYDRA (SMT, Wakhariawadi, India) are two self-expanding nitinol frame valves with bovine pericardial leaflets. Their use is limited to high surgical risk patients and the evidence of safety and efficacy are quietly poor.

4.3 Device choice

So far, there is insufficient evidence to claim the superiority of a prosthesis or another. Each TAVI device has a unique design, and certain elements may slightly favor one or another prosthesis. Among the factors to consider when choosing a valve for TAVI, those that may favor BEV are short or narrow sinus of Valsalva, the presence of conduction disturbances (right bundle branch block or 1st degree AV block), and the anticipated need for future coronary re-access and a horizontal aorta. In small annuli and in case of severe LV outflow tract calcification, SEV may be preferred [52, 54].

The intra-annular design is associated with higher trans-prosthetic gradients and more frequent patient-prosthesis mismatch (an effective orifice area too small in comparison to patient's body surface area) [55]. Patient-prosthesis mismatch is associated with a worse prognosis in surgical prosthesis; however, the clinical relevance of TAVI remains uncertain [56].

Only few randomized trials directly compared different TAVI devices. Direct comparisons are difficult because the small number of events makes necessary the use of composite endpoints. Furthermore, data from early generations TAVI devices cannot be automatically extrapolated to current-generation prosthesis. The Comparison of Transcatheter Heart Valves in High-Risk Patients With Severe Aortic Stenosis (CHOICE; NCT01645202) trial, which randomized high-risk patients to receive a BEV (Sapien XT) or a SEV (Core Valve), showed a greater rate of device success with early generation BEV. The greater device success of BEV in comparison to SEV (95.9% vs. 77.5%; relative risk, 1.24; 95% CI, 1.12–1-37; $p < 0.001$) was driven by a significantly lower frequency of significant aortic regurgitation and less frequent need for the implant of a second valve. Placement of a new permanent pacemaker was less frequent in the BEV group (17.3% vs. 37.6%, $P = 0.001$). A randomized trial compared the SAPIEN 3 valve with the ACURATE Neo valve (Safety and efficacy of the Symetis ACURATE Neo/TF Compared to the Edwards SAPIEN 3 Bioprosthesis - SCOPE 1; NCT03011346) [57]. The non-inferiority of the ACURATE Neo was not met in a composite endpoint. In the SCOPE 2 trial (NCT03192813), the ACURATE Neo valve did not meet the non-inferiority criteria in comparison with Core Valve Evolut prosthesis. Nevertheless, the ACURATE neo showed a significative reduction in permanent pacemaker implantation (PPI) (10.5% vs. 18%) [58]. Data from observational analysis seem to favor BEV [59, 60], but should be interpreted with caution.

5. Minimizing complications

5.1 Paravalvular leaks

Paravalvular leak (PVL) consists of a residual gap between the native calcified aortic valve, aortic annulus, and the prosthesis. PVL can be identified during the TAVI procedure using invasive hemodynamics and cine-angiography, while echocardiography is the most diffusely used technique to detect, grade, and follow PVL [61].

The hemodynamic effects of a significant residual regurgitation have a negative clinical impact. Moderate to severe PVL are independent predictors of short-term and long-term mortality, while the impact of mild PVL is unclear [62].

Calcification of the aortic valve, leaflet asymmetry, prosthesis malposition and under-sizing, and the use of SEV is associated with the development of PVL [63].

SEV is more influenced by the calcium burden, as they exert less radial force than BEV, therefore they are more often under-expended or eccentrically shaped. On the other side, the higher radial force exerted by BEV could lead to annular rupture [63, 64].

The first-generation devices had a 30-day incidence of moderate to severe PVL of 9.0% and 11.8% (respectively for SEV and BEV) in high-risk patients [65, 66]. Newer-generation devices were designed with features aimed to reduce PVL, such as external skirt of the SAPIEN 3 Valve and the external sealing system of the Evolut PRO Valve. In the more recent PARTNER III trial, the SAPIEN 3 valve had a decreased incidence of moderate to severe PVL in low-risk patients (0.6%) and of note that was similar to residual PVL of SAVR (0.5%) [8]. In the Evolut Low-Risk Trial, there was a greater incidence of moderate to severe PVL: 3,5% in TAVI vs. 0,5% in SAVR [10]. This discrepancy is consistent with the different designs of prosthesis.

A significant PVL may benefit from several treatment options, which includes balloon post-dilatation of the prosthesis, percutaneous closure with plugs, and TAVI-in-TAVI to exert a superior radial force against the PVL, and surgical intervention.

5.2 Coronary obstruction and coronary re-access

Almost half of the patients undergoing TAVI have coronary artery disease, and about a third of the patients are in a low-risk population [8, 67]. TAVI may influence coronary in two ways: the prosthetic valve struts may prevent the selective catheterization of coronaries during PCI and the prosthesis or the dislodged native leaflets may cause acute coronary obstruction.

The coronary re-access following TAVI is influenced by several anatomical factors (sino-tubular junction dimensions, sinus height, leaflet length and bulkiness, sinus of Valsalva width, and coronary ostial height) and device-related and procedural factors (commissural tab orientation, sealing skirt height, and valve implantation depth) [68]. Prosthesis with higher frame design hinders coronary re-access more than those with a lower frame due to the barrier of the stent frame in allowing coronary catheters to directly engage the coronary ostia (**Figure 6**). Therefore, selective coronary angiography after TAVI with some SEV could be more challenging than with BEV [68].

Otherwise, some SEVs, such as ACURATE NEO (Boston Scientific, MA, USA), are characterized by lower stent frame, which could allow for easy coronary engagement.

The alignment of the TAVI valve commissures with the native aortic valve commissures is a promising modifiable factor to facilitate coronary re-access. TAVI differs from aortic valve replacement in the fact that the orientation of commissural posts relative to the coronary ostia is random. It has been shown that specific orientations of the Evolut and ACURATE neo at initial deployment could improve commissural alignment [69]. Of note, a commissural alignment is particularly helpful in high-frame SEV in avoiding coronary artery overlap; this may be fundamental in coronary artery access and redo TAVR.

Acute or delayed coronary obstruction after TAVI is a rare but life-threatening complication, with an incidence inferior to 1% [70, 71]. Coronary obstruction is usually caused by the displacement of the calcified native valve leaflet over the coronary ostium or by the direct occlusion of the coronary ostium by the covered skirt of the transcatheter aortic prosthesis. Anatomical factors associated with coronary obstruction are low coronary ostia height and shallow sinuses of Valsalva. Procedural-related elements include BEV and valve-in-valve (VIV) for surgical bioprosthesis [70]. To prevent this complication some coronary protection techniques may be used, such

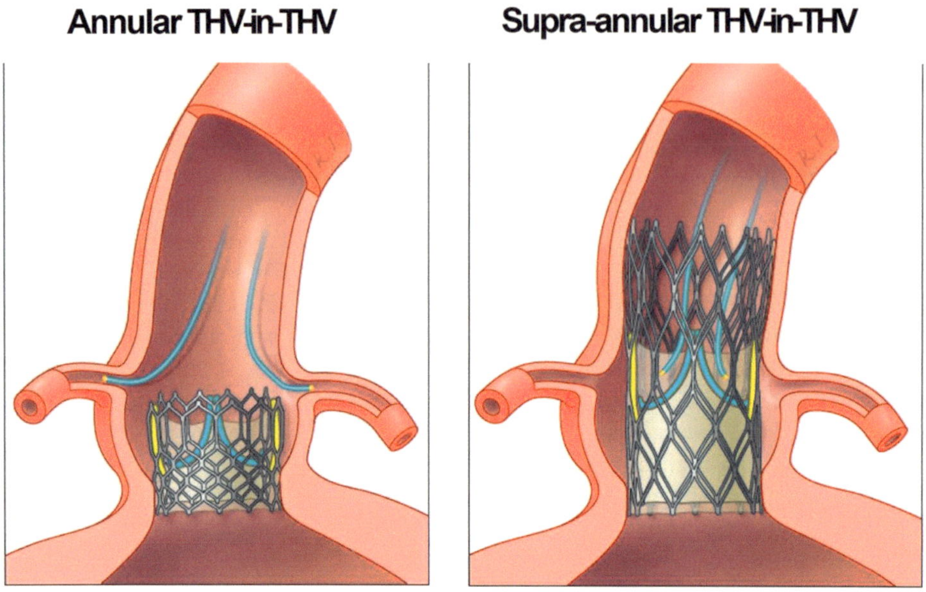

Figure 6.
Difference between TAVI device profile in coronary re-engagement. Device with low profile could theoretically guarantee a easier coronary cannulation.

as preventive coronary wiring or positioning of an undeployed stent in high-risk patients. If the coronary blood flow is compromised during or after TAVI release, the stent is retracted and deployed to create a channel for coronary perfusion between the displaced leaflets and the aortic wall (chimney technique) [72, 73].

5.3 Pacemaker implantation

High-grade atrioventricular block requiring permanent pacemaker implantation (PPI) is one of the most common complications following TAVI, with an incidence ranging from 2 to 36%, depending on the patient population in exam and the prosthesis design [74]. Notably, the rate of PPI remains high even in recent trials with newer generation devices compared with previous trials [74, 75]. SEV is associated with higher risk of PPI than BEV, probably because of the increased radial force exerted on the left ventricle outflow tract (**Figure** 7). In the Core Valve High-Risk trial, PPI was significantly more frequent in the TAVI group than in the SAVR group (19.8% vs. 7.1%, $p < 0.001$) [65]. A more frequent occurrence of PPI in TAVI patients was also observed in the Evolut Low-Risk trial [10]. In the PARTNER III trial, the rate of PPI-associated TAVI was similar to that of surgical patients (6.6% vs. 4.1%, hazard ratio 1.65; 95% CI, 0.92 to 2.95), although the onset of a new left bundle block was more common after TAVI (22.0% vs. 8.0%; hazard ratio 3.17; 95% CI 2.13 to 4.72) [8].

The link between the occurrence of conduction disturbances and the TAVI procedure is explained by the proximity between the aortic valve and the structures of the cardiac conduction system. The atrioventricular node is situated in the right atrium, continues as the Bundle of His, and then splits into the left and the right bundle branches. The Bundle of His emerges at the level of the interventricular membranous septum, caudally to the commissure between the right and noncoronary cusp. The course of the Bundle of His may be within the right half of the membranous sept, within the left half, or under the endocardium; conduction disorders during TAVI are lower with the first anatomic variant [76, 77]. During TAVI, the conduction system can be injured by the insertion of guidewires, balloon pre-dilation, and valve deployment.

The conduction disturbances after TAVI range from new-onset complete atrioventricular blockade to left bundle branch block and transient complete atrioventricular block. The presence of baseline right bundle branch block (RBBB) is the strongest predictor of need for PPI. Other predictors for PPI after TAVI are PR-interval prolongation, left anterior hemiblock, older age, presence of left ventricle outflow tract calcifications, severe mitral annular calcification, and the length of the membranous septum. Procedural predictors are the use of SEV, deeper valve implantation, balloon pre- and post-dilation, and prosthesis oversizing (**Figure 8**) [74, 78–80].

As per standard of care, PPI is recommended when the patient develops a persistent complete or high-grade atrioventricular block after TAVI. It is also recommended in case of new-onset alternating bundle branch block, while it may be considered in

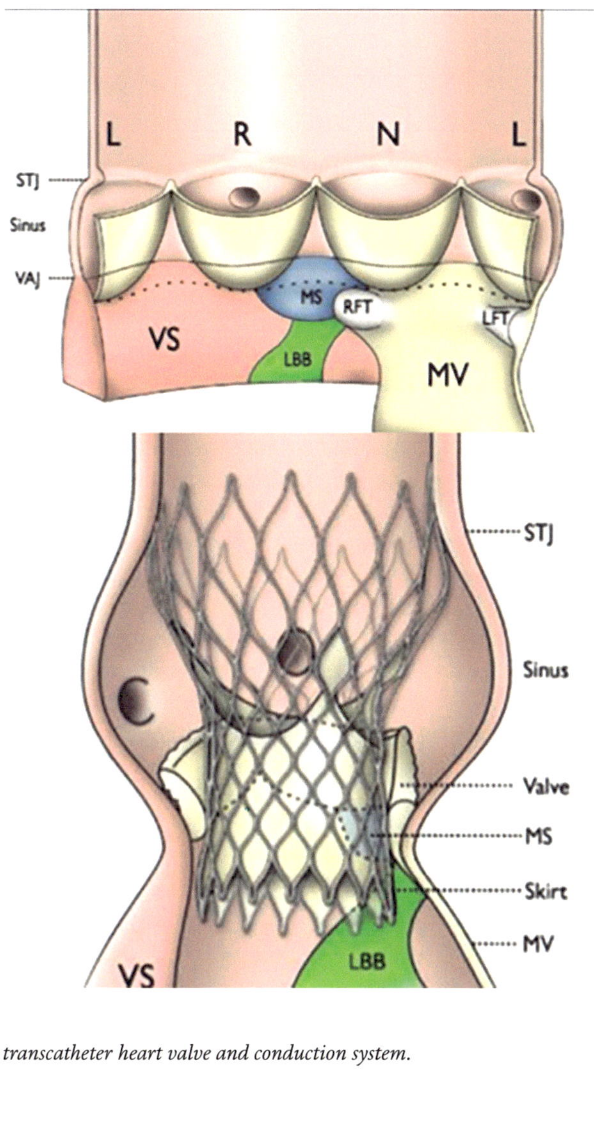

Figure 7.
Relationship between transcatheter heart valve and conduction system.

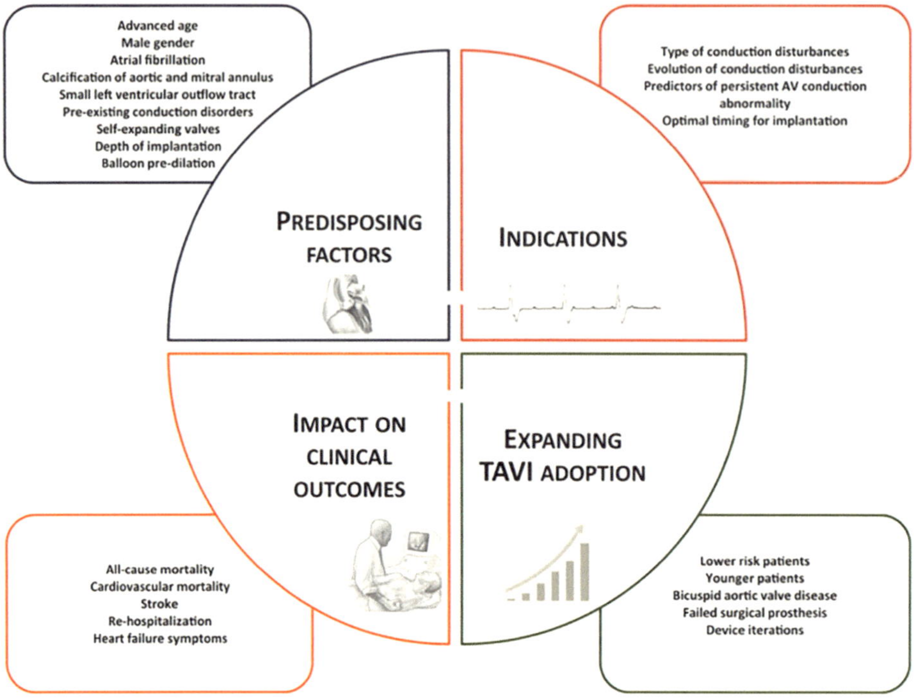

Figure 8.
Major factors associated with permanent pacemaker implantation after TAVI.

patients with pre-existing right bundle branch block who develop new post-procedure conduction disturbance. There is not yet consensus about the optimal strategy for patients with other conduction abnormalities [78].

PPI after TAVI has been associated with increased mortality and rehospitalization, as the need for RV pacing may lead to decreased LV function and heart failure, yet there is still conflicting evidence [78, 81]. Risk factors that should be assessed in the preoperative TAVI evaluation are preexisting conduction disturbances and LVOT calcification. There may be a trade-off between the reduction of PVL and the risk of PPI, as a greater radial force may reduce the regurgitation, but it may damage the conduction system [52]. A BEV may be preferred in patients with baseline conduction disorders. A higher implantation strategy may minimize the contact between the valve and membranous septum, reducing conduction defects after the implantation [82]. In this context, an angiographic view providing an accurate visualization of the implantation depth (the cusp overlap view, as the right coronary cusp and the non-coronary cusp appear overlapping) demonstrates to reduce the rate of PPI [83].

6. Particular cases

6.1 Pure aortic regurgitation

Moderate to severe aortic regurgitation has a prevalence of 0.5%. The course of chronic aortic regurgitation leads to left ventricular dilation and heart failure. Primary aortic regurgitation may be caused by infective endocarditis, rheumatic disease, or degenerative/calcific valve disease. Bicuspid aortic valve, while more commonly associated with stenosis, may cause pure aortic regurgitation or a mixed disease. Aortic regurgitation may also be secondary to marked dilation of the ascending aorta [84].

The gold standard treatment is surgery, with both aortic valve replacement or aortic valve-sparing root replacement. Currently, the role of TAVI is limited to selected patients with aortic regurgitation deemed ineligible for SAVR [13, 85].

The commercially available TAVI devices have been designed for the treatment of degenerative calcific aortic stenosis. The presence of a rigid frame of calcium in the annulus provides an anchoring point for device deployment. The lack of calcium poses thus a significant challenge, as there is increased risk of device malposition, dislodgment, and embolization. The lack of calcification may also lead to higher rates of PVL. Another issue is the risk of implanting undersized devices, as regurgitant aortic valves are more elastic than calcific stenotic valves and can expand to a greater degree during valve deployment. Furthermore, the concomitant presence of a certain degree of aortic disease with dilation and friable tissues poses a further degree of risk for the procedure [85, 86].

Registry data show that TAVI in pure aortic regurgitation has worse outcome than TAVI in aortic stenosis. A 331 patients registry showed a 3% rate of procedure-related death, a 3.6% conversion to open surgery, a 1.2% rate of coronary obstruction, a 1.5% of aortic root injury, and a 16.6% need for second valve implantation. Newer generations valves scored better, as device success went from 61.3% to 81.1% ($p < 0.001$) and moderate to severe aortic regurgitation decreased from 18.8 to 4.2% ($p < 0.001$). [85] In another registry, also including patients with failing bioprosthesis, device success was achieved in 85% of patients with new-generation devices [87].

New prosthesis specifically designed for aortic regurgitation are currently being investigated, such as the Trilogy Heart Valve (Trilogy; Jena Valve Technology), which features anchor rings to clasp the native aortic leaflets [88]. While TAVI may be an alternative for selected patients deemed at high risk for surgical aortic valve replacement, it is currently an off-label indication; randomized control trials and long-term data are still needed.

6.2 Bicuspid aortic valve stenosis

The bicuspid aortic valve is the most common congenital heart defect, with an incidence of around 1% [89]. Almost half of the patients undergoing isolated aortic valve replacement have a bicuspid aortic valve, with a higher incidence in younger patients [90]. In the contemporary practice, up to 10% of patients with bicuspid aortic valve stenosis are referred to TAVI [91].

Echocardiography often underestimates the prevalence of bicuspid valves in calcified aortic stenosis [91]. CT scan provides a more accurate diagnosis and visualization of the bicuspid morphology [92]. Bicuspid aortic valve encompasses a wide range of morphologies; the most common classification categorizes it according to the number of raphes [93].

Aortic annuli in patients with bicuspid valve tends to be larger than in patients with a tricuspid valve. The annulus size may be outside of the range for the currently available devices. Furthermore, the aortic valve complex may have a non-tubular geometry, such as tapered or funnel anatomy. This adds complexity to the selection of a compatible prosthesis [94].

Bicuspid valves have a higher calcific burden than tricuspid stenotic valves. The calcium involves the leaflets in an asymmetrical way and often extends to the LV outflow tract. The majority of the bicuspid valves have a fibrotic and calcified raphe. These anatomic elements hinder the optimal expansion of the valve during TAVI. The asymmetric expansion of the prosthesis increases the risk of PVL. The presence of a highly calcified raphe, if localized between right coronary cusp and non-coronary cusp, increases the risk of conduction disturbances. Calcified raphe and excess leaflet calcification have been found to predict all-cause mortality in TAVI, and when both were present patients had higher rates of aortic root injury and PVL [94, 95].

In addition, coronary anomalies are more frequent in patients with bicuspid aortic valve, and 20 to 30% of them have concomitant aortic disease [89, 94]. Many patients may need aortic root surgery in addition to the valve replacement.

Data about the outcome of TAVI in bicuspid valve anatomy are limited to observational studies, as it was an exclusion criterion in all the randomized trials confronting TAVI with SAVR. In patients at increased surgical risk included in the STS/ACC transcatheter valve therapy registry (STS/ACC TVT Registry; NCT01737528), TAVI for bicuspid aortic valve stenosis showed acceptable safety outcomes with low complications rates [96]. When current-generation devices were used, device success was higher (96.3 vs. 93.5; $P = 0.001$) and the incidence of moderate to severe PVL was lower (2.7% vs. 14.0%; $P < 0.001$) in comparison with older-generation devices. With current-generation devices, device success was slightly lower in the bicuspid valve group (96.3% vs. 97.4%; $P = 0.07$) in comparison with tricuspid stenosis, with a slightly higher incidence of residual moderate or severe PVL. A comparable 1-year mortality was observed, with no increase in the risk of stroke [97]. Results of TAVI in low-risk patients with bicuspid valve anatomy seem similar to those patients with tricuspid aortic valve. In the PARTNER 3 bicuspid registry, with a population of 169 patients, a propensity score matching with TAVI patients showed no difference in the primary endpoint and in the individual components (death, strokes, cardiovascular rehospitalization). Of note, almost half of the patients submitted (47%) were not treated, being excluded because of anatomic or clinical criteria [98]. Another small prospective trial showed good short-term outcomes in low-risk patients with bicuspid aortic valve [99]. Despite the good outcomes in selected patients with favorable anatomies those results cannot be inferred for all the patients with bicuspid aortic valve.

Technical recommendations for TAVI include more frequent balloon valvuloplasty and post-dilation, a low degree of oversizing, and the use of repositioning prosthesis. In tapered anatomies, a supra-annular positioning of the prosthesis has been suggested [94].

7. Conclusions

In recent years the treatment of severe aortic stenosis has been deeply transformed by the introduction of the transcatheter approach. We have reported an overview of the more relevant clinical and technical aspects of the TAVI procedure. As the indications extend to younger patients and with lower surgical risk, it is even more crucial to optimize the results and reduce the complication rate. Further improvements in both technologies and techniques are needed before expanding indications in aortic stenosis in bicuspid valve and in aortic regurgitation.

DOI: http://dx.doi.org/10.5772/intechopen.105860

Author details

Francesco Gallo[1*], Alberto Barolo[2], Enrico Forlin[2] and Marco Barbierato[1]

1 Department of Cardiology, Ospedale dell'Angelo, Venezia Mestre, Italy

2 Department of Cardiology, University of Padua, Azienda Ospedaliera di Padova, Padua, Italy

*Address all correspondence to: galfra87@gmail.com

References

[1] Iung B, Arangalage D. Community burden of aortic valve disease. Heart. 2021;**107**(18):1446-1447. DOI: 10.1136/HEARTJNL-2021-319560

[2] D'Arcy JL, Coffey S, Loudon MA, et al. Large-scale community echocardiographic screening reveals a major burden of undiagnosed valvular heart disease in older people: The OxVALVE population cohort study. European Heart Journal. 2016;**37**:3515-3522

[3] Nkomo VT, Gardin JM, Skelton TN, Gottdiener JS, Scott CG, Enriquez-Sarano M. Burden of valvular heart diseases: A population-based study. Lancet. 2006;**368**(9540):1005-1011. DOI: 10.1016/S0140-6736(06)69208-8

[4] O'Brien KD. Epidemiology and genetics of calcific aortic valve disease. Journal of Investigative Medicine. 2007;**55**:284-291

[5] Vahanian A, Alfieri O, Andreotti F, et al. Guidelines on the management of valvular heart disease (version 2012) the joint task force on the management of Valvular heart disease of the European Society of Cardiology (ESC) and the European Association for Cardio-Thoracic Surgery (EACTS). European Heart Journal. 2013;**66**(2):E1-E42

[6] Kapadia SR, Leon MB, Makkar RR, Tuzcu EM, Svensson LG, Kodali S, et al. 5-year outcomes of transcatheter aortic valve replacement compared with standard treatment for patients with inoperable aortic stenosis (PARTNER 1): A randomised controlled trial. The Lancet. 2015;**385**(9986):2485-2491. DOI: 10.1016/S0140-6736(15)60290-2

[7] Leon MB, Smith CR, Mack MJ, Makkar RR, Svensson LG, Kodali SK, et al. Transcatheter or surgical aortic-valve replacement in intermediate-risk patients. New England Journal of Medicine. 2016;**374**(17):1609-1620. DOI: 10.1056

[8] Mack MJ, Leon MB, Thourani VH, Makkar R, Kodali SK, Russo M, et al. Transcatheter aortic-valve replacement with a balloon-expandable valve in low-risk patients. New England Journal of Medicine. 2019;**380**(18):1695-1705. DOI: 10.1056

[9] Reardon MJ, Van Mieghem NM, Popma JJ, Kleiman NS, Søndergaard L, Mumtaz M, et al. Surgical or Transcatheter aortic-valve replacement in intermediate-risk patients. New England Journal of Medicine. 2017;**376**(14):1321-1331. DOI: 10.1056/NEJMOA1700456/SUPPL_FILE/NEJMOA1700456_DISCLOSURES.PDF

[10] Popma JJ, Deeb GM, Yakubov SJ, Mumtaz M, Gada H, O'Hair D, et al. Transcatheter aortic-valve replacement with a self-expanding valve in low-risk patients. New England Journal of Medicine. 2019;**380**(18):1706-1715. DOI: 10.1056/NEJMOA1816885/SUPPL_FILE/NEJMOA1816885_DATA-SHARING.PDF

[11] Coylewright M, Forrest J, McCabe J, et al. TAVR in low-risk patients. Journal of the American College of Cardiology. 2020;**75**(10):1208-1211. DOI: 10.1016/j.jacc.2019.12.057

[12] Baron SJ, Magnuson EA, Michael L, et al. Health status after Transcatheter vs. surgical aortic valve replacement in lowrisk patients with aortic stenosis. Journal of the American College of Cardiology. 2019;**74**(23):2833-2842. DOI: 10.1016/j.jacc.2019.09.007

[13] Vahanian A, Beyersdorf F, Praz F, Milojevic M, Baldus S, Bauersachs J, et al.

2021 ESC/EACTS guidelines for the management of valvular heart disease: Developed by the task force for the management of valvular heart disease of the European Society of Cardiology (ESC) and the European Association for Cardio-Thoracic Surgery (EACTS). European Heart Journal. 2022;**43**(7):561-632. DOI: 10.1093/eurheartj/ehab395

[14] Pellikka PA, Nishimura RA, Bailey KR, Tajik AJ. The natural history of adults with asymptomatic, hemodynamically significant aortic stenosis. Journal of the American College of Cardiology. 1990;**15**(5):1012-1017

[15] Kelly TA, Rothbart RM, Cooper CM, Kaiser DL, Smucker ML, Gibson RS. Comparison of outcome of asymptomatic to symptomatic patients older than 20 years of age with valvular aortic stenosis. The American Journal of Cardiology. 1988;**61**(1):123-130

[16] Rosenhek R, Zilberszac R, Schemper M, Czerny M, Mundigler G, Graf S, et al. Natural history of very severe aortic stenosis. Circulation. 2010;**121**:151-156

[17] Ross J Jr, Braunwald E. Aortic stenosis. Circulation. 1968;**38**(Suppl. 1):61-67

[18] Bonow RO, Greenland P. Population-wide trends in aortic stenosis incidence and outcomes [editorial]. Circulation. 2015;**131**(11):969-971

[19] Otto CM, Prendergast B. Aortic-valve stenosis from patients at risk to severe valve obstruction. The New England Journal of Medicine. 2014;**371**(8):744-756

[20] Otto CM, Nishimura RA, Bonow RO, Carabello BA, Erwin JP, Gentile F, et al. 2020 ACC/AHA guideline for the Management of Patients with Valvular Heart Disease: A report of the American College of Cardiology/American Heart Association joint committee on clinical practice guidelines. Circulation. 2021;**143**(5):E72-E227. DOI: 10.1161/CIR.0000000000000923

[21] Ben-Dor I, Gaglia MA Jr, Barbash IM, et al. Comparison between Society of Thoracic Surgeons score and logistic EuroSCORE for predicting mortality in patients referred for transcatheter aortic valve implantation. Cardiovascular Revascularization Medicine. 2011;**12**(6):345-349

[22] D'Ascenzo F, Ballocca F, Moretti C, Barbanti M, Gasparetto V, Mennuni M, et al. Inaccuracy of available surgical risk scores to predict outcomes after transcatheter aortic valve replacement. Journal of Cardiovascular Medicine (Hagerstown, Md.). 2013;**14**(12):894-898. DOI: 10.2459/JCM.0b013e3283638e26

[23] Baron SJ, Wang K, House JA, Magnuson EA, Reynolds MR, Makkar R, et al. Cost-effectiveness of Transcatheter versus surgical aortic valve replacement in patients with severe aortic stenosis at intermediate risk. Circulation. 2019;**139**(7):877-888. DOI: 10.1161/CIRCULATIONAHA.118.035236

[24] Otto CM, Kumbhani DJ, Alexander KP, Calhoon JH, Desai MY, Kaul S, et al. 2017 ACC expert consensus decision pathway for Transcatheter aortic valve replacement in the Management of Adults with Aortic Stenosis: A report of the American College of Cardiology Task Force on clinical expert consensus documents. Journal of the American College of Cardiology. 2017;**69**(10):1313-1346. DOI: 10.1016/J.JACC.2016.12.006

[25] Afilalo J, Lauck S, Kim DH, Lefèvre T, Piazza N, Lachapelle K, et al. Frailty in older adults undergoing aortic valve replacement: The FRAILTY-AVR study. Journal of the American College of

Cardiology. 2017;**70**(6):689-700. DOI: 10.1016/J.JACC.2017.06.024

[26] Barbanti M, Webb JG, Gilard M, Capodanno D, Tamburino C. Transcatheter aortic valve implantation in 2017: State of the art. EuroIntervention. 2017;**13**:AA11-AA21. DOI: 10.4244/EIJ-D-17-00567

[27] Arnold SV, Petrossian G, Reardon MJ, Kleiman NS, Yakubov SJ, Wang K, et al. Five-year clinical and quality of life outcomes from the Core valve US pivotal extreme risk trial. Circulation: Cardiovascular Interventions. 2021;**14**:620-627. DOI: 10.1161/CIRCINTERVENTIONS.120.010258

[28] Barbanti M, Petronio AS, Ettori F, Latib A, Bedogni F, De Marco F, et al. 5-year outcomes after Transcatheter aortic valve implantation with Core valve prosthesis. JACC: Cardiovascular Interventions. 2015;**8**(8):1084-1091. DOI: 10.1016/J.JCIN.2015.03.024

[29] Xiong TY, Liao YB, Zhao ZG, et al. Causes of death following Transcatheter aortic valve replacement: A systematic review and meta-analysis. Journal of the American Heart Association. 2015;**4**(9):e002096. Published 2015 Sep 21. DOI: 10.1161/JAHA.115.002096

[30] Stortecky S, Schoenenberger AW, Moser A, Kalesan B, Jüni P, Carrel T, et al. Evaluation of multidimensional geriatric assessment as a predictor of mortality and cardiovascular events after transcatheter aortic valve implantation. JACC. Cardiovascular Interventions. 2012;**5**(5):489-496. DOI: 10.1016/j.jcin.2012.02.012

[31] Green P, Woglom AE, Genereux P, Daneault B, Paradis JM, Schnell S, et al. The impact of frailty status on survival after transcatheter aortic valve replacement in older adults with severe aortic stenosis: A single-center experience. JACC. Cardiovascular Interventions. 2012;**5**(9):974-981. DOI: 10.1016/j.jcin.2012.06.011

[32] Bashore TM, Berman AD, Davidson CJ, et al. Percutaneous balloon aortic valvuloplasty. Acute and 30-day follow-up results in 674 patients from the NHLBI balloon Valvuloplasty registry. Circulation. 1991;**84**:2383-2397

[33] Arnold SV, Afilalo J, Spertus JA, et al. Prediction of poor outcome after transcatheter aortic valve replacement. Journal of the American College of Cardiology. 2016;**68**:1868-1877. DOI: 10.1016/j.jacc.2016.07.762

[34] Elmariah S, Palacios IF, McAndrew T, et al. Outcomes of transcatheter and surgical aortic valve replacement in high-risk patients with aortic stenosis and left ventricular dysfunction: Results from the placement of aortic Transcatheter valves (PARTNER) trial (cohort a). Circulation. Cardiovascular Interventions. 2013;**6**:604-614. DOI: 10.1161/CIRCINTERVENTIONS.113.000650

[35] Muratori M, Fusini L, Tamborini G, et al. Mitral valve regurgitation in patients undergoing TAVI: Impact of severity and etiology on clinical outcome. International Journal of Cardiology. 2020;**299**:228-234. DOI: 10.1016/j.ijcard.2019.07.060

[36] Mok M, Nombela-Franco L, Dumont E, et al. Chronic obstructive pulmonary disease in patients undergoing transcatheter aortic valve implantation: Insights on clinical outcomes, prognostic markers, and functional status changes. JACC. Cardiovascular Interventions. 2013;**6**:1072-1084. DOI: 10.1016/j.jcin.2013.06.008

[37] Sinning JM, Hammerstingl C, Chin D, et al. Decrease of pulmonary hypertension impacts on prognosis after

transcatheter aortic valve replacement. EuroIntervention. 2014;**9**:1042-1049. DOI: 10.4244/EIJV9I9A177

[38] Mangner N, Woitek FJ, Haussig S, et al. Impact of active cancer disease on the outcome of patients undergoing transcatheter aortic valve replacement. Journal of Interventional Cardiology. 2018;**31**:188-196. DOI: 10.1111/joic.12458

[39] Saia F, Marrozzini C, Moretti C, Ciuca C, Taglieri N, Bordoni B, et al. The role of percutaneous balloon aortic valvuloplasty as a bridge for transcatheter aortic valve implantation. EuroIntervention. 2011;**7**(6):723-729

[40] Saia F, Moretti C, Dall'Ara G, Ciuca C, Taglieri N, Berardini A, et al. Balloon aortic valvuloplasty as a bridge-to-decision in high risk patients with aortic stenosis: A new paradigm for the heart team decision making. Journal of Geriatric Cardiology. 2016;**13**(6):475-482. DOI: 10.11909/j.issn.1671-5411.2016.06.002

[41] Dall'Ara G, Santarelli A, Marzocchi A, Bacchi Reggiani ML, Sabattini MR, Moretti C, et al. Vascular complications after balloon aortic valvuloplasty in recent years: Incidence and comparison of two hemostatic devices. Catheterization and Cardiovascular Interventions. 2018;**91**(6):E49-E55. DOI: 10.1002/ccd.27328 Epub 2017 Oct 5

[42] Tumscitz C, Campo G, Tebaldi M, Gallo F, Pirani L, Biscaglia S. Safety and feasibility of Transradial mini-invasive balloon aortic Valvuloplasty: A pilot study. JACC. Cardiovascular Interventions. 2017;**10**(13):1375-1377. DOI: 10.1016/j.jcin.2017.05.007

[43] Lauten A, Zahn R, Horack M, Sievert H, Linke A, Ferrari M, et al. German Transcatheter aortic valve interventions registry investigators. Transcatheter aortic valve implantation in patients with low-flow, low-gradient aortic stenosis. JACC. Cardiovascular Interventions. 2012;**5**(5):552-559. DOI: 10.1016/j.jcin.2012.04.001

[44] Hachicha Z, Dumesnil JG, Bogaty P, Pibarot P. Paradoxical low-flow, low-gradient severe aortic stenosis despite preserved ejection fraction is associated with higher afterload and reduced survival. Circulation. 2007;**115**(22):2856-2864. DOI: 10.1161/CIRCULATIONAHA.106.668681 Epub 2007 May 28

[45] Minners J, Allgeier M, Gohlke-Baerwolf C, Kienzle RP, Neumann FJ, Jander N. Inconsistencies of echocardiographic criteria for the grading of aortic valve stenosis. European Heart Journal. 2008;**29**(8):1043-1048 [Internet]. [cited 2022 Apr 10] Available from: https://academic.oup.com/eurheartj/article/29/8/1043/420517

[46] Niederberger J, Schima H, Maurer G, Baumgartner H. Importance of pressure recovery for the assessment of aortic stenosis by Doppler ultrasound: Role of aortic size, aortic valve area, and direction of the stenotic jet in vitro. Circulation. 1996;**94**(8):1934-1940

[47] Garcia D, Dumesnil JG, Durand LG, Kadem L, Pibarot P. Discrepancies between catheter and doppler estimates of valve effective orifice area can be predicted from the pressure recovery phenomenon: Practical implications with regard to quantification of aortic stenosis severity. Journal of the American College of Cardiology. 2003;**41**(3):435-442

[48] Hatle L, Angelsen B. Doppler Ultrasound in Cardiology: Physical Principles and Clinical Applications.

2nd ed. Philadelphia, Pa: Lea & Febiger; 1986. p. 78

[49] Jilaihawi H, Kashif M, Fontana G, et al. Cross-sectional computed tomographic assessment improves accuracy of aortic annular sizing for Transcatheter aortic valve replacement and reduces the incidence of paravalvular aortic regurgitation. Journal of the American College of Cardiology. 2012;**59**(14):1275-1286. DOI: 10.1016/j.jacc.2011.11.045

[50] Willson AB, Webb JG, Labounty TM, Achenbach S, Moss R, Wheeler M, et al. 3-dimensional aortic annular assessment by multidetector computed tomography predicts moderate or severe paravalvular regurgitation after transcatheter aortic valve replacement: A multicenter retrospective analysis. Journal of the American College of Cardiology. 2012;**59**(14):1287-1294. DOI: 10.1016/j.jacc.2011.12.015 Epub 2012 Feb 22

[51] Toggweiler S, Webb JG. Challenges in transcatheter aortic valve implantation. Swiss Medical Weekly. 2012;**142**:w13735. DOI: 10.4414/smw.2012.13735

[52] Claessen BE, Tang GHL, Kini AS, Sharma SK. Considerations for optimal device selection in Transcatheter aortic valve replacement: A review. JAMA Cardiology. American Medical Association. 2021;**6**:102-112

[53] Kim WK, Hengstenberg C, Hilker M, Schäfer U, Rudolph TK, Toggweiler S, et al. Transcatheter aortic valve implantation with the ACURATE neo valve: Indications, procedural aspects and clinical outcomes. EuroIntervention. Europa Group. 2020;**15**:E1571-E1579

[54] Kapadia SR, Krishnaswamy A. Valve choice in TAVR: A complex equation to solve. Journal of the American College of Cardiology. Elsevier Inc. 2021;**77**:2216-2218

[55] Hahn RT, Leipsic J, Douglas PS, Jaber WA, Weissman NJ, Pibarot P, et al. Comprehensive echocardiographic assessment of Normal Transcatheter valve function. JACC: Cardiovascular Imaging. 2019;**12**(1):25-34

[56] Ternacle J, Pibarot P, Herrmann HC, Kodali S, Leipsic J, Blanke P, et al. Prosthesis-patient mismatch after aortic valve replacement in the PARTNER 2 trial and registry. JACC: Cardiovascular Interventions. 2021;**14**(13):1466-1477

[57] Lanz J, Kim WK, Walther T, Burgdorf C, Möllmann H, Linke A, et al. Safety and efficacy of a self-expanding versus a balloon-expandable bioprosthesis for transcatheter aortic valve replacement in patients with symptomatic severe aortic stenosis: A randomised non-inferiority trial. The Lancet. 2019;**394**(10209):1619-1628

[58] Tamburino C, Bleiziffer S, Thiele H, Scholtz S, Hildick-Smith D, Cunnington M, et al. Comparison of self-expanding bioprostheses for Transcatheter aortic valve replacement in patients with symptomatic severe aortic stenosis: SCOPE 2 randomized clinical trial. Circulation. 2020;**142**(25):2431-2442

[59] Deharo P, Bisson A, Herbert J, Lacour T, Etienne CS, Grammatico-Guillon L, et al. Impact of Sapien 3 balloon-expandable versus Evolut R self-expandable Transcatheter aortic valve implantation in patients with aortic stenosis: Data from a Nationwide analysis. Circulation. 2020;**141**(4):260-268

[60] van Belle E, Vincent F, Labreuche J, Auffret V, Debry N, Lefèvre T, et al. Balloon-expandable versus self-expanding Transcatheter aortic valve replacement: A propensity-matched comparison from the FRANCE-TAVI registry. Circulation. 2020;**141**(4):243-259

[61] Van Belle E, Vincent F, Labreuche J, Auffret V, Debry N, Lefèvre T, et al. Balloon-expandable versus self-expanding Transcatheter aortic valve replacement: A propensity-matched comparison from the FRANCE-TAVI registry. Circulation. 2020;**141**(4):243-259

[62] Jerez-Valero M, Urena M, Webb JG, Tamburino C, Munoz-Garcia AJ, Cheema A, et al. Clinical impact of aortic regurgitation after Transcatheter aortic valve replacement insights into the degree and acuteness of presentation. JACC: Cardiovascular Interventions. 2014;**7**(9):1022-1032

[63] Almeida JG, Ferreira SM, Fonseca P, Dias T, Guerreiro C, Barbosa A, et al. Comparison of self-expanding and balloon-expandable transcatheter aortic valves morphology and association with paravalvular regurgitation: Evaluation using multidetector computed tomography. Catheterization and Cardiovascular Interventions. 2018;**92**(3):533-541

[64] Spears J, Al-Saiegh Y, Goldberg D, Manthey S, Goldberg S. TAVR: A review of current practices and considerations in low-risk patients. Journal of Interventional Cardiology. Hindawi Limited. 2020;**2020**

[65] Adams DH, Popma JJ, Reardon MJ, Yakubov SJ, Coselli JS, Deeb GM, et al. Transcatheter aortic-valve replacement with a self-expanding prosthesis. New England Journal of Medicine. 2014;**370**(19):1790-1798

[66] Smith CR, Leon MB, Mack MJ, Craig D, Moses JW, Svensson LG, et al. Transcatheter versus surgical aortic-valve replacement in high-risk patients. The New England Journal of Medicine. 2011;**364**(23):2187-2198

[67] Faroux L, Guimaraes L, Wintzer-Wehekind J, Junquera L, Ferreira-Neto AN, del Val D, et al. Coronary artery disease and Transcatheter aortic valve replacement: JACC state-of-the-art review. Journal of the American College of Cardiology. Elsevier USA. 2019;**74**:362-372

[68] Yudi MB, Sharma SK, Tang GHL, Kini A. Coronary angiography and percutaneous coronary intervention after Transcatheter aortic valve replacement. Journal of the American College of Cardiology. Elsevier USA. 2018;**71**:1360-1378

[69] Tang GHL, Zaid S, Fuchs A, Yamabe T, Yazdchi F, Gupta E, et al. Alignment of Transcatheter aortic-valve neo-commissures (ALIGN TAVR): Impact on final valve orientation and coronary artery overlap. JACC: Cardiovascular Interventions. 2020;**13**(9):1030-1042

[70] Ribeiro HB, Webb JG, Makkar RR, Cohen MG, Kapadia SR, Kodali S, et al. Predictive factors, management, and clinical outcomes of coronary obstruction following transcatheter aortic valve implantation: Insights from a large multicenter registry. Journal of the American College of Cardiology. 2013;**62**(17):1552-1562

[71] Jabbour RJ, Tanaka A, Finkelstein A, Mack M, Tamburino C, van Mieghem N, et al. Delayed coronary obstruction after Transcatheter aortic valve replacement. Journal of the American College of Cardiology. 2018;**71**(14):1513-1524

[72] Mercanti F, Rosseel L, Neylon A, Bagur R, Sinning JM, Nickenig G, et al. Chimney stenting for coronary occlusion during TAVR: Insights from the chimney registry. JACC: Cardiovascular Interventions. 2020;**13**(6):751-761

[73] Abramowitz Y, Chakravarty T, Jilaihawi H, Kashif M, Kazuno Y,

Takahashi N, et al. Clinical impact of coronary protection during transcatheter aortic valve implantation: First reported series of patients. EuroIntervention. 2015;**11**(5):572-581

[74] Van Rosendael PJ, Delgado V, Bax JJ. Pacemaker implantation rate after transcatheter aortic valve implantation with early and new-generation devices: A systematic review. European Heart Journal. Oxford University Press. 2018;**39**:2003-2013

[75] Mas-Peiro S, Fichtlscherer S, Walther C, Vasa-Nicotera M. Current issues in transcatheter aortic valve replacement. Journal of Thoracic Disease. AME Publishing Company. 2020;**12**:1665-1680

[76] Kawashima T, Sato F. Visualizing anatomical evidences on atrioventricular conduction system for TAVI. International Journal of Cardiology. Elsevier Ireland Ltd. 2014;**174**:1-6

[77] Lilly SM, Deshmukh AJ, Epstein AE, Ricciardi MJ, Shreenivas S, Velagapudi P, et al. 2020 ACC expert consensus decision pathway on Management of Conduction Disturbances in patients undergoing Transcatheter aortic valve replacement: A report of the American College of Cardiology Solution set Oversight Committee. Journal of the American College of Cardiology. 2020;**76**(20):2391-2411

[78] Glikson M, Nielsen JC, Kronborg MB, Michowitz Y, Auricchio A, Barbash IM, et al. ESC guidelines on cardiac pacing and cardiac resynchronization therapy. European Heart Journal. Oxford University Press. 2021;**42, 2021**:3427-3520

[79] Sammour Y, Krishnaswamy A, Kumar A, Puri R, Tarakji KG, Bazarbashi N, et al. Incidence, predictors, and implications of permanent pacemaker requirement after Transcatheter aortic valve replacement. JACC: Cardiovascular Interventions. Elsevier Inc. 2021;**14**:115-134

[80] Rodés-Cabau J, Ellenbogen KA, Krahn AD, Latib A, Mack M, Mittal S, et al. Management of Conduction Disturbances Associated with Transcatheter Aortic Valve Replacement: JACC scientific expert panel. Journal of the American College of Cardiology. Elsevier USA. 2019;**74**:1086-1106

[81] Aljabbary T, Qiu F, Masih S, Fang J, Elbaz-Greener G, Austin PC, et al. Association of Clinical and Economic Outcomes with Permanent Pacemaker Implantation after Transcatheter Aortic Valve Replacement. JAMA Network Open. 2018;**1**(1):e180088

[82] Jilaihawi H, Zhao Z, Du R, Staniloae C, Saric M, Neuburger PJ, et al. Minimizing permanent pacemaker following repositionable self-expanding Transcatheter aortic valve replacement. JACC: Cardiovascular Interventions. 2019;**12**(18):1796-1807

[83] Tang GHL, Zaid S, Michev I, et al. "Cusp-overlap" view simplifies fluoroscopy-guided implantation of selfexpanding valve in transcatheter aortic valve replacement. JACC: Cardiovascular Interventions. Elsevier Inc. 2018;**11**:1663-1665

[84] Maurer G. Aortic regurgitation. Heart. 2006;**92**:994-1000

[85] Yoon SH, Schmidt T, Bleiziffer S, Schofer N, Fiorina C, Munoz-Garcia AJ, et al. Transcatheter aortic valve replacement in pure native aortic valve regurgitation. Journal of the American College of Cardiology. 2017;**70**(22):2752-2763

[86] Markham R, Ghodsian M, Sharma R. TAVR in patients with pure aortic regurgitation: Ready to use? Current Cardiology Reports. Springer. 2020;**22**(9):98

[87] Sawaya FJ, Deutsch MA, Seiffert M, Yoon SH, Codner P, Wickramarachchi U, et al. Safety and efficacy of Transcatheter aortic valve replacement in the treatment of pure aortic regurgitation in native valves and failing surgical bioprostheses results from an international registry study. JACC: Cardiovascular Interventions. 2017;**10**(10):1048-1056

[88] Hensey M, Murdoch DJ, Sathananthan J, Alenezi A, Sathananthan G, Moss R, et al. First-in-human experience of a new-generation transfemoral transcatheter aortic valve for the treatment of severe aortic regurgitation: The J-valve transfemoral system. EuroIntervention. Europa Group. 2019;**14**:E1553-E1555

[89] Michelena HI, della Corte A, Prakash SK, Milewicz DM, Evangelista A, Enriquez-Sarano M. Bicuspid aortic valve aortopathy in adults: Incidence, etiology, and clinical significance. International Journal of Cardiology. Elsevier Ireland Ltd. 2015;**201**:400-407

[90] Roberts WC, Ko JM. Frequency by decades of unicuspid, bicuspid, and tricuspid aortic valves in adults having isolated aortic valve replacement for aortic stenosis, with or without associated aortic regurgitation. Circulation. 2005;**111**(7):920-925

[91] Kim WK, Liebetrau C, Fischer-Rasokat U, Renker M, Rolf A, Doss M, et al. Challenges of recognizing bicuspid aortic valve in elderly patients undergoing TAVR. International Journal of Cardiovascular Imaging. 2020;**36**(2):251-256

[92] Blanke P, Weir-McCall JR, Achenbach S, Delgado V, Hausleiter J, Jilaihawi H, et al. Computed tomography imaging in the context of Transcatheter aortic valve implantation (TAVI)/Transcatheter aortic valve replacement (TAVR): An expert consensus document of the Society of Cardiovascular Computed Tomography. JACC: Cardiovascular Imaging. 2019;**12**(1):1-24

[93] Sievers HH, Schmidtke C. A classification system for the bicuspid aortic valve from 304 surgical specimens. Journal of Thoracic and Cardiovascular Surgery. 2007;**133**(5):1226-1233

[94] Vincent F, Ternacle J, Denimal T, Shen M, Redfors B, Delhaye C, et al. Transcatheter aortic valve replacement in bicuspid aortic valve stenosis. Circulation. Lippincott Williams and Wilkins. 2021;**143**(10):1043-1061

[95] Yoon SH, Kim WK, Dhoble A, Milhorini Pio S, Babaliaros V, Jilaihawi H, et al. Bicuspid aortic valve morphology and outcomes after Transcatheter aortic valve replacement. Journal of the American College of Cardiology. 2020;**76**(9):1018-1030

[96] Forrest JK, Kaple RK, Ramlawi B, Gleason TG, Meduri CU, Yakubov SJ, et al. Transcatheter aortic valve replacement in bicuspid versus tricuspid aortic valves from the STS/ACC TVT registry. JACC: Cardiovascular Interventions. 2020;**13**(15):1749-1759

[97] Halim SA, Edwards FH, Dai D, Li Z, Mack MJ, Holmes DR, et al. Outcomes of transcatheter aortic valve replacement in patients with bicuspid aortic valve disease: A report from the Society of Thoracic Surgeons/American College of Cardiology Transcatheter valve therapy registry. Circulation. 2020;**141**(13):1071-1079

[98] Williams MR, Jilaihawi H, Makkar R, O'Neill WW, Guyton R, Malaisrie SC, et al. The PARTNER 3 bicuspid registry for Transcatheter aortic valve replacement in low-surgical-risk patients. JACC: Cardiovascular Interventions. 2022;**15**(5):523-532

[99] Waksman R, Craig PE, Torguson R, Asch FM, Weissman G, Ruiz D, et al. Transcatheter aortic valve replacement in low-risk patients with symptomatic severe bicuspid aortic valve stenosis. JACC: Cardiovascular Interventions. 2020;**13**(9):1019-1027